D0214285

ESCHERICHIA COLI IN DOMESTIC ANIMALS AND HUMANS

ESCHERICHIA COLI IN DOMESTIC ANIMALS AND HUMANS

Edited by

C.L. GYLES

Department of Veterinary Microbiology and Immunology
Ontario Veterinary College
University of Guelph
Guelph, Ontario
Canada

CAB INTERNATIONAL

CAB INTERNATIONAL
Wallingford
Oxon OX10 8DE
UK

Tel: Wallingford (0491) 832111
Telex: 847964 (COMAGG G)
Telecom Gold/Dialcom: 84: CAU001
Fax: (0491) 833508

A catalogue entry for this book is available from the British Library.

ISBN 0 85198 921 7

Typeset by Colset Pte Ltd, Singapore
Printed and bound in the UK at Biddles Ltd, Guildford

Contents

Contributors

ALEXANDER, T.J.L. *Department of Clinical Veterinary Medicine, University of Cambridge, Madingly Road, Cambridge CB3 0ES, UK*

BERTSCHINGER, H.U. *Institut für Veterinärbakteriologie der Universität Zurich, Winterthurerstrasse 270, 8057 Zurich, Switzerland*

BESSER, T. *Department of Microbiology and Pathology, College of Veterinary Medicine, Washington State University, Pullman, Washington 99164–6610, USA*

BETTELHEIM, K.A. *School of Agriculture, La Trobe University, Bundoora, Victoria 3083, Australia*

BUTLER, D.G. *Department of Clinical Studies, University of Guelph, Guelph, Ontario, Canada N1G 2W1*

CLARKE, B.R. *Department of Microbiology, University of Guelph, Guelph, Ontario, Canada N1G 2W1*

CLARKE, R.C. *Health of Animals Laboratory, Agriculture and Agri-Food Canada, Guelph, Ontario, Canada N1G 3W4*

FAIRBROTHER, J.M. *Swine Infectious Disease Research Group (Groupe de Recherche sur les Maladies Infectieuses du Porc: GREMIP), Faculty of Veterinary Medicine, University of Montreal, CP 5000, St-Hyacinthe, Quebec, Canada J2S 7C6*

GAY, C.C. *Department of Veterinary Clinical Sciences, College of Veterinary Medicine, Washington State University, Pullman, Washington 99164–6610, USA*

GRIFFITHS, E. *National Institute for Biological Standards and Control, Blanche Lane, South Mimms, Potters Bar, Hertfordshire EN6 3QG, UK*

GROSS, W.G. *1509 Lark Lane, Blacksburg, Virginia 24060, USA*

GYLES, C.L. *Department of Veterinary Microbiology and Immunology, University of Guelph, Guelph, Ontario, Canada N1G 2W1*

HAMPSON, D.J. *School of Veterinary Studies, Murdoch University, Murdoch, Western Australia 6150*

HANCOCK, R.E.W. *Department of Microbiology and Immunology, University of British Columbia, Vancouver, BC, Canada V6T 1W5*

HILL, A.W. *AFRC Institute for Animal Health, Compton, Newbury, Berkshire RG16 0NN, UK*

HODGSON, J.C. *Moredun Research Institute, 408 Gilmerton Road, Edinburgh EH17 7JH, UK*

ISAACSON, R.E. *Department of Veterinary Pathobiology, University of Illinois, College of Veterinary Medicine, Urbana, Illinois 61801, USA*

KEENLEYSIDE, W.J. *Department of Microbiology, University of Guelph, Guelph, Ontario, Canada N1G 2W1*

KNUTTON, S. *Institute of Child Health, University of Birmingham, The Nuffield Building, Francis Road, Birmingham B16 8ET, UK*

LEVINE, M.M. *Center for Vaccine Development, School of Medicine, University of Maryland at Baltimore, 10 South Pine Street, Baltimore, Maryland 21201, USA*

LIOR, H. *Laboratory Centre for Disease Control, Health Canada, Tunney's Pasture, Ottawa, Ontario, Canada K1A OL2*

MARRON, M. *Department of Microbiology, Moyne Institute, University of Dublin, Trinity College, Dublin 2, Ireland*

NATARO, J.P. *Center for Vaccine Development, School of Medicine, University of Maryland at Baltimore, 10 South Pine Street, Baltimore, Maryland 21201, USA*

NGELEKA, M. *Swine Infectious Disease Research Group (Groupe de Recherche sur les Maladies Infectieuses du Porc: GREMIP), Faculty of Veterinary Medicine, University of Montreal, CP 5000, St-Hyacinthe, Quebec, Canada J25 7C6*

PEETERS, J.E. *National Instituut voor Diergeneeskundig Onderzoek, Department of Small Stock Pathology and Parasitology, Groeselenberg 99, B 1180 Brussels, Belgium*

PIERS, K. *Department of Microbiology and Immunology, University of British Columbia, Vancouver, BC, Canada V6T 1W5*

SMITH, S.G.J. *Department of Microbiology, Moyne Institute, University of Dublin, Trinity College, Dublin 2, Ireland*

SMYTH, C.J. *Department of Microbiology, Moyne Institute, University of Dublin, Trinity College, Dublin 2, Ireland*

WHITFIELD, C. *Department of Microbiology, University of Guelph, Guelph, Ontario, Canada N1G 2W1*

WOODWARD, M.J. *Bacteriology Department, Central Veterinary Laboratory, Woodham Lane, New Haw, Addlestone, Surrey KT15 3NB, UK*

WRAY, C. *Bacteriology Department, Central Veterinary Laboratory, Woodham Lane, New Haw, Addlestone, Surrey KT15 3NB, UK*

Preface

Ever since *Escherichia coli* was first isolated from the intestine of humans and animals at the dawn of bacteriology in 1885, its possible role as an enteric pathogen has been of considerable interest. As early as 1892, the Danish worker C.O. Jensen used *E. coli* isolates to experimentally reproduce diarrhoea in calves, but a major effort to implicate *E. coli* as an agent of diarrhoeal disease did not come until the 1940s, when serological typing of the organism was placed on a sound footing and was used to implicate certain serotypes in outbreaks of diarrhoea in human infants.

The late 1950s and early 1960s witnessed a resurgence of interest in *E. coli* as an animal pathogen. The pioneering studies of H. Williams Smith at the Animal Health Trust, Stock, Essex, and Walter Sojka's group at the Central Veterinary Laboratory, Weybridge, led to important discoveries about the role of *E. coli* in enteric and septicaemic diseases in animals. Serotyping emerged as a major tool in understanding the association of specific groups of *E. coli* with disease in various animal species and its use by Sojka and the Orskovs resulted in the discovery of the first fimbrial *E. coli* antigen (K88) shown to be responsible for intestinal colonization. Much of the excitement of the era, as well as the unsolved puzzles, were lucidly captured by Walter Sojka in his 1965 book Escherichia coli *in Domestic Animals and Poultry*, although no one had any idea that *E. coli* would later be revealed to be such a remarkably diverse and versatile pathogen.

Since 1965, there has been impressive progress in our understanding of virulence factors of *E. coli* and their contributions to the increasingly wide variety of disease recognized to be caused by *E. coli*. Demonstration of the critical role of K88 fimbriae in *E. coli* diarrhoea in pigs led to a search for other fimbriae that could confer intestinal colonizing ability and to the discovery by Sojka and Williams Smith of K99 fimbriae on *E. coli* from calf diarrhoea. Later, Evans and co-workers reported the first colonizing fimbriae (CFA/I) on *E. coli* from human diarrhoeal disease.

In 1967, Smith and Halls made the important discovery that *E. coli* produced a heat-stable enterotoxin that could account for the fluid disturbances in the intestine of pigs and calves with *E. coli* diarrhoea. Not long after, Gyles and Barnum described a heat-labile enterotoxin, antigenically related to cholera toxin, that was produced by porcine diarrhoeagenic *E. coli*. These findings paved the way for recognition of the category of enterotoxigenic *E. coli* (ETEC). Considered with the earlier findings on colonizing fimbriae, these observations encouraged a way of thinking about *E. coli* as a pathogen in the intestinal tract, namely, that it requires a colonization mechanism and a separate method for causing fluid and electrolyte disturbances. This has led to understanding of mechanisms of enteric disease caused by several other categories of *E. coli*. The brilliant research and extraordinary insight of H. Williams Smith established the transmissibility of the genes for a wide range of *E. coli* virulence factors including the enterotoxins, adherence antigens and haemolysin. These studies involved novel approaches for evaluating putative virulence factors by genetic manipulations of the organism; they still form the basis of much of today's investigations of bacterial virulence. His work on antibiotic resistance plasmids in *E. coli* demonstrated the effect of human interventions in the spread of genetically changed bacteria and led to major changes in antibacterial drug usage in animals.

During the 1970s and 1980s fimbriae and enterotoxins of ETEC were purified, characterized and exploited as vaccines. These developments were greatly aided by techniques of molecular genetics, by which the genes for all the common colonization fimbriae of animal and human ETEC and for the *E. coli* enterotoxins were cloned and sequenced. Vaccines, based primarily on fimbriae, were developed for ETEC diseases in pigs and calves. Highlights towards the end of this period included the discovery of *E. coli* verotoxin (Shiga-like toxin) by Konawalchuk and colleagues in 1977 and the subsequent implication of this toxin in haemorrhagic colitis in humans and animals. A major related discovery by Karmali and co-workers in 1983 was that verotoxigenic *E. coli* (VTEC) were involved in the haemolytic uraemic syndrome in humans. Furthermore, it soon became clear that cattle were a major source of VTEC for humans. Following the demonstration that the toxin produced by oedema disease strains of *E. coli* was a verotoxin, there was renewal of interest in oedema disease of swine. Later, the discovery and characterization of colonizing fimbriae on strains of *E. coli* from oedema disease and postweaning diarrhoea of pigs added valuable new information to our understanding of these diseases.

In contrast to the substantial amount of research on *E. coli* in diseases of food animals, there has only been a limited amount of research on

E. coli diseases of pet and sporting animals, and this area is clearly ripe for investigation. There has also been much less investigation of extraintestinal compared with intestinal *E. coli* infections, although there have been many studies on septicaemic *E. coli* infections in poultry.

This book describes the major advances in knowledge of *E. coli* as a pathogen of animals and humans. It is unique in bringing these advances together in a single source. Many aspects of the disease processes are the same irrespective of the host species and veterinary and human medicine have learnt a lot from each other in the field of pathogenesis of *E. coli* infections. The emphasis of the book is on the role of *E. coli* in animal disease, but substantial portions are either common to human and veterinary medicine, or are devoted to human diseases. The comprehensive nature of the book is evident from the table of contents. In Part I of the book, a discussion of the biochemical and serologic characteristics of the organism lays the foundation for an understanding of *E. coli* as a pathogen. The following section discusses pathogenesis of intestinal and extra-intestinal disease in animals and humans. The third section is devoted to detailed discussions of established or putative virulence factors of *E. coli* and the final section discusses diagnostic laboratory tests and the use of vaccines against *E. coli* diseases.

In Escherichia coli *in Domestic Animals and Humans*, common themes are described for different hosts, but host species specificity is clear and fascinating variations on the themes are frequent. The genetic versatility of the bacterium is evident throughout: plasmid or phage-encoded virulence genes are common and toxins are borrowed from obliging neighbours. Characteristics of the organism are presented by experts on its biochemistry, antigenicity, surface structures, toxins, and metabolism, and interactions of the bacterium with the host are discussed at levels varying from animal, tissue; cells to molecules. The book will be valuable to researchers with a special interest in diseases caused by *E. coli*, to veterinary and medical clinicians, to graduate veterinary and medical students, and as a reference for senior undergraduate students.

I

Characteristics of *Escherichia coli*

Biochemical Characteristics of *Escherichia coli*

1

K.A. Bettelheim
School of Agriculture, La Trobe University, Bundoora, Victoria 3083, Australia

Introduction

The organisms isolated from the faeces of neonates and first described by Escherich as *Bacterium coli commune* (Escherich, 1885, 1988; Bettelheim, 1986) have become the most fully documented organisms currently known. Most studies on bacterial metabolism and biochemical processes have been conducted on *Escherichia coli*.

Initially, *E. coli* were considered commensal organisms and most of the investigations on these organisms at the turn of the century were concerned with the problems of distinguishing the 'agents of typhoid fever' and other types of *Salmonella* from them. During the first few decades of this century it was predominantly these investigations which led to the development of the biochemical tests which are the basis of modern bacterial taxonomy. The demonstration that there were a number of types and subtypes of these organisms, which could easily be distinguished from the typhoid bacillus by these tests, became the basis of the taxonomy of the Enterobacteriaceae in general and *E. coli* in particular.

Metabolism

Growth requirements

Carbon and energy sources

E. coli are typical members of the Enterobacteriaceae, which are characterized by being able to grow aerobically and anaerobically. They are able to utilize simple carbon and nitrogen sources for all their metabolic and energy needs. Thus *E. coli* can multiply effectively in a medium containing only glucose, ammonium and mineral salts. While a variety of other carbon-containing substrates can be similarly utilized, glucose is by far the preferred substrate. Glucose is transported across the cytoplasmic membrane via the phosphoenolpyruvate-dependent sugar phosphotransferase system (PTS) (Konings *et al.*, 1981). Glucose competitively inhibits the uptake of other sugars using this transport mechanism and employs a variety of mechanisms to inhibit the uptake of sugars not using this system.

There is also control by glucose at the level of initiation of transcription of the enzymes required to metabolize other substrates. In *E. coli*, cyclic AMP (cAMP) in a complex with the catabolite-gene activator protein (CAP) must bind to the promoter region of an operator on the genome, to enable the binding of the RNA polymerase and the subsequent initiation of transcription to occur (Botsford, 1981). The metabolism of glucose decreases the intracellular concentration of cAMP, causing a repression of the various operons that require activation by the cAMP–CAP complex. This phenomenon, which was termed catabolite repression as long ago as 1961 (Magasanik, 1961), appears to have an important role for a phosphorylated enzyme of the PTS. These two linked mechanisms, the exclusion of the inducer and prevention of induction of the catabolic enzymes by lowered cAMP concentration, cause the preferential utilization of glucose and the phenomenon of diauxic growth of *E. coli* on mixtures of glucose and another carbohydrate substrate.

E. coli can also utilize fatty acids and acetate as sole carbon and energy sources (Nunn, 1986). Apart from acetate, fatty acids must be at least 12 carbon atoms long in order to be able to act as sole carbon and energy source, and their use in this manner is characterized by a distinct lag phase. There is a requirement for the coordinated induction of the synthesis of at least five fatty acid-oxidative enzymes. In addition, when *E. coli* grows on acetate or fatty acids, the glyoxylate shunt is required to be in operation and the two unique enzymes of the shunt, isocitrate lyase and malate synthetase A, are induced (Kornberg, 1966).

Nitrogen sources

Ammonium sulfate is the preferred nitrogen source for *E. coli*. The products of genes closely linked to the structural gene for glutamine synthetase are associated with the regulation of the various genes involved in the control of nitrogen metabolism. While a number of Enterobacteriaceae including *Klebsiella pneumoniae* can grow well aerobically with nitrate or nitrite as sole source of nitrogen (Nagatani *et al.*, 1971), this has not been demonstrated in *E. coli*, which lacks the ability to form an assimilatory nitrate reductase. *E. coli* produces an NADH-nitrite reductase (Kemp and

Atkinson, 1966), whose induction is not controlled by the availability of ammonia, but by anaerobiosis. Nitrite derived from nitrate by reduction can also serve as inducer of NADH-nitrite reductase synthesis but at high concentrations nitrate suppresses nitrite reductase synthesis (Cole and Wimpenny, 1968) and *E. coli* grown anaerobically in high concentrations of nitrate may not be able to utilize the resultant nitrite effectively. The ammonia formed by the anaerobic reduction of nitrite can be utilized by *E. coli* as a source of nitrogen in the usual way. *E. coli* can grow anaerobically on nitrate as sole nitrogen source.

Approximately a quarter of the total nitrite reductase activity in *E. coli* is linked to formate oxidation (Abou-Jaoude *et al.*, 1979). This pathway may be involved in energy conservation. Nitrate respiring cells resemble aerobic cells by generating NAD^+ through a respiratory chain. In addition, they contain low levels of alcohol dehydrogenase and formate-hydrogen lyase. Unlike anaerobic cells they have an incomplete tricarboxylic acid cycle and excrete acetate.

Responses of **E. coli** *to the environment*

Like most microorganisms, *E. coli* is well able to respond to changes in the environment by controlling the activities of existing enzymes. Three types of such rapid control mechanisms have been identified: modulation, covalent modification and selective inactivation. Modulation is based on the fact that many enzymes are allosteric and their activities can be changed by the presence of low-molecular-weight effector molecules (Baumberg, 1981). The accumulation of endproducts in biosynthetic pathways, such as those for amino acids, often leads to specific inhibition of the first enzyme involved in the pathway. This has also been described as feedback inhibition. Another example of this mechanism can be taken from the tricarboxylic acid cycle enzymes of *E. coli*. Citrate synthetase activity is inhibited when the concentrations of nicotinamide adenine dinucleotide (NADH) and α-ketoglutarate are reduced. Conversely, there is activation of pyruvate kinase by fructose-1,6-biphosphate. The enzyme phosphofructokinase is subject to inhibition by phosphoenolpyruvate and activation by adenosine 5′-diphosphate (Baumberg, 1981).

An example of enzyme regulation by the covalent conversion of an enzyme is the biochemistry of glutamine synthetase, which catalyses the ATP-dependent production of glutamine from ammonia and glutamate. This enzyme consists of 12 identical subunits and is subject to reversible adenylation of a specific tyrosyl residue on each subunit. The biosynthetic activity of the enzyme is maximal when it is completely unadenylated, and the fully adenylated enzyme is biosynthetically inactive, while activity varies over a wide range depending on the degree of adenylation (Tyler, 1978). This enzyme is also subject to feedback inhibition and its activity is controlled by the concentrations of divalent cations.

When an organism has to adapt to a major change in the availability of nutrients, there is selective inactivation of enzymes, particularly those that are no longer required or ones which might be harmful in the new conditions. This is known as selective inactivation. It can proceed either by modification of the enzyme protein or by its degradation (Switzer, 1977), as is the case with lysine-sensitive aspartokinase of *E. coli*.

E. coli will grow more rapidly with glucose as carbon source than with acetate. It will grow even more rapidly if the glucose is supplemented with vitamins, amino acids, nucleotide precursors, etc. With changes in growth rate, there are also internal changes within each cell, which becomes larger in fast growing cultures and has more replication forks on the chromosome. There is a parallel increase in the RNA/mass ratio with growth rate as more ribosomes are formed in the fast growing cells. The DNA/mass and protein/mass ratios remain fairly constant at different growth rates. When *E. coli* are subjected to a nutritional downshift, there occurs the so-called stringent response (Baracchini and Bremer, 1988) linked with a cessation of stable RNA accumulation. Examples of such nutritional downshifts are the changing of the carbon source from glucose to acetate or the removing of amino acids from the medium.

Glucose can support a far higher growth rate than acetate (Ingraham *et al.*, 1983). It is presumed that the energy requirement per unit molecule of pumping one molecule of acetate into the cell is the same as for one molecule of glucose. Acetate contains only two carbon atoms compared to the six of glucose, thus a significant amount of the energy obtained by the metabolism of these substrates must be used for their actual pumping into the cell. From these and similar observations it has been found that an equal amount of energy per unit time is consumed by *E. coli* over a wide range of doubling times with a wide variety of substrates (Andersen and von Meyenburg, 1980).

The growth rate of an organism like *E. coli* will increase the more the medium is supplemented with the various utilizable biosynthetic building blocks such as amino acids, nucleosides, bases and vitamins. When the available carbon sources and energy do not have to be used for the synthesis of these building blocks, they can be used to form the more activated precursors for the biosynthesis of macromolecules. In a rich medium *E. coli* can grow very fast, because the genes coding for products contributing to the macromolecular apparatus of protein and RNA synthesis have very high maximal rates of expression. This makes the cell dependent on a large pool of precursors, which is not available when the organisms grow in minimal conditions, and then the rate of growth decreases according to the availability of these precursors.

The *E. coli* cell has been described as an unsaturated system designed for rapid growth, but limited by the 'feeder reactions' and the medium

(Jensen and Pedersen, 1990). Several growth-related phenomena might be explicable as resulting from medium-induced changes in the elongation kinetics during protein and RNA synthesis. By affecting the availability of free ribosomes and free RNA polymerase, the chain elongation reactions, which consume substrates, may control the rates of chain initiation, which do not consume substrates.

An important factor for the growth of an organism like *E. coli* in an animate environment is the availability of iron. *E. coli* has the ability to absorb iron from the environment (Chart *et al.*, 1988). Law *et al.* (1992) showed that the iron-uptake abilities of enteropathogenic and control *E. coli* were similar, as were the incidence of aerobactin and enterochelin production. In contrast to the data for *E. coli* in the intestinal environment, there is substantial evidence that ability to compete with the host for limited iron may be critical for invasive *E. coli* (Chapter 19).

In their natural environment *E. coli* cells survive a variety of environmental challenges. Natural populations of *E. coli* have extensive genetic diversity and studies involving multilocus enzyme electrophoresis, carbohydrate fermentation patterns, and serotyping have shown that *E. coli* may be organized into a limited number of genetically distinct clones (Whittam, 1989). Whittam further suggests that many such clones are sufficiently stable to have achieved a broad geographic distribution. While this is particularly noted for some of the pathogenic types, it may also occur with the non-pathogenic forms. Within a restricted environment, such as the intestinal tract of a host animal, a diversity of clones will be maintained as new clones enter the system and may establish and some even become dominant, while others may become extinct.

The ability of *E. coli* to carry virulence factor genes probably is of selective advantage for growth in a host animal, however it is probably not advantageous in the inanimate environment. Martins *et al.* (1992) demonstrated that 13% of *E. coli* isolates from treated and raw waters carried DNA sequences for one or more virulence factors including the Shiga-like toxins, the heat-labile and heat-stable enterotoxins, and the adherence factors EAF and Eae. This clearly indicates the ability of the pathogenic *E. coli* clones to survive in the environment. For such factors, which are often encoded on plasmids, to survive and be maintained in their host populations, they must confer some selective advantage on their host (Gordon, 1992). *E. coli* O157:H7, which had been associated with a water-borne outbreak of haemorrhagic colitis, was shown to be easily obtained after many days from water (Rice *et al.*, 1992).

E. coli is a typical facultative anaerobe; it can grow both in the presence and absence of oxygen. It is partly responsible for maintaining the strictly anaerobic conditions prevailing in the intestines, which permit the strict anaerobes to grow. The ability of *E. coli* to grow aerobically must provide distinct ecological advantages. In the intestinal environment it would permit *E. coli* to multiply close to epithelial cells, where oxygen may be available from the blood after passage through the cells to the attached microbial mat (Savage, 1977). Ability to multiply aerobically must provide *E. coli* with a distinct selective advantage in the natural environment outside the intestinal tracts of humans or animals. *E. coli* and only a few other bacterial species synthesize menaquinone (vitamin K), which is a component of the respiratory chain as well as a precursor of prothrombin in the host liver (Clarke and Bauchop, 1977). By being able to survive on a relatively limited number of low-molecular-weight compounds, *E. coli* is particularly well adapted to its environment (Koch, 1976). As these substances may only be present in low amounts and often transiently, this scavenging role must be maintained by potent active transport systems, the energy of which must be provided by oxidoreduction reactions, which must be able to utilize a variety of different electron donors and acceptors.

E. coli are widely distributed in waters including natural waters, particularly in tropical regions. High densities of both total and faecal coliforms have been detected in pristine streams and in groundwater samples (Hazen, 1988) in many parts of the world. They have even been found in epiphytic vegetation 10 m above ground in rain forests. Nucleic acid analyses have shown that many of these isolates are identical to clinical isolates. Apart from these culturable forms of *E. coli*, a number of studies from many parts of the world have shown the presence of viable *E. coli*, which cannot be cultured on the media currently available (Xu *et al.*, 1982; Flint, 1987). Plasmid DNA is stably maintained in these viable but non-culturable forms of *E. coli* in a variety of waters (Flint, 1987; Caldwell *et al.*, 1989; Byrd and Colwell, 1990). These non-culturable forms, which develop as a result of starvation conditions, may revert to culturable forms following ingestion into human or animal intestinal tracts. The survival of the *E. coli* DNA including the virulence and resistance plasmids in such non-culturable forms has serious ecological implications (McKay, 1992).

Biochemical reactions of **E. coli**

Taxonomy of E. coli

The complexity of the metabolism of *E. coli* described above should be taken into account when the biochemical and other tests which are used to identify and characterize these organisms are considered. *E. coli* are members of the family Enterobacteriaceae. The characteristics of the family have recently been defined by Brenner (1992) and the type genus is *Escherichia*. *E. coli* is only one species of the genus *Escherichia* but it is the major species. There have been a number of definitions of the genus but the most useful is the one given by Ewing (1986).

Other species of the genus *Escherichia* include *E. adecarboxylata*,

E. blattae, *E. fergusonii*, *E. hermanii* and *E. vulneris*. *E. adecarboxylata*, a yellow pigmented organism, was described by Leclerc in 1962. It has now been suggested that this organism may be part of the *Enterobacter agglomerans–Erwinia* group (Farmer *et al.*, 1985a) and it has been transferred to the new genus *Leclercia* (Tamura *et al.*, 1986).

Strains of *E. blattae* were first isolated from the cockroach intestine (Burgess *et al.*, 1973) and do not seem to have been isolated from any other sources. The species *E. fergusonii* was only recently named (Farmer *et al.*, 1985b) and characterized and strains of this species have been isolated mainly from human faeces, blood and urine as well as various domestic animals, including cows, pigs, horses and turkeys. They were previously listed as Enteric Group 10.

The species now designated as *E. hermannii*, which had previously been listed as Enteric Group 11, are yellow pigmented. Most have been isolated from human wounds and faeces, but there have also been a few isolations from spinal fluid and blood (Brenner *et al.*, 1982a). Strains of the species *E. vulneris*, previously Enteric Group 1 (also known as API Group 2, Alma Group 1), while similar to *Enterobacter agglomerans*, were placed in the new species in the genus *Escherichia* in 1982 (Brenner *et al.*, 1982b). These strains were mainly isolated from wounds and faeces. The main biochemical characteristics of these species are given in Table 1.1.

Biochemical basis of taxonomic tests

The ability to ferment glucose with the production of acid and gas is a basic characteristic of *E. coli*. Furthermore the ability of *E. coli* to ferment other carbohydrate substrates is generally dependent on its ability to convert them to glucose or to derivatives of glucose on the fermentation pathway. *E. coli* belongs to the group of organisms in which acids such as acetic, formic, lactic and succinic, as well as ethanol, predominate. Hence these organisms are able to reduce the pH to levels at which methyl red changes colour (methyl red positive). *E. coli* does not produce 2,3-butanediol and acetoin, which are characteristic of the fermentation of *Enterobacter aerogenes*. These are measured by the Voges–Proskauer (VP) test, in which *Ent. aerogenes* is positive and *E. coli* is negative. The gas produced by *E. coli* is generally a mixture of almost equal amounts of hydrogen and carbon dioxide produced by the breakdown of formic acid by the action of the enzyme formate hydrogen lyase. Anaerogenic strains of *E. coli* and most strains of *Shigella* lack this enzyme.

The basis of the ability of *E. coli* to ferment lactose, which generally has distinguished it from strains of *Salmonella* and *Shigella*, is that most strains carry the enzyme β-galactosidase, which splits lactose into glucose and galactose. These sugars are then fermented in the usual way. Le Minor and Ben Hamida (1962) developed a test for the presence of β-galactosidase

Table 1.1. Main biochemical characteristics of the genus *Escherichia*.

Test	Percentage of isolates positive in the test				
	E. coli	*E. blattae*	*E. fergusonii*	*E. hermanii*	*E. vulneris*
Indole	98	0	98	99	0
Methyl Red	99	100	100	100	100
Voges–Proskauer	0	0	0	0	0
Citrate (Simmons')	1	50	17	1	0
Hydrogen sulfide (TSI)	1	0	0	0	0
Urease	1	0	0	0	0
Phenylalanine deaminase	0	0	0	0	0
Lysine decarboxylase	90	100	95	6	85
Arginine dihydrolase	17	0	5	0	30
Ornithine decarboxylase	65	100	100	100	0
Motility (36 °C)	95	0	93	99	100
Gelatin hydrolysis (22 °C)	0	0	0	0	0
Growth in KCN	3	0	0	94	15
Malonate utilization	0	100	35	0	85
D-Glucose, acid	100	100	100	100	100
D-Glucose, gas	95	100	95	97	97
Lactose fermentation	95	0	0	45	15
Sucrose fermentation	50	0	0	45	8
D-Mannitol fermentation	98	0	98	100	100
Dulcitol fermentation	60	0	60	19	0
Salicin fermentation	40	0	65	40	30
Adonitol fermentation	5	0	98	0	0
myo-Inositol fermentation	1	0	0	0	0
D-Sorbitol fermentation	94	0	0	0	1
L-Arabinose fermentation	99	100	98	100	100

Raffinose fermentation	50	0	0	40	99
L-Rhamnose fermentation	80	100	92	97	93
Maltose fermentation	95	100	96	100	100
D-Xylose fermentation	95	100	96	100	100
Trehalose fermentation	98	75	96	100	100
Cellobiose fermentation	2	0	96	97	100
α-Methyl-D-glucoside fermentation	0	0	0	0	25
Erythritol fermentation	0	0	0	0	0
Aesculin hydrolysis	35	0	46	40	20
Mellibiose fermentation	75	0	0	0	100
D-Arabitol fermentation	5	0	100	8	0
Glycerol fermentation	75	100	20	3	25
Mucate fermentation	95	50	0	97	78
Tartrate, Jordan's	95	50	96	35	2
Acetate utilization	90	0	96	78	30
Lipase (corn oil)	0	0	0	0	0
DNase at 25 °C	0	0	0	0	0
Nitrate → nitrite	100	100	100	100	100
Oxidase, Kovac's	0	0	0	0	0
ONPG	95	0	83	98	100
Yellow pigment	0	0	0	98	50
D-Mannose fermentation	98	100	100	100	100

based on the ability of this enzyme to split the colourless *ortho*-nitrophenyl β-D-galactopyranoside to the yellow *ortho*-nitrophenol. Addition of an inducer of β-galactosidase such as isopropyl β-D-thiogalactopyranoside has been found to enhance the technique for the detection of *E. coli* (Diehl, 1991). When an organism can ferment either melibiose, or sucrose, or both, it is also able to ferment raffinose (Buissiére *et al.*, 1977). This is because raffinose is α-galactosido-(1-6)-glucosido-β-(1-2)-fructofuranoside and galactose can be removed by the α-galactosidase which splits melibiose and the fructose can be removed by the β-fructosidase (invertase), which splits sucrose.

A number of the characteristics used in Table 1.1, such as growth in potassium cyanide (KCN) and Kovac's oxidase test, are reflected in the respiratory chain of the organism. *E. coli* is negative in the KCN test, which means it is unable to grow in the presence of ≈1 mM KCN (Møller, 1954). Also, in common with all Enterobacteriaceae, *E. coli* is 'oxidase-negative'. The basis of this test is the ability of the organism to catalyse the oxidation of di- or tetramethyl-*p*-phenylenediamine plus α-naphthol to indophenol blue. A positive reaction, which usually occurs within 30 seconds, is due to the presence of a membrane-bound high-potential cytochrome *c* linked to an active cytochrome oxidase (Jurtshuk *et al.*, 1975). This is frequently also an indicator of the presence of 'energy coupling site 3' which may reflect the fact that oxidase-negative organisms like *E. coli* tend to occupy ecological niches where there is a relative abundance of energy and reducing power (Jones *et al.*, 1977; Jones, 1980).

Many strains of *E. coli* are able to decarboxylate ornithine and/or arginine. These abilities are used in the taxonomic differentiation of the Enterobacteriaceae and have been used to biotype strains of *E. coli*. Tabor and Tabor (1985) noted that under semianaerobic conditions at low pH, 'inducible' ornithine and arginine decarboxylases can appear if there is an excess of those amino acids present. These inducible enzymes are distinct from the biosynthetic ones and are involved in pH control of the organisms. Neither enzyme is inhibited by physiological concentrations of polyamines. When *E. coli* ferments a carbohydrate such as glucose, the resulting acid reduces the pH of the medium. In the presence of an amino acid such as arginine, lysine or ornithine, the basic amines agmatine, cadaverine and putrescine, respectively, are formed with the loss of CO_2, reversing the pH effect of the fermentation of glucose. This is the basis of the decarboxylase tests designed by Møller (1955). The decomposition of other amino acids with the production of ammonia has also been suggested as a useful diagnostic tool for *E. coli* (Serény, 1963/4). The production of indole by the action of tryptophanase on tryptophan is one of the characteristic features of *E. coli*.

Recently a new chromogenic compound, 5-bromo-4-chloro-3-indoxyl-β-D-glucuronide, was found to be useful for the rapid differentiation of

E. coli (Watkins *et al.*, 1988). The cyclohexylammonium salt of 5-bromo-4-chloro-3-indoxyl-β-D-glucuronic acid (BCIG) was incorporated into media for the isolation of *E. coli* and compared with media containing the other recently described compound for the differentiation of *E. coli*, 4-methylumbelliferyl-β-D-glucuronide (MUG) (Feng and Hartman, 1982). Overall it was found that reactions in MUG and BCIG were in agreement. These compounds can be used to identify strains as *E. coli*. In 1991, Sarhan and Foster introduced a new medium incorporating MUG for the isolation and identification of *E. coli*, but the enterohaemorrhagic *E. coli* O157:H7 are generally negative in this reaction (Thompson *et al.*, 1990).

The production of haemolysins by *E. coli* has been known since 1903 and most studies on them have been concerned mainly with their possible role as virulence factors. Haemolysin production can also be used as a differentiating characteristic for *E. coli*. Smith (1963) distinguished strains producing α-haemolysin, which occurs free in culture fluid filtrates from β-haemolysin, which is cell bound. *E. coli* may produce either one or both. Of a number of other haemolysins, which have been described since, enterohaemolysin (Beutin *et al.*, 1988) was found associated with *E. coli* isolated from infants with gastroenteritis. The *E. coli* haemolysins have recently been reviewed (Beutin, 1991) and are discussed in Chapter 15.

It is important to realize that, following subculture, strains of *E. coli* may become altered in their biochemical characteristics. In a recent study both loss and gain of biochemical activity were observed following subculture (Katouli *et al.*, 1990). However, strains stored at −70°C or 4°C did not show any changes.

Typing *E. coli*

Micro and rapid methods for typing E. coli

Micromethods for identification

The classical or conventional tests for the identification of microorganisms, which have been in use for up to a century, are based on the ability of a given microorganism to use various carbon sources or to produce various metabolic endproducts. Initially, different laboratories used different formulations of media and different categories of tests for their identification procedures, making interlaboratory comparisons difficult. However, during the first half of this century some international agreement was reached. Later, the concept of miniaturizing some of these conventional procedures was developed (Hartman, 1968). The basis for these tests was the assumption that a sufficient concentration of preformed bacterial enzymes was present after primary growth, to perform the metabolic conversions of taxonomic relevance. On the basis of these concepts, commercially produced reagent-impregnated strips became available in the 1960s.

The lessons learnt in these developments led to a return to the use of conventional tests but now organized in a series of miniaturized tubes containing individual substrates, multicompartment tubes or plates with multiple substrates, and paper strips or discs impregnated with dehydrated substrates. Each of these tubes or reacting systems contains substrates carefully selected by the manufacturer such that reproducibility and speed of reaction were insured. Identifications were then based on percentage tables such as those published by Edwards and Ewing (1972). These systems not only differed from each other in the sets of substrates provided, but also in the specific formulations of substrate media. These formulations and the conditions of incubation often differed from those used in the classical tests on which the percentage tables of Edwards and Ewing (1972) and similar data were based. Thus, a strong potential for misidentification existed in these early systems.

In the more recent systems, the manufacturers have compiled sets of highly sophisticated computer-generated identification data bases uniquely designed for each system. Large numbers of strains identified by classical means and by the system in question are placed in these data bases, which are regularly updated. Based on the results obtained with a given strain, a biochemical profile is obtained and compared with the data base, which gives an identification and a level of confidence in the identification. The computer also indicates whether further tests are needed to confirm the identity of the isolate.

The Enterobacteriaceae were among the first groups of organisms for which such systems were developed. One of the earliest systems, which is still being used very successfully throughout the world, is the API system (API, Bio Mérieux SA, Lyon, France; Analytab Products, Plainview, New York, USA), which was first described in 1972 (Bartoli *et al.*, 1972; Smith *et al.*, 1972). The API system comprises a series of plastic pockets containing dehydrated media into which is transferred a suspension of the organism to be tested. Some of the tests are covered with mineral oil to maintain anaerobic conditions. The tests include the ONPG test; tests for dehydrolysis of arginine and decarboxylation of lysine and ornithine; utilization of citrate; production of H_2S, indole and acetoin; urease, tryptophan deaminase and gelatinase activities; and fermentation of glucose, mannitol, inositol, sorbitol, rhamnose, sucrose, melibiose, amygdalin and arabinose. After overnight incubation at 37°C in a humid chamber the results of the tests are determined on the basis of the colour changes. Specific reagents have to be added to three tests: indole, Voges–Proskauer and tryptophan deaminase. On the basis of the test results a profile is established and identification is made by consulting a computer-generated list.

Recently, a more rapid method of identifying strains was developed based on the API system. This is the ATB 32E system (API), which includes 32 wells corresponding to the various biochemical tests (Freney *et al.*, 1991). Both conventional as well as some newly developed tests are included and it is considered very suitable for the rapid identification of Enterobacteriaceae including *E. coli*.

A system has also been developed using strips of plastic wells, like microtitre trays (Microbact System, Disposable Products Pty Ltd, Technology Park, SA, Australia). These are inoculated with a suspension of the organism to be tested. Anaerobic conditions are applied to some tests by use of mineral oil and the strips are sealed with plastic tape. Following overnight incubation, the colour changes are recorded. In addition the three tests requiring additional reagents are performed as for the API and again a profile for the test organism is obtained and compared with the list provided. In comparative studies with API the Microbact system has performed well (Mugg and Hill, 1981).

A more rapid method for identifying Enterobacteriaceae is the Micro-ID system (General Diagnostics, Organon Teknika Corporation, Morris Plains, New Jersey, USA). This system is based on the principle that the inoculated organisms contain preformed enzyme systems, whose levels can be detected within 4 hours. The system uses filter paper discs impregnated with reagents designed to detect the presence of specific enzyme systems or metabolic products. There are 15 different discs in 15 chambers in a molded styrene tray. Apart from the Voges–Proskauer test, all substrate and detection reagents which are required are present. A suspension of a colony from a primary isolation plate can be used and only 0.2 ml of suspension is required. The suspension is pipetted into the tray which is then incubated for 4 hours. A 20% solution of KOH is added to the Voges–Proskauer test well and the colour changes in all 15 wells are recorded. In evaluation studies this system has performed well (Barry and Badal, 1979).

The use of preformed enzymes and their action on fluorogenic substrates was also investigated by Godsey *et al.* (1981). They found that using overnight growth suspended in saline to a standard density and added to the substrates gave a reproducible enzyme profile within 30 minutes.

Recently the Cobas Micro (Becton Dickinson, Meylan, France), a computer-controlled apparatus which performs automatic identification and sensitivity testing using specially designed rotors, has been put on the market. The principle of the system is that the inoculated rotor is centrifuged, which allows distribution of an exact sample volume to each of the chambers and a photometer measures absorbance values in each rotor chamber. The rotor for the identification of Enterobacteriaceae (ID-E/NF) is comprised of 33 chambers of which two are control chambers, providing

31 tests per sample. Depending on inoculum density, results are determined after incubation periods of 5 or 17–24 hours. The system gave good identification of a variety of Gram-negative organisms including nonfermenters (Geiss and Geiss, 1992). All 110 strains of *E. coli* were correctly identified.

The Vitek system (Vitek Systems, Inc., Hazelwood, MO, USA) has been commercially available since 1976. A plastic card containing dehydrated media is filled with a standard sample suspension and loaded into a reader/incubator, which is connected to a computer and prints out a complete form at 4 or 18 hours, giving an identification as compared with a data base. Knight *et al.* (1990) found that 97% of *E. coli* were correctly identified by this method.

The Enterotube (Roche Diagnostics, Nutley, New Jersey, USA) consists of a plastic tube, which is subdivided into a number of compartments containing agar-based media. Through the centre of the tube runs a metal wire. With the bare, sterile tip of the wire the colony to be tested is touched, the wire is then drawn through the tube, inoculating each of the media as it passes through. The tube is then incubated overnight at 37°C and the characteristic colour changes determined. A profile is determined and identification is made by comparison with a computer-generated list of profiles.

Biotyping and subtyping of E. coli

For any type of epidemiological investigation involving microorganisms it is important to be able to distinguish strains and show relatedness. While serotyping which employs an internationally accepted scheme is the method of choice, the requirement for a large number of fully characterized antisera largely restricts this method of differentiation to a reference laboratory. As there are some biochemical reactions in which some strains of *E. coli* will be positive while others will be negative, including some fermentation and the decarboxylase reactions (Table 1.1), these would lend themselves particularly for use in biotyping. In addition, drug resistance provides another useful set of markers which can be used to differentiate strains of *E. coli*. The value of these discriminatory tests for distinguishing strains of *E. coli* has been demonstrated for a number of years (Mushin and Ashburner, 1964; Bettelheim *et al.*, 1974). While these techniques have yielded valuable epidemiological results, caution has to be exercised with them, as with all means of differentiating microorganisms. The fact that drug resistances are frequently plasmid mediated is well known; it should also be realized that fermentation reactions which are the main backbone of these biotyping methods can also be plasmid mediated (Shinebaum *et al.*, 1977). In this study it was shown that by transmitting a plasmid coding for the enzyme invertase, a strain of *E. coli* could ferment both sucrose and raffinose and that this ability was lost by treatment with ethidium bromide. The ability to ferment raffinose but not sucrose was also found to be transmissible and in this case it was linked to tetracycline resistance and H_2S production, which is rare in *E. coli* (Ørskov and Ørskov, 1973). Biotyping was also found to be a useful method of distinguishing haemolytic strains of *E. coli* belonging to serogroups O138, O139 and O141, which had been isolated from pigs (Månson, 1962). Månson particularly noted that some strains were atypical in being urease and KCN positive as well as having unusual decarboxylase patterns.

Extensive studies have been reported by Crichton and Old (1979, 1980, 1982) on the development of biotyping schemes for *E. coli*. Tests for the ability of strains to ferment dulcitol, raffinose and sorbose and to decarboxylate ornithine gave optimal discrimination among strains. With these four tests they were able to establish 16 primary biotypes, which could be further subdivided by means of a secondary set of tests, which included the fermentation of rhamnose, decarboxylation of lysine, hydrolysis of aesculin, motility within 24 hours, production of type 1 fimbriae, requirement for nicotinamide, thiamine and/or another factor for growth on minimal medium. Based on the biotyping and resistotyping methods developed over the previous decade, Crichton and Old (1992) produced a discriminatory index for *E. coli*. When strains from a variety of sources were tested then good discrimination was achieved, however when the sources were limited discrimination was not so good, suggesting that strains may well be related within clones or subclones.

Biotyping systems can be developed for a variety of strains of different sources depending on the type of answer that the study is designed to obtain. Generally they must be simple, not require complex reagents and give maximum discrimination. A set using six tests: fermentation of dulcitol, raffinose, sorbose and 5-ketogluconate, motility and production of β-haemolysis, was successfully used in conjunction with the API20E identification system to differentiate strains of *E. coli* (Gargan *et al.*, 1982).

With the development of rapid methods for identifying Enterobacteriaceae, some of these provide a ready-made set of biochemical tests which can be used for biotyping as well as for identifying strains of *E. coli*. Kühn *et al.* (1990) examined the value of two systems for the purposes of discriminating between strains of *E. coli*. They not only used biotyping but also biochemical fingerprinting, in which a quantitative measurement of the metabolism of the various substrates is obtained by measuring the speed and intensity of each reaction (Kühn, 1985). The systems examined in these studies were the PhP-EC (BioSys Inova, Stockholm, Sweden) and the API 50 CH (La Balme, Les Grottes, France). The former uses 24 biochemical tests selected to give high discrimination. The dehydrated reagents are kept in flat-bottomed microtitre trays, such that there are four sets of 24 reagents per tray. The bacterial suspensions in 0.2% peptone and

0.1% bromothymol blue are dispensed into each well and the light absorbance is read after 4, 7, 24 and 48 hours. By linking the optical reader to a computer a quantitative result depending on the speed and intensity of each reaction can be obtained.

The API 50 CH system consists of 49 carbohydrates and one negative control. The dehydrated reagents, including phenol red as a pH indicator, are provided in specially designed plastic trays, into which the bacterial suspension is dispensed. The reactions are read visually after 3, 6, 24 and 48 hours' incubation scoring the indicator colour change from zero (no reaction) to 4 (full positive reaction).

In their analysis of the results using epidemiologically unrelated strains of *E. coli* Kühn *et al.* (1990) applied a variety of techniques to enhance the discriminatory capabilities of the systems. They concluded that the PhP-EC was superior as it is specifically designed for *E. coli* while the API 50 CH was a more general system designed to study carbohydrate metabolism among Enterobacteriaceae in general.

While these commercial systems will give good differentiation, it is important in some cases to be able to limit oneself to only a few tests or perhaps to include some substrates which in general do not give high discrimination but are nevertheless useful to discriminate certain groups of strains. It has been shown (Buckwold *et al.*, 1979) that by designing one's own set of tests far greater discrimination could be achieved than with commercial systems. They used the following nine tests: fermentation of melibiose, adonitol, rhamnose, lactose, raffinose and sucrose, β-haemolysis, production of lysine decarboxylase and motility. The system developed by Yap and Barton (1985) is totally flexible in that any fermentable carbohydrate can be used. By increasing both the agar concentration and pH of the base medium, diffusion of acidity was minimized so that a large number of strains could be tested per plate. They tested as many as 52 strains, using a multiple-inoculation technique on one 90-mm plate.

Like many organisms, *E. coli* produce a variety of esterases, which hydrolyse multiple substrates. The electrophoretic diversity of these esterases can give reliable information for both the specific as well as the subspecific differentiation of the Enterobacteriaceae and be successfully used to differentiate strains of *E. coli* (Goullet, 1973, 1980; Goullet and Picard, 1984). A large number of strains of both human and animal origin have been studied for their esterase patterns (Goullet and Picard, 1986a) and good discrimination between strains was achieved. Certain pathogenic forms were shown to produce distinctive carboxylesterases (Goullet and Picard, 1986b).

Extensive studies have also shown that polymorphism among the outer membrane proteins (OMP) of *E. coli* can be used to differentiate strains and characterize specific clones (Achtman *et al.*, 1986) and these investigations have demonstrated that OMP patterns discriminate among the genetically different clonal groups within the serogroups O2 and O78, which are associated with avian disease (Kapur *et al.*, 1992).

Bettelheim and Carlile (1976) demonstrated that the Dienes phenomenon, which had been described some time ago for swarming strains of *Proteus*, could also be observed among *E. coli* if they were cultured on semisolid agar. They termed this general phenomenon 'colony incompatibility' and further studies found that by permitting strains to swarm towards each other and determining whether they are compatible or not, they could be subdivided (Bettelheim, 1980).

Development of Drug Resistance by *E. coli*

While native *E. coli* unexposed to antibiotic pressures tend to be fully sensitive to a wide spectrum of antibiotics and other antimicrobial agents, exposure to such substances will select for resistance. This resistance development in *E. coli* has been observed from the earliest times of the use of these agents and there is an extensive literature on the subject.

Plasmid encoded β-lactamases acquired by *E. coli* constitute a major weapon against an important class of antibiotics. Plasmid-mediated extended-spectrum β-lactamases (ESβs), which cause resistance to most penicillins, cephalosporins and aztreonam have been described (Philippon *et al.*, 1989; Weber *et al.*, 1990). Strains which produce ESβs are often resistant to currently available β-lactamase inhibitor/β-lactam drug combinations as well.

At least six chromosomally mediated β-lactamases have been distinguished in ampicillin-resistant *E. coli* by isoelectric focusing (Matthew and Harris, 1986). While most ampicillin-resistant strains of *E. coli* produce a chromosomal β-lactamase as well as a plasmid-mediated enzyme, which is responsible for the resistance, this latter enzyme is not present in about a fifth of them (Medeiros, 1984). These strains probably hyperproduce a chromosomal β-lactamase. Such chromosomal β-lactamases have always been associated with cephalosporin resistance and these organisms should thus not be considered cephalosporin sensitive (Marre and Aleksic, 1990).

By increasing the number of gene copies encoding for the production of a β-lactamase, *E. coli* can increase the level of β-lactamase leading to drug resistance. By altering the promoter or attenuator regions affecting gene transcription or by changing the complex regulatory apparatus involved in inducible β-lactamase expression, the levels of these enzymes can similarly be increased (Lindberg and Normark, 1986; Sanders, 1992). *E. coli* which were high-level producers of the broad spectrum β-lactamase TEM-1, and were resistant to the various β-lactamase inhibitor/β-lactam drug combinations, have been isolated from clinical conditions.

The basis for the organisms' resistance to the drug clavulanate, despite the enzyme being clavulanate sensitive, is the production of high levels of β-lactamase due to a high copy number of the structural gene. Levels of resistance increase with rising enzyme levels (Thomson *et al.*, 1990). The development of resistance in these *E. coli* can be explained on the basis of the interplay between permeation and the activity of the β-lactamase. It is considered that both the β-lactam drug and the β-lactamase inhibitor of the drug/inhibitor combinations would be permeating through the same pathway. If the *E. coli* only produce low levels of β-lactamase then the presence of the inhibitor would be sufficient to inactivate the β-lactamase. If the *E. coli* strain is a high level producer of β-lactamase then the amount of inhibitor permeating into the cells would be insufficient to inactivate all the β-lactamase. As the level of permeation of both the inhibitor and the drug is generally limited by the outer membrane of the *E. coli*, simply raising the level of β-lactamase will cause resistance to the drug/inhibitor combination. Further mutations causing decreases in permeability will augment the resistance of *E. coli* (Reguera *et al.*, 1991).

Mutants of *E. coli* which overproduce AmpC β-lactamase have been isolated from clinical situations and can be resistant to inhibitor/β-lactam combinations, second and third generation cephalosporins and cephamycins (Marre and Aleksic, 1990). It seems that, in the clinical isolates, enhanced expression of AmpC β-lactamase appears to arise predominantly through a mutation of the *amp*D gene, whose product prevents the transcription of the structural *amp*C gene, resulting in stable high-level production of β-lactamase (Lindberg *et al.*, 1988).

The observed β-lactam resistance among clinical *E. coli* isolates appears to be mainly mediated by TEM β-lactamase. The observed varied spectrum of resistances is probably determined by a number of additional strain-dependent factors (Cooksey *et al.*, 1990). The TEM-1 enzyme has been found in up to 50% of *E. coli* isolates and up to 85% of ampicillin-resistant *E. coli*. It was even present in 42% of commensal *E. coli* isolated from the faeces of healthy volunteers in Scotland (Thomson and Amyes, 1992).

Studies on carriage of antibiotic-resistant *E. coli* by children in a day care centre found that such strains frequently acquire trimethoprim resistance compared to strains from children not attending such centres (Reves *et al.*, 1990). Plasmid profile analysis of these isolates demonstrated that these *E. coli* were unique to each day care centre, indicating that these would likely be transmitted from the children to other members of the households and thus into the community. Fornasini *et al.* (1992) investigated this spread into households. The prevalence was highest in mothers (35%) and siblings (30%) and least in fathers (12%). In general, trimethoprim-resistant strains with the same plasmid profile isolated from the children were also found among the household members. There appeared to be no link between antibiotic use in a household and the spread of trimethoprim-resistant strains of *E. coli* within the household.

The resistance in one strain was associated with alterations in outer membrane proteins and not with the TEM-1 β-lactamase, which the strain also carried. Although potassium clavulanate enhanced the activity of ceftazidime against this strain of *E. coli*, it was due to a direct effect on the outer membrane proteins of the strain rather than to β-lactamase inhibition. Similar high levels of trimethoprim resistance were also found associated with *E. coli* isolated from children with diarrhoea in Nigeria, with over half the isolates being able to transfer their resistance into a sensitive strain of *E. coli* (Lamikanra *et al.*, 1990). Nearly half the enterotoxigenic strains able to transfer the drug resistance were also able to transfer their toxigenic characteristics. The transferability of drug resistance linked to enterotoxigenicity plasmids has been demonstrated by several researchers (Gyles *et al.*, 1977; Scotland *et al.*, 1979; Echeverria and Murphy, 1980; Singh *et al.*, 1992).

Similarly, norfloxacin-resistant mutants of *E. coli* have been shown to have altered outer membrane proteins, thereby affecting the uptake of the drug (Aoyama *et al.*, 1987). They also exhibited an alteration of the A subunit of the DNA gyrase. *E. coli* has developed two major mechanisms of resistance to the quinolone drugs. A major mechanism is the development of DNA gyrase with altered subunit structure (Wolfson *et al.*, 1989), while another is decreased outer membrane permeability arising from a reduced number of porins (Bedard *et al.*, 1989). The fluoroquinolones probably cross the outer membrane through the OmpF porin (Chapman and Georgopapadakou, 1988). Rough mutants, which are deficient in the lipopolysaccharide structures, were more susceptible to the hydrophobic quinolones than were the smooth wild-type strains, indicating that the porins are not the only mechanism by which these drugs enter *E. coli* cells. The drugs tosufloxacin and sparfloxacin appear to be more efficiently accumulated by *E. coli* porin-deficient mutants than by the parent strains (Mitsuyama *et al.*, 1992), indicating another mechanism of uptake. These drugs may permeate through the phospholipid bilayers and this ability may be independent of the hydrophobicity of the molecule.

The important role of outer membrane permeability for the introduction of drugs into *E. coli* has recently also been demonstrated for imipenem and the new related drug meropenem (Cornaglia *et al.*, 1992). There was no evidence of specific porin pathways for these drugs. Meropenem penetrated through the outer membrane of *E. coli* five times faster than cephaloridine but twice as slowly as imipenem. Although meropenem penetrated *E. coli* cells more slowly it was significantly more active against *E. coli* strains, both wild type as well as mutant strains, which were porin defective, and irrespective of whether they carried the CphA β-lactamase or not. Meropenem may have a higher affinity for the penicillin-binding proteins than imipenem.

With increasing use of drugs such as zidovidine (AZT), a thymine analogue, which is active against the human immunodeficiency virus, it has been found that organisms such as *E. coli* can readily become resistant to it. The mechanisms have been shown to be associated with the loss of thymidine kinase, which is required to convert AZT to the active triphosphate form (Lewin *et al.*, 1990).

For plasmids such as those conferring antibiotic resistance, to be maintained in *E. coli* in the natural environment selective advantage to their host bacterium must be provided (Gordon, 1992). A great diversity was found (Cooksey *et al.*, 1990) when the carriage of plasmids conferring β-lactam resistance was studied among hospital isolates of *E. coli*. This suggests that a wide distribution of such strains occurs in nature. Similar observations were made with the carriage of trimethoprim-resistant *E. coli* by children in day care centres and their family members (Fornasini *et al.*, 1992). Such studies demonstrate that there is extensive interchange of plasmids and other genetic material among *E. coli* in nature.

Concluding Remarks

This chapter has discussed the complexity of metabolism in *E. coli* and has illustrated the contribution to adaptability made by plasmids. It is not surpising, therefore, that this bacterium has been effective in surviving in a variety of environments inside and outside animal and human hosts. *E. coli* is also capable of producing a wide range of metabolic products, which cause damage to host organisms. These aspects of metabolism will be dealt with in subsequent chapters.

References

Abou-Jaoude, A., Chippaux, M. and Pascal, M.-C. (1979) Formate-nitrite reduction in *Escherichia coli* K12. 1 Physiological study of the system. *European Journal of Biochemistry* 95, 309–314.

Achtman, M., Heuzenroeder, M., Kusecek, B., Ochman, H., Caugant, D., Selander, R.K., Visanen-Rhen, V., Korhonen, T., Stuart, S., Ørskov, F. and Ørskov, I. (1986) Clonal analysis of *Escherichia coli* O2:K1 isolated from diseases humans and animals. *Infection and Immunity* 51, 268–276.

Andersen, K.B. and von Meyenburg, K. (1980) Are growth rates of *Escherichia coli* in batch culture limited by respiration? *Journal of Bacteriology* 144, 114–123.

Aoyama, H., Sato, K., Kato, T., Hirai, K. and Mitsuhashi, S. (1987) Norfloxacin resistance in a clinical isolate of *Escherichia coli*. *Antimicrobial Agents and Chemotherapy* 31, 1640–1641.

Baracchini, E. and Bremer, H. (1988) Stringent and growth control of rRNA synthesis in *Escherichia coli* are both mediated by ppGpp. *Journal of Biological Chemistry* 263, 2597–2602.

Barry, A.L. and Badal, R.E. (1979) Rapid identification of Enterobacteriaceae with the Micro-ID System versus API 20E and conventional media. *Journal of Clinical Microbiology* 10, 293–298.

Bartoli, M., Chouteau, J., Ettori, D., Bonnet, D. and Payen, G. (1972) Utilisation en pratique journalière d'une galerie d'intefication des Enterobacteréries. A propos de 671 souches. *Lyon Pharmaceutique* 23, 269–275.

Baumberg, S. (1981) The evolution of metabolic regulation. In: Carlile, M.J., Collins, J.F. and Moseley, B.E.B. (eds) *Molecular and Cellular Aspects of Microbial Evolution, Symposium of the Society for General Microbiology*. Cambridge University Press, Cambridge, pp. 229–272.

Bedard, J., Chamberland, S., Wong, S., Schollaardt, T. and Bryan, L.E. (1989) Contribution of permeability and susceptibility to inhibition of DNA synthesis in determining susceptibilities of *Escherichia coli*, *Pseudomonas aeruginosa*, and *Alcaligenes faecalis* to ciprofloxacin. *Antimicrobial Agents and Chemotherapy* 33, 1457–1464.

Bettelheim, K.A. (1980) Colony incompatibility among strains of *Escherichia coli* isolated during an outbreak of gastroenteritis in one ward. *Journal of Medical Microbiology* 13, 463–468.

Bettelheim, K.A. (1986) Commemoration of the publication 100 years ago of the papers by Dr. Th. Escherich in which are described for the first time the organisms that bear his name. *Zentralblatt für Bakteriologie, Parasitenkunde und Hygiene, I Abteilung Originale A* 261, 255–265.

Bettelheim, K.A. and Carlile, M.J. (1976) Colony incompatibility in bacteria. *Nature, London* 264, 757.

Bettelheim, K.A., Teoh-Chan, C.H., Chandler, M.E., O'Farrell, S.M., Rahamin, L., Shaw, E.J. and Shooter, R.A. (1974) Further studies of *Escherichia coli* in babies after normal delivery. *Journal of Hygiene, Cambridge* 73, 277–285.

Beutin, L. (1991) The different hemolysins of *Escherichia coli. Medical Microbiology and Immunology* 180, 167–182.

Beutin, L., Prada, J., Zimmermann, S., Stephan, R., Ørskov, I. and Ørskov, F. (1988) Enterohemolysin, a new type of hemolysin produced by some strains of enteropathogenic *E. coli* (EPEC). *Zentralblatt für Bakteriologie, Parasitenkunde und Hygiene, I Abteilung Originale A* 267, 576–588.

Botsford, J.L. (1981) Cyclic nucleotides in procaryotes. *Microbiolological Reviews* 45, 620–642.

Brenner, D.J. (1992) Introduction to the family Enterobacteriaceae. In: Balows, A., Truper, H.G., Dworkin, M., Harder, W. and Schleifer, K.-H. (eds) *The Procaryotes*. Springer-Verlag, New York, pp. 2673–2695.

Brenner, D.J., Davis, B.R., Steigerwalt, A.G., Riddle, C.F., McWorter, A.C., Allen, S.D., Farmer, J.J. III, Saitoh, Y. and Fanning, G.R. (1982a) Atypical biogroups of *Escherichia coli* found in clinical specimens and descriptions of *Escherichia hermannii* sp. nov. *Journal of Clinical Microbiology* 15, 703–713.

Brenner, D.J., McWorter, A.C, Knutson, J.K.L. and Steigerwalt, A.G. (1982b) *Escherichia vulneris*: a new species of Enterobacteriaceae associated with human wounds. *Journal of Clinical Microbiology* 15, 1133–1140.

Buckwold, F.J., Ronald, A.R., Harding, G.K.M., Marrie, T.J., Fox, L. and Cates, C. (1979) Biotyping of *Escherichia coli* by a simple multiple inoculation agar plate technique. *Journal of Clinical Microbiology* 10, 275–278.

Buissiére, J., Coynault, C. and Le Minor, L. (1977) Étude des conditions d'expression du caractère raffinose chez les *Escherichia* et *Salmonella. Annales Microbiologie (Institut Pasteur)* 128, 167–183.

Burgess, N.R.H., McDermott, S.N. and Whiting, J. (1973) Aerobic bacteria occurring in the hind-gut of the cockroach, *Blatta orientalis. Journal of Hygiene (Cambridge)* 71, 1–7.

Byrd, J.J. and Colwell, R.R. (1990) Maintenance of plasmids pBR322 and pUC8 in non-culturable *Escherichia coli* in the marine environment. *Applied and Environmental Microbiology* 56, 2104–2107.

Caldwell, B.A., Ye, C., Griffiths, R.P., Moyer, C.L. and Morita, R.Y. (1989) Plasmid expression and maintenance during long-term starvation-survival of bacteria in well water. *Applied and Environmental Microbiology* 55, 1860–1864.

Chapman, J.S. and Georgopapadakou, N.H. (1988) Route of quinolone permeation in *Escherichia coli. Antimicrobial Agents and Chemotherapy* 32, 438–442.

Chart, H., Stevenson, P. and Griffiths, E. (1988) Iron-regulated outer-membrane proteins of *Escherichia coli* strains associated with enteric extraintestinal diseases of man and animals. *Journal of General Microbiology* 134, 1549–1559.

Clarke, R.T.J. and Bauchop, T. (eds) (1977) *Microbial Ecology of the Gut.* Academic Press, London.

Cole, J.A. and Wimpenny, J.W.T. (1968) Metabolic pathways for nitrate reduction in *Escherichia coli. Biochimica et Biophysica Acta* 162, 39–48.

Cooksey, R., Swenson, J., Clark, N., Gay, E. and Thornsberry, C. (1990) Patterns and mechanisms of β-lactam resistance among isolates of *Escherichia coli* from hospitals in the United States. *Antimicrobial Agents and Chemotherapy* 34, 739–745.

Cornaglia, G., Guan, L., Fontana, R. and Satta, G. (1992) Diffusion of meropenem and imipenem through the outer membrane of *Escherichia coli* K-12 and correlation with their antibacterial activities. *Antimicrobial Agents and Chemotherapy* 36, 1902–1908.

Crichton, P.B. and Old, D.C. (1979) Biotyping of *Escherichia coli. Journal of Medical Microbiology* 12, 473–485.

Crichton, P.B. and Old, D.C. (1980) Differentiation of strains of *Escherichia coli*: multiple typing approach. *Journal of Clinical Microbiology* 11, 635–640.

Crichton, P.B. and Old, D.C. (1982) A biotyping scheme for the subspecific discrimination of *Escherichia coli. Journal of Medical Microbiology* 15, 233–242.

Crichton, P.B. and Old, D.C. (1992) Numerical index of the discriminatory ability of biotyping and resistotyping for strains of *Escherichia coli. Epidemiology and Infection* 108, 279–286.

Diehl, J.D., Jr (1991) Improved method for coliform verification. *Applied and Environmental Microbiology* 57, 604–605.

Echeverria, P. and Murphy, J.R. (1980) Enterotoxigenic *Escherichia coli* carrying plasmids coding for antibiotic resistance and enterotoxin production. *Journal of Infectious Diseases* 142, 273–278.

Edwards, P.R. and Ewing, W.H. (1972) *Identification of Enterobacteriaceae*. Burgess, Minneapolis.

Escherich, Th. (1885) Die Darmbakterien des Neugeboren und Sauglings. *Fortschritte der Medizin* 3, 515–522, 547–554.

Escherich, Th. (Translated, Bettelheim, K.A.) (1988) The intestinal bacteria of the neonate and breast-fed infant. *Review of Infectious Diseases* 10, 1220–1225.

Ewing, W.H. (1986) *Edwards and Ewing's Identification of Enterobacteriaceae*, 4th edn. Elsevier Science, New York.

Farmer, J.J. III, Davis, B.R., Hickman-Brenner, F.W., McWorter, A., Huntley-Carter, G.P., Asbury, M.A., Riddle, C., Wathe-Grady, H.G., Elias, C., Fanning, G.R., Steigerwalt, A.G., O'Hara, C.M., Morris, G.K., Smith, P.B. and Brenner, D.J. (1985a) Biochemical identification of new species and biogroups of Enterobacteriaceae isolated from clinical specimens. *Journal of Clinical Microbiology* 21, 46–76.

Farmer, J.J. III, Fanning, G.R., Davis, B.R., O'Hara, C.M., Riddle, C., Hickman-Brenner, F.W., Asbury, M.A., Lowery, V.A III and Brenner, D.J. (1985b) *Escherichia fergusonii* and *Enterobacter taylorae*, two new species of Enterobacteriaceae isolated from clinical specimens. *Journal of Clinical Microbiology* 21, 77–78.

Feng, P.C.S. and Hartman, P.A. (1982) Fluorogenic assays for immediate confirmation of *Escherichia coli*. *Applied and Environmental Microbiology* 43, 1320–1329.

Flint, K.P. (1987) The long-term survival of *Escherichia coli* in river water. *Journal of Applied Bacteriology* 63, 261–270.

Fornasini, M., Reves, R.R., Murray, B.E., Morrow, A.L. and Pickering, L.K. (1992) Trimethoprim-resistant *Escherichia coli* in households of children attending day care centers. *Journal of Infectious Diseases* 166, 326–330.

Freney, J., Herve, C., Desmonceaux, M., Allard, F., Boeufgras, J.M., Monget, D. and Fleurette, J. (1991) Description and evaluation of the semiautomated 4-hour ATB 32E method for identification of members of the family Enterobacteriaceae. *Journal of Clinical Microbiology* 29, 138–141.

Gargan, R., Brumfitt, W. and Hamilton-Miller, J.M.T. (1982) A concise biotyping system for differentiating strains of *Escherichia coli*. *Journal of Clinical Pathology* 35, 1366–1369.

Geiss, H.K. and Geiss, M. (1992) Evaluation of a new commercial system for the identification of Enterobacteriaceae and non-fermentative bacteria. *European Journal of Clinical Microbiology and Infectious Diseases* 11, 610–616.

Godsey, J.H., Matteo, M.R., Shen, D., Tolman, G. and Gohlke, J.R. (1981) Rapid identification of Enterobacteriaceae with microbial enzyme activity profiles. *Journal of Clinical Microbiology* 13, 483–490.

Gordon, D.M. (1992) Rate of plasmid transfer among *Escherichia coli* strains isolated from natural populations. *Journal of General Microbiology* 138, 17–21.

Goullet, P. (1973) An esterase zymogram of *Escherichia coli*. *Journal of General Microbiology* 77, 27–35.

Goullet, P. (1980) Esterase electrophoretic pattern relatedness between *Shigella* species and *Escherichia coli*. *Journal of General Microbiology* 117, 493–500.

Goullet P. and Picard, B. (1984) Typage électrophorétique des ésterase d'*Escherichia coli* au cours de septicémies. *Presse Médicale* 13, 1079–1081.

Goullet P. and Picard, B. (1986a) Comparative esterase electrophoretic polymorphism of *Escherichia coli* isolates obtained from animal and human sources. *Journal of General Microbiology* 132, 1843–1851.

Goullet P. and Picard, B. (1986b) Highly pathogenic strains of *Escherichia coli* revealed by the distinct electrophoretic patterns of carboxylesterase B. *Journal of General Microbiology* 132, 1853–1858.

Gyles, C.L., Palchaudhuri, S. and Maas, W.K. (1977) Naturally occurring plasmid carrying genes for enterotoxin production and drug resistance. *Science* 198, 198–199.

Hartman, P.A. (1968) *Miniaturized Microbiological Methods*. Academic Press, New York.

Hazen, T.C. (1988) Fecal coliforms as indicators in tropical waters: a review. *Toxicity Assessment: An International Journal* 3, 461–477.

Ingraham, J.L., Maaløe, O. and Neidhardt, F.C. (1983) *Growth of the Bacterial Cell*. Sinauer Associates, Sunderland, Massachusetts.

Jensen, K.F. and Pedersen, S. (1990) Metabolic growth rate control in *Escherichia coli* may be a consequence of subsaturation of the macromolecular biosynthetic apparatus with substrates and catalytic components. *Microbiological Reviews* 54, 89–100.

Jones, C.W. (1980) Cytochrome patterns in classification and identification including their relevance to the oxidase test. *Society of Applied Bacteriology, Symposium Series* 8, 127–138.

Jones, C.W., Brice, J.M. and Edwards, C. (1977) The effect of respiratory chain composition on the growth efficiencies of aerobic bacteria. *Archives in Microbiology* 115, 85–93.

Jurtshuk, P., Mueller, T.J. and Acord, W.C. (1975) Bacterial terminal oxidases. *Critical Reviews in Microbiolology* 3, 399–468.

Kapur, V., White, D.G., Wilson, R.A. and Whittam, T.S. (1992) Outer membrane protein patterns mark clones of *Escherichia coli* O2 and O78 strains that cause avian septicaemia. *Infection and Immunity* 60, 1687–1691.

Katouli, M., Kühn, I. and Möllby, R. (1990) Evaluation of the stability of biochemical phenotypes of *Escherichia coli* upon subculturing and storage. *Journal of General Microbiology* 136, 1681–1688.

Kemp, J.D. and Atkinson, D.E. (1966) Nitrite reductase of *Escherichia coli* specific for reduced nicotinamide adenine dinucleotide. *Journal of Bacteriology* 92, 628–634.

Knight, M.T., Wood, D.W., Black, J.F., Gosney, G., Rigney, R.O. and Agin, J.R. (1990) Gram-negative identification card for identification of *Salmonella*, *Escherichia coli*, and other Enterobacteriaceae isolated from foods: collaborative study. *Journal of the Association of Official Analytical Chemists* 73, 729–733.

Koch, A.L. (1976) How bacteria face depression, recession and derepression. *Perspectives in Biology and Medicine* 20, 44–63.

Konings, W.N., Hellingwerf, K.J. and Robillard, G.T. (1981) Transport across bacterial membranes. In: Bonting, S.L. and de Pont, J.J.H.H.M. (eds) *Membrane Transport*. Elsevier, North Holland, pp. 257–283.

Kornberg, H.L. (1966) The role and control of the glyoxylate cycle in *Escherichia coli*. *Biochemical Journal* 99, 1–11.

Kühn, I. (1985) Biochemical fingerprinting of *Escherichia coli*. A simple method for epidemiological investigations. *Journal of Microbiological Methods* 3, 159–170.

Kühn, I., Brouner, A. and Möllby, R. (1990) Evaluation of numerical typing systems for *Escherichia coli* using the API 50 CH and the PhP-EC systems as models. *Epidemiology and Infection* 105, 521–531.

Lamikanra, A., Ako-Nai, A.K. and Ola, J.B. (1990) Transmissible trimethoprim resistance of *Escherichia coli* isolated from cases of infantile diarrhoea. *Journal of Medical Microbiology* 32, 159–162.

Law, D., Wilkie, K.M., Freeman, R. and Gould, F.K. (1992) The iron uptake mechanisms of enteropathogenic *Escherichia coli*: the use of haem and haemoglobin during growth in an iron-limited environment. *Journal of Medical Microbiology* 37, 15–21.

Leclerc, H. (1962) Etude biochimique d'Enterobacteriaceae pigmentees. *Annales de l'Institut Pasteur* (*Paris*) 102, 726–741.

Le Minor, L. and Ben Hamida, F. (1962) Advantages de la recherche de la β-galactosidase sur cell de la fermentation du lactose en milieux dans le diagnostic bacteriologique, en particulier des Enterobacteriaceae. *Annales de l'Institut Pasteur* (*Paris*) 102, 267–277.

Lewin, C.S., Allen, R. and Amyes, A.G.B. (1990) Zidovidine-resistance in *Salmonella typhimurium* and *Escherichia coli*. *Antimicrobial Agents and Chemotherapy* 25, 706–708.

Lindberg, F. and Normark, S. (1986) Contribution of chromosomal β-lactamases to β-lactam resistance in enterobacteria. *Review of Infectious Diseases* 8 (Supplement 3), S292–S304.

Lindberg, F. Lindquist, S. and Normark, S. (1988) Genetic basis of induction and overproduction of chromosomal class I β-lactamase in nonfastidious gram-negative bacili. *Review of Infectious Diseases* 10, 782–785.

Magasanik, B. (1961) Catabolite repression. *Cold Spring Harbor Symposia on Quantitative Biology* 26, 245–256.

Månson, I. (1962) Biochemical properties of haemolytic *E. coli* strains belonging to O-groups 138, 139 and 141. *Acta Veterinaria Scandinavica* 3, 79–87.

Marre, R. and Aleksic, S. (1990) Beta-lactamase types and beta-lactam resistance of *Escherichia coli* strains with chromosomally mediated ampicillin resistance. *European Journal of Clinical Microbiology and Infectious Diseases* 1, 44–46.

Martins, M.T., Rivera, I.G., Clark, D.L. and Olson, B.H. (1992) Detection of virulence factors in culturable *Escherichia coli* isolates from water samples by DNA probes and recovery of toxin-bearing strains in minimal *o*-nitrophenol-β-D-galactopyranoside-4-methylumbelliferyl-β-D-glucuronide media. *Applied and Environmental Microbiology* 58, 3095–3100.

Matthew, M. and Harris, A.M. (1986) Identification of β-lactamase by analytical isoelectric focussing: correlation with bacterial taxonomy. *Journal of General Microbiology* 94, 55–67.

McKay, A.M. (1992) Viable but non-culturable forms of potentially pathogenic bacteria in water. *Letters in Applied Microbiology* 14, 129–135.

Medeiros, A.A. (1984) Beta-lactamases. *British Medical Bulletin* 40, 18–27.

Mitsuyama, J.-I., Itoh, Y., Takahata, M., Okamoto, S. and Yasuda, T. (1992) *In vitro* antibacterial activities of tosufloxacin against and uptake of tosufloxacin by outer membrane mutants of *Escherichia coli*, *Proteus mirabilis*, and *Salmonella typhimurium*. *Antimicrobial Agents and Chemotherapy* 36, 2030–2036.

Møller, V. (1954) Diagnostic use of the Braun KCN test within the Enterobacteriaceae. *Acta Pathologica et Microbiologica Scandinavia* 34, 115–116.

Møller, V. (1955) Simplified tests for some amino acid decarboxylases and for the arginine dihydrolase system. *Acta Pathologica et Microbiologica Scandinavia* 36, 158–172.

Mugg, P. and Hill, A. (1981) Comparison of the Microbact 12E and 24E systems and the API 20E system for the identification of Enterobacteriaceae. *Journal of Hygiene, Cambridge* 87, 287–297.

Mushin, R. and Ashburner, F.M. (1964) Ecology and epidemiology of coliform infections: II. The biochemical reactions and drug sensitivity of coliform organisms. *Medical Journal of Australia* 1, 303–308.

Nagatani, H., Shimizu, M. and Valentine, R.C. (1971) The mechanism of ammonia assimilation in nitrogen fixing bacteria. *Archiv für Mikrobiologie* 79, 164–175.

Nunn, W.D. (1986) A molecular view of fatty acid catabolism in *Escherichia coli*. *Bacteriological Reviews* 50, 179–192.

Ørskov, I. and Ørskov, F. (1973) Plasmid-determined H_2S character in *Escherichia coli* and its relation to plasmid-carried raffinose fermentation and tetracycline resistance characters. *Journal of General Microbiology* 77, 487–499.

Philippon, A., Labia, R. and Jacoby G. (1989) Extended spectrum β-lactamases. *Antimicrobial Agents and Chemotherapy* 34, 1131–1136.

Reguera, J.A., Baquero, F., Pérez-Diaz, J.C. and Martinez, J.L. (1991) Factors determining resistance to β-lactam combined with β-lactamase inhibitors in *Escherichia coli*. *Journal of Antimicrobial Agents and Chemotherapy* 27, 569–575.

Reves, R.R., Fong, M., Pickering, L.K., Bartlett, A., III, Alvarez, M. and Murray, B.E. (1990) Risk factors for fecal colonization with trimethoprim- and multiresistant *Escherichia coli* among children in day care centers in Houston. *Antimicrobial Agents and Chemotherapy* 34, 1429–1434.

Rice, E.W., Johnson, C.H., Wild, D.K. and Reasoner, D.J. (1992) Survival of *Escherichia coli* O157:H7 in drinking water associated with a waterborne disease outbreak of hemorrhagic colitis. *Letters in Applied Microbiology* 15, 38–40.

Sanders, C.C. (1992). β-Lactamases of gram-negative bacteria: new challenges for new drugs. *Clinical Infectious Diseases* 14, 1089–1099.

Sarhan, H.R. and Foster, H.A. (1991) A rapid fluorogenic method for the detection of *Escherichia coli* by the production of β-glucuronidase. *Journal of Applied Bacteriology* 70, 394–400.

Savage, D.C. (1977) Microbial ecology of the gastrointestinal tract. *Annual Review of Microbiology* 31, 107–133.

Scotland, S.M., Gross, R.J., Cheasty, T. and Rowe, B. (1979) The occurrence of plasmids carrying genes for both enterotoxin production and drug resistance in *Escherichia coli* of human origin. *Journal of Hygiene* 83, 531–538.

Serény, B. (1963/4) Breakdown of amino-acids by Enterobacteriaceae: its use as a routine diagnostic test. *Acta Microbiologica, Academiae Scientiarum Hungarica* 10, 403–407.

Shinebaum, R., Shaw, E.J., Bettelheim, K.A. and Dickerson, A.G. (1977) Transfer of invertase production from a wild strain of *Escherichia coli. Zentralblatt für Bakteriologie, Parasitenkunde und Hygiene, I Abteilung Originale A* 2, 189–195.

Singh, M., Sanyal, S.C. and Yadav, J.N.S. (1992) Enterotoxigenic drug resistant plasmids in animal isolates of *Escherichia coli* and their zoonotic importance. *Journal of Tropical Medicine and Hygiene* 95, 316–321.

Smith, H.W. (1963) The haemolysins of *Escherichia coli. Journal of Pathology and Bacteriology* 85, 197–211.

Smith, P.B., Tomfohrde, K.M., Rhoden, D.L. and Balows, A. (1972) API System: a multitube micromethod for identification of Enterobacteriaceae. *Applied Microbiology* 24, 449–452.

Switzer, R.L. (1977) The inactivation of microbial enzymes *in vivo. Annual Review of Microbiology* 31, 135–157.

Tabor, C.W. and Tabor, H. (1985) Polyamines in microorganisms. *Microbiological Reviews* 49, 81–99.

Tamura, K., Sakazaki, R., Kosako, Y. and Yoshizaki, E. (1986) *Leclercia adecarboxylata* gen. nov., comb. nov., formerly known as *Escherichia adecarboxylata*. Current Microbiology 13, 179–184.

Thompson, J.S., Hodge, D.S. and Borczyk, A.A. (1990) Rapid biochemical test to identify verocytotoxin-positive strains of *Escherichia coli* serotype O157. *Journal of Clinical Microbiology* 28, 2165–2168.

Thomson, C.J. and Amyes, S.G.B. (1992) Prospects for expanding the use of β-lactamase inhibitors. *Journal of Medical Microbiology* 37, 297–298.

Thomson, K.S. Weber, D.A., Sanders, C.C. and Sanders, W.E., Jr (1990) β-Lactamase production in members of the family Enterobacteriaceae and resistance to β-lactam-enzyme inhibitor combinations. *Antimicrobial Agents and Chemotherapy* 34, 622–627.

Tyler, B. (1978) Regulation of the assimilation of nitrogen compounds. *Annual Review of Biochemistry* 47, 1127–1162.

Watkins, W.D., Rippey, S.R., Clavet, C.R., Kelly-Reitz, D.J. and Burkhardt, W., III (1988) Novel compound for identifying *Escherichia coli*. Applied and Environmental Microbiology 54, 1874–1875.

Weber, D.A., Sanders, C.C., Bakken, J.S. and Quinn, J.P. (1990) A novel chromosomal TEM derivative and alterations in outer membrane proteins together mediate selective ceftazidime resistance in *Escherichia coli. Journal of Infectious Diseases* 162, 460–465.

Whittam, T.S. (1989) Clonal dynamics of *Escherichia coli* in its natural habitat. *Antonie van Leeuwenhoek* 55, 23–32.

Wolfson, J.S., Hooper, D.C. and Swartz, M.N. (1989) Mechanisms of action of and resistance to quinolone antimicrobial agents. In: Wolfson, J.S. and Hooper, D.C. (eds) *Quinolone Antimicrobial Agents*. American Society for Microbiology, Washington, DC pp. 5–34.

Xu, H.S., Robert, N., Singleton, F.L., Attwell, R.W., Grimes, D.J. and Colwell,

R.R. (1982) Survival and viability of non-culturable *Escherichia coli* and *Vibrio cholerae* in estuarine and marine environment. *Microbial Ecology* 8, 313–323.

Yap, K.W. and Barton, A.P. (1985) Biotyping of *Escherichia coli* by a multiple inoculation agar technique. *Medical Laboratory Sciences* 42, 287–288.

Classification of *Escherichia coli* 2

H. Lior
Laboratory Centre for Disease Control, Health Canada, Tunney's Pasture, Ottawa, Ontario, Canada K1A OL2

Introduction

The species *Escherichia coli* is composed of bacteria that have similar biochemical reactions but can be separated into groups on the basis of association with different types of disease and hosts, antigenic composition, plasmid profiles, production of haemolysins and colicins, enzyme polymorphism, and patterns of susceptibility to bacteriophages. This chapter will consider all these bases for subdividing the species but will place greatest emphasis on serotyping, which is a well-established and widely used scheme for identifying *E. coli* associated with diseases.

Serological Characteristics of *E. coli*

In 1885, Theodor Escherich, a German paediatrician working in Austria, described slim, slightly curved rods which grew when the faeces of infants was cultured on artificial media. Escherich called this organism *Bacterium coli commune*, which is now known as *Escherichia coli*. In 1889, Laurelle suggested an association of *Bacterium coli commune* with diarrhoeal disease and vomiting and, in 1897, Le Sage showed that serum from an acute case of diarrhoea agglutinated the organisms from other cases in an epidemic but not the organisms from healthy children. Subsequently, substantial effort was directed at differentiation of pathogenic and non-pathogenic strains. In 1923, Adam in Germany studied infantile gastro-enteritis and, having tried and failed to identify a serological method for identifying *E. coli* types associated with disease, was able to identify biochemically distinct groups of *E. coli*. In 1933, Goldschmidt continued

Adam's work and showed by serological typing in a slide agglutination technique that 'dyspepsiekoli' could be identified. Using this technique she studied the epidemiology of infantile gastroenteritis in institutions and pointed out the importance of healthy carriers of epidemic strains.

Later, Bray (1945) investigated an outbreak of enteritis in babies in a London hospital and showed the association of an antigenically homogeneous *E. coli* serological type with the epidemic. Bray's observations were confirmed (Giles and Sangster, 1948; Giles *et al.*, 1949) during the investigation of an outbreak of diarrhoea in Aberdeen in which two serological types were identified and were named Aberdeen alpha and beta. In 1949 Taylor *et al.* investigated epidemics in nurseries in London and identified the epidemic strain as *E. coli* D433. Kauffmann (1947), having started a systematic approach to the serological classification of *E. coli*, showed that Bray's Aberdeen alpha strain and Taylor's D433 strain were identical and belonged to the newly established serogroup *E. coli* O111:B4; the Aberdeen beta strain belonged to the O55:B5 serogroup.

Kauffmann (1944) was the first to classify *E. coli* by serological methods; he described 20 'O' groups based on agglutination of boiled culture suspensions. Knipschildt (1945) added another five 'O' antigens and in 1947 Kauffmann published an antigenic schema which consisted of 25 'O' antigens, 55 'K' antigens and 19 'H' antigens. During his investigations, Kauffmann observed that some freshly isolated strains were not agglutinated in antisera prepared against boiled antigens. This inhibition of agglutinability could be destroyed by heating the bacterial suspension at 100°C. The reason for the inhibition of agglutinability was due to a 'L' (labile) antigen inactivated by heat. Since then the *E. coli* antigenic scheme has been extended (Table 2.1) and now consists of 167 'O' antigen groups numbered O1–O173 (seven serogroups – O31, O47, O67, O72, O93, O94 and O122 have been deleted from the scheme) (see Ewing, 1986).

The serotyping of *E. coli* is based on the identification of O antigens, K antigens (where applicable) and H antigen factors. The serological characteristics of *E. coli* are based on the determination of 'O', 'K', 'H' and 'F' (fimbrial) antigens (Ørskov and Ørskov, 1983).

Somatic antigens

Polysaccharide antigens

'O' ANTIGENS (LIPOPOLYSACCHARIDE ANTIGENS)

The 'O' antigens are somatic factors composed of phospholipid–polysaccharide complexes and it is the nature of the terminal groups and the order in which they occur in the repeating units of the polysaccharide chain that define the specificity of various 'O' antigens. The 'O' antigens are heat stable, not inactivated by heating at 100°C or 121°C and divisible into

Table 2.1. *E. coli* antigenic scheme comprising all O-, K- and H-antigenic test strains.

O	K	H	Culture number
1	1	7	U5-41
1	*51*	—	A183a
2	*1*	*4*	U9-41
2	*7(56)*	7	H17b
2	1	*6*	A2oa
2	2	*1*	Su1242
2	ne	*8*	Ap32oc
3	*2ab*	2	U14-41
3	ne	*31*	K15 (=HW33)
3	ne	*44*	781-55
4	*3*	*5*	U4-41
4	*6*	5	Bi7457-41
4	12	—	Su65-42
4	*52*	—	A103
5	*4*	4	U1-41
6	2a	1	Bi7458-41
6	*13*	1	Su4344-41
6	*15*	*16*	F8316-41
6	53	—	PA236
6	54	10	A12b
6	13	*49*	2147-59
7	1	—	Bi7509-41
7	*7*	4	Pus 3432-41
8	*8*	4	G3404-41
8	*25*	9	Bi7575-41
8	*27*(A)	—	E56b
8	*40*	9	A51d
8	41	11	A433a
8	*42*(A)	—	A295b
8	43	11	A195a
8	*44*(A)	—	A168a
8	*45*	9	A169a
8	*46*	30	A236a
8	*47*	2	A282a
8	*48*	9	A290a
8	*49*	21	A180a
8	*50*	—	PA80c
8	84(A)	—	H308b[a]
8	87	19	D277(=G:7, K:88−)
8	*102*(A)	—	6CB10-1
8	ne	*20*	H330b
8	ne	*21*	U11a-44
8 (60)	ne	*51*	C218-70
9	*9*	*12*	Bi316-42
9a	*26*(A)	—	Bi449-42
9ab	*28*(A)	—	K14a
9	*29*(A)	—	Bi161-42

Table 2.1. *continued*

O	K	H	Culture number
9	*30*(A)	12	E69
9	*31*(A)	—	Su3973-41
9	*32*(A)	19	H36
9	*33*(A)	—	Ap289
9	*34*(A)	—	E759
9	*35*(A)	—	A140a
9	*37*(A)	—	A84a
9	*38*(A)	—	A262a
9	*39*(A)	9	A121a
9	*55*	—	N24c
9	*57*	32	H509d
9	ne	*19*	A18d
10	*5*	*4*	Bi8337-41
11	*10*	*10*	Bi623-42
11	ne	*33*	K181 (=HW35)
11	ne	*52*	C2187-69
12	5	—	Bi626-42
13	*11*	*11*	Su4321-41
14[b]	*7*	—	Su4411-41
15	*14*	4	F7902-41
15	ne	*17*	P12b
15	ne	*25*	N234 (=HW26)
15	ne	*27*	K50 (=HW28)
16	1	—	F11119-41
16	ne	48	P4
17	*16*	*18*	K12a
18ab	*(76)*	*14*	F10018-41
18ac	5(77)	*7*	D-M3219-54
19ab	ne	7	F8188-41
20	*17*	—	P7a
20	*83*	26	CDC134-51
20	*84*	26	CDC2292-55
20	*101*	—	1413
21	*20*	—	E19a
22	13	1	E14a
23	*18*	*15*	E39a
23	*(21)*[c]	15	H38
23	*22*	15	H67
24	+	—	E41a
25	*19*	12	E47a
25	*23*	1	H54
26	(60)	—	H311b
26	*(60)*	—	F41
26	*(60)*	*46*	5306-56
27	—	—	F9884-41
28	—	—	K1a
28	(73)	—	Kattwijk
29	—	10	Su4338-41

Table 2.1. *continued*

O	K	H	Culture number
30	—	—	P2a
32	—	19	P6a
33	—	—	E40
34	—	10	H304
35	—	10	E77a
36	—	9	H502a
37	—	10	H510c
38	—	26	F11621-41
38	ne	*30*	N157 (=HW32)
39	—	—	H7
40	—	4	H316
41	—	40	H710c
42	—	*37*	P11a
43	—	*2*	Bi7455-41
44	*74*	18	H702c
45	*1*	10	H61
45	ne	*23*	K42 (=HW23)
46	—	16	P1c
48	—	—	U8-41
49	+	12	U12-41
50	—	4	U18-41
51	—	24	U19-41
51	ne	*24*	K72 (=HW25)
52	—	10	U20-41
52	ne	*45*	4106-54
53	—	*3*	Bi7327-41
54	—	2	Su3972-41
55	(59)	—	Su3912-41
55	(59)	6	Aberdeen 1064
56	+	—	Su3684-41
57	—	—	F8198-41
58	—	27	F8962-41
59	—	19	F9095-41
60	—	33	F10167a-41
61	—	19	F10167b-41
62	—	30	F10524-61
63	—	—	F10598-41
64	—	—	K6b
65	—	—	K11a
66	—	25	P1a
68	—	4	P7d
69	—	*38*	P9b
70	ne	*42*	P9c
71	—	12	P10a
73	—	31	P12a
73	*92*	34	6181-66
74	—	*39*	E3a
75	*95*	5	E3b75

Table 2.1. *continued*

O	K	H	Culture number
75	100	5	F147
76	—	8	E5d
77	*96*	—	E10
78	*(80)*	—	E38
79	—	*40*	E49
80	—	26	E71
81	*97*	—	H5
82	—	—	H14
83	—	31	H17a
83	*24*	31[d]	H45
84	—	21	H19
85	—	1	H23
86	—	25	H35
86	*(61)*	—	E990
86	2ab*(62)*	2	F1961
86	(64)	*36*	5017-53
86	(61)	*34*	BP12665
86	ne	*47*	1755-58
87	—	12	H40
88	—	25	H53
89	—	16	H68
90	—	—	H77
91	—	—	H307b
92	—	33	H308a
95	+	33	H311a
96	—	19	H319
97	—	—	H320a
98	—	8	H501d
99	—	33	H504c
100	—	2	H509a
101	—	33	H510a
101	99 = F:5	—	B41
101	*103*(A)	—	8CE275-6
102	—	40	H511
103	+	8	H515b
104	—	12	H519
105	—	8	H520b
106	—	33	H521a
107	*98*	27	H705
108	—	10	H708b
109	—	19	H709c
110	—	39	H711c
111	*(58)*	—	Stoke W
112ab	*(68)*	18	1411-50
112ac	*(66)*	—	Guanabara (1685)
113	*(75)*	21	6182-50
114	*(90)*	*32*	26w (= K10 = HW34)
115	—	18	27w

Table 2.1. *continued*

O	K	H	Culture number
116	+	10	28w
117	98	4	30w
118	—	—	31w
119	*(69)*	27	34w
120	+	6	35w.
121	—	10	39w
123	—	16	43w
124	*(72)*	30	Ew277
125ab	*(70)*	19	Canioni
125ac	*(70)*	6	Ew2129-54
126	*(71)*	2	E611
127a	*(63)*	—	4932-53
127ab	*(65)*	4	2160-53
128	*(67)*	2	Cigleris
129	—	11	Seeliger 178-54
130	—	9	Ew4866-53
131	—	*26*	S239 (=HW27)
132	+	*28*	N87 (=HW30)
133	—	*29*	N282 (=HW31)
134	—	*35*	4370-53
135	—	—	Coli Pecs
136	*(78)*	—	1111-55
137	*(79)*	*41*	RVC1787
138	*(81)*	—	CDC62-57
139	12*(82)*	1	CDC63-57
139	—	*56*	SN3N/1
140	—	43	CDC149-51
141	*(85)*	4	RVC2907
141	(85ab), 88ab = F:4ab	4	E68
142	*(86)*	6	C771
143	—	—	4608-58
144	—	—	1624-56
145	—	—	E1385(3)
146	—	21	CDC2950-54
147	(89)	19	D357 (=G1253), K:88$^-$
147	(89), *88ac* = F:4ac	19	G1253
148	—	28	E519-66
148a	ne	*53*	E480-68
149	*(91)*, 88ac = F:4ac	10	Abbotstown A
150	*93*	6	1935
151	—	10	880-67
152	—	—	1184-68
153	—	7	14097
154	*94*	4	E1541-68

Table 2.1. *continued*

O	K	H	Culture number
155	—	9	E1529-68
156	—	47	E1585-68
157	88ac = F:4ac	19	A2
158	—	23	E1020-72
159	—	20	E2476-72
160	—	34	E110-69
161	—	*54*	E223-69
162	—	10	10B1/1
163	—	19	SN3B/1
164	—	—	145/46
165	—	—	E78634
166	—	4	3866-54
167	—	5	E10702
168	—	16	E10710
169	—	8	1792-54
170	—	1	745-54
171	—	—	244-55
172	—	—	3288-85
173	—	—	L119B-10

ne, not examined.
[a] Former test strain O:93 (Ørskov *et al.*, 1977).
[b] 14 does not contain S-LPS but R-LPS.
[c] Strain H:38 has lost its K:21-antigen, K:21 has therefore been deleted.
[d] Test strain for K:24 ('H:45'), formerly assigned to O-group 22.
Numbers in italics are test (reference) antigens. Numbers in italics in parentheses are former reference antigens, now deleted. These numbers will not be used in the future. The following polysaccharide K-antigens are closely related or identical (Semjén *et al.*, 1977): K:2ab ~ K:2ac ~ K:*62*, K:7 = K:*56*, K:*12* ~ K:*82*, K:*13* ~ K:*23*, K*18* ~ K:*22*, K:*16* ~ K:*37* ~ K:*97*, K:*53* ~ K:*93*, K:*54* ~ K:*96*. This scheme only contains the serotype formulae of the reference strains used at the WHO Collaborative Centre for Reference and Research on *Escherichia* antigens. The strains have been collected over more than 30 years and many different considerations have determined the selection.
Source: Ørskov and Ørskov, 1984.

two groups on the basis of mobility in an electric field. The 'O' antigens of one group are immobile, because of a lack of acidic components in the lipopolysaccharide (LPS) moiety, and are mostly found in *E. coli* implicated in extraintestinal disease. The 'O' antigens of the second group contain acidic components and migrate towards the anode during electrophoresis; they are usually associated with strains which cause dysentery-like disease (Ørskov and Ørskov, 1972).

Various techniques have been proposed for the determination of 'O' antigens. In general bacterial suspensions are heated at 100 °C or in special instances, autoclaved at 121 °C for 2 hours for the inactivation of heat-resistant capsular antigens (see 'K' antigens). In most laboratories the 'O' antigen determination is carried out using antisera produced in rabbits inoculated with heated (100 °C or 121 °C) antigen suspensions on a slide, tube, microtitre tray system which could be automated (Guinee *et al.*, 1972; Bettelheim *et al.*, 1975), and by passive haemagglutination (Neter *et al.*, 1956). Using this technique, Kunin *et al.* (1962) reported the existence of an enterobacterial common antigen (ECA) among *E. coli* isolated from urinary tract infections. These investigators reported that an antiserum against *E. coli* O14 cross-reacted with an antigen common to all *E. coli* strains. This ECA (or Kunin antigen) was also found in several other members of the family Enterobacteriaceae (Kunin *et al.*, 1962) but was not present among *Pseudomonas* or *Brucella* species or in any Gram-positive bacteria. Low levels of anti-common antigen antibodies may be present in normal human sera and antibodies to ECA were also found in sera from horses, cattle, dogs and pigs (Kunin and Beard, 1963). No antibodies were detected in normal rabbit serum at a dilution of 1 : 10. Mäkelä and Mayer (1976) reviewed extensively the chemistry, immunogenicity and genetic aspects of ECA. Brodhage (1962) reported another cross-reactive antigen (the C antigen) in urea extracts of bacteria.

Other factors such as common LPS of Gram-negative bacteria and outer membrane proteins can lead to cross-reactivity. Rabbit antisera prepared against whole cells of *E. coli*, *Salmonella* and *Shigella* have been shown to contain antibodies to a common lipoprotein (Braun *et al.*, 1976).

Many cross-reactions among the 'O' antigens of *E. coli* have been reported (Ørskov *et al.*, 1977; Ewing, 1986), indicating that in spite of the fact that cultures belonging to certain 'O' antigenic groups react specifically, strong reciprocal and unilateral 'O' antigenic relationships exist among 'O' antigen groups. Precise serotyping of these strains requires absorption of antisera with cross-reacting antigens (Ørskov and Ørskov, 1984; Ewing, 1986). Certain antigenic relationships occurring within an 'O' group were described such as a,b–a,c and a–a,b variety in which the letter 'a' represents the common factor responsible for the cross-reactivity, while the specific factors are b and c respectively. The a,b–a,c, a–a,b and a–a,c variation has been identified in several serogroups such as O111 a,b, O111 a,c and others associated with diarrhoeal disease (Ewing, 1986).

In addition to cross-reactions among *E. coli* 'O' groups, 'O' antigens of *E. coli* may share antigenic specificity with shigellae consistent with the well-known close relationship between the two groups of organisms (Table 2.2). Cross-reactions with the 'O' antigens of salmonella have also been reported (Ørskov and Ørskov, 1984) (Table 2.3). Winkle *et al.* (1972) described *O*-antigenic relationships between *Vibrio cholerae*, and some *E. coli*, *Salmonella* and *Citrobacter* strains.

Table 2.2. Cross-reactions between O-antigens of enteroinvasive *E. coli* and *Shigella*.[a]

E. coli	*Shigella*
O28ac (Kattwijk)	*S. boydii* 13
O112ac (Guanabara)	*S. dysenteriae* 2, identical
O124	*S. dysenteriae* 3, identical
O143	*S. boydii* 8, identical
O144	*S dysenteriae* 10
O152	Not examined

From Edwards and Ewings, 1972.
[a] Other strong O-antigen cross-relations between *E. coli* and *Shigella* are O32/*S. boydii* 14, O53/*S. boydii* 4, O58/*S. dysenteriae* 5, O79/*S. boydii* 5, O87ab/*S. boydii* 2, O105ab/*S. boydii* 11, O112ab/*S. boydii* 15, O129/*S. flexneri* 5, O55/*S. flexneri* 4b and O167/*S. boydii* 3.
Source: Ørskov and Ørskov, 1984.

Table 2.3. Cross-relations between O-antigens of *E. coli* and *Salmonella*.

E. coli	*Salmonella*
O1	$O42_1$
O2	55
O6	$O40_1$, 40_3
O15	O59
O21	O38
O23	O51
O44, O62, O68 O70, O73, O99 O106 and O129	O6, 14
O55	$O50_1$, 50_2, 50_4
O75	O11
O85	O17
O86, O90	O43
O111	O35
O132	O17
O134	O36

Source: Ørskov and Ørskov, 1984.

'O' antigens may undergo variations from smooth (S) O^+ to rough (R) O^- due to mutations in genes for the synthesis of O-specific polysaccharide chains or the basal core. O^- (rough strains which have lost their antigenic specificity) autoagglutinate in saline and therefore cannot be serotyped by the usual procedures in the laboratory.

'K' ANTIGENS (ACIDIC POLYSACCHARIDE FACTORS)

In investigating the serological characteristics of *E. coli*, Kauffmann noticed that many live bacteria were not agglutinated by the corresponding O antiserum. The inhibition of agglutinability in O sera could be resolved by heating the bacterial suspension. Kauffmann and his collaborators (Kauffmann, 1947) introduced the term 'K' antigen from the word 'Kapsel' (capsular or envelope antigen), and divided K antigens into three classes: L, A and B. L type K antigens were heat labile and lost their antigenicity and antibody-binding activity after heating at 100°C for 1 hour. The A type K antigens were unaffected by heating at 100°C but lost their antigenicity and inhibition of agglutinability in O sera after heating at 121°C for 2 hours, while still being able to bind antibody (Table 2.4).

Evidence for the existence of B antigens has been inadequate, although for many years these have been part of antigenic formulae of the EPEC strains such as O26:B6 and O111:B4. The presence of B antigens was inferred in cases of inagglutinability of unheated cultures in O sera.

It should also be noted that this kind of inagglutinability may be caused by flagella, fimbriae or perhaps other surface structures. Given

Table 2.4. Schematic presentation of the agglutination results on which earlier definitions of K-antigens (A, B and L) were based.

			Agglutination in OK antiserum	
K-type	Antigen preparation	Agglutination in anti-O serum	Absorbed by culture heated to 100°C for 1 hour	Unabsorbed
A	Live	–	–	+
	Boiled/autoclaved	–/+	–	+
B	Live	'–'	–	+
	Boiled	+	–	+
L	Live	'–'	+	+
	Boiled (100°C for 1 hour)	+	–	+

'–', Negative or significantly lower than that of the boiled culture; –, no agglutination; +, agglutination.
Source: Ørskov and Ørskov, 1984.

the difficulties encountered by many in trying to determine these antigens, Ørskov *et al.* (1977) proposed giving up the L, A, B nomenclature and restricting the nomenclature of K antigens to acidic polysaccharide antigens.

Some K antigens may be associated specifically with O groups 8, 9, 20 and 101 which render these inagglutinable in O sera after heating at 100°C, but will agglutinate after heating at 121°C for 2 hours. The designation K (A) will apply to these antigens. Due to several deletions of B antigens, the present scheme recognizes 74 K antigens (numbered 1–103), among them two fimbrial protein antigens (K88 and K99). The remaining K antigens are acidic polysaccharides which consist of oligosaccharide repeating units (Jann and Jann, 1990). Recently, the capsular polysaccharides have been placed into two groups on the basis of their amino sugar component and the nature of their acid components (Jann and Jann, 1992).

K antigens have been determined by slide or tube agglutination of live cultures in OK sera (whole cell antisera) and two-dimensional gel electrophoresis with Cetavlon precipitation of acidic polysaccharides using extracts obtained by heating bacteria at 60°C and 100°C, or only at 60°C. Similar heat extracts were used in counter-current immunoelectrophoresis, a technique which allows a clear differentiation of K antigens which show an anodic precipitation in the presence of O and OK antisera (Semjen *et al.*, 1977; Ørskov and Ørskov, 1990b). The patterns obtained by immunoelectrophoresis in agar allowed the determination of five groups (1A, 1Ba, 1Bb, 2a and 2b), which are discussed in Chapter 16. Groups 1A and 1Ba contain the K(A) antigens of O8, O9, O20 and O101; patterns 1Bb and 2b include the majority of the strains which do not show the presence of K antigens and have been associated with diarrhoeal disease. As a result of these studies, the existence and value of most K antigen determinations have been questioned and most reference laboratories rarely attempt the identification of these antigens, except for a few such as K1 and K5, which play significant roles in disease in humans.

K1 antigen is immunologically identical to the meningococcal group b polysaccharide and can be detected by agglutination with antiserum to group b meningococci followed by confirmation, using five specific capsular phages (Gross *et al.*, 1977). K1 antigen has been associated with serotypes O1:K1:H$^-$, O1:K1:H7, O2:K1:H4, O2:K1:H6, O7:K1:H1, O16:K1:H6, O18ac:K1:H7 and O83:K1:H4. Ørskov *et al.* in 1979 described form variation in *E. coli* K1 cultures where two types of colonies were found: one giving a strong agglutination with the antiserum (K1$^+$) and another showing a weak agglutination (K1$^-$). K1 polysaccharide is a very poor immunogen and antiserum has not been successfully raised in rabbits. Monoclonal antibodies have been described against K1 antigen (Frosch *et al.*, 1985) and also against other poor immunogens such as K5

(Bitter-Suermann *et al.*, 1986), K12 (Abe *et al.*, 1988) and K13 (Söderström *et al.*, 1983).

The K18 and K100 antigens are polyribosyl-ribitol phosphates (Rodriguez *et al.*, 1988) and are closely related to the capsular polysaccharide of *Haemophilus influenzae* type b. K92 cross-reacts with *Neisseria meningitidis* group c (Robbins *et al.*, 1975), K93 with *N. meningitidis* group a (Guirguis *et al.*, 1985) and K2 with *N. meningitidis* group h (Adlam *et al.*, 1985). Antigens K1, K2, K3, K5, K12 and K13 are K antigens that are found at high frequency in extraintestinal infections in humans (Robbins *et al.*, 1974; Kaijser *et al.*, 1977; Ørskov and Ørskov, 1985).

Protein antigens

K ANTIGENS – K88, K99

K88 and K99 antigens are fimbrial antigens associated with diarrhoeal disease in pigs (K88) (Jones and Rutter, 1972) and calves, lambs and pigs (K99) (Smith and Linggood, 1972). K88 antigens are associated with O serogroups 8, 45, 138, 141, 147, 149 and 157 and are expressed in three antigenic forms: K88a,b; K88a,c; K88a,d (Guinee and Jansen, 1979). K99 antigens have been detected on strains belonging to O serogroups 8, 9, 20, 64 and 101. Many strains carrying K99 antigen, especially strains of serogroups O9 and O101, also produce another adhesin, called F41 (Morris *et al.*, 1982).

FLAGELLAR ANTIGENS

Flagellar 'H' antigens represent distinct serological determinants found on flagellin, the protein which constitutes the flagella of motile organisms. Fifty-three 'H' antigens have been described for *E. coli*. In many instances freshly isolated strains of *E. coli* may display a sluggish motility which makes them unsuitable for 'H' serological determination. In such cases, the strains should be passaged one or more times in fluid or semisolid agar media, until motility is well developed. Unlike typical 'O' antigen agglutinates which are granular, the 'H' agglutinates are fluffy and loose floccular, easily dispersible upon tapping the tubes.

Most *E. coli* 'H' antigens are specific and show little or no significant cross-reactivity (Ewing, 1986). It was generally believed that *E. coli* strains possessed a single structural gene encoding flagellar 'H' antigen specificity and were therefore monophasic, manifesting only one antigen specificity. However, Ratiner (1982) reported that *E. coli* 'H' antigens H3 and H17 can spontaneously change their antigens to H16 and H4 respectively. It is possible that the change in specificity may depend on the presence and functioning of a special genetic system resembling that of diphasic salmonella, which displays two alternative types of 'H' antigens (Ewing,

1986). As H antigens may occur in association with any of the O antigen groups, the determination of 'H' antigens is extremely important alongside with the determination of 'O' antigen factors ('OH' serotypes) as markers of pathogenicity of many *E. coli* in diarrhoeal and extraintestinal disease.

FIMBRIAE

Fimbriae or pili are thread-like structures projecting from the bacterial surface of many Gram-negative bacteria, including *E. coli*. These non-flagellar, filamentous appendages were recognized in *E. coli* by Houwink and van Iterson in 1950. The most documented role for pili is in bacterial adherence to epithelial cell surfaces (Beachey, 1981). Strains of *E. coli* which cause enteric or urinary tract infections can be distinguished by their ability to colonize the intestinal or urinary tract of humans and animals (Moon, 1990) and the most important event in the colonization of epithelial cells process is the ability to attach to mucosal surfaces of the intestinal tract or urinary tract.

In addition to type 1 fimbriae, pathogenic *E. coli* may possess other fimbriae. Fimbriae and adhesins have been classified on the basis of morphology and ability to agglutinate erythrocytes of various animals (Duguid *et al.*, 1966) and the nature of the receptors to which they adhere (Duguid *et al.*, 1966; Klemm, 1985; De Graaf and Mooi, 1986). Ørskov and Ørskov (1983) proposed the use of serological characteristics of the fimbrial adhesins as a fourth group of surface antigens designated by the prefix 'F' in addition to O:K:H antigens (O:K:H:F).

Bacterial agglutinations are not always suitable for demonstrating fimbrial antigens, since one strain may display several fimbriae of different antigenic types. Ørskov and Ørskov (1983), using bacterial extracts of isolates from urinary tract infections, demonstrated six fimbrial antigens (F7 to F12) among P fimbriated uropathogenic strains. The designations F1 to F6 were applied to established fimbrial antigens: Type 1 fimbriae = F1; colonization factor antigen (CFA)/I = F2; CFA/II = F3; K88 = F4; K99 = F5; 987P = F6.

The number of F antigens has increased from 12 to 17 and serotyping of these antigens appears complicated, given the fact that not only major but also minor fimbrial antigens should be determined (Van Die *et al.*, 1988; Ørskov and Ørskov, 1990a). Furthermore, new F antigens are being discovered. Gulati *et al.* (1992) reported the isolation of *E. coli* associated with diarrhoea in calves which possessed F17 fimbriae. Bertschinger *et al.* (1990) and Imberechts *et al.* (1992) described a new colonization factor, fimbrial antigen F107, in about 85% of *E. coli* strains that belong to serogroups O138, O139 and O141 and produce the oedema disease verotoxin.

Fimbrial adhesion may be sensitive or resistant to inhibition by D-mannose and is referred to as mannose sensitive (MS) or mannose resistant

MR). Adhesion by type 1 fimbriae is MS, whereas adherence mediated by most fimbriae associated with pathogenic *E. coli* is MR and is usually demonstrable with strains of *E. coli* grown at 37°C but not at 18°C.

As *E. coli* strains carrying a particular type of MR haemagglutinin appear to bind erythrocytes from a number of species, Evans *et al.* (1979, 1980) proposed a haemagglutination typing system for the presumptive identification of enterotoxigenic *E. coli* possessing colonization factor antigens CFA/I and CFA/II. Seven haemagglutination types were described, designated HA type I to HA type VII but this system is not in general use.

Classification of Enteric *E. coli* Pathogens

In 1955, Neter applied the term enteropathogenic *E. coli* (EEC or EPEC) to indicate characterized strains associated epidemiologically with enteric rather than extraintestinal infections. For many years the name EPEC represented a variety of serogroups and serotypes of *E. coli* associated with diarrhoeal disease and with unknown pathogenic mechanisms. More recently, characteristics implicated in pathogenesis of EPEC infections have been identified and it is now possible to classify EPEC and other types of enteric pathogenic *E. coli* on the basis of virulence properties. The scheme has been developed primarily for *E. coli* in human disease, but applies equally well to *E. coli* in animal diseases. Five classes of *E. coli* implicated in diarrhoeal diseases have been recognized as follows: enteropathogenic (EPEC), enterotoxigenic (ETEC), enteroinvasive (EIEC), enterohaemorrhagic (EHEC) and enteroaggregative (EAggEC). Details of the characteristics of these groups of organisms and their involvement in disease are presented in Chapter 13. This chapter will emphasize the serotypes that are involved with each group.

Enteropathogenic E. coli *(EPEC)*

Over the years the number of serogroups of EPEC expanded from the few recognized in the 1940s to a long list (Table 2.5) of which the most prevalent are O20, O26 (now mostly associated with the enterohaemorrhagic group), O44, O55, O86, O111, O114, O119, O125, O126, O127, O128, O142 and O158 (Sussman, 1985).

EPEC may also be divided on the basis of adherence to HEp-2 cells in tissue culture (Cravioto *et al.*, 1979). The classical enteropathogenic *E. coli* group can be divided into two classes. Class I contains the most common O serogroups O55, O86, O111, O119, O125, O126, O127, O128ab and O142 which adhere to HEp-2 cells and possess a 60 MDa plasmid (the EPEC adherence factor or EAF) encoding adhesiveness to HEp-2 cells.

Table 2.5. Serogroups and serotypes of *E. coli* isolated from humans with intestinal infections.

Classification of *E. coli*	Principal serogroups and serotypes involved		
Enteropathogenic	O18a, 18c:H7	O111a, 111b:NM	O127:NM
	O20a, 20b:H26	O111a, 111b:H2	O127:H9
	O26:NM	O111a, 111b:H12	O127:H21
	O28a, 28c:NM	O114:H10	O128a, 128b:H2
	O44:H34	O114:H32	O128a, 128c:H12
	O55:NM	O119:NM	O158:H23
	O55:H6	O119:H6	O142:H6
	O55:H7	O125a, 125c:H21	O159
	O86:H34	O126:NM	
	O86a:NM	O126:H27	
Enterotoxigenic	O6:H16	O25:H42	O148:H28
	O8:H9	O27:H7	O149:H10
	O11:H27	O63	O159:H20
	O15:H11	O78:H11	O16, O148:H28
	O20:NM	O78:H12	O173:H^{-}
	O25:NM	O128:H7	

Enteroinvasive	O28a:28c:NM	O112a, 112c,:NM	O124:NM
	O124:H30	O124:H32	O136:NM
	O143:NM	O144:NM	O152:NM
	O159:H2	O164	
	O167:H4	O167:H5	
Enterohaemorrhagic	O26:H11, H21, H32, H^{-}		O113:H21
	O111a, b:H^{-}, H8	O117:H14	O172:H^{-}
	O111a, c	O128a, b	O157:H7
Enteroaggregative	O7:H^{-}	O86:H^{-}	O127:$H2^{-}$
	O77:H18	O126:H27	

Modified from Ewing (1986).

Class II consists of less common serogroups such as O18, O44, O112 and O114 which are not adherent to HEp-2 cells (are EAF$^-$, or may be only rarely EAF$^+$) (Baldini *et al.*, 1983; Levine, 1987).

Recently, other EAF$^+$ EPEC serogroups not belonging to the classical serogroups (O88, O145 and O153) have been detected and have been shown to produce localized adherence (LA) to HeLa cells (Pedroso *et al.* 1993). Nataro *et al.* (1985) have developed a sensitive and specific DNA probe for the detection of EPEC carrying the EAF plasmid.

Enterotoxigenic E. coli *(ETEC)*

The second major group of *E. coli* to be associated with diarrhoea, the ETEC, was described in India by Gorbach *et al.* (1971) and Sack (1980). Enterotoxigenic *E. coli* colonize the small intestine, where they produce one or both of two enterotoxins, heat-labile (LT) and heat-stable (ST) toxins. ETEC of human origin belong to a limited number of serogroups (Table 2.5) and are associated with a small number of fimbrial types.

The first fimbrial colonization factor CFA/I in an ETEC strain of human origin was described by Evans *et al.* (1975) and subsequently associated with strains of serogroups O15, O25, O63, O78, O128 and O153. Evans and Evans (1978) reported a second colonization factor CFA/II associated with serogroups O6, O8, O80, O85 and O139 (Evans and Evans, 1983). Cravioto *et al.* (1982) and Smyth (1982) showed that CFA/II represented combinations of distinct antigens which were referred to as CS1, CS2 and CS3. Thomas *et al.* (1982) described a new putative colonization factor fimbria in strain E8775, serogroup O25, and also in serogroups O115 and O167. E8775 consisted of three distinct antigens CS4, CS5 and CS6. These factors were identified among strains belonging to serogroups O27 and O148. Tacket *et al.* (1987) reported that unlike other colonization factor fimbriae, strains belonging to serotype O159:H4 have fimbriae which do not show mannose-resistant haemagglutination activity.

Enteroinvasive E. coli *(EIEC)*

The third class of *E. coli* associated with diarrhoeal disease (EIEC) resemble shigellae in the disease they cause (DuPont *et al.*, 1971) and share somatic antigens with shigellae (Table 2.2). EIEC are frequently non-motile and are less active biochemically than typical *E. coli*, fail to produce gas from glucose and do not decarboxylate lysine (Toledo and Trabulsi, 1983). Like some species of *Shigella*, these invasive strains possess large plasmids 140 MDa, which encode critical virulence factors (Harris *et al.*, 1982; Hale *et al.*, 1983). In the laboratory, invasiveness of EIEC is indicated by a positive Sereny test for ability to induce keratoconjunctivitis in the guinea-pig or rabbit (Sereny, 1957) or by invasion of HeLa tissue culture cells (La Brec *et al.*, 1964).

EIEC can be identified by serotyping as they belong to a restricted range of serogroups (mostly non-motile and without K antigens) which differ from classical serotypes found among ETEC and EPEC (Table 2.5). Serotypes most often encountered are O28:H$^-$, O124:H30, O136:H$^-$, O144:H$^-$ and O173:H$^-$ (Rowe, 1979; Ørskov *et al.*, 1991).

Enterohaemorrhagic E. coli *(EHEC)*

A major recent development in the field of enteric infections due to *E. coli* has been the recognition of a new group of pathogenic *E. coli* that produce verotoxin or Shiga-like toxin. In 1982 two outbreaks of bloody diarrhoea in Oregon and Michigan (Riley *et al.*, 1983) and another outbreak in Ottawa, Canada (Stewart *et al.*, 1983) led to the recognition of a new pathogenic serotype, *E. coli* O157:H7. This serotype had previously been isolated from one case of bloody diarrhoea in California in 1975. In Canada the first isolation was made in 1978 and by the end of 1981, five strains of this serotype were identified. Johnson *et al.* (1983) were the first to report that *E. coli* O157:H7 produce verotoxins.

It was soon recognized that other *E. coli* serotypes produce verotoxins and since 1983, the association of verotoxigenic *E. coli* (VTEC) or Shiga-like toxin producing *E. coli* (SLTEC) with bloody diarrhoea, haemorrhagic colitis and haemolytic uraemic syndrome has been further supported by reports from a number of countries.

E. coli O157:H7, unlike most *E. coli*, do not ferment sorbitol after 24 hours' incubation (Johnson *et al.*, 1983), and their identification was facilitated by the availability in 1985 of culture media such as Sorbitol–MacConkey agar which allowed the screening of sorbitol-negative colonies at 24 hours' incubation. It should be noted, however, that about 6% of other *E. coli* may be sorbitol negative and about 10–15% of human diarrhoeal stool specimens may contain non-sorbitol fermenting species. Stool cultures should be performed early in the disease, within 3–5 days after the onset of symptoms, as cultures taken later are often negative for *E. coli* O157:H7 (Pai *et al.*, 1988). Agglutination in O157 antiserum alone is not sufficient for identification as other *E. coli* may be sorbitol negative (Borczyk *et al.*, 1989) and non-toxigenic strains belonging to *E. coli* O157 serogroup possessing H antigens H8, H16, H19, H39, H42, H43 and H45 may also be found in stools. *Escherichia hermanii*, another sorbitol-negative species, may agglutinate in O157 antisera (Lior and Borczyk, 1987). Since O157:H7 is the only motile O157 associated with production of verotoxins, false-positive reports can be avoided by routine determination of H7, flagellar antigen. Non-motile, verotoxigenic O157:H$^-$ do occur and their identification may rely on another characteristic of these strains, lack of beta-glucuronidase production (MUG test negative) (Thompson *et al.*, 1990). Confirmation of verotoxin production however must be made for all isolates.

Recently, strains of verotoxin-producing O157:H$^-$ isolated in Germany, have been shown to ferment sorbitol in 24 hours and are MUG positive, features which may complicate the identification of this serotype (Gunzer *et al.*, 1992). Atypical strains of verotoxigenic *E. coli* O157:H7 which are urease positive, have been occasionally encountered.

E. coli O157:H7 represents but one serotype among more than 100 serotypes of *E. coli* which may produce verotoxins, but identification of other verotoxigenic *E. coli* (VTEC) is more difficult as there are no special markers which will allow easy identification and diagnostic antisera are not commercially available. Other *E. coli* serotypes involved belong to a variety of serotypes such as O4:H$^-$, O5:H$^-$, O16:H6, O26:H11 or H$^-$, O55:H7, O91:H21, O111:H8, O113:H21, O118:H12, O119:H6, O125:H$^-$, O126:H8, O128:H2, O145:H$^-$, and many others.

The production of verotoxins is mediated by lysogenic (temperate) phages which code for the production of verotoxin 1 (VT1) or Shiga-like toxin I (SLT-I) and verotoxin 2 (VT2) or Shiga-like toxin II (SLT-II). These phages represent potentially mobile genetic elements which may explain the increasing number of toxin-producing strains. Conversely strains of *E. coli* O157:H7 have been encountered which lost the ability to produce verotoxins.

In view of the wide range of serotypes of verotoxigenic *E. coli*, their identification by serological procedures is possible only in specialized laboratories such as reference centres. The typing of the numerous serogroups is labour intensive and other methodologies may be required for the detection of VTEC in clinical material and in foods (Padhye and Doyle, 1992).

The detection of VTEC colonies may be greatly simplified by protocols such as immunoblots or colony-blots to detect toxin-producing colonies or by detection of verotoxin genes using DNA probes (Smith and Scotland, 1993), or by the polymerase chain reaction (PCR) amplification procedure. The PCR technique is very sensitive and allows the rapid, specific, detection of the five different toxin genes directly in the stool or from primary enrichment broths used in food microbiology (Johnson *et al.*, 1990; Pollard *et al.*, 1990; Tyler *et al.*, 1991). Recently proposed protocols for the isolation of *E. coli* O157:H7 from foods and faeces are based on immunomagnetic separation of these organisms from heavily contaminated materials, followed by culture, direct fluorescent antibody procedure or by PCR amplification of the toxin genes (Fratamico *et al.*, 1992).

Verotoxins can also be demonstrated in tissue culture assays such as the Vero cell or HeLa cell assay. The Vero cell assay is preferred because some verotoxins such as VT2e and other VT2 variants show little or no activity on HeLa cells. Direct detection of free faecal verotoxin can be accomplished using tissue culture assays followed by neutralization of the toxins with specific antitoxins (Smith and Scotland, 1993). Other methods for the detection of verotoxins include ELISA, counter-immunoelectrophoresis on faecal filtrates and indirect immunofluorescence on colony blots.

In Canada, laboratory surveillance of isolations of *E. coli* O157:H7 and VTEC in all 10 provinces has been in place since 1982 and the number of isolations reported increased yearly from 25 reports in 1982 to 1643 isolations in 1992. This increase is due in part to the introduction in clinical laboratories of the Sorbitol–MacConkey agar in 1985, increased awareness of these pathogens and routine culture in practically all laboratories.

The investigation of outbreaks requires epidemiological markers which will allow clustering of strains. Traditionally serotyping, biotyping and phagetyping have been successfully applied to the differentiation of enteric pathogens such as salmonella, and more recently campylobacters. Molecular techniques such as plasmid profile analysis, restriction endonuclease patterns, multilocus enzyme electrophoresis, pulsed-field gel electrophoresis and the use of PCR with random amplified polymorphic DNA (RAPD) have become tools of choice in the investigation of foodborne outbreaks. Attempts to biotype *E. coli* O157:H7 have failed because of lack of reproducibility, and plasmid profile analysis revealed not unexpectedly a variety of patterns which did not allow accurate tracing of infections. A phagetyping scheme has been developed for the differentiation of *E. coli* O157:H7 and has proven extremely valuable in epidemiological investigations.

In some cases, pulsed-field gel electrophoresis may be less informative than phagetyping and the use of PCR and RAPD may prove to be an important tool in the provision of molecular epidemiological markers. Genetyping by PCR and restriction endonuclease patterns provides additional molecular markers for the tracing of infections of humans to foods.

Enteroaggregative **E. coli** *(EAggEC)*

A recently recognized class of diarrhoeagenic *E. coli*, the enteroaggregative *E. coli* (EAggEC), are defined by their distinctive, 'stacked-brick-like' aggregative pattern of adherence to HEp-2 cells *in vitro*, caused by formation of microcolonies on tissue culture cell surface (Vial *et al.*, 1988). Studies in Chile, India, Brazil and Mexico have shown a strong association of EAggEC with diarrhoea in children and especially with persistent episodes lasting more than 14 days. Baudry *et al.* (1990) described a specific DNA probe for the detection of EAggEC, a 1.0 kb fragment derived from the 55–65 MDa virulence plasmid (Vial *et al.*, 1988). Baldwin *et al.* (1992) reported that non-haemolytic EAggEc produce a heat-labile toxin antigenically related to *E. coli* haemolysin. Savarino *et al.* (1993) have shown that EAggEC secrete a plasmid-encoded, heat-stable toxin (EAST1), immunologically and genetically different from the heat-stable toxin (STa) of other human enterotoxigenic isolates. Yamamoto *et al.* (1991) reported that a strain of EAggEC serotype O127a:H2 isolated from a diarrhoea case, formed bacterial clumps and a thick scum when grown in broth. Albert *et al.* (1993) described a rapid test for the screening of EaggEc in which positive strains produce a scum on the surface of Mueller–Hinton broth incubated at 37°C. Other serotypes that were isolated were O7:H$^-$, O77:H8, O86:H$^-$ and O126:H27 (Albert *et al.*, 1993) (Table 2.5).

E. coli Serotypes in Normal Stools

In Western populations human faeces contain 10^2–10^9 *E. coli* g^{-1}. The organisms are found shortly after birth and become normal intestinal inhabitants representing a multitude of serotypes. Bettelheim *et al.* in 1972 examined 1580 *E. coli* strains isolated from 90 sites of nine faecal specimens and found that in eight stools there was a single predominant serotype constituting more than half of the colonies. More than one serotype was isolated from seven stools and from one stool 11 different serotypes were distinguished. Another sampling study of the normal *E. coli* flora of the human intestinal tract based on statistical analysis showed that by picking five colonies two different serotypes could be identified; for each additional serotype multiples of five colonies were required (Hedges *et al.*, 1977).

There appears to be a consistent fluctuation of serotypes among the intestinal flora with some residential types and some transient in nature (Sears and Brownlee, 1952).

Serogroups of *E. coli* in Animal Diseases

E. coli have been associated with a variety of enteric and septicaemic diseases in animals. Diseases in the various animal species are discussed in subsequent chapters in this book. Tables 2.6, 2.7 and 2.8 show the major serogroups of *E. coli* implicated in diseases in calves, pigs and poultry, respectively.

Plasmid Profiles as a Means of Classification

Plasmids are circular pieces of DNA that exist independently of the chromosome in the cytosol of many prokaryotic and a few eukaryotic cells. Some unusual biochemical characteristics of *E. coli*, such as citrate utilization (Sato *et al.*, 1978; Ishiguro and Sato, 1979), urease production

Table 2.6. Serogroups of *E. coli* implicated in septicaemic and enteric colibacillosis in calves.

	Enteric isolates		
		Fimbrial antigens	
Septicaemic isolates[a]	OK serogroups[b]	K99	F41
O15:K	O8:K25	+	
O26:K60	O8:K28	+	
O78:K80	O8:K85	+	
O35:K	O9:K	+	+
O86:K61	O9:K30[c]	+	+
O115:K	O9:K35	+	+
O117:K98	O20:K	+	
O119:K	O20:K17	+	
	O101:K		+
	O101:K	+	+
	O101:K28	+	+
	O101:K30[c]	+	+
	O101:K30	+	+
	O101:K32	+	+

[a] Based on Sojka (1965), Renault (1979) and Ørskov (1978).
[b] Based on Ørskov *et al.* (1975), Ørskov and Ørskov (1978) and H. Lior (unpublished).
[c] Most commonly encountered OK groups.

Table 2.7. Serotypes of enterotoxigenic *E. coli* from pig diseases.[a]

Serotype	Fimbrial antigens
O8:K87:H19	F4 (K88)
O9:K35:H$^-$	F5 (K99)
O9:K103:H$^-$	F6 (987P)
O20:K101:H$^-$	F6 (987P)
O45:H$^-$	F4 (K88)
O101:K30:H$^-$	F5 (K99)
O138:H14	F4 (K88)
O141:H4	F4 (K88)
O147:H19	F4 (K88)
O149:H10	F4 (K88)
O138:H$^-$[b]	
O139:K82:H1[b]	
O141:K85:H4[b]	

[a] Ørskov and Ørskov (1984).
[b] Associated with oedema disease.

Table 2.8. Some *E. coli* O-groups from poultry.[a]

Sources	O serogroups
Septicaemia (pericarditis, air sacculitis)	O1, O2, O8, O71, O73, O78
Cellulitis[b]	O2, O78, O115
Hjärre's disease (coli granuloma disease)	O8, O9, O16
Faeces	O3, O8, O9, O18, O44, O77, O83, O103, O114

[a] Ørskov and Ørskov (1984).
[b] S.M. Peighambari and C.L. Gyles, 1993, University of Guelph, unpublished.

(Wachsmuth *et al.*, 1979), production of hydrogen sulfide (Braunstein and Mladineo, 1974) are all characteristics encoded by plasmids. These may complicate the identification of these organisms because of the ease with which plasmids may be lost or transferred.

Several virulence factors of *E. coli* are encoded by plasmids. The role of plasmids in the carriage and transmission of virulence in *E. coli* was first demonstrated by Ørskov and Ørskov in 1966, and Smith and Halls in 1968 were the first to show that toxin production in *E. coli* was transmissible by conjugation. Subsequently, it has been shown that genes for fimbrial adhesins of human ETEC and most types of animal ETEC are plasmid encoded (see Chapter 16). The genes for heat-labile enterotoxin (LT) and the heat-stable enterotoxins, STa and STb, produced by ETEC are also carried by plasmids (Chapter 14). Other plasmid-encoded virulence properties include localized adherence by EPEC encoded by the EAF plasmid, adherence of *E. coli* strain RDEC-1 by AF/RI fimbriae (Wolf *et al.*, 1988), heat-stable enterotoxin EASTI of EAggEC (Savarino *et al.*, 1991) and invasiveness of EIEC (Silva *et al.*, 1982).

In addition to virulence factors, plasmids often carry genes for antimicrobial resistance. The presence of resistance and virulence plasmids in bacterial cells can lead to the formation of hybrid plasmids. Gyles *et al.* (1977) reported the isolation of a strain of *E. coli* from a pig with diarrhoea in which antibiotic resistance and enterotoxigenicity were on the same plasmid. Scotland *et al.* (1979) and Echeverria and Murphy (1980) reported transfer of drug resistance and enterotoxigenicity on the same plasmid. The use of antibiotics as feed additives for therapeutic purposes and disease prevention in food animals, may select not only for the maintenance of antibiotic resistance factors but also for virulence determinants.

Plasmid fingerprinting has been used in many instances where the differentiation of the strains was not possible because of lack of serotyping or phagetyping schemes. Plasmid DNA is extracted by established techniques and bands are separated by electrophoresis in agarose, stained with ethidium bromide, and visualized by exposure to ultraviolet light (Maniatis *et al.*, 1982). The migration rate of the plasmid DNA is proportional to the logarithm of its molecular size. A problem with this method is the presence of open-circular forms of plasmids which migrate independently of the covalently closed circular form (Tenover, 1985).

Plasmid fingerprinting has been used in outbreaks involving community acquired infections and also in the follow-up of the spread of nosocomial pathogens in institutions (Wachsmuth, 1986; Mayer, 1988). When large numbers of isolates are investigated, it is often that organisms are found which harbour only a single plasmid. If there is little epidemiologic data to link the isolates, another method confirming the identity of such strains is to use restriction endonucleases to cleave the plasmid into a series of fragments (usually 4 to 8), that can be compared using agarose gel electrophoresis.

Classification on the Basis of Haemolysins

E. coli may produce at least four types of haemolysins and strains may be characterized by the presence or absence of haemolysis as well as by the kind(s) of haemolysin they produce. Smith (1963) and Smith and Halls (1967) identified alpha-haemolysin as a heat-labile, extracellular product that was sometimes plasmid mediated in strains of *E. coli* from pigs. Beta-haemolysin was cell associated and not well characterized. Both types produced clear lysis zones and were indistinguishable on blood agar plates. Subsequently, alpha-haemolysin associated with strains of *E. coli* implicated in extraintestinal infections in humans was shown to be frequently chromosomally encoded (Muller *et al.*, 1983). Beutin *et al.* (1986) reported that, among human EPEC isolates of serogroups O114 and O126, the *hly* genes were chromosomally located, while among O26 strains the *hly* genes were carried on a 100 MDa plasmid. Berger *et al.* (1982) reported chromosomally encoded *hly* genes in *E. coli* of O serogroups 4, 6, 18 and 75.

Strains of alpha-haemolytic *E. coli* are frequently isolated from the faeces of normal pigs at weaning, pigs with oedema disease, and pigs with diarrhoea (Sojka, 1965). Early studies of haemolysin production by *E. coli* (Dudgeon *et al.*, 1921) showed a high incidence in strains causing urinary tract infections in man. Cavalieri *et al.* (1984) reported that up to 50% of *E. coli* strains isolated from extraintestinal infections carried alpha-haemolysin determinants, and suggested that haemolysins may play a role in the pathogenicity of *E. coli* by releasing iron required for bacterial growth, by killing the host defence cells, or by their cytotoxic effects on kidney cells.

In examining haemolysin production in EPEC strains, Beutin *et al.* (1988) found that some strains of serogroups O26, O111 and other 'O' groups, produced a different type of haemolysin, which they called enterohaemolysin. This type of haemolysin was detectable only on media containing washed sheep, rabbit or human red cells.

A fourth type of haemolysin, gamma haemolysin, described by Walton and Smith in 1969, is active on horse, guinea-pig and sheep red cells but in contrast to enterohaemolysin does not lyse human or rabbit red cells.

Colicin Typing

The name colicin was first used by Gratia in 1925 in Belgium and later by Gratia and Frederiq in 1946 to describe a distinctive class of antibiotic substances produced by strains of *E. coli* which in contrast to other antibiotics acted only on strains of the same or closely related species. Similar substances have been described in other species under the name bacteriocins.

Colicins are 40–60 KDa, plasmid-encoded proteins that are released extracellularly (Pugsley, 1984a, b). The killing action of colicins is a multistep process in which they first bind specifically to particular receptors on the outer membrane of sensitive cells followed by translocation across the outer membrane. Once inside the cell, colicins exert their killing activity by enzymatic cleavage of DNA or 16S rRNA (colicins E2, E3) or by de-energization of the cytoplasmic membrane (colicins E1, A, B, Ia, Ib, K). The major group of colicins, E1, A, B, N, Ia, Ib and K may kill sensitive cells by forming ion channels in the cytoplasmatic membrane (Cramer *et al.*, 1983). One colicin molecule is able to kill one bacterium – a molecularity of one.

Colicin V

Gratia in 1925 first described colicin V (Col V) calling it 'principle V' after a collibacillus strain virulent for animals designated 'Coli V'. Unlike other colicins, Col V is found primarily among virulent bacteria implicated in extraintestinal infections in humans and animals. Fernandez-Beros *et al.* (1990) showed that the colicin V genotype was predominantly plasmid encoded in bacteraemic isolates but among diarrhoeal isolates was predominantly chromosomal.

Col V is a small molecule which, unlike other colicins, is not released from the bacterial cells by lysis, but by an export mechanism (Gilson *et al.*, 1987). The Col V plasmids, in addition to colicin V, encode other virulence factors such as the aerobactin iron uptake system (Braun, 1981), increased serum survival (Binns *et al.*, 1979), altered motility (Tewari *et al.*,

1986), changes in hydrophobicity, and bacterial surface proteins that facilitate attachment to appropriate host cells (Tewari *et al.*, 1985) and intestinal epithelial cell adherence (Clancy and Savage, 1981). Smith (1974) observed in experimental animals that *E. coli* strains that had acquired the Col V plasmid became more virulent and that the virulence decreased after loss of the plasmid. Significant correlation between Col V plasmid carriage and septicaemia in calves and chickens was reported by Smith and Huggins in 1976. Milch *et al.* in 1984 reported the isolation of *E. coli* strains producing Col V from cases of meningitis in newborn infants. In a study of 474 *E. coli* strains belonging to 70 different serogroups, 39% produced Col V.

The first demonstration of the epidemiological relevance of colicin typing of *E. coli* was by Shannon in 1957 who identified six colicin types among isolates of O group 55. McGeachie (1965) applied colicin typing to *E. coli* strains isolated from urinary tract infection. Hettiaratchy *et al.* (1973) reported on the usefulness of colicin typing as an epidemiological tool in conjunction with serotyping and observed that there was no relationship between colicin type and serotype. Most serotypes could be subdivided into several colicin types. However lack of reproducibility, variation in colicin types noted on some strains after 6 months' storage, and low typability of the strains, have detracted from the usefulness of this method in epidemiological investigations.

Electrophoretic Typing

Multilocus enzyme electrophoresis or electrophoretic typing is yet another method for identifying similarities and differences among *E. coli* isolates. This system is based on the existence of several alleles for each locus that encodes a bacterial enzyme. The genetic variations result in production of no enzyme or of enzymes with different mobilities during electrophoresis in gels. In order to determine the electrophoretic types (ETs), overnight cultures of the organism are disrupted and protein extracts are subjected to horizontal starch gel electrophoresis, followed by staining for selected enzymes (Whittam and Wilson, 1988). Each enzyme that is used in the analysis is assayed individually for variation in mobility, and scores are assigned, based on the rate of anodal migration. A zero score is assigned if the enzyme is not produced. The pattern of scores for each enzyme may be used to assign the isolate to an electrophoretic type.

By using a selection of 20 enzymes, for example, similarities and differences among isolates are readily recognized (White *et al.*, 1990). This method allows detection of differences among isolates of the same serogroup as well as of similarities among isolates of different serogroups (White *et al.*, 1990; Kapur *et al.*, 1992). It has been used extensively in investigations of clones associated with specific disease syndromes. For example, White *et al.* (1990) found that among a selection of 22 *E. coli* isolates from swollen head syndrome in chickens, polymorphisms were present in 14 of 20 alleles, with an average of 2.6 alleles per locus. In a collection of 115 isolates from *E. coli* diseases in chickens, these researchers detected polymorphisms in 17 of 20 enzymes and an average of 3.5 alleles per locus.

Electrophoretic typing may provide clues about pathogenic features of *E. coli* isolates from various disease syndromes. Seelander *et al.* (1986) used electrophoretic typing to analyse 63 *E. coli* isolates from septicaemia and meningitis in infants. They determined that 63% of these isolates belonged to a cluster and that production of aerobactin, K1 antigen and type 1 pili were characteristic of members of this cluster. White *et al.* (1990) showed that isolates from swollen head syndrome in chickens were genetically diverse, as indicated by electrophoretic typing. This diversity was also evident on the basis of serotyping. Such diversity may arise from horizontal transfer of genes for virulence factors or may indicate that at least some of the isolates represent opportunistic infections. Isolates of O serogroups 2 and 78, recovered from avian colibacillosis, constitute a group which belong to only two O antigenic types but show considerable genetic diversity. Whittam and Wilson (1988) identified 14 ETs, belonging to three major clone clusters among 48 O2 and O78 isolates from chickens and noted that one of the clones had isolates from both O serogroups. Kapur *et al.* (1992) observed that there was a high concordance (93.8%) between outer membrane protein patterns and ETs among O2 and O78 strains of *E. coli* from avian septicaemia. They suggested that the outer membrane patterns may be useful for rapid discrimination among the major clones of *E. coli* of these two O serogroups.

The clonal relationship of 16 serotypes of verotoxigenic *E. coli* was investigated by Whittam *et al.* (1993) by multilocus enzyme electrophoresis. Multiple electrophoretic types were identified among isolates of each serotype and 72% of the 1300 strains that were tested were found to belong to 15 major electrophoretic types, each representing a clone with a wide geographical distribution.

Phagetyping

Phages are bacterial viruses that have the ability to lyse certain but not all bacteria of a given species. Typing schemes have been developed on the basis of variation in susceptibility of *E. coli* isolates to a battery of phages. Phagetyping has been successfully used for a number of years for the differentiation and subdivision of bacterial species and it has become very useful, especially in epidemiological investigations.

A major advantage of phagetyping as an epidemiological tool is its ability to detect differences among strains belonging to the same species, serotype and biotype. With the recognition of certain serogroups of EPEC such as O26, O55 and O111 in the late 1940s and early 1950s, Nicolle *et al.* (1952) proposed phage typing schemes for these *E. coli* serogroups isolated from 300 diarrhoeal cases in children. Using 14 phages, some isolated from the stools of the patients, the authors subdivided *E. coli* O111 into seven phagetypes, *E. coli* O55 also into seven phagetypes, and *E. coli* O26 into five phagetypes. This scheme provided good discrimination amongst strains from different geographic regions.

Milch and Gyenes (1972) developed a phagetyping scheme based on 28 phages and reported a close association of certain serotypes with phagetypes such as a serogroup O4 with phage types 4, 17, 20, 22 and serogroup O18 with types 4, 12, 13, 16, 17 and 18. Serogroup O111 could be subdivided into eight phagetypes, O26 into 10 types and O55 into 11 types. Other enteropathogenic serogroups could also be subdivided by this scheme. (For a review see Milch, 1978.)

Phagetyping of *E. coli* strains isolated from urinary tract infections was reported by Brown and Parisi (1966) who were able with eight phages to differentiate 74 of 90 isolates *E. coli*, belonging to seven different serogroups. Pande *et al.* (1976) investigated 108 isolates of enteropathogenic *E. coli* from sporadic cases of acute and chronic diarrhoea. With the aid of seven phages, 15 phagetypes were identified but only 61% of the strains from acute and 46% of the chronic diarrhoea were typeable.

Sterne *et al.* (1970) examined 571 strains of *E. coli* isolated from diarrhoeal and healthy pigs and found 61% of the strains susceptible to phages but were unable to show any differences in phage patterns between isolates from healthy and sick pigs. A typing scheme for *E. coli* isolated from calves (Smith and Crabb, 1956) recognized 71 types among isolates from healthy and diseased calves. The phagetypes of the strains from the sick calves were different from those obtained from healthy animals. Bhatia (1977), using 10 phages isolated from sewage, investigated 101 isolates from poultry and found that 94 strains were lysed by one or more phages.

Interest in the phagetyping of *E. coli* has been sporadic and this method has not become a routine tool in the investigation of *E. coli* infections. Several factors may be responsible for this. Some phagetyping schemes were designed for specific EPEC serogroups (O111, O26, O55), which for some years ceased to pose serious public health problems and were no longer associated with the outbreaks observed in the early 1940s and 1950s. Also, although phagetyping is easy to perform, it requires propagation and standardization protocols which have become areas of expertise in specialized laboratories.

With the recognition in 1982 of outbreaks involving a newly recognized pathogenic *E. coli* O157:H7 and subsequent increased isolations of

Table 2.9. Phage types of *E. coli* O157:H7 identified in 151 outbreaks.

Phage type	Outbreaks[a] (no.)	Cases (no.)
1	32	86
2	13	40
4	29	87
8	17	64
14	16	32
21	2	5
23	3	11
31	14	39
32	9	27
34	1	2
40	1	3
43	1	2
48	1	3
1 and 2	1	25
1 and 4	4	45
1 and 8	3	11
1 and 23	1	7
1, 4, 14 and 31	1	13
1, 4, 21 and 31	1	16
8, 23 and 31	1	38
Total	151	556

[a] Settings of the outbreaks studied: nursing home outbreaks, 19; community outbreaks (day care, field, trips, banquets), 12; non-specified outbreaks, 5; hospital outbreaks, 3; family outbreaks, 112.

this serotype from sporadic and outbreak cases of bloody and watery diarrhoea, Ahmed *et al.* (1987) described a phagetyping scheme which using 16 phages recognized 14 types. Khakhria *et al.* (1990) investigated 6946 isolates of *E. coli* O157:H7 isolated from sporadic cases and from 151 outbreaks in Canada and extended the typing scheme from 14 phagetypes to 62 types (Table 2.9).

Epidemiologically related strains from an outbreak showed the same phagetype, and in 12 outbreaks multiple types were encountered indicating the presence of more than one bacterial strain in the contaminated food. This phagetyping scheme has provided excellent epidemiological markers in the other 139 outbreaks in which phagetypes 4, 8, 2, 1 and 31 were encountered most frequently.

Concluding Comments

Serotyping remains an effective means of classifying *E. coli* isolates into groups of closely related organisms. The existence of an international scheme has facilitated comparison of data from laboratories all over the world. The major drawback of this method is that it demands substantial resources in antisera and time and is therefore limited to a small number of reference laboratories. Electrophoretic typing holds considerable promise and is likely to be used more extensively in the future for the study of relationships among *E. coli* isolates. Unlike serotyping, this technique is within the competence of many research laboratories. Nucleic-acid-based methodologies, especially those for identifying specific virulence factors, have been used extensively in identification of various types of pathogenic *E. coli*. Such techniques are likely to see more extensive use, as simple kits become available.

References

Abe, C., Schmitz, S., Jann, B. and Jann, K. (1988) Monoclonal antibodies against O and K antigens of uropathogenic *Escherichia coli* O4:K12:H$^-$ as opsonins. *Federation of European Microbiological Societies Microbiological Letters* 51, 153–158.

Adam, A. (1923) Uber die biologie der dyspepsiekoli und ihre beziehungen zur pathogenese der dyspepsie und intoxication. *Jahrbuch für Kinderheilkunde und Physiche Erziehung* 101, 295–314.

Adlam, C., Knights, J.M., Mugridge, A., Lindon, J.C., Williams, J.M. and Beesley, J.E. (1985) Purification, characterization and immunological properties of the capsular polysaccharide of *Pasteurella haemolytica* capsule T15: its identity with K62 (K2ab) capsular polysaccharide of *Escherichia coli* and the capsular polysaccharide of *Neisseria meningitidis* serogroup H. *Journal of General Microbiology* 131, 1963–1972.

Ahmed, R., Bopp, C., Borczyk, A. and Kasatiya, S. (1987) Phage-typing scheme for *Escherichia coli* O157:H7. *Journal of Infectious Diseases* 155, 806–809.

Albert, M.J., Qadri, F., Haque, A. and Bhuiyan, N.A. (1993) Bacterial clump formation at the surface of liquid culture as a rapid test for identification of enteroaggregative *Escherichia coil. Journal of Clinical Microbiology* 31, 1397–1399.

Baldini, M.M., Kaper, J.B., Levine, M.M., Candy, D.C.A. and Moon, H.W. (1983) Plasmid mediated adhesion in enteropathogenic *Escherichia coli. Journal of Pediatric Gastroenterology* 2, 534–538.

Baldwin, T.J., Knutton, S., Sellers, L., Manharrez Hernandez, H.A., Aitken, A. and Williams, P.H. (1992) Enteroaggregative *Escherichia coli* strains secrete a heat-labile toxin antigenically related to *E. coli* hemolysin. *Infection and Immunity* 60, 292–295.

Baudry, B., Savarino, S.J., Vial, P., Kaper, J.B. and Levine, M.M. (1990) A sensitive and specific DNA probe to identify enteroaggregative *Escherichia coli*, a recently discovered diarrheal pathogen. *Journal of Infectious Diseases* 161, 1249–1251.

Beachey, E.H. (1981) Bacterial adherence: adhesin–receptor interactions mediating the attachment of bacteria to mucosal surfaces. *Journal of Infectious Diseases* 143, 325–345.

Berger, H., Hacker, J., Juarez, A., Hughes, C. and Goebel, W. (1982) Cloning of the chromosomal determinants encoding hemolysin production and mannose-resistant hemagglutination in *Escherichia coli*. *Journal of Bacteriology* 152, 1241–1247.

Bertschinger, H.U., Bachmann, M., Mettler, C., Pospischil, A., Schraner, E.M., Stamm, M., Sydler, T. and Wild, P. (1990) Adhesive fimbriae produced *in vivo* by *Escherichia coli* O139:K12 (B):H1 associated with enterotoxaemia in pigs. *Veterinary Microbiology* 25, 267–281.

Bettelheim, K.A., Faiers, M. and Shooter, R.A. (1972) Serotypes of *Escherichia coli* in normal stools. *Lancet* ii, 1223–1224.

Bettelheim, K.A., Bushrod, F.M., Chandler, M.E., Trotman, R.E. and Byrne, K.C. (1975) An automatic method for serotyping *Escherichia coli*. *Zentralblatt für Bakteriologie, Parasitenkunde, Infektionskranheiten und Hygiene – erste abteilung originale – Reihe A: Medizinische Mikrobiologie und Parasitologie* 230, 443–445.

Beutin, L., Montenegro, M., Zimmermann, S. and Stephan, R. (1986) Characterization of hemolytic strains of *Escherichia coli* belonging to classical enteropathogenic O-serogroups. *Zentralblatt für Bakteriologie und Hygiene A* 261, 266–279.

Beutin, L., Zimmermann, S., Stephan, R., Ørskov, I. and Ørskov, F. (1988) Enterohemolysin, a new type of hemolysin produced by some strains of enteropathogenic *E. coli* (EPEC). *Zentralblatt für Bakteriologie und Hygiene, I Abteilung Originale A* 267, 576–588.

Bhatia, T.R.S. (1977) Phagetyping of *Escherichia coli* isolated from chickens. *Canadian Journal of Microbiology* 23, 1151–1153.

Binns, M.M., Davies, D.L. and Hardy, K.G. (1979) Cloned fragments of the plasmid Col V, I-K94 specifying virulence and serum resistance. *Nature (London)* 279, 778–781.

Bitter-Suermann, D., Goergen, I. and Frosch, M. (1986) Monoclonal antibodies to weak immunogenic *Escherichia coli* and meningococcal polysaccharide. In: Lark, D.L., Normark, S., Uhlin, B.-E. and Wolf-Watz, H. (eds) *Protein Carbohydrate Interactions in Biological Systems*. Academic Press, London, pp. 395–396.

Borczyk, A.A., Lior, H. and Thompson, S. (1989) Sorbitol negative *Escherichia coli* other than H7. *Journal of Infection* 18, 198–199.

Braun, V. (1981) *Escherichia coli* cells containing the Col V plasmid produce iron ionophore aerobactin. *Federation of European Microbiological Societies Microbiology Letters* 11, 225–228.

Braun, V., Bosch, V., Klumpp, E.R., Neff, I., Mayer, H. and Schlecht, S. (1976) Antigenic determinant of murein-lipoprotein and its exposure at the surface of Enterobacteriaceae. *European Journal of Biochemistry* 62, 555–566.

Braunstein, M. and Mladineo, M.A. (1974) *Escherichia coli* strains producing hydrogen sulfide in iron-agar medium. *American Journal of Clinical Pathology* 62, 420–424.

Bray, J. (1945) Isolation of antigenically homogeneous strain of *Bacterium coli Neapolitanum* from summer diarrhoea of infants. *Journal of Pathology and Bacteriology* 57, 239–247.

Brodhage, R.E. (1962) Urea-treated gram negative bacilli in the indirect hemagglutination reaction. *Nature (London)* 193, 501–502.

Brown, W.J. and Parisi, J.T. (1966) Bacteriophage typing of *Bacterium coli* (30751). *Proceedings of the Society of Experimental Biology and Medicine (New York)* 121, 259–262.

Cavalieri, S.J., Bohach, A. and Snyder, I.S. (1984) *Escherichia coli* alpha-hemolysin: characteristics and probable role in pathogenicity. *Microbiological Reviews* 48, 326–343.

Clancy, J. and Savage, D.C. (1981) Another Colicin V phenotype: *in vitro* adhesion of *Escherichia coli* to mouse intestinal epithelium. *Infection and Immunity* 32, 343–352.

Cramer, W.A., Dankert, J.R. and Uratani, Y. (1983) The membrane channel-forming bacteriocidal protein, Colicin E1. *Biochimica et Biophysica Acta* 737, 173–193.

Cravioto, A., Gross, R.J., Scotland, S.M. and Rowe, B. (1979) An adhesive factor found in strains of *Escherichia coli* belonging to the traditional infantile enteropathogenic serotypes. *Current Microbiology* 3, 95–99.

Cravioto, A., Scotland, S.M. and Rowe, B. (1982) Haemagglutination activity and colonization factor antigens I and II in enterotoxigenic and non-enterotoxigenic strains of *Escherichia coli* isolated from humans. *Infection and Immunity* 36, 189–197.

De Graaf, F.K. and Mooi, F.R. (1986) The fimbrial adhesins of *Escherichia coli. Advances in Microbiology and Physiology* 28, 65–143.

Dudgeon, L.S., Wordley, E. and Bawtree, F. (1921) On *Bacillus coli* infections of the urinary tract, especially in relation to haemolytic organisms. *Journal of Hygiene (Cambridge)* 20, 137–164.

Duguid, J.P., Anderson, E.S. and Campbell, I. (1966) Fimbrial and adhesive properties in *Salmonella. Journal of Pathology and Bacteriology* 92, 107–138.

DuPont, J.L., Formal, S.B., Hornick, R.B., Snyder, M.J., Libonati, J.P., Sheahan, D.G., Labrec, E.H. and Kalas, J.P. (1971) Pathogenesis of *Escherichia coli* diarrhea. *New England Journal of Medicine* 285, 1–9.

Echeverria, P. and Murphy, J.R. (1980) Enterotoxigenic *Escherichia coli* carrying plasmids coding for antibiotic resistance and enterotoxin production. *Journal of Infectious Diseases* 142, 273–278.

Escherich, T. (1885) Die darmbakterien des neugeborenen und sauglings. *Fortschrifte Der Medizin* 3, 515–522, 542–544.

Evans, D.G. and Evans, D.J., Jr (1978) New surface-associated heat-labile colonization factor antigen (CFA/II) produced by enterotoxigenic *Escherichia coli* of serogroups O6 and O8. *Infection and Immunity* 21, 638–647.

Evans, D.G., Silver, R.P., Evans, D.J., Chase, D.G. and Gorbach, S.L. (1975) Plasmid-controlled colonization factor associated with virulence in *Escherichia coli* enterotoxigenic for humans. *Infection and Immunity* 12, 656–667.

Evans, D.G., Evans, D.J., Jr, Tjoa, W.S. and DuPont, H.L. (1978) Detection and characterization of colonization factor of enterotoxigenic *Escherichia coli* isolated from adults with diarrhea. *Infection and Immunity* 19, 727–736.

Evans, D.J., Jr and Evans, D.G. (1983) Classification of pathogenic *Escherichia coli* according to serotype and the production of virulence factors with special reference to colonization-factor antigens. *Reviews of Infectious Diseases* 5 (Suppl. 4), S692–S701.

Evans, D.J., Jr, Evans, D.G. and DuPont, H.L. (1979) Hemagglutinating patterns of enterotoxigenic and enteropathogenic *Escherichia coli* determined with human, bovine, chicken, and guinea pig erythrocytes in the presence and absence of mannose. *Infection and Immunity* 23, 336–346.

Evans, D.J., Jr, Evans, D.G., Young, L.S. and Pitt, J. (1980) Hemagglutination typing of *Escherichia coli*: definition of seven hemagglutination types. *Journal of Clinical Microbiology* 12, 235–242.

Ewing, W.H. (1986) *Edwards and Ewing's Identification of Enterobacteriaceae*, 4th edn. Elsevier Science, New York.

Fernandez-Beros, M.E., Kissel, V., Lior, H. and Cabello, F.C. (1990) Virulence-related genes in Col V plasmids of *Escherichia coli* isolated from human blood and intestines. *Journal of Clinical Microbiology* 28, 742–746.

Fratamico, P.M., Schutz, F.J. and Buchanan, R.L. (1992) Rapid isolation of *Escherichia coli* O157:H7 from enrichment cultures of foods using an immunomagnetic separation method. *Food Microbiology* 9, 105–113.

Frosch, M., Gorgen, I., Boulnois, G.J., Timmins, K.N. and Bitter-Suermann, D. (1985) NZB mouse system for production of monoclonal antibodies to weak bacterial antigens: isolation of an IgG antibody to the polysaccharide capsules of *Escherichia coli* K1 and group B meningococci. *Proceedings of the National Academy of Sciences of the United States of America* 82, 1194–1198.

Giles, D.C. and Sangster, G. (1948) An outbreak of infantile gastro-enteritis in Aberdeen. The association of a special type of *Bacterium coli* with the infection. *Journal of Hygiene* 46, 1–9.

Giles, C., Sangster, G. and Smith, J. (1949) Epidemic gastro-enteritis of infants in Aberdeen during 1947. *Archives of Diseases of Childhood* 24, 45–53.

Gilson, L., Mahanty, H.K. and Kolter, R. (1987) Four plasmid genes are required for Colicin V synthesis, export and immunity. *Journal of Bacteriology* 169, 2466–2470.

Goldschmidt, R. (1933) Untersuchungen zur aetiologie der durchfallserkrankungen der sauglings. *Jahrbuch für Kinderheilkunde und Physiche Erziehung* 139, 318–358.

Gorbach, S.L., Banwell, J.G., Chatterjee, B.D., Jacobs, B. and Sack, R.B. (1971) Acute undifferentiated human diarrhea in the tropics. I. Alterations in intestinal microflora. *Journal of Clinical Investigation* 50, 881–889.

Gratia, A. (1925) Sur un remarquable exemple d'antagonisme entre deux souches de colibaccile. *Comptes Rendus des Séances de la Societé de Biologie* 93, 1041–1042.

Gratia, A. and Fredericq, P. (1946) Diversité des souches antibiotiques de *B. coli* et étendue variable de leur champ d'action. *Comptes Rendus des Séances de la Societé de Biologie* 140, 1032–1033.

Gross, R.J., Cheasty, T. and Rowe, B. (1977) Isolation of bacteriophages specific for K1 polysaccharide antigen of *Escherichia coli. Journal of Clinical Microbiology* 6, 548–550.

Guinee, P.A.M. and Jansen, W.H. (1979) Behaviour of *Escherichia coli* K antigens K88ab, K88ac, and K88ad in immunoelectrophoresis, double diffusion and hemagglutination. *Infection and Immunity* 23, 700–705.

Guinee, P.A.M., Agterberg, C.M. and Jansen, W.H. (1972) *Escherichia coli* O antigen typing by means of a mechanized microtechnique. *Applied Microbiology* 24, 127–131.

Guirguis, N.R., Schneerson, R., Bax, A., Egan, W., Robbins, J.B., Shiloah. J. and Ørskov, I. (1985) *Escherichia coli* K51 and K93 capsular polysaccharides are cross-reactive with capsular polysaccharide of *Neisseria meningitidis. Journal of Experimental Medicine* 162, 1837–1851.

Gulati, B.R., Sharma, V.K. and Taku, A.K. (1992) Occurrence and enterotoxigenicity of F17 fimbriae bearing *Escherichia coli* from calf diarrhoea. *Veterinary Record* 131, 348–349.

Gunzer, F., Bohm, H., Russmann, H., Bitzan, M., Aleksic, S. and Karch, H. (1992) Molecular detection of sorbitol-fermenting *Escherichia coli* O157 in patients with hemolytic-uremic syndrome. *Journal of Clinical Microbiology* 30, 1807–1810.

Gyles, C.L., Palchaudhuri, S. and Maas, W.K. (1977) Naturally occurring plasmids carrying genes for enterotoxin production and drug resistance. *Science* 198, 198–199.

Hale, T.L., Sansonetti, P.J., Schad, P.A., Austin, S. and Formal, S.B. (1983) Characterization of virulence plasmids and plasmid-associated outer membrane proteins in *Shigella flexneri*, *Shigella sonnei*, and *Escherichia coli. Infection and Immunity* 40, 340–350.

Harris, J.R., Wachsmuth, I.K., Davis, B.R. and Cohen, M.L. (1982) High molecular-weight plasmid correlates with *Escherichia coli* enteroinvasiveness. *Infection and Immunity* 37, 1295–1298.

Hedges, A.J., Howe, K. and Linton, A.H. (1977) Statistical considerations in the sampling of *E. coli* from intestinal sources for serotyping. *Journal of Applied Bacteriology* 43, 271–280.

Hettiaratchy, I.G., Cooke, E.M. and Shooter, R.A. (1973) Colicine production as an epidemiological marker of *Escherichia coli. Journal of Medical Microbiology* 6, 1–11.

Houwink, A.L. and Van Iterson, W. (1950) Electron microscopical observations on bacterial cytology. II. A study on flagellation. *Biochimica et Biophysica Acta* 5, 10–44.

Imberechts, H., De Greve, H., Schlicker, C., Bouchet, H., Pohl, P., Charlier, G., Bertschinger, H., Wild, P., Vandekerckhove, J., Van Damme, J., Van Montagu, M. and Lintermans, P. (1992) Characterization of F107 fimbriae of *Escherichia coli* 107/86 which causes edema disease in pigs, and nucleotide sequence of the major fimbrial subunit gene, *fed*A. *Infection and Immunity* 60, 1963–1971.

Ishiguro, N. and Sato, G. (1979) The distribution of plasmids determining citrate utilization in citrate-positive variants of *Escherichia coli* from human, domestic animals, feral birds and environments. *Journal of Hygiene Cambridge* 83, 331–344.

Jann, B. and Jann, K. (1990) Structure and biosynthesis of the capsular antigens of *Escherichia coli. Current Topics in Microbiology and Immunology* 150, 19–42.

Jann, K. and Jann, B. (1992) Capsules of *Escherichia coli* and biological significance. *Canadian Journal of Microbiology* 38, 705–710.

Johnson, W.M., Lior, H. and Bezanson, G.S. (1983) Cytotoxic *Escherichia coli* O157:H7 associated with haemorrhagic colitis in Canada. *Lancet* i, 76.

Johnson, W.M., Pollard, D.R., Lior, H., Tyler, S.D. and Rozee, K.R. (1990) Differentiation of genes coding for *Escherichia coli* verotoxin 2 and the verotoxin associated with porcine edema disease (VTe) by the polymerase chain reaction. *Journal of Clinical Microbiology* 28, 2351–2353.

Jones, G.W. and Rutter, J.M. (1972) Role of the K88 antigen in the pathogenesis of neonatal diarrhea caused by *Escherichia coli* in piglets. *Infection and Immunity* 6, 918–927.

Kaijser, B., Hanson, L.A., Jodel, U., Lidin-Janson, G. and Robbins, J.B. (1977) Frequency of *E. coli* K antigens in urinary tract infection. *Lancet* i, 663–666.

Kapur, V., White, D.G., Wilson, R.A. and Whittam, T.S. (1992) Outer membrane protein patterns mark clones of *Escherichia coli* O2 and O78 that cause avian septicemia. *Infection and Immunity* 60, 1687–1691.

Kauffmann, F. (1944) Zur serologie der coli-grouppe. *Acta Pathologica Microbiologica Scandinavica* 21, 20–45.

Kauffmann, F. (1947) The serology of the coli group. *Journal of Immunology* 57, 71–100.

Khakhria, R., Duck, D. and Lior, H. (1990) Extended phage-typing scheme for *Escherichia coli* O157:H7. *Epidemiology and Infection* 105, 511–520.

Klemm, P. (1985) Fimbrial adhesins of *Escherichia coli. Reviews in Infectious Diseases* 7, 321–340.

Knipschildt, H.E. (1945) *Untersøgelser over Coligruppens Serologi*. Nyt Nordisk Forlag Arnold Busck, Kobenhavn.

Kunin, C.M. and Beard, M.V. (1963) Serological studies of O antigens by means of the hemagglutination test. *Journal of Bacteriology* 85, 541–548.

Kunin, C.M., Beard, M.V. and Halmagyi, N. (1962) Evidence for a common hapten associated with endotoxin fractions of *E. coli* and other Enterobacteriaceae. *Proceedings of the Society for Experimental Biology and Medicine* 111, 160–166.

La Brec, E.H., Schneider, H., Magnani, T.J. and Formal, S.B. (1964) Epithelial cell penetration as an essential step in the pathogenesis of bacillary dysentery. *Journal of Bacteriology* 88, 1503–1518.

Laurelle, L. (1889) L'Etude bacteriologique sur les peritonites par perforation. *La Cellule* 5, 60–123.

Le Sage, A.A. (1897) Contribution a l'etude des enterites infantiles-sero-diagnostic des races de *Bacterium coli. Comptes Rendus des Séances de la Societé de Biologie* 49, 900–901.

Levine, M.M. (1987) *Escherichia coli* that cause diarrhea: enterotoxigenic, enteropathogenic, enteroinvasive, enterohemorrhagic and enteroadherent. *Journal of Infectious Diseases* 155, 377–389.

Lior, H. and Borczyk, A.A. (1987) False-positive identifications of *Escherichia coli* O157:H7. *Lancet* i, 333.

Mäkelä, P.H. and Mayer, H. (1976) Enterobacterial common antigen. *Bacteriological Reviews* 40, 591–632.

Maniatis, T., Fritsch, E.F. and Sambrook, J. (1982) *Molecular Cloning: A Laboratory Manual*. Cold Spring Harbor Laboratory, Cold Spring Harbor, New York.

Mayer, L.W. (1988) Use of plasmid profiles in epidemiologic surveillance of disease outbreaks and in tracing the transmission of antibiotic resistance. *Clinical Microbiology Reviews* 1, 228–243.

McGeachie, J. (1965) Bacteriocin typing in urinary infection. *Zentralblatt für Bakteriologie Parasitenkunde, Infektionskrankheiten und Hygiene* 196, 377–384.

Milch, H. (1978) Phagetyping of *Escherichia coli*. In: Bergan, T. and Norris, J.R. (eds) *Methods In Microbiology*. Academic Press, New York, pp. 87–155.

Milch, H. and Gyenes, M. (1972) Subdivision and correlation studies of serologically grouped *Escherichia coli* strains by phagetyping, colicinogeny, lysogeny and biochemical test. *Acta Microbiologica Academicae Scientiarum Hungaricae* 19, 213–244.

Milch, H., Nikolnikov, S. and Czirok, E. (1984) *Escherichia coli* Col V plasmids and their role in pathogenicity. *Acta Microbiologica Hungarica* 31, 117–125.

Moon, H.W. (1990) Colonization factor antigens of enterotoxigenic *Escherichia coli* in animals. *Current Topics in Microbiology and Immunology* 151, 147–165.

Morris, J.A., Thorns, C.J., Scott, A.C., Sojka, W.J. and Wells, G.A.H. (1982) Adhesion *in vitro* and *in vivo* associated with an adhesive agent (F41) produced by a $K99^-$ mutant of the reference strain *Escherichia coli* B41. *Infection and Immunity* 36, 1146–1153.

Muller, D., Hughes, C. and Goebel, W. (1983) Relationship between plasmid and chromosomal hemolysin determinants of *Escherichia coli*. *Journal of Bacteriology* 153, 846–851.

Nataro, J.P., Baldini, M.M., Kaper, J.B., Black, R.E., Bravo, N. and Levine, M.M. (1985) Detection of an adherence factor of enteropathogenic *Escherichia coli* with a DNA probe. *Journal of Infectious Diseases* 152, 560–565.

Neter, E., Westphal, O., Luderitz, O. and Gorzynski, E.A. (1955) Demonstration of antibodies against enteropathogenic *Escherichia coli* in sera of children of various ages. *Journal of Pediatrics* 16, 801–807.

Neter, E., Westphal, O., Luderitz, O. and Gorzynski, E.A. (1956) The bacterial hemagglutination test for the demonstration of antibodies to Enterobacteriaceae. *Annals of the New York Academy of Science* 66, 141–156.

Nicolle, P., Le Minor, L., Buttaux, R. and Ducrest, P. (1952) Phagetyping of *Escherichia coli* isolated in infantile gastroenteritis. *Bulletin de L'academie Nationale de Medecine (Paris)* 136, 480–485.

Ørskov, I. and Ørskov, F. (1966) Episome-carried surface antigen K88 of *Escherichia coli*. I. Transmission of the determinant of the K88 antigen and influence on the transfer of chromosomal markers. *Journal of Bacteriology* 91, 69–75.

Ørskov, F. and Ørskov, I. (1972) Immunoelectrophoretic patterns of extracts from *Escherichia coli* O antigen test strains O1 to O157 examinations in homologous OK sera. Further comments on the classification of *Escherichia* K antigens. *Acta Pathologica et Microbiologica Scandinavica (Section B) Microbiology and Immunology* 80, 905–910.

Ørskov, I. and Ørskov, F. (1983) Serology of *Escherichia coli* fimbriae. *Progress in Allergy* 33, 80–105.

Ørskov, F. and Ørskov, I. (1984) Serotyping of *E. coli*. In: Bergan, T. and Norris, J.R. (eds) *Methods In Microbiology*. Academic Press, New York, pp. 43–112.

Ørskov, I. and Ørskov, F. (1985) *Escherichia coli* in extraintestinal infections. *Journal of Hygiene* 95, 551–575.

Ørskov, I. and Ørskov, F. (1990a) Serologic classification of fimbriae. *Current Topics in Microbiology and Immunology* 151, 71–90.

Ørskov, F. and Ørskov, I. (1990b) The serology of capsular antigens. *Current Topics in Microbiology and Immunology* 150, 43–63.

Ørskov, I., Ørskov, F., Jann, B. and Jann, K. (1977) Serology, chemistry, and genetics of O and K antigens of *Escherichia coli. Bacteriological Reviews* 41, 667–710.

Ørskov, F., Ørskov, I., Sutton, A., Schneerson, R., Lin, W., Egan, W., Hoff, G.E. and Robbins, J.B. (1979) Form variation in *Escherichia coli* K1: determined by *O*-acetylation of the capsular polysaccharide. *Journal of Experimental Medicine* 149, 669–685.

Ørskov, I., Wachsmuth, I.K., Taylor, D.N., Echeverria, P., Rowe, B., Sakazaki, R. and Ørskov, F. (1991) Two new *Escherichia coli* O Groups: O172 from 'Shigella-like' toxin producing strains (EHEC) and O173 from enteroinvasive *E. coli* (EIEC). *Acta Pathologica Microbiologica et Immunologica Sandinavica* 90, 30–32.

Padhye, N.V. and Doyle, M.P. (1992) *Escherichia coli* O157:H7: epidemiology, pathogenesis and methods for detection in food. *Journal of Food Protection* 55, 555–565.

Pai, C.H., Ahmed, N., Lior, H., Johnson, W.M., Sims, H.V. and Woods, D.E. (1988) Epidemiology of sporadic diarrhea due to verocytotoxin-producing *Escherichia coli*: a two year prospective study. *Journal of Infectious Diseases* 157, 1054–1057.

Pande, R.C., Rajvanshi, V.S., Mehrotra, T.N. and Gupta, S.C. (1976) Phage typing of enteropathogenic serotypes of *Escherichia coli* from sporadic cases of acute and chronic diarrhoea and gastroenteritis in Allahabad. *Indian Journal of Medical Research* 64, 841–846.

Pedroso, M.Z., Freymuller, E., Trabulsi, L.R. and Gomes, T.A.T. (1993) Attaching-effacing lesions and intracellular penetration in HeLa cells and human duodenal mucosa by two *Escherichia coli* strains not belonging to the classical enteropathogenic *E. coli* serogroups. *Infection and Immunity* 61, 1152–1156.

Pollard, D.R., Johnson, W.M., Lior, H., Tyler, S.D. and Rozee, K.R. (1990) Rapid and specific detection of verotoxin genes in *Escherichia coli* by the polymerase chain reaction. *Journal of Clinical Microbiology* 28, 540–545.

Pugsely, A.P. (1984a) The ins and outs of colicins. Part 1: Production, and translocation across membranes. *Microbiological Sciences* 1, 168–175.

Pugsley, A.P. (1984b) The ins and outs of colicins. Part 2: Lethal action, immunity and ecological implications. *Microbiological Sciences* 1, 203–205.

Ratiner, Y.A. (1982) Phase variation of the H antigen in *Escherichia coli* strain Bi7327-41 the standard strain of *Escherichia coli* flagellar antigen H3. *Federation of European Microbiological Societies Microbiology Letters* 15, 33–36.

Riley, L.W., Remis, R.S., Helgerson, S.D., McGee, H.B., Wells, J.G., Davis, B.R., Hebert, R.J., Olcott, E.S., Johnson, L.M., Hargrett, N.T., Blake, P.A. and Cohen, M.L. (1983) Hemorrhagic colitis associated with a rare *Escherichia coli* serotype. *New England Journal of Medicine* 308, 681–685.

Robbins, J.B., McCraken, G.H. and Gotschlich, E.C. (1974) *Escherichia coli* K1 capsular polysaccharide associated with neonatal meningitis. *New England Journal of Medicine* 290, 1216–1220.

Robbins, J.B., Schneerson, R., Liu, T.Y., Schiffer, M.S., Schiffman, G., Myerowitz, R.L. and McCraken, G.H. (1975) Cross-reacting bacterial antigens and immunity to disease caused by encapsulated bacteria. In: Neter, E. and Milgram, F. (eds) *The Immune System and Infectious Diseases*. 4th International Convocation on Immunology, Buffalo, New York, pp. 218–241.

Rodriguez, M.L., Jann, B. and Jann, K. (1988) Comparative structural elucidation of the K 18, K 22, and K 100 antigens of *Escherichia coli* as related ribosylribitol phosphates. *Carbohydrate Research* 173, 243–253.

Sack, R.B. (1980) Enterotoxigenic *Escherichia coli*: identification and characterization. *Journal of Infectious Diseases* 142, 279–286.

Sato, G., Asagi, M., Oka, C., Ishiguro, N. and Terakado, N. (1978) Transmissible citrate-utilizing ability in *Escherichia coli* isolated from pigeons, pigs and cattle. *Microbiology and Immunology* 22, 357–360.

Savarino, S.J., Fasano, A., Robertson, D.C. and Levine, M.M. (1991) Enteroaggregative *Escherichia coli* elaborate a heat-stable enterotoxin demonstrable in an *in vitro* rabbit intestinal model. *Journal of Clinical Investigation* 87, 1450–1455.

Savarino, S.J., Fasano, A., Watson, J., Martin, B.M., Levine, M.M., Guandalini, S. and Guerry, P. (1993) Enteroaggregative *Escherichia coli* heat-stable enterotoxin 1 represents another subfamily of *E. coli* heat-stable toxin. *Proceedings of the National Academy of Sciences of the United States of America* 90, 3093–3097.

Scotland, S.M., Gross, R.J., Cheasty, T. and Rowe, B. (1979) The occurrence of plasmids carrying genes for both enterotoxin production and drug resistance in *Escherichia coli* of human origin. *Journal of Hygiene (Cambridge)* 83, 531–538.

Sears, H.J. and Brownlee, I. (1952) Further observations on the resistance of individual strains of *Escherichia coli* in the intestinal tract of man. *Journal of Bacteriology* 63, 47–57.

Seelander, R.K., Korhonen, T.K., Väisänen-Rhen, V., Williams, P.H., Pattison, P. and Caugant, D.A. (1986) Genetic relationships and clonal structure of strains of *Escherichia coli* causing neonatal septicemia and meningitis. *Infection and Immunity* 52, 213–222.

Semjén, G.I., Ørskov, I. and Ørskov, F. (1977) K antigen determination of *Escherichia coli* by counter-current immunoelectrophoresis (CIE). *Acta Pathologica Microbiologica Scandinavica Section B* 85, 103–107.

Sereny, B. (1957) Experimental keratoconjuctivitis shigellosa. *Acta Microbiologica Academiae Scientiarum Hungaricae* 4, 367–376.

Shannon, R. (1957) Colicin production as a method for typing *Bact. coli* O55 B5. *Journal of Medical Laboratory Technology* 14, 199–214.

Silva, R.M., Toledo, M.R. and Trabulsi, L.R. (1982) Correlation of invasivness with plasmid in enteroinvasive strains of *Escherichia coli. Journal of Infectious Diseases* 146, 706.

Smith, H.W. (1963) The haemolysins of *Escherichia coli. Journal of Pathology and Bacteriology* 85, 197–211.

Smith, H.W. (1974) A search for transmissible pathogenic characters in invasive strains of *Escherichia coli*. The discovery of plasmid-controlled toxin and a plasmid-controlled lethal character closely associated or identical with colicin V. *Journal of General Microbiology* 83, 95–111.

Smith, H.W. and Crabb, W.E. (1956) The typing of *E. coli* by bacteriophage: its application in the study of the *E. coli* population of the intestinal tract of healthy calves and of calves suffering from white scours. *Journal of General Microbiology* 15, 556–574.

Smith, H.W. and Halls, S. (1967) The transmissible nature of the genetic factor in *E. coli* that controls haemolysin production. *Journal of General Microbiology* 47, 301–312.

Smith, H.W. and Halls, S. (1968) The transmissible nature of the genetic factor in *Escherichia coli* that controls enterotoxin production. *Journal of General Microbiology* 52, 319–334.

Smith, H.W. and Huggins, M.B. (1976) Further observation on the association of the Colicin V plasmid of *Escherichia coli* with pathogenicity and with survival in the alimentary tract. *Journal of General Microbiology* 92, 335–350.

Smith, H.W. and Linggood, M.A. (1972) Further observation on *Escherichia coli* enterotoxins with particular regard to those produced by atypical piglet strain and by calf and lamb strains. The transmissible nature of these enterotoxins and of a K antigen possessed by calf and lamb strains. *Journal of Medical Microbiology* 5, 243–250.

Smith, H.R. and Scotland, S.M. (1993) Isolation and identification methods for *Escherichia coli* O157 and other vero cytotoxin producing strains. *Journal of Clinical Pathology* 46, 10–17.

Smyth, C.J. (1982) Two mannose-resistant haemagglutinins on enterotoxigenic *Escherichia coli* of serotype O6:K15:H16 or H^{-} isolated from travellers' and infantile diarrhoea. *Journal of General Microbiology* 128, 2081–2096.

Söderström, T., Stein, K., Brinton, C.C., Hosea, S., Burch, C., Hansson, H.A., Karpas, A., Schneerson, R., Sutton, A., Vann, W.I. and Hanson, L.A. (1983) Serological and functional properties of monoclonal antibodies to *Escherichia coli* type I pilus and capsular antigens. *Progress in Allergy* 33, 259–274.

Sojka, W.J. (1965) Escherichia coli *in Domestic Animals and Poultry*. Commonwealth Agricultural Bureaux, Farnham Royal, UK.

Sterne, R.B., Wescott, R.B. and Parisi, J.T. (1970) Phage types of *Escherichia coli* isolated from swine. *American Journal of Veterinary Research* 31, 2101–2103.

Stewart, P.J., Desormeaux, W. and Chene, J. (1983) Hemorrhagic colitis in a home for the aged – Ontario. *Canada Diseases Weekly Report* 9, 29–32.

Sussman, M. (1985) *Escherichia coli* in human and animal disease. In: Sussman, M. (ed.) *The Virulence of* Escherichia coli. Academic Press, London, pp. 7–45.

Tacket, C.O., Maneval, D.R. and Levine, M.M. (1987) Purification, morphology and genetics of a new fimbrial colonization factor of enterotoxigenic *Escherichia coli* O159:H4. *Infection and Immunity* 55, 1063–1066.

Taylor, J., Powell, B.W. and Wright, J. (1949) Infantile diarrhoea and vomiting. A clinical and bacteriological investigation. *British Medical Journal* 2, 117–125.

Tenover, F.C. (1985) Plasmid fingerprinting: a tool for bacterial strain identification and surveillance of nosocomial and community-acquired infections. *Clinics in Laboratory Medicine* 5, 413–436.

Tewari, R., Smith, D.G. and Rowbury, R.J. (1985) Effect of Col V plasmids on the hydrophobicity of *Escherichia coli. Federation of European Microbiological Societies Microbiology Letters* 29, 245–249.

Tewari, R., Smith, D.G. and Rowbury, R.J. (1986) A motility lesion in Col V^+ *Escherichia coli* strains and its possible clinical significance. *Annales de L'Institut Pasteur – Microbiologie* 137, 223–237.

Thomas, L.V., Cravioto, A., Scotland, S.M. and Rowe, B. (1982) New fimbrial antigenic type (E8775) that may represent a colonization factor in enterotoxigenic *Escherichia coli* in humans. *Infection and Immunity* 35, 1119–1124.

Thompson, J.S., Hodge, D.S. and Borczyk, A.A. (1990) Rapid biochemical test to identify verocytotoxin-positive strains of *Escherichia coli* serotype O157:H7. *Journal of Clinical Microbiology* 28, 2165–2168.

Toledo, M.R.F. and Trabulsi, L.R. (1983) Correlation between biochemical and serological characteristics of *Escherichia coli* and results of the Sereny test. *Journal of Clinical Microbiology* 17, 419–421.

Tyler, S.D., Johnson, W.M., Lior, H., Wang, G. and Rozee, K.R. (1991) Identification of verotoxin type 2 variant B subunit genes in *Escherichia coli* by the polymerase chain reaction and restriction fragment length polymorphism analysis. *Journal of Clinical Microbiology* 29, 1339–1343.

Van Die, I., Riegman, N., Gaykema, O., Van Megen, I., Hoekstra, W., Bergman, H., De Ree, H. and Van Der Bosch, H. (1988) Localization of antigenic determinants of P-fimbriae of uropathogenic *Escherichia coli. Federation of European Microbiological Societies Microbiology Letters* 49, 95–100.

Vial, P.A., Robins-Browne, R., Lior, H., Prado, V., Kaper, J.B., Nataro, J.P., Maneval, D., ElSayed, A. and Levine, M.M. (1988) Characterization of entero-adherent-aggregative *Escherichia coli*, a putative agent of diarrheal disease. *Journal of Infectious Diseases* 158, 70–79.

Wachsmuth, I.K. (1986) Molecular epidemiology of bacterial infections: examples of methodology and of investigations of outbreaks. *Reviews of Infectious Diseases* 8, 682–692.

Wachsmuth, I.K., Davis, B.R. and Allen, S.D. (1979) Ureolytic *Escherichia coli* of human origin: serological, epidemiological and genetic analysis. *Journal of Clinical Microbiology* 10, 897–902.

Walton, J.R. and Smith, D.H. (1969) New hemolysin (gamma) produced by *Escherichia coli. Journal of Bacteriology* 98, 304–305.

White, D.G., Wilson, R.A., San Gabriel, A., Saco, M. and Whittam, T.S. (1990) Genetic relationships among strains of avian *Escherichia coli* associated with swollen-head syndrome. *Infection and Immunity* 58, 3613–3620.

Whittam, T.S. and Wilson, R.A. (1988) Genetic relationships among pathogenic strains of avian *Escherichia coli. Infection and Immunity* 56, 2458–2466.

Whittam, T.S., Wolfe, M.L., Wachsmuth, I.K., Orskov, F., Orskov, I. and Wilson, R.A. (1993) Clonal relationships among *Escherichia coli* strains that cause hemorrhagic colitis in infantile diarrhea. *Infection and Immunity* 61, 1619–1629.

Winkle, S.M., Refai, M. and Rhode, R. (1972) On the antigenic relationship of *Vibrio cholerae* to Enterobacteriaceae. *Annales de L'Institut Pasteur* 123, 775–781.

Wolf, M.K., Andrews, G.P., Fritz, D.L., Sjogren, R.W. and Boedeker, E.C. (1988) Characterization of the plasmid from *Escherichia coli* RDEC-1 that mediates expression of adhesin AF/R1 and evidence that AF/R1 pili promote but are not essential for enteropathogenic disease. *Infection and Immunity* 56, 1846–1857.

Yamamoto, Y., Endo, S., Yokota, T. and Echeverria, P. (1991) Characteristics of adherence of enteroaggregative *Escherichia coli* to human and animal mucosa. *Infection and Immunity* 59, 3722–3739.

II

Diseases Caused by *Escherichia coli*

Escherichia coli Septicaemia in Calves

3

C.C. Gay[1] and T.E. Besser[2]

[1]*Department of Veterinary Clinical Sciences and* [2]*Department of Microbiology and Pathology, College of Veterinary Medicine, Washington State University, Pullman, Washington 99164–6610, USA*

Septicaemic disease of calves caused by *E. coli* (septicaemic colibacillosis, colisepticaemia) occurs predominantly in dairy calves under 1 week of age. There are two determinants for the occurrence of septicaemic colibacillosis. The primary determinant is a deficiency in circulating immunoglobulins in the calf resulting from a failure in passive transfer of colostral immunoglobulins. The second determinant is the exposure of such a calf to a strain of *E. coli* with the ability to invade and multiply in the blood and internal organs, producing a bacteraemia and finally an overwhelming septicaemia and endotoxaemia. Septicaemic colibacillosis is usually a sporadic disease but on larger farms may occur in clusters or as an outbreak. Outbreaks are the result of farm practices of feeding colostrum in a manner that leads to a high prevalence of failure of passive transfer of colostral immunoglobulins, coupled with calf management systems that promote transmission of infection within groups of susceptible neonatal calves.

Early Studies on Colisepticaemia

E. coli has been recognized as a cause of mortality in newborn calves for over 100 years. The initial description of *E. coli* as a cause of septicaemia and diarrhoea in calves that was given by Jensen in 1893 (cited by Sojka, 1965) was the first attempt to associate *E. coli* with a specific disease syndrome in any species (Ørskov and Ørskov, 1984). Following Jensen's original descriptions, and through the period up to the 1960s, there were a number of significant studies that laid a considerable grounding to the current understanding of *E. coli*-associated disease in neonatal calves. Prominent among these are observations in America by Theobald Smith and his co-workers in the 1920s and a series of experiments conducted in the 1950s by Aschaffenburg and his co-workers at the National Institute for Research in Dairying and the Royal Veterinary College in England. These studies defined the nature of passive transfer of colostral immunoglobulins to the calf and also established that, although both colostrum-deprived and colostrum-fed calves could succumb to colibacillosis, the calf that was deprived of colostrum was especially susceptible to colisepticaemia.

The protection afforded the calf by colostrum was believed to be related to its specific antibody content, particularly to the presence of antibody directed against the K antigen of *E. coli* incriminated in the disease. During this period there were also a number of reports from Europe, England and North America, dealing with serological examinations of isolates of *E. coli* from colisepticaemia. These established that specific serotypes, OK groups and O groups were associated with this disease. It was generally considered that enteric colibacillosis and septicaemic colibacillosis were varying manifestations of the same *E. coli* infection. Septicaemic colibacillosis, in most instances, was thought to be a consequence of a preceding colienteritis and to occur when a calf was exposed to a pathogenic strain of *E. coli* against which it had received no colostral antibody. Consequently, the thrust in the prevention of colisepticaemia following these early studies evolved towards attempts to increase the specific antibody content in colostrum against the predominant *E. coli* associated with the disease. These and other studies prior to the 1960s, which defined the association of *E. coli* with neonatal calf disease and the mechanisms of passive transfer of colostral immunoglobulins, have been extensively reviewed elsewhere (Lovell, 1955; Pierce, 1961; Gay, 1965; Sojka, 1965; Butler, 1969; Fey, 1971, 1972; Bourne, 1977).

Two related observations in the 1960s led to a major advance in the understanding of this disease. The first observation was that natural cases of colisepticaemia were restricted to calves that were agammaglobulinaemic or markedly hypogammaglobulinaemic despite having been fed colostrum. The second was that a deficiency in circulating immunoglobulins was a relatively common occurrence in calves that had supposedly received colostrum (Fey and Margadant, 1961a; Fey, 1962; Smith, 1962; Gay *et al.*, 1964, 1965). This led to the recognition that failure of passive transfer was the prime determinant of the occurrence of colisepticaemia and that colisepticaemia had a pathogenesis quite distinct from enteric forms of colibacillosis (Gay, 1965; Smith and Halls, 1968; Fey, 1972; Smith and Huggins, 1979).

Pathogenesis and Transmission

Knowledge of the pathogenesis and transmission of colisepticaemia derives both from observations on natural cases and from experimental infections. Colisepticaemia can be reproduced experimentally in colostrum-deprived calves by oral challenge with invasive strains of *E. coli* isolated from natural cases of colisepticaemia. In contrast, calves that have been fed colostrum, and that have absorbed immunoglobulins, are resistant to the equivalent challenge (Fey, 1962; Gay *et al.*, 1964; Smith and Halls, 1968; Smith and Huggins, 1979; Contrepois *et al.*, 1986; Wickstrom *et al.*, 1987). On the farm, spontaneous cases occur only in calves that are deficient in circulating immunoglobulins (Gay *et al.*, 1965; McEwan *et al.*, 1970; Penhale *et al.*, 1970;, Fey, 1972; McGuire *et al.*, 1976). Experimental infections indicate several potential routes of invasion. Invasion across the intestinal epithelium is a common route of infection (Smith and Halls, 1968) and pinocytosis of *E. coli* with transepithelial migration to the mesenteric lymph node has been observed in neonatal calves during the period of intestinal permeability to large proteins (Corley *et al.*, 1977). Intestinal infection and colonization are not essential for the development of the disease, as the organism can also invade through the nasal and oropharyngeal mucosa. This was demonstrated in calves in which the oesophagus was ligated prior to challenge to preclude intestinal infection (Fey, 1962, 1972; Fey *et al.*, 1962). Invasion can also occur via the umbilicus and umbilical veins (Fey, 1972).

Following oral challenge of colostrum-deprived calves with an invasive strain of *E. coli* the challenge strain is demonstrable in the retropharyngeal and intestinal mesenteric lymph nodes 2–4 hours postchallenge (Smith and Halls, 1968). Bacteraemia is evident by 6–8 hours (Smith and Halls, 1968; Fey, 1972; Wickstrom *et al.*, 1987) and progresses to the development of clinical signs of septicaemia as early as 18–24 hours postchallenge. Endotoxaemia contributes significantly to the rapidly fatal course (Cullor, 1992). The period of bacteraemia is more protracted in calves infected with less virulent strains of *E. coli*, and in calves that have acquired small amounts of immunoglobulin from colostrum. The protracted bacteraemia allows localization of the infection and the occurrence of polyarthritis, meningitis and, less commonly, uveitis and nephritis. Localization of infection, with or without subsequent septicaemia, can also occur in calves that are bacteraemic at the time they absorb antibodies from a late-fed colostrum (Fey and Margadant, 1962).

The primary routes of excretion of the organism are via nasal and oral secretions, urine and faeces. The organism can be isolated from oral and nasal secretions throughout the time period between challenge and death. It is present in the urine shortly following the onset of bacteraemia and is excreted in urine in increasing numbers through the period of clinical illness. The organism may be present in the nasal secretions and urine of bacteraemic calves prior to the onset of obvious clinical illness. Its presence in faeces is variable. With strains that establish in the intestinal tract, the faeces are an important source of infection for other calves and the septicaemic strain is commonly present in the faeces at the terminal stages of the disease (Smith and Halls, 1968). However, in some cases of colisepticaemia the septicaemic strain is not detected in the faeces or the intestine of the calf at death (Fey, 1972).

The relative importance of these routes of invasion and excretion to the transmission of the disease and the occurrence of multiple cases varies with the management of the calves and the potential for exposure. Failure of passive transfer of colostral immunoglobulins is a common occurrence in dairy calves and on many farms there can be a large proportion of calves susceptible to colisepticaemia (McGuire and Adams, 1982). However, the disease does not invariably occur in calves that are susceptible; rather it occurs in clusters, or temporally restricted outbreaks, suggesting that strains of *E. coli* with the invasive potential to produce colisepticaemia are rare in the environment of the calf. Only a few studies carried out in the 1960s and early 1970s have directly examined the epidemiology of transmission of colisepticaemia in outbreaks. Fey and Margadant (1961b) sampled the environment of calves on 18 farms for the presence of *E. coli* O78:K80 during periods of mortality associated with this serogroup. They found that it was present in areas such as the walls of the calf pens, on buckets, on the hands or in the faeces of farm workers and in the faeces and nasal cavity of clinically normal calves and cows on 14 farms. The detection of this serogroup on farms was temporarily closely related to the outbreak of colisepticaemia associated with it and isolations from the environment were rare at times where there were no calf deaths. This serogroup of *E. coli* and other O groups associated with colisepticaemia are not commonly found in the intestinal flora of healthy cattle (Gay, 1965).

The occurrence of a sporadic case of colisepticaemia probably reflects the chance encounter of a susceptible calf with an invasive strain of *E. coli* present in its environment. Outbreaks in communally housed calves can result from exposure to a contaminated environment. There is also the potential for transmission of infection between calves by faecal–oral contact, by direct nose to nose contact, via urinary and respiratory aerosols, and oral or umbilical infection following navel sucking. In groups of communally housed calves, calves that are in the bacteraemic phase of infection prior to the development of clinical disease can be unrecognized sources of infection to other calves in their environment, and can precipitate outbreaks of colisepticaemia in large herds where colostral transfer of immunoglobulins is inadequate. This may result in the clustering of a single serotype of *E. coli* seen in association with outbreaks of the disease (Fey, 1972).

Clinical Disease and Laboratory Findings

Colisepticaemia occurs during the first week of life, most commonly in calves between 2 and 5 days of age, although cases, especially those with localizing signs, can occur up to 2 weeks of age. Clinical abnormality is not evident during the early bacteraemic phase of the disease; the calves remain bright and alert until they develop septic shock. The clinical course is short, varying from 3 to 8 hours and there are no diagnostic clinical findings. The case fatality approaches 100%. Initial signs are listlessness and early loss of interest in sucking followed by depression, poor response to external stimuli and eventual collapse, recumbency and coma. Pyrexia is not a feature in the acute form of the disease, but there is tachycardia, a prolonged capillary refill time and evidence of cardiovascular collapse. Commonly there is the passage of loose, mucoid faeces in the terminal stages of the disease. Diarrhoea is not a feature of uncomplicated cases but may be present as the immunodeficiency that predisposes to colisepticaemia also can predispose to separate enteric infections (Gay, 1984). In the early stages of colisepticaemia there is a moderate but significant leucocytosis and neutrophilia which is followed by a marked leucopenia in the terminal stages. Hypoproteinaemia is a constant finding and is due to the deficiency in circulating immunoglobulins (Tennant *et al.*, 1975; Green and Smith, 1992). Endotoxaemia contributes significantly to the fatal course of the disease. The clinical, biochemical and physiological responses of newborn calves to infusion with endotoxin have been described and reviewed (Morris *et al.*, 1986; Cullor, 1992).

Cases of colisepticaemia with a more prolonged clinical course may show clinical evidence of localized infection in the joints and meninges. Polyarthritis is manifest with palpable fluid in the larger joints of the limbs and joint fluid obtained by arthrocentesis has increased inflammatory cells and protein content. Clinical signs of meningitis include tremor, hyperaesthesia, opisthotonos and convulsion but many calves with meningitis manifest primarily with stupor and coma. Analysis of the cerebrospinal fluid is a valuable adjunct to diagnosis; pleocytosis and elevated protein concentration are evident and organisms may be observed on microscopic examination (Green and Smith, 1992).

The gross findings at postmortem examination are minor. With peracute septicaemic deaths there are usually petechial haemorrhages on the epicardium and serosal surfaces and there may be some enlargement of the spleen and evidence of pulmonary oedema and haemorrhage. Dehydration is minimal unless there is a concurrent enteric infection. More chronic cases show fibrinous polyarthritis and meningitis (Wray and Thomlinson, 1974). On bacteriological examination of cases of colisepticaemia a single strain of *E. coli* can be isolated with profuse growth and in pure culture from heart blood, bone marrow and all internal organs. Depending upon the case the septicaemic strain may be dominant in isolates from different levels of the intestine, may be present only in the upper small intestine, or may not be detectable at any level of the intestine (Fey, 1972). It is always present in high numbers in the urine (Smith and Halls, 1968; Fey, 1972).

Virulence Attributes of *E. coli* Associated with Colisepticaemia

The serological associations of isolates of *E. coli* from cases of colisepticaemia have been examined in several countries in studies prior to the 1970s. These studies established that isolates from colisepticaemia that could be typed possess K antigens and belong to a relatively small number of O groups, most commonly O groups 8, 9, 15, 26, 35, 45, 78, 86, 101, 115, 117 and 137 (Gay, 1965; Sojka, 1965; Glantz, 1971; Fey, 1972; Morris and Sojka, 1985; Contrepois *et al.*, 1986). The relative importance of individual serogroups varies between countries. Thus O78:K80 has high prevalence in several serological studies in Europe but has low prevalence in North America. Similarly O137:K79 is recorded as an important serogroup in England but has low prevalence in other countries. Within a given geographical area the same serogroups tend to predominate over time although the relative prevalence changes (Fey, 1972; Pohl and Thomas, 1972; Schoenaers and Kaeckenbeeck, 1974; Contrepois *et al.*, 1986). However, OK antigen type is not a definitive method of identification and several different serotypes and characteristics have been identified in *E. coli* O78:K80 isolates from colisepticaemia (Fey, 1972; Dassouli-Mrani-Belkebir *et al.*, 1988).

The association of particular *E. coli* serotypes with calf septicaemia suggests that specific factors linked to these serotypes (or in some cases the specific serotype determinants themselves) are necessary for virulence. Virulence of septicaemic *E. coli* requires that the organism reaches the portal of entry into the body (which may require competition with other bacteria for a mucosal niche), invades the host, survives in the face of specific and non-specific host defences (phagocytosis, the bactericidal effects of serum), and has a mechanism for injuring the host. The results of investigations into virulence factors associated with septicaemic *E. coli* are consistent with a view that septicaemic strains of *E. coli* are diverse and that the capability to cause septicaemia is multifactorial.

Specific traits which have been linked to septicaemic strains of *E. coli* include the aerobactin iron acquisition system (Linggood *et al.*, 1987; Wittig *et al.*, 1988), colicin V production (Waters and Crosa, 1991), increased serum survival (Binns *et al.*, 1979), resistance to phagocytosis (Waters and Crosa, 1991) and intestinal epithelial cell adherence (Morris *et al.*, 1982; Contrepois *et al.*, 1986; Girardeau *et al.*, 1988). The aerobactin-regulated iron uptake system is strongly associated with extraintestinal infections by

E. coli, presumably because it is necessary for the bacterium to obtain iron in the presence of serum transferrin. Experimentally, simultaneous iron injections negated the virulence differences otherwise apparent between aerobactin-containing and -lacking *E. coli* strains (Williams, 1979). In some cases, the lack of aerobactin may be compensated for by iron released from erythrocytes lysed by bacterial haemolysins (Opal *et al.*, 1990), but *E. coli* implicated in septicaemia in calves are typically non-haemolytic.

In addition to low iron concentrations, there are other specific and non-specific mechanisms of host defence which bacteria must overcome to survive in serum, including specific antibodies (Wiemer *et al.*, 1985), lysozyme, complement (Binns *et al.*, 1982; Goldman *et al.*, 1984) and phagocytosis. While the ability to resist these factors is clearly multifactorial and difficult to characterize clearly in many cases, there is a clear association between the ability to survive in serum and the ability of *E. coli* to cause extraintestinal infections.

The ability of septicaemic *E. coli* to compete at the mucosal surface prior to invasion and entry into the blood may also be an important determinant of virulence. This ability may be provided both by adhesins which enable the organism to adhere to the mucosal surface, and by colicins which adversely affect competing microflora. Adherence at the mucosal surface may be mediated by fimbrial adhesins homologous to other known adhesin molecules, or by simpler interactions such as hydrophobicity differences which promote adherence to the epithelium. Specific molecules postulated to effect the adherence of *E. coli* strains to the epithelium include a Vir plasmid product (which may be related to the fimbrial adhesin F17a (Smith, 1974; Oswald *et al.*, 1991)) and the surface antigen CS31a (Contrepois *et al.*, 1986).

Several genera of pathogenic, invasive bacteria share the characteristic that large plasmids present in low copy number are associated with virulence. The best characterized of these plasmids in *E. coli* are Col V plasmids (recently reviewed by Waters and Crosa, 1991). A plasmid encoding the production of colicin V, a molecule which results in the lysis of other *E. coli* strains, was observed to be carried twice as frequently in pathogenic, invasive strains than in non-pathogenic strains. Later investigations demonstrated that the colicin encoding portion of Col V was less essential to virulence in an intraperitoneal challenge model than were other regions of the Col V plasmid (Binns *et al.*, 1979; Quackenbush and Falkow, 1979). A major Col V encoded virulence trait was subsequently identified as the aerobactin iron transport system (Williams and Warner, 1980; Warner *et al.*, 1981), which enables Col V^+ strains to grow in the low iron concentrations found in serum. It is now known that Col V plasmids are heterogeneous, and that in addition to aerobactin and colicin production, other traits potentially related to virulence are encoded by, and coordinately regulated in, Col V plasmids (Waters and Crosa, 1991). Multiple virulence related traits, coordinately regulated in a plasmid which also carries the capability of effecting its own transfer to other *E. coli* strains, may represent a combination closely associated with extraintestinal virulence of *E. coli* in a range of host species.

The Role of Colostrum in Septicaemic Colibacillosis

Calves are born virtually devoid of circulating immunoglobulins and those that subsequently fail to acquire immunoglobulins from colostrum are susceptible to colisepticaemia. Individual cases of colisepticaemia can occur as a result of occasional failures of this transfer process but multiple cases and outbreaks in a herd are due to inadequate management practices. These practices include methods of feeding colostrum that lead to a high prevalence of failure of passive transfer of colostral immunoglobulins and management systems that promote transmission of infection within groups of susceptible neonatal calves. The amount of immunoglobulin required for protection against colisepticaemia is minimal and less than that required for protection against other neonatal infectious diseases. Calves that absorb sufficient immunoglobulin to acquire blood serum concentrations of $5\,mg\,ml^{-1}$ IgG1 and $0.22\,mg\,ml^{-1}$ IgM or greater are resistant (Gay, 1984). Protection appears to be predominantly associated with the IgM fraction and 1.5 g of bovine IgM administered intravenously will protect against the experimental disease (Logan and Penhale, 1971; Penhale *et al.*, 1971).

Experimental studies have shown that small amounts of hyperimmune serotype-specific antibody will protect against infection with the homologous strain (Fey, 1971). However, the nature of natural immunity against this disease is compatible with antibody that is non-serotype specific and universally present in colostral immunoglobulins so that all calves that acquire a minimal concentration of immunoglobulin are protected against the disease (Gay, 1975). Colisepticaemia in calves is therefore an outcome of management systems that result in the failure of the normal passive transfer of colostral immunoglobulins rather than the result of a deficiency in specific antibody in an otherwise normogammaglobulinaemic calf.

Several factors can impact the passive transfer of colostral immunoglobulins (Selman, 1973; Gay, 1984; Besser and Gay, 1985; Boyd, 1987) but the time after birth when colostrum is ingested and the mass of immunoglobulin ingested are the most critical. The time from birth to the intake of colostrum is crucial, as the ability to absorb intact immunoglobulin from colostrum across the intestinal wall to the blood stream decreases rapidly in the period immediately following birth. Any delay beyond the first few hours of life significantly reduces the amount of immunoglobulin absorbed and complete loss of the ability to absorb immunoglobulin (closure) occurs by 24–36 hours after birth (Selman *et al.*, 1971; Penhale *et al.*, 1973; Stott *et al.*, 1979a). In all breeds of cattle, but especially in dairy breeds, there can be considerable variation in the time after birth that individual calves first suckle colostrum from the cow. This may be due to differences in cow behaviour, calf vitality or physical problems with access to the udder. The result is that some calves fail to ingest adequate colostrum volumes before onset of the closure process, and therefore absorb insufficient colostral immunoglobulin (Selman *et al.*, 1970; Stott *et al.*, 1979b; Edwards, 1982; Ventorp and Michanek, 1992). Delayed nursing and decreased immunoglobulin absorption frequently accompany perinatal asphyxia or acidosis due to the greatly decreased vigour of the calf in the first few hours of life (Eigenmann *et al.*, 1983; Besser *et al.*, 1990).

The mass of immunoglobulin ingested by the calf during the period of maximal absorption is the other major determinant of successful passive transfer and is determined by the immunoglobulin concentration in the colostrum and the volume that is ingested. Some breeds of cattle, including American Holsteins, produce colostrum that shows considerable cow to cow variation, and, on average, has relatively low immunoglobulin concentration (Penhale and Christie, 1969; Devery-Pocius and Larson, 1983; Pritchett *et al.*, 1991). A significant proportion of calves that suckle cows of these breeds ingest an inadequate mass of immunoglobulin (Brignole and Stott, 1979; Besser *et al.*, 1991). Immunoglobulin concentration in colostrum is at its highest in first-milking colostrum and is influenced by breed, parity, the volume of the colostrum, pre-milking and leaking of colostrum prior to calving (Devery-Pocius and Larson, 1983; Besser and Gay, 1985; Pritchett *et al.*, 1991).

Treatment and Prevention of Colisepticaemia

Traditional approaches to the treatment of colisepticaemia include antibiotics to combat the infecting *E. coli* (Wilcke, 1991) and fluid and electrolyte therapy to combat endotoxic shock. Currently there is considerable interest in the potential of anti-endotoxic drugs and antisera for therapy in Gram-negative sepsis. The models tested for colisepticaemia in calves have been calves infused with endotoxin. The cyclooxygenase inhibitor flunixin meglumine mitigates early endotoxin-induced alterations in haematological and biochemical variables (Templeton *et al.*, 1988) and when combined with dexamethasone prevents many of the metabolic derangements of endotoxic shock (Margolis *et al.*, 1987). The lazorid drug, tirilazad mesylate, mitigates the clinical signs and many of the pathophysiological responses associated with endotoxaemia and also shows promise for the treatment of endotoxic shock (Rose and Semrad, 1992).

The use of anti-endotoxin antisera is also under investigation as an adjunct for the treatment of septic shock. The J-5 strain of *E. coli* has a mutation in the gene for uridine diphosphate galactose 4-epimerase, resulting in incomplete synthesis of its O antigen side-chains and exposure of lipopolysaccharide core epitopes common to other Gram-negative bacteria. Antiserum to *E. coli* strain J-5 has shown promise in the treatment of endotoxaemia associated with some Gram-negative septic diseases in animals (Tyler *et al.*, 1990). However, administration of antiserum to J-5 has little mitigating effect on the activity of infused endotoxin in neonatal calves (Morris *et al.*, 1986) and, while delaying the onset of bacteraemia and clinical signs, has no effect on the final outcome in experimentally produced colisepticaemia (Wickstrom *et al.*, 1987). There is, as yet, no effective treatment for colisepticaemia and the case fatality still approaches 100%. In large part this may be because there are no early indications of infection, and treatment is initiated following the onset of clinical disease, by which time there is already a significant and irreversible septicaemia and endotoxaemia.

The disease can be totally prevented by ensuring an adequate transfer of colostral immunoglobulins. The mass of ingested immunoglobulin required to achieve protection against colisepticaemia is quite small and even commercially available colostrum substitutes, prepared from cheese whey and containing approximately 25 g of immunoglobulins, confer protection (Hunt and Hunt, 1991). However, although the concentration of circulating immunoglobulins required for protection against colisepticaemia is minimal, higher concentrations of circulating immunoglobulins are associated with decreased susceptibility to other neonatal infectious diseases (Hancock, 1985). Strategies for prevention aim to achieve increased protection against a wide spectrum of infectious neonatal calf diseases by ensuring the early ingestion of an adequate volume of colostrum containing a high concentration of immunoglobulins. The optimal strategy will vary between herds and breeds.

Available evidence suggests that with beef breeds the vigour of the newborn calf, coupled with the clearly superior immunoglobulin concentrations in colostrum, favour the practice of natural suckling as the optimal method of colostrum delivery, unless the dam is observed to refuse nursing or the calf's viability and sucking drive are compromised (Petrie, 1984; Bradley and Niilo, 1985). In these instances artificial feeding of colostrum is indicated. At the other extreme, with the American Holstein and other dairy breeds, the frequent occurrence of delayed suckling coupled with a high prevalence of colostrum with a low immunoglobulin concentration results in very high rates of failure of passive transfer with natural suckling. In these breeds, assisted suckling or artificial feeding is the preferred method of feeding colostrum. Artificial feeding systems should ensure the early feeding of an adequate volume of a colostrum with a high concentration of immunoglobulin so as to ensure adequate passive transfer of immunoglobulins. However, artificial feeding systems will only be superior to natural sucking practices if there is a clear commitment by farmers to optimal calf feeding systems. This will most likely be achieved if the colostrum is a first-milking colostrum of low volume from an older parity cow that has not leaked milk prior to calving and if the colostrum is fed by a nipple bottle or oesophageal probe within the first 2 hours after birth. With dairy breeds that produce colostrum of low immunoglobulin concentration, large volumes of colostrum need to be fed if the calf is to receive the immunoglobulin mass required for increased resistance against the common calfhood infectious diseases. It has been determined for the American Holstein that feeding the traditional volume of 2 quarts or 2 litres at first feeding will fail to provide an adequate mass of immunoglobulin in over 70% of feedings (Besser *et al.*, 1991; Pritchett *et al.*, 1991).

Alternative strategies for prophylaxis have been reported. Hyperimmune serum, raised against the common serotypes of *E. coli* associated with colisepticaemia, has been shown to be protective when administered to calves prior to experimental challenge with those serotypes (Fey, 1971). This could be indicated for prophylaxis in calves known to be at risk for failure of passive transfer in areas where there are dominant serotypes of *E. coli* associated with this disease. Protection engendered by hyperimmune serum appears to require serotype specificity as hyperimmune serum raised to the core lipopolysaccharide of *E. coli* (anti J5 sera) only delays the onset of bacteraemia but does not affect the final outcome of experimental challenge in colostrum-deprived calves (Wickstrom *et al.*, 1987). Field trials of the immunization of late pregnant cows with vaccines incorporating the common serotypes of *E. coli* associated with colisepticaemia have shown a significant reduction in mortality (Fey, 1971). Presumably this reduction is due to an increase in serotype-specific antibodies in the colostrum suckled by calves that obtained otherwise marginal concentrations of circulating immunoglobulins. Non-serotype-specific protection against experimental challenge of colostrum-deprived calves has also been achieved by the *in utero* immunization of prenatal calves but the procedure has a risk of inducing premature birth (Gay, 1975). Whereas strategies of immunoprophylaxis can be effective, it is difficult to justify this approach in view of the universal protection that can be achieved by ensuring an adequate passive transfer of colostral immunoglobulins.

References

Besser, T.E. and Gay, C.C. (1985) Septicemic colibacillosis and failure of passive transfer of colostral immunoglobulin in calves. *Veterinary Clinics of North America, Food Animal Practice* 1, 445–459.

Besser, T.E., Szenci, O. and Gay, C.C. (1990) Decreased colostral immunoglobulin absorption in calves with postnatal acidosis. *Journal of the American Veterinary Medical Association* 196, 1239–1243.

Besser, T.E., Gay, C.C. and Pritchett, L. (1991) Comparison of three methods of feeding colostrum to dairy calves. *Journal of the American Veterinary Medical Association* 198, 419–422.

Binns, M.M., Davies, D.L. and Hardy, K.G. (1979) Cloned fragments of the plasmid ColV,I-K94 specifying virulence and serum resistance. *Nature (London)* 279, 778–781.

Binns, M.M., Mayden, J. and Levine, R.P. (1982) Further characterization of complement resistance conferred by *Escherichia coli* by the plasmid genes *traT* of R100 and *iss* of ColV,I-K94. *Infection and Immunity* 35, 654–659.

Bourne, F.J. (1977) The mammary gland and neonatal immunity. *Veterinary Science Communications* 1, 141–151.

Boyd, J.W. (1987) Computer model of the absorption and distribution of colostral immunoglobulins in the newborn calf. *Research in Veterinary Science* 43, 291–296.

Bradley, J.A. and Niilo, L. (1985) Immunoglobulin transfer and weight gain in suckled beef calves force-fed stored colostrum. *Canadian Veterinary Journal* 26, 118–119.

Brignole, T.J. and Stott, G.H. (1979) Effect of suckling followed by bottle feeding colostrum on immunoglobulin absorption and calf survival. *Journal of Dairy Science* 63, 451–456.

Butler, J. E. (1969) Bovine immunoglobulins. A review. *Journal of Dairy Science* 52, 1895–1909.

Contrepois, M., Dubourguier, H.C., Parodi, A.L., Girardeau, J.P. and Ollier, J.L. (1986) Septicemic *Escherichia coli* and experimental infection of calves. *Veterinary Microbiology* 12, 109–118.

Corley, L.D., Staley, T.E., Bush, L.J. and Jones, E.W. (1977) The influence of colostrum on the transepithelial movement of *Escherichia coli* 055. *Journal of Dairy Science* 60, 1416–1421.

Cullor, J.S. (1992) Shock attributable to bacteremia and endotoxemia in cattle: clinical and experimental findings. *Journal of the American Veterinary Medical Association* 200, 1894–1902.

Dassouli-Mrani-Belkebir, A., Contrepois, M., Girardeau, J.P. and Vartanian, M. (1988) Characters of *Escherichia coli* 078 isolated from septicemic animals. *Veterinary Microbiology* 17, 345–356.

Devery-Pocius, J.E. and Larson, B.L. (1983) Age and previous lactation as factors in the amount of bovine colostral immunoglobulins. *Journal of Dairy Science* 66, 221–228.

Edwards, S.A. (1982) Factors affecting the time to first suckling in dairy calves. *Animal Production* 34, 339–346.

Eigenmann, V.U.J.E., Zaremba, W., Luetgebrune, K. and Grunert, E. (1983) Untersuchungen über die Kolostrumaufnahme und die Immunoglobulinabsorption bei Kälbern mit und ohne geburtsazidose. *Berliner Münchener Tierärztliche Wochenshrift* 96, 109–113.

Fey, H. (1962) Neuere Untersuchungen über die Colisepsis des Kalbes. *Schweizer Archiv für Tierheilkunde* 104, 1–12.

Fey, H. (1971) Immunology of the newborn calf: its relationship to colisepticemia. *Annals of the New York Academy of Sciences* 176, 49–63.

Fey, H. (1972) *Colibacillosis in Calves*. Hans Huber, Bern, Switzerland.

Fey, H. and Margadant, A. (1961a) Hypogammaglobulinämie bei der Colisepsis des Kalbes. *Pathologia et Microbiolgia* 24, 970–976.

Fey, H. and Margadant, A. (1961b) Zur Pathogenese der Kälber-Colisepsis. II. Umgebungsuntersuchungen in Sepsisbestanden. *Zentralblatt für Bakteriologie, Parasitenkunde, Abt. I, Originale* 182, 465–472.

Fey, H. and Margadant, A. (1962) Zur Pathogenese der Kälber-Colisepsis. V.Versuche zur kunstlichen Infection neugeborener Kalber mit dem Colityp 78:80B. *Zentralblatt für Veterinarmedizin* 9, 767–778.

Fey, H., Lanz, E., Margadant, A. and Nicolet, J. (1962) Zur Pathogenese der Kälber-Colisepsis. VI. Experimentelle Infection zum Beweis der parenteralen Genese. *Deutsche Tierärztliche Wochenschrift* 69, 581–586.

Gay, C.C. (1965) *Escherichia coli* and neonatal disease in calves. *Bacteriological Reviews* 29, 75–101.

Gay, C.C. (1975) *In utero* immunization of calves against colisepticemia. *American Journal of Veterinary Research* 36, 625–630.

Gay, C.C. (1984) Failure of passive transfer of colostral immunoglobulin and neonatal disease in calves: a review. In: Acres, S. (ed.) *Proceedings of the Fourth International Symposium on Neonatal Diarrhea*. Veterinary Infectious Diseases Organization, Saskatoon, Saskatchewan, pp. 346–364.

Gay, C.C., McKay, K.A. and Barnum, D.A. (1964) Studies of colibacillosis of calves. III. Experimental reproduction of colibacillosis. *Canadian Veterinary Journal* 5, 314–325.

Gay, C.C., Anderson, N., Fisher, E.W. and McEwan, A.D. (1965) Gammaglobulin levels and neonatal mortality in market calves. *Veterinary Record* 77, 148–149.

Girardeau, J.P., Der-Vartanian, M., Ollier, J.L. and Contrepois, M. (1988) CS31A, a new K88-related fimbrial antigen on bovine enterotoxigenic and septicemic *Escherichia coli* strains. *Infection and Immunity* 56, 2180–2188.

Glantz, P.J. (1971) Neonatal gastrointestinal disease: epidemiological and microbiological aspects: serotypes of *Escherichia coli* isolated with colibacillosis in neonatal animals. *Annals of the New York Academy of Sciences* 176, 67–69.

Goldman, R.C., Joiner, K. and Leive, L. (1984) Serum-resistant mutants of *Escherichia coli* O111 contain increased lipopolysaccharide, lack an O antigen-containing capsule, and cover more of their lipid A core with O antigen. *Journal of Bacteriology* 159, 877–882.

Green, S.L. and Smith, L.L. (1992) Meningitis in neonatal calves: 32 cases (1983–1990). *Journal of the American Veterinary Medical Association* 201, 125–128.

Hancock, D.D. (1985) Assessing efficiency of passive immune transfer in dairy herds. *Journal of Dairy Science* 68, 163–183.

Hunt, E. and Hunt, L.D. (1991) *Escherichia coli* challenge in agammaglobulinemic calves fed colostrum supplements. *Proceedings 9th American College Veterinary Internal Medicine Forum* 543–545.

Linggood, M.A., Roberts, M., Ford, S., Parry, S.H. and Williams, P.H. (1987)

Incidence of the aerobactin iron uptake system among *E. coli* isolates from infection of farm animals. *Journal of General Microbiology* 133, 835–842.

Logan, E.F. and Penhale, W.J. (1971). The prevention of experimental colisepticaemia by the intravenous administration of a bovine serum IgM-rich fraction. *Veterinary Record* 89, 663–667.

Lovell, R. (1955) Intestinal disease of young calves with special reference to infection with *Bacterium coli. Veterinary Reviews and Annotations* 1, 1–31.

Margolis, J.H., Bottoms, G.D. and Fessler, J.F. (1987) The efficacy of dexamethasone and fluxinin meglumine in treating endotoxin-induced changes in calves. *Veterinary Research Communications* 11, 479–491.

McEwan, A.D., Fisher, E.W. and Selman, I.E. (1970) Observations on the immune globulin levels of neonatal calves and their relationship to disease. *Journal of Comparative Pathology* 80, 259–265.

McGuire, T.C. and Adams, D.S. (1982) Failure of colostral immunoglobulin transfer in calves: prevalence and diagnosis. *Compendium of Continuing Education for the Practicing Veterinarian* 4, S35–S39.

McGuire, T.C., Pfeiffer, N.E., Weikel, J.M. and Bartsch, R.C. (1976) Failure of colostral immunoglobulin transfer in calves dying from infectious disease. *Journal of the American Veterinary Medical Association* 169, 713–720.

Morris, D.D., Cullor, J.S., Whitlock, R.H., Wickstrom, M. and Corbeil, L.B. (1986) Endotoxemia in neonatal calves given antiserum to mutant *Escherichia coli* (J-5). *American Journal of Veterinary Research* 47, 2554–2565.

Morris, J.A. and Sojka, W.J. (1985) Escherichia coli as a pathogen in animals. In: Sussman, M. (ed.) *The Virulence of* Escherichia coli. Academic Press, London, pp. 47–77.

Morris, J.A., Thorns, C.J., Scott, A.C. and Sojka, W.J. (1982) Adhesive properties associated with strains of invasive *Escherichia coli. Journal of General Microbiology* 128, 2097–2103.

Opal, S., Cross, A.S., Gemski, P. and Lyhte, L.W. (1990) Aerobactin and alphahemolysin as virulence determinants in *Escherichia coli* isolated from human blood, urine, and stool. *Journal of Infectious Diseases* 161, 794–796.

Ørskov, F. and Ørskov, I. (1984) Serotyping of *Escherichia coli. Methods in Microbiology* 14, 43–112.

Oswald, E., de-Rycke, J., Lintermans, P., van-Muylem, K., Mainil, J., Daube, G. and Pohl, P. (1991) Virulence factors associated with cytotoxic necrotizing factor type two in bovine diarrheic and septicemic strains of *Escherichia coli. Journal of Clinical Microbiology* 29, 2522–2527.

Penhale, W.J. and Christie, G. (1969) Quantitative studies on bovine immunoglobulins. *Research in Veterinary Science* 10, 493–501.

Penhale, W.J., Christie, G., McEwan, A.D., Fisher, E.W. and Selman, I.E. (1970) Quantitative studies on bovine immunoglobulins. II. Plasma immunoglobulin levels in market calves and their relationship to neonatal infection. *British Veterinary Journal* 126, 30–37.

Penhale, W.J., Logan, E.F. and Stenhouse, A. (1971) Studies on the immunity of the calf to colibacillosis. II. Preparation of an IgM-rich fraction from bovine serum and its prophylactic use in experimental colisepticemia. *Veterinary record* 89, 623–628.

Penhale, W.J., Logan, E.F., Selman, I.E., Fisher, E.W. and McEwan, A.D. (1973)

Observations on the absorption of colostral immunoglobulins by the calf and their significance in colibacillosis. *Annales de Recherches Veterinaires* 4, 223–233.

Petrie, L. (1984) Maximising the absorption of colostral immunoglobulins in the newborn dairy calf. *Veterinary Record* 114, 157–163.

Pierce, A.E. (1961) Antigens and antibodies in the newborn. In: Grunsell, C.S. and Wright, A.I. (eds) *Animal Health and Production. Proceedings of the 13th Symposium of the Colston Research Society*. Butterworths, London, pp. 189–206.

Pohl, P. and Thomas, J. (1972) Antigenes somatiques des colibacilles resposables des septiemies du veau en Belgique de 1967 à 1971. *Annales de Medecine Veterinaire* 116, 661–668.

Pritchett, L., Gay, C.C., Besser, T.E. and Hancock, D.D. (1991) Management and production factors influencing immunoglobulin G_1 concentration in colostrum from Holstein cows. *Journal of Dairy Science* 74, 2336–2341.

Quackenbush, R.L. and Falkow, S. (1979) Relationship between colicin V activity and virulence in *Escherichia coli. Infection and Immunity* 24, 562–564.

Rose, M.L. and Semrad, S. D. (1992) Clinical efficacy of tirilazad mesylate for the treatment of endotoxemia in neonatal calves. *American Journal of Veterinary Research* 53, 2305–2310.

Schoenaers, F. and Kaeckenbeeck, A. (1974) Septicemie colibacillaire du veau nouveau-ne. Antigenes somatiques des colibacilles isoles en Belgique de 1960 a 1966. *Annales de Medecine Veterinaire* 118, 1–17.

Selman, I.E. (1973) The absorption of colostral globulins by newborn calves. *Annales de Recherches Veterinaires* 4, 213–221.

Selman, I.E., McEwan, A.D. and Fisher, E.W. (1970) Studies on natural suckling in cattle during the first 8 hours post partum. II. (Calves) behavioral studies. *Animal Behavior* 18, 284–289.

Selman, I.E., McEwan, A.D. and Fisher, E.W. (1971) Studies on dairy calves allowed to suckle their dams at fixed times post-partum. *Research in Veterinary Science* 12, 1–6.

Smith, H.W. (1962) Observations on the aetiology of neonatal diarrhoea (scours) in calves. *Journal of Pathology and Bacteriology* 84, 147–168.

Smith, H.W. (1974) A search for transmissible pathogenic characters in invasive strains of *Escherichia coli*. The discovery of a plasmid-controlled toxin and plasmid-controlled lethal character closely associated, or identical with colicine V. *Journal of General Microbiology* 83, 95–111.

Smith, H.W. and Halls, S. (1968) The experimental infection of calves with bacteraemia-producing strains of *Escherichia coli*: the influence of colostrum. *Journal of Medical Microbiology* 1, 61–78.

Smith, H.W. and Huggins, M.B. (1979) Experimental infection of calves, piglets and lambs with mixtures of invasive and enteropathogenic strains of *Escherichia coli. Journal of Medical Microbiology* 12, 500–510.

Sojka, W.J. (1965) Escherichia coli *in Domestic Animals and Poultry*. Commonwealth Agricultural Bureaux, Farnham Royal, UK.

Stott, G.H., Marx, D.B., Menefee, B.E. and Nightengale, G.T. (1979a) Colostral immunoglobulin transfer in calves: I. Period of absorption. *Journal of Dairy Science* 62, 1632–1638.

Stott, G.H., Marx, D.B., Menefee, B.E. and Nightengale, G.T. (1979b) Colostral immunoglobulin transfer in calves. IV. Effect of suckling. *Journal of Dairy Science* 62, 1908–1913.

Templeton, C.B., Bottoms, G.D. and Feesler, J.F. (1988) Hemodynamics, plasma eicosanoid concentrations, and plasma biochemical changes in calves given multiple injections of *Escherichia coli* endotoxin. *American Journal of Veterinary Research* 49, 90–95.

Tennant, B., Harrold, D. and Reina-Guerra, M. (1975) Hematology of the neonatal calf. II. Response associated with acute enteric infections, gram-negative septicemia, and experimental endotoxemia. *Cornell Veterinarian* 65, 457–475.

Tyler, J.W., Cullor, J.S., Spier, S.J. and Smith, B.P. (1990) Immunity targeting common core antigens of Gram-negative bacteria. *Veterinary Internal Medicine* 4, 17–25.

Ventorp, M. and Michanek, P. (1992) The importance of udder and teat conformation for teat seeking by the newborn calf. *Journal of Dairy Science* 75, 262–268.

Warner, P.J., Williams, P.H., Bindereif, A. and Neilands, J.B. (1981) ColV plasmid-specified aerobactin synthesis by invasive strains of *Escherichia coli. Infection and Immunity* 33, 540–545.

Waters, V.L. and Crosa, J.H. (1991) Colicin V virulence plasmids. *Microbiological Reviews* 55, 437–450.

Wickstrom, M.L., Gay, C.C., Hodgson, J.L., Widders, P.R., Schaeffer, D., Lee, R. and Corbeil, L.B. (1987) Cross-reactive antibody in immunity to colisepticemia in calves. *Veterinary Microbiology* 13, 259–271.

Wiemer, C.W., Kubens, B. and Opferkuch, W. (1985) Influence of imipenem on the serum resistance of Enterobacteriaceae. *Review of Infectious Diseases* 7 (Suppl. 3), S426–S431.

Wilcke, J.R. (1991) Clinical pharmacology of antimicrobial drugs for the treatment of septic neonatal calves. *Veterinary Clinics of North America: Food Animal Practice* 7, 695–711.

Williams, P.H. (1979) Novel iron uptake system specified by ColV plasmids: an important component in the virulence of invasive strains of *Escherichia coli. Infection and Immunity* 26, 925–932.

Williams, P.H. and Warner, P.J. (1980) ColV plasmid-mediated, colicin V-independent iron uptake system of invasive strains of *Escherichia coli. Infection and Immunity* 29, 411–416.

Wittig, W., Prager, R., Tietze, E., Seltmann, G. and Tschape, H. (1988) Aerobactin-positive *Escherichia coli* as causative agents of extra-intestinal infections among animals. *Archiv für Experimentelle Veterinärmedizin* 2 (Suppl.), 221–229.

Wray, C. and Thomlinson, J.R. (1974) Lesions and bacteriologic findings in colibacillosis of calves. *British Veterinary Journal* 130, 189–199.

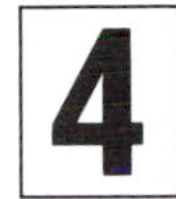

Diarrhoea and Dysentery in Calves

D.G. BUTLER[1] AND R.C. CLARKE[2]

[1]*Department of Clinical Studies, University of Guelph, Guelph, Ontario, Canada NIG 2WI and* [2]*Health of Animals Laboratory, Agriculture and Agri-Food Canada, Guelph, Ontario, Canada N1G 3W4*

Diarrhoea in the neonatal calf (first 4 weeks after birth) is a very common clinical sign of digestive upset. It occurs as a part of symptom complexes now referred to as calf scour complex (Besser and Gay, 1985) or acute or chronic neonatal calf diarrhoea (NCD) (Blood and Radostits, 1989). NCD involves an interaction between one or more pathogenic microorganisms (bacterial, viral or protozoal agents), the immune status of the calf, and one or more environmental factors (Blood and Radostits, 1989). It is estimated that enterotoxigenic *E. coli* (ETEC), rota and corona viruses and *Cryptosporidium* spp. together account for 75–95% of all cases of NCD, worldwide (Acres, 1985; Tzipori, 1985). More recently, verotoxigenic *E. coli* (VTEC) have been implicated in diarrhoea and dysentery in 2- to 8-week-old calves. This review will be restricted to the role of ETEC and VTEC in diarrhoea and dysentery in calves. Diarrhoea is defined as soft to watery faeces containing <10% dry matter and dysentery as the frequent passage of stools containing frank blood and mucus.

Historical Overview

Until the late 1960s, what is now called acute or chronic NCD was without foundation frequently attributed to certain strains of *E. coli*. Affected calves were considered to have one of three clinical syndromes: colisepticaemia, enterotoxaemic colibacillosis or enteric colibacillosis (Gay, 1965).

Septicaemic colibacillosis was documented in the late 1960s as a specific disease entity in calves less than 5 days old suffering from partial to complete failure of transfer of maternal antibody in the colostrum (Fey, 1971). Affected calves sometimes suffered from diarrhoea. This infection was reviewed in the preceding chapter. Nonetheless, it is appropriate here to recognize that documentation of the distinction between septicaemic colibacillosis and enteric colibacillosis enabled veterinary clinicians to refine their diagnostic, therapeutic and prophylactic approaches to acute and chronic enteric colibacillosis.

Enteric colibacillosis, also referred to as white scours or colibacillosis, represented the very common clinical syndrome of acute or chronic NCD as opposed to the very uncommon enterotoxaemic form of colibacillosis characterized by peracute collapse and death. The detection of *E. coli* enterotoxin (Smith and Halls, 1967a) provided the first evidence that enterotoxin-producing *E. coli* (ETEC) had an aetiological role in enteric colibacillosis. In the early 1980s, a new class of *E. coli* causing enteric disease in cattle (VTEC) was identified (Chanter *et al.*, 1984). This evolution in the understanding of the role of *E. coli* in enteric disease of cattle has been paralleled by similar developments in other species including humans. These developments have complicated the terminology associated with *E. coli* diarrhoea in calves, since enteric colibacillosis used to be synonymous with diarrhoea Due to ETEC but must now take account of diarrhoea due to VTEC. In this chapter, the terms ETEC-mediated diarrhoea and VTEC-mediated disease will be used to distinguish diseases associated with these distinctly different types of *E. coli*.

Diarrhoea Due to Enterotoxigenic *E. coli*

Enterotoxigenic E. coli

ETEC associated with enteric disease in calves possess two important virulence attributes: they colonize the intestine and produce enterotoxin. Detailed discussions of pilus (fimbrial) adhesins that permit colonization and of the characteristics of *E. coli* enterotoxins are presented in Chapters 16 and 14, respectively. These aspects of bovine ETEC will therefore be dealt with only briefly in this chapter.

Several studies have investigated colony morphology, biochemical properties, O, K and F antigens, and toxins of bovine ETEC. Characteristically, bovine ETEC produce non-haemolytic, mucoid colonies. Culture of faeces from a calf with ETEC diarrhoea usually shows this type of colony as the dominant or sole colony type. Biochemical characterization has proven incapable of distinguishing bovine ETEC from non-enterotoxigenic *E. coli* (Braaten and Myers, 1977; Isaacson *et al.*, 1978).

Serotyping has shown that these organisms are restricted to a few serotypes. Prior to the discovery of fimbriae and enterotoxin as virulence factors of bovine ETEC (Smith and Halls, 1967a; Smith and Linggood, 1971), there was no method for identification of ETEC. Furthermore, failure to distinguish between septicaemic disease accompanied by diarrhoea and diarrhoeal disease with terminal invasion of organs meant that *E. coli* strains from 'colibacillosis' often included both septicaemic and enterotoxigenic types. Wramby (1948) compared the frequency of various serogroups in association with diseased and normal calves and noted that strains of O groups 8 and 9 occurred more frequently in the intestine compared with the extraintestinal organs of calves that had died of colibacillosis. He was the first to present epidemiological evidence to support a role for these O groups in diarrhoeal disease. Other early reports of *E. coli* implicated in diarrhoeal disease in calves were based largely on simple recovery of the organism from calves with diarrhoea. It is not surprising, therefore, that a retrospective examination shows that the reports included both ETEC and non-ETEC. Strains of O serogroups 8, 9, 20 and 101 (along with O serogroups 1, 2, 4, 7, 15, 17, 20, 26, 38, 78, 88, 115, 117, 136, 119) were among the isolates from diarrhoea typed by a number of researchers (Wramby, 1948; Ulbrich, 1954; Glantz *et al.*, 1959; Gosling *et al.*, 1964). Fey (1972) has an excellent review of the early studies on serological characterization of *E. coli* from calves with diarrhoea.

Experimental oral infection of newborn calves constituted a useful method for determining pathogenicity of isolates. Glantz *et al.* (1959) used an O8:K?:NM isolate from a calf with diarrhoea to reproduce the disease in 17 of 19 colostrum-deprived calves. Later, Smith and Halls (1967b) reproduced a syndrome of severe diarrhoea in colostrum-fed calves less than 20 hours of age that were fed *E. coli* strains of O groups 8, 9 and 101. Interestingly, Moll and Ingalsbe (1955) had failed to induce diarrhoea with strains of O groups 8 and 9 recovered from calves with diarrhoea when they used colostrum-fed calves older than 1 day of age. This is consistent with the observation that as the calf ages its resistance to experimental infection increases dramatically. Several researchers have noted that it was not possible to induce disease in calves older than 1 day of age (Smith and Halls, 1967b; Tzipori *et al.*, 1981). Tzipori *et al.* (1981) fed ETEC to gnotobiotic, colostrum-deprived and sucking calves which ranged in age from a few hours to 26 days and were able to induce diarrhoea only in calves less than 24 hours old. There is considerable evidence to show that ETEC infections in calves older than 3 days are usually associated with a concurrent viral infection (Tzipori *et al.*, 1981; Krogh, 1983). Experimental studies have demonstrated that combinations of ETEC and rotavirus produce more severe illness than does either agent alone and induce disease in 1–2-week-old calves which are resistant to infection with either agent alone (Tzipori *et al.*, 1983). Snodgrass *et al.* (1982) found that previous or simultaneous infection with rotavirus was necessary for colonization of the intestine of 6-day-old calves by ETEC.

It is now well established that the most common O serogroups of bovine ETEC are 8, 9, 20 and 101 (Acres *et al.*, 1977; Braaten and Myers,

1977; Wolk *et al.*, 1992). K antigens 25, 28, 30 and 35 are often found on bovine ETEC. These K antigens are similar to the K antigens of *Klebsiella* and are associated with abundant capsular polysaccharide and a mucoid colony. Hadad and Gyles (1982) found that a spontaneous capsule-minus mutant of a virulent ETEC failed to colonize the intestine of newborn calves and to induce diarrhoea, whereas the capsule-producing parent colonized and induced severe diarrhoea. It is possible that the capsular polysaccharide enhances colonization initiated by the K99 fimbriae.

The most common OK combinations associated with calf diarrhoea are O8:K25, O8:K85, O9:K35, O20:K?, O101:K28 and O101:K30 (Myers and Guinee, 1976; Braaten and Myers, 1977; Chapter 2, Table 2.6). Strains of O26 were associated with calf diarrhoea in early studies (Ulbrich, 1954; Gosling *et al.*, 1964). However, strains of this serogroup have been shown to be non-ETEC, but sometimes verotoxigenic.

K99 (F5) pili mediate adherence of ETEC primarily to the bovine ileum (Isaacson *et al.*, 1978). This fimbrial antigen is almost always present on bovine ETEC. For example, Braaten and Myers (1977) found that 172 of 177 bovine ETEC possessed the K99 antigen. Isaacson *et al.* (1978) found that all 37 clinically significant ETEC that were isolated from calves produced the K99 antigen. Krogh (1983) reported that all 289 ETEC isolates from calves possessed the K99 antigen. Unless special care is taken with respect to the medium on which ETEC are grown, expression of K99 pili may be repressed and isolates may be falsely identified as lacking this antigen. Tests for the genes coding for this antigen have been effective in overcoming this problem. Immunological tests for the K99 antigen are often used to screen for bovine ETEC (Thorns *et al.*, 1992) because there is a high correlation between enterotoxigenicity and possession of the K99 antigen (Shimizu *et al.*, 1987).

K99 mediates attachment of ETEC primarily to the posterior small intestine. Pearson and Logan (1979) experimentally reproduced neonatal diarrhoea in seven calves less than 14 hours old by oral inoculation of an O101:K30:K99 ETEC. By killing the calves at varying times from 6 to 43 hours postinfection they followed the progress of intestinal colonization. They showed that adhesion of the ETEC started in the lower ileum and progressed anteriorly to involve over half the small intestine. Fig. 4.1 illustrates the colonization of villi in the intestine of a calf experimentally infected by a K99-positive bovine ETEC.

Although K99 occupies a dominant position among colonizing pili of bovine ETEC, other pili are also associated with this type of ETEC. F41 fimbriae are often found along with K99 fimbriae on bovine ETEC of O serogroups 9 and 101 (Morris *et al.*, 1980, 1982). Occasionally, strains are found that produce F41 but not K99 and these strains appear to be capable of causing diarrhoeal disease (To, 1984). Some K99-negative ETEC isolated from calves possess the 987P (F6) pili but these isolates fail to proliferate

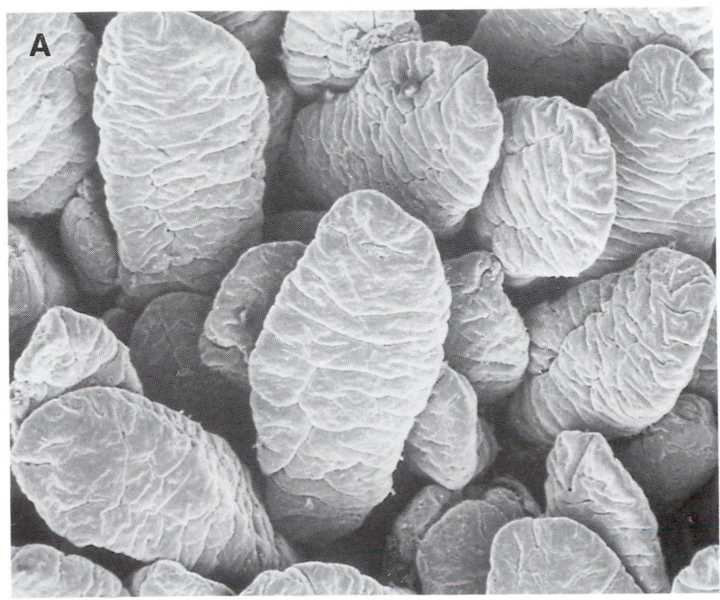

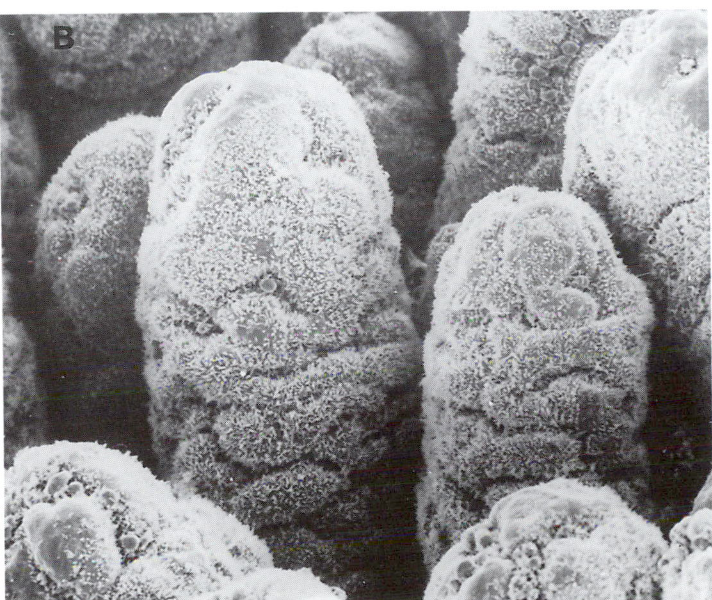

Fig. 4.1. A, Scanning electron micrograph showing the appearance of villi in the jejunum of a normal calf. No bacteria are visible on the surface of the villi. **B**, Scanning electron micrograph of villi in the jejunum of a calf infected with an enterotoxigenic *E. coli*. The surface of the villi is covered with bacteria. (Reprinted with permission from Hadad and Gyles, 1982.)

in the calf intestine and do not induce diarrhoea in calves (Isaacson *et al.*, 1978; Smith and Huggins, 1978). Pilus antigen F17 has been found alone or in association with K99 or F41 on bovine ETEC (Gulati *et al.*, 1992). CS31A is a new pilus antigen which is related to K88 and has been associated with bovine *E. coli* from diarrhoea as well as from septicaemia (Girardeau *et al.*, 1988) but its role in disease is not clear. Shimizu *et al.* (1987) recovered non-enterotoxigenic CS31A-positive *E. coli* strains from diarrhoeic calves and provided experimental evidence to suggest that these strains increase the severity of diarrhoea due to K99-positive ETEC. These workers reported similar findings for the pilus antigen FY (Att 25).

Bovine ETEC typically produce only heat-stable enterotoxin STa (Smith and Gyles, 1970; Sivaswamy and Gyles, 1976; Blanco *et al.*, 1988). This toxin causes fluid distention in ligated calf intestine (Smith and Halls, 1967a) and is also demonstrable by oral inoculation of infant mice (Dean *et al.*, 1972; Gianella, 1976). Strains of bovine ETEC may vary considerably with respect to the amount of STa produced *in vitro* (Saeed *et al.*, 1986) but it is not known whether a similar variation occurs *in vivo*. Of paramount clinical importance is the fact that STa does not damage the intestinal mucosa. Rather, it induces increased intracellular concentrations of cyclic guanosine 3′,5′-monophosphate in gut epithelial cells causing hypersecretion (Field *et al.*, 1978) and concomitant losses of water and electrolyte. This STa-induced dysfunction of the intestinal epithelium of the lower small intestine (distal jejunum/ileum) produces the cardinal clinical abnormalities associated with ETEC-induced enteric colibacillosis, namely diarrhoea, dehydration and acidaemia. Only occasionally have LT-producing *E. coli* been recovered from calves with diarrhoea (Ellis and Kienholz, 1977; Isaacson *et al.*, 1978).

Susceptibility of calves to ETEC is affected by a number of factors. Age is an important one and has been referred to above. It is likely that high gastric pH associated with newborn animals increases susceptibility. It should also be noted that gastric pH increases markedly following feeding with milk replacer. Hadad (1980) determined that whereas the pH values of abomasal contents of 2-day-old calves ranged from 2.1 to 3.0, the values rose to 6.1 to 6.6 within 30 min of feeding milk replacer and did not return to the prefeeding levels until approximately 6 hours. Presence of specific anti-capsular or anti-K99 antibodies in the lumen of the intestines has a major inhibitory effect on colonization of the intestine by ETEC and development of diarrhoea (Acres *et al.*, 1982).

There have only been a limited number of studies on infectious dose, shedding and persistence of ETEC in calves. van Zijderveld *et al.* (1982) infected calves with graded doses of an O9:K35:K99 strain of ETEC and found that severe disease with mortality could be obtained with as few as 7000 organisms. Calves excreted high numbers of the organism in their faeces and shedding persisted for as long as 7 weeks. Prophylactic use of polymyxin in all newborn calves combined with improvements in hygiene and management resulted in disappearance of the ETEC from a herd with a longstanding ETEC diarrhoea problem. Infected calves were considered to be the major source of persistent infections with ETEC in the herd.

In summary, a susceptible calf ingests ETEC from the environment, contaminated feeding utensils or feed, and the organism successfully reaches the small intestine. K99 fimbrial adhesin on the ETEC attaches the bacteria to specific receptors on the villus enterocyte, thereby overcoming the flushing action of peristalsis and facilitating colonization of the small intestine. The organisms proliferate and release STa which induces a profuse watery diarrhoea in the absence of structural damage to the intestinal epithelium. The extreme electrolyte and water losses from the calf rapidly lead to dehydration, metabolic acidosis, collapse and death unless fluid and electrolytes are replaced.

Clinical findings in ETEC-mediated diarrhoea

As indicated earlier, there is strong experimental evidence and field data to show that the peak time of occurrence of uncomplicated ETEC diarrhoea is in the first 3 days of life of the calf. Mixed infections involving ETEC do occur in calves up to 14 days of age and undifferentiated NCD occurs in calves up to 21 days of age (Blood and Radostits, 1989).

Calves with ETEC-induced enteric colibacillosis produce profuse amounts of foul-smelling pasty to watery faeces of variable colour (pale yellow to white) which occasionally contains flecks of blood. The frequent effortless passage of large volumes of faeces leads to extensive soiling of the buttocks and loss of extracellular fluid and electrolyte. This results in progressive dehydration and acidaemia evidenced clinically by a loss of skin elasticity and sinking of the eyes into the head, lassitude, reduced feed intake, and generalized muscle wasting. In acute cases, the rapid and extensive loss of body water accounts for a marked decrease in body weight which can exceed 10% of preinfection body weight within 6–8 hours of the onset of diarrhoea. In more chronic cases of diarrhoea body weight loss can be attributed to a combination of body water loss (dehydration) and generalized muscle wasting, the latter associated with protein catabolism induced by an inadequate caloric intake or maldigestion of the diet. The more rapid the loss of water and salt, the more rapid and life threatening the clinical deterioration. Overwhelming disease may induce a state of collapse characterized by severe weakness, recumbency and hypothermia which unless treated promptly, progresses rapidly to death with or without terminal convulsions. Periodically this progression to death occurs without diarrhoea being apparent. However, the astute clinician will recognize that excess fluid (including body water and electrolytes) is sequestered in the digestive tract causing gross abdominal distension. This observation which can be confirmed by the detection of excess fluid on abdominal succussion provides an explanation for the severely dehydrated and acidotic state of the animal and the apparent absence of diarrhoea.

Untreated calves with mild to moderate disease or calves with severe ETEC-induced diarrhoea but which are supplemented with adequate volumes of an appropriate electrolyte solution may exhibit diarrhoea for several days without evidence of dehydration, weakness or loss of appetite. During an outbreak of ETEC-induced enteric colibacillosis on a farm, 15–30% of affected calves will often gradually deteriorate over a few days and require rehydration therapy. In beef calves, the morbidity rate in unimmunized herds can reach 50% and, in confined dairy calves, 75% (Haggard, 1985). Depending on the virulence of the ETEC strain, extent of exposure and environmental contamination, presence and virulence of other enteropathogens, non-specific and specific immune resistance of the calves and quality of herd management, case fatality rate can vary from 5% to 50% (Blood and Radostits, 1989).

Diagnosis of ETEC-mediated diarrhoea

The age of the calf may indicate the probable involvement of ETEC, since the peak of ETEC-induced diarrhoea is in calves less than 3 days of age, whereas rotavirus and corona virus affect calves 3 days to 2 weeks old, and *Cryptosporidium* causes diarrhoea in calves from 5 days to 6 weeks of age (Tzipori, 1985). However, it is not possible to make a clinical diagnosis of enteric colibacillosis. Rather the diagnosis is undifferentiated NCD until an *E. coli* is isolated from the faeces or intestinal content of an affected calf and classified as a calf enteropathogen. This process is optimized by sacrificing an untreated calf within a few hours of the onset of diarrhoea for pathological and microbiological examination. Although the small and large bowel are distended with fluid and gas in NCD, with ETEC the intestinal mucosa is shiny (intact) to the naked eye and appears normal by light microscopy. This finding, although subtle, can help an experienced pathologist rule out other common causes of NCD such as corona virus, *Salmonella* spp. and coccidia. Ultimately, the diagnosis of ETEC-induced NCD depends on the isolation or identification of a $K99^+$, STa-producing strain of *E. coli* in large numbers from the distal small intestine (Tzipori, 1985). A commercial, enzyme-linked immunosorbent assay is reported to be capable of detecting ETEC in the faeces of calves within an hour (Marshall *et al.*, 1986).

Diarrhoea and Dysentery Due to Verotoxigenic *E. coli*

Verotoxigenic E. coli

The name enterohaemorrhagic *E. coli* (EHEC) has been applied to verotoxigenic *E. coli* (VTEC) implicated in haemorrhagic colitis in humans (Levine, 1987). These organisms belong principally to serotypes O157:H7 and O26:H11 (see Chapters 2, 13 and 20) and are characterized by their ability to produce verotoxins (Chapter 15) and to induce attaching and effacing lesions (Chapter 20). Organisms with these characteristics have been recovered from calves with bloody diarrhoea and will be referred to as bovine EHEC.

VTEC belonging to a wide variety of serogroups have been recovered from the faeces of healthy cattle in countries all over the world (Mohamad *et al.*, 1986; Bulte *et al.*, 1990; Montenegro *et al.*, 1990; Wilson *et al.*, 1992, 1993; Beutin *et al.*, 1993). Table 4.1 lists serotypes of VTEC

Table 4.1. VTEC serotypes isolated from cattle and beef products.[a]

O1:H20	O49:NM	O113:H21	O153:NM
O2:H29	O69:H11	O113:NM	O156:H7
O2:H39	O74:H?	O115:H8	O156:H25
O2:NM	O76:H25	O115:H18	O156:NM
O5:NM	O76:H?	O116:H21	O156:H?
O6:H3	O80:NM	O116:NM	O157:H7
O6:H34	O82:H8	O117:H4	O163:H2
O6:H?	O84:NM	O118:H16	O165:NM
O7:H4	O84:H?	O118:NM	O171:H2
O8:H19	O91:H14	O121:H7	O172:NM
O15:H27	O91:H21	O126:H8	O?:H2
O15:NM	O98:H25	O126:H27	O?:H4
O18:H11	O98:NM	O128:H35	O?:H7
O22:H8	O103:H2	O132:NM	O?:H8
O22:H16	O103:H?	O136:H12	O?:H10
O26:H11	O103:NM	O136:H16	O?:H16
O26:NM	O111:H8	O139:H19	O?:H19
O38:H21	O111:H11	O145:H8	O?:H21
O40:H8	O111:NM	O145:H16	O?:H25
O43:H2	O111:H?	O145:NM	O?:H32
O46:H38	O113:H2	O153:H21	O?:H?
O46:H?	O113:H4	O153:H25	

[a] Isolates from Canadian surveys conducted by Health of Animals Laboratory, Guelph, 1985–93. Serotyping was carried out by the Laboratory Centres for Disease Control, Ottawa.

recovered from cattle in Ontario, Canada. However, as is the case in humans, only a few serotypes have been implicated in haemorrhagic colitis in cattle. The common bovine EHEC serotypes which have been identified to date are O5:NM, O26:H11, O103:H2, O111:NM, O111:H8, O111:H11 and O118:H16 (Chanter *et al.*, 1986; Moxley and Francis, 1986; Schoonderwoerd *et al.*, 1988; Gonzalez and Blanco, 1989; R.C. Clarke, Guelph, Ontario, unpublished). Interestingly, cattle appear to be a reservoir of the human EHEC O157:H7, but this serotype is not known to be associated with disease in cattle.

The first report of EHEC in calves appeared in 1984 (Chanter *et al.*, 1984). The researchers described the experimental reproduction of a dysenteric syndrome in gnotobiotic calves to which an O5:NM isolate had been administered orally. The organism had been recovered from an outbreak of dysentery in 8- to 21-day-old calves in the UK. Subsequently there have been several reports of outbreaks of haemorrhagic colitis in calves from which EHEC were isolated. The O5:NM strains were the first to be associated with dysentery in calves and were found to be urease positive and anaerogenic. Moxley and Francis (1986) in the USA isolated an O5:K4:NM, urease-positive *E. coli* from a 2-day-old calf in a herd with an outbreak of diarrhoea and reproduced bloody diarrhoea in some gnotobiotic calves and non-bloody diarrhoea in others. Schoonderwoerd *et al.* (1988) in Canada investigated an outbreak of dysentery in a group of 20 veal calves in which there was 100% morbidity and 20% mortality. They isolated an O111:NM strain of *E. coli* from affected calves and attempted to reproduce the disease in a colostrum-deprived calf. The calf did not develop diarrhoea or dysentery but attaching-effacing lesions were demonstrated in association with patchy colonization of the colon by the infecting strain. The AE lesions that developed in the colon are illustrated in Fig. 4.2. Wray *et al.* (1989) experimentally infected calves with a VT1-positive O26:H11 and a VT2-positive O8:H9 strain of *E. coli* and reproduced diarrhoea, dysentery and attaching and effacing lesions. Janke *et al.* (1990) recovered EHEC of serotypes O5:NM, O26:NM and O111:NM from 31 calves in a group of 60 calves involved in outbreaks of diarrhoea and dysentery in the USA. The mean age of affected calves was approximately 2 weeks.

Verotoxin (VT) is considered to be a virulence factor for bovine EHEC. The pattern of production of VTs by bovine EHEC is similar to that seen in human strains; isolates may produce VT1, VT2, or both VT1 and VT2 (Dorn *et al.*, 1989; Tokhi *et al.*, 1993). Further discussion of verotoxins may be found in Chapter 15. Serological studies in cattle have shown that a high proportion of adult cattle (78.4%) have neutralizing antibodies to VT1, and a much lower proportion have antibodies to VT2 (5.6%) (Borman-Eby *et al.*, 1993). These findings indicate that cattle mount a good serum antibody response to VT1. The high percentage of animals

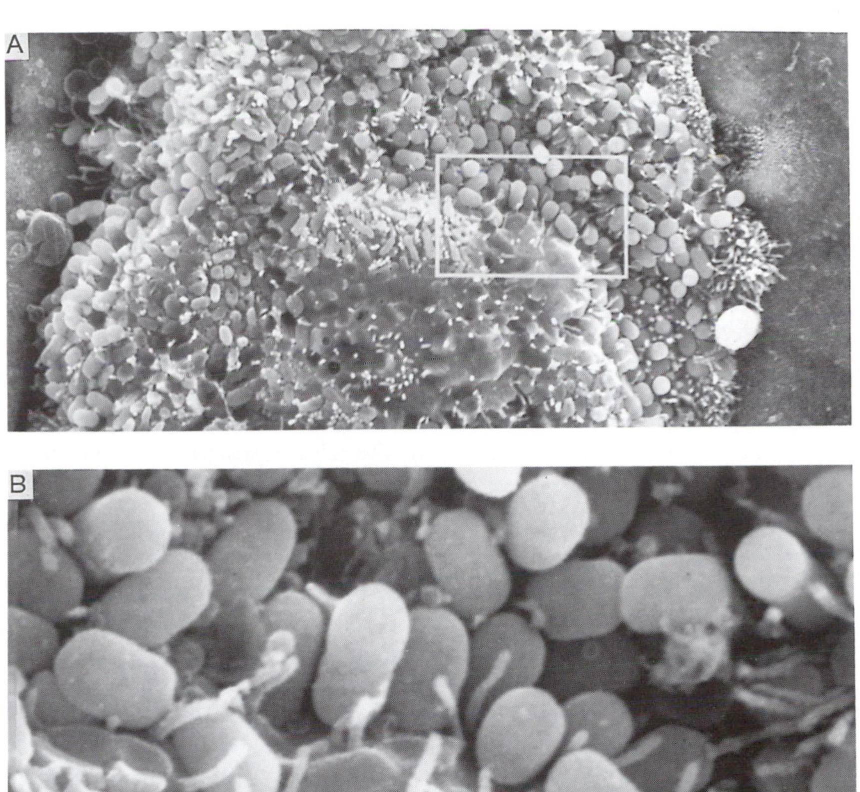

B

Fig. 4.2. Scanning electron micrograph of verotoxigenic *E. coli* in the colon of a calf. **A**, Extensive colonization of the epithelial surface; an extensive area from which bacteria were detached is evident. **B**, Higher magnification showing damaged microvilli and cup-like depressions which accommodate bacteria on the surface. (Schoonderwoerd *et al.*, 1988, reprinted with permission, *Canadian Journal of Veterinary Research*.)

with antibody to VT1 is consistent with the frequent carriage of VTEC by cattle. However, it is not clear why there is a disproportionate response to VT1, since VT1 and VT2 are represented to similar degrees among VTEC isolated from cattle (Tokhi *et al.*, 1993). Tokhi *et al.* (1993) reported that in some calves there was a serological response to VT1, but in no case was there a serological response to VT2. Interestingly, this apparently poor serum antibody response to VT2 following exposure to VT2-producing *E. coli* is also a feature in humans (Ashkenazi *et al.*, 1988) and pigs (Gannon *et al.*, 1988). The common occurrence of neutralizing antibody to VT in cattle may explain the restriction in occurrence of disease to calves 2 weeks and older. Production of anti-VT1 antibodies did not prevent persistence of faecal excretion of VT1-positive VTEC (Tokhi *et al.*, 1993).

Attempts have been made to detect biochemical markers for EHEC (Read *et al.*, 1990). However, except for the urease-positive reaction of O5 strains, there are no distinctive biochemical features of bovine EHEC. Ability to produce enterohaemolysin is one characteristic that has been associated with a high percentage of bovine VTEC. Beutin *et al.* (1989) found that 57.6% of bovine VTEC produced enterohaemolysin and that all O5 : NM VT-positive strains (26) from cattle were enterohaemolysin positive. Wieler *et al.* (1992) reported that 70.8% of VT1-positive *E. coli* from calves produced enterohaemolysin.

Attaching and effacing lesions have already been mentioned as a characteristic associated with bovine EHEC. A detailed discussion of bacterial and host factors involved in development of attaching and effacing lesions is presented in Chapter 20. One contributor to the attaching and effacing (AE) lesion is the product of a chromosomal gene called *eae*. There are conserved regions of the *eae* gene among bovine EHEC, but some regions are variable. Although the precise role of the *eae* gene product in disease is not known, there is an intriguing association between this gene and EHEC. The *eae* A gene is found in approximately 30% of bovine VTEC (K. Sandhu and R.C. Clarke, Guelph, Ontario, 1992, unpublished) but in most bovine EHEC and in 100% of strains of O157 : H7, the most prevalent human EHEC. However, when the *eae* gene is disabled, O157 : H7 organisms retain their pathogenicity for experimental animals, indicating that the *eae* gene is not essential for virulence of O157 : H7 strains (Donnenberg *et al.*, 1993). Furthermore, the fact that O157 : H7 strains possess the *eae* gene, but lack pathogenicity for cattle indicates that the possession of this gene does not make a strain virulent for cattle. Mainil *et al.* (1993) found that of 70 *E. coli* isolates from calves with diarrhoea that were positive with an *eae* probe, 60 produced VT and attaching effacing lesions and 10 did not produce VT but were attaching-effacing *E. coli*. Interestingly, 56 of the 60 *eae*-positive VTEC produced VT1 only.

EHEC appear to be closely related to enteropathogenic *E. coli* (EPEC) in a number of respects. In particular, both EPEC and EHEC induce attaching and effacing lesions. However, the lesions are found in the small intestine in the case of EPEC and predominantly in the large intestine in the case of EHEC. Bundle-forming pili (Girón *et al.*, 1991) have been reported to be responsible for initial attachment of EPEC to intestinal epithelial cells, but no such pili have been detected for EHEC.

Several studies have reported the prevalence of VTEC in cattle faeces. Reports from the UK (Sherwood *et al.*, 1985) and Sri Lanka (Mohammad *et al.*, 1986) were among the first to identify a large number of serogroups of VTEC from calves with diarrhoea. The Sri Lankan study identified 27 O groups of VTEC. Since then many additional serotypes of VTEC have been identified among *E. coli* from cattle (Table 4.1) and new serotypes continue to be discovered. Prevalence rates of VTEC in cattle faeces vary from 10.8% (Montenegro *et al.*, 1990) to 21.1% (Beutin *et al.*, 1993) in Germany, to 9.5% in adult cattle and 24.7% in calves (Wilson *et al.*, 1992) in Canada. A significant percentage of the serotypes of bovine VTEC are serotypes that are also recovered from humans. However, little is known about the pathogenicity of most of these VTEC for either cattle or humans.

Several studies have compared the prevalence of VTEC in the faeces of normal and diarrhoeic calves. In Sri Lanka, Mohammad *et al.* (1985) found that the percentage of faecal samples which yielded VTEC was significantly higher in diarrhoeic compared with normal calves. VTEC were found in 28% of calves with diarrhoea compared with 4% of healthy calves. In the UK, Sherwood *et al.* (1985) found VTEC in nine of 306 diarrhoeic calves, but did not investigate healthy calves. In Germany, Wieler *et al.* (1992) recovered VTEC from 17.8% of calves with diarrhoea compared with 5.0% of healthy calves. They noted that VT1-positive *E. coli* were present in 8.9% of non-diarrhoeic calves but in only 4.1% of diarrhoeic calves. Tokhi *et al.* (1993) conducted a longitudinal study on VTEC in calves in Sri Lanka. They reported that faecal VTEC were significantly associated with diarrhoea in calves less than 10 weeks of age. Not all studies showed such an association. Blanco *et al.* (1993) found no difference in the association of VTEC with diarrhoeic compared with healthy calves in Spain.

VTEC of serotype O157:H7, although not pathogenic for cattle, have assumed enormous significance for regulatory and public health purposes. Serotype O157:H7 is the most common VTEC implicated in outbreaks of disease due to VTEC in humans (Karmali, 1989; Griffin and Tauxe, 1991). There is impressive evidence that cattle and their products are important sources of human infection. This serotype is worldwide in its distribution in both cattle and human populations. Prevalence rates of serotype O157:H7 in cattle have been estimated to be low. Recovery rates from samples of faeces have been reported as 10 of 3750 (0.28%) from dairy cattle and 10 of 1412 from beef cattle (0.14%) in Washington State, USA (Hancock *et al.*, 1994). In Canada, the rates have varied from 0 to 2%

(Wilson *et al.*, 1992; Clarke *et al.*, 1993). Factors such as age of animals, type of farm operation, herd size and season appear to influence the frequency of recovery of this organism from cattle. There appears to be an increase in shedding during the warm months. Because shedding is usually transient, trace back to a source animal is difficult. The organism may be shed for up to 5 weeks by animals challenged with large doses.

There has been a strong association between outbreaks of VTEC disease in humans and consumption of improperly cooked ground beef and other foods (including apple cider and vegetables) contaminated by bovine faecal organisms (Griffin and Tauxe, 1991; Cieslak *et al.*, 1993). During the summer months, increased reports of human disease due to O157:H7 may be due to the higher rates of excretion of the organisms by cattle, and higher rates of multiplication of the organisms in meats and the environment.

Bovine EHEC are distributed in cattle ranging in age from newborn to adult. However, disease occurs naturally in a fairly narrow age range, from 2 to 8 weeks, although experimental disease has been produced in the first week of life following inoculation of 1-day-old colostrum-deprived calves (Wray *et al.*, 1989). These observations suggest that predisposing factors play a significant part in development of disease. Furthermore, the occurrence of severe disease in only a few animals at risk suggests that individual animal factors may be critical.

EHEC isolates from severely ill calves are often multiply resistant to antibiotics (Schonderwoerd *et al.*, 1988; R.C. Clarke, Guelph, Ontario, unpublished). This may be a reflection of a reliance on antimicrobials rather than good management on farms with outbreaks, or it may reflect an advantage of drug-resistant organisms in colonization of the intestine in the face of antibacterial agents.

Clinical findings in VTEC disease

The clinical picture associated with VTEC in calves can be constructed from studies of VTEC isolations from healthy calves (Wilson *et al.*, 1992), and from outbreaks of disease and experimental infections (Chanter *et al.*, 1984, 1986; Hall *et al.*, 1985; Moxley and Francis, 1986; Schoonderwoerd *et al.*, 1988; Pearson *et al.*, 1989; Wray *et al.*, 1989; Janke *et al.*, 1989, 1990). Infection with VTEC may result in a range of clinical appearances from normal, through mild watery diarrhoea, to severe bloody diarrhoea, with deaths occurring in a small percentage of calves.

Most naturally occurring cases of VTEC-induced disease have been reported in calves 2–8 weeks of age. Dysentery, pyrexia, depression and a tendency to chronicity with less marked dehydration in calves in this age range raise the clinician's index of suspicion that VTEC, as opposed to ETEC, are the aetiological cause of the NCD problem. However other common causes of diarrhoea and dysentery in this age range of calf must be excluded including infection with corona and adenovirus, *Salmonella* spp. and coccidia spp. using appropriate diagnostic techniques (Blood and Radostits, 1989).

Diagnosis of VTEC disease

Definitive diagnosis of VTEC-mediated diarrhoea or dysentery depends on isolation of a VTEC from the faeces of a (usually 2 to 8 weeks old) calf with diarrhoea or dysentery. If the isolate belongs to one of the known EHEC serotypes this increases confidence in the significance of the isolate. Assistance from a reference laboratory equipped to detect production of verotoxins or presence of genes coding for VT and to carry out serological typing is needed. In cases of diarrhoea, it may be useful to determine whether ETEC are present. In cases of dysentery, bacteriological culture should be conducted to determine whether *Salmonella* are present in the faecal sample. A good indication of VTEC-mediated disease may be obtained from gross and microscopic examination of the mucosa of the large and distal small intestine. Despite dysentery being a common finding in VTEC-induced disease, grossly visible mucosal lesions in uncomplicated VTEC infection primarily involve hyperaemia of the mucosa of the distal small and large intestine. Histologically, however, focal (distal small intestine) and diffuse (large intestine) colonization of the mucosa with Gram-negative rods associated with attaching and effacing lesions is readily apparent and pathognomonic (Moxley and Francis, 1986; Schoonderwoerd *et al.*, 1988; Wray *et al.*, 1989). The characteristic AE lesions will not be seen if autolysis has begun.

Treatment of Diseases Due to ETEC and VTEC

The main effects of ETEC diarrhoea are dehydration, acidosis, uraemia and hyponatraemia (Groutides and Michell, 1990a). These effects in general and dehydration in particular appear to be much less important in disease associated with VTEC. Regardless of whether ETEC or VTEC is the cause of diarrhoea, correction of body water, electrolyte and acid–base abnormalities with 2 to 5 litres of an oral or intravenous rehydration solution formulated for the treatment of calf diarrhoea constitutes the single most important therapy (Phillips, 1985; Groutides and Michell, 1990a, b; Michell *et al.*, 1992). In the treatment of VTEC-induced diarrhoea, the response to fluid therapy does not appear to be as dramatic or as efficacious as in ETEC-induced diarrhoea. Acute, severely dehydrated cases of ETEC diarrhoea often show remarkable responses within 1–2 hours of initiating such therapy. Calves previously too weak and ill to stand regain their ability to stand, become bright and alert and regain their appetite even though the diarrhoea may continue unabated. Further, as long as the calf continues to be supplemented with such fluids in adequate volume to compensate for the losses occurring in the faeces, the animal will likely remain bright and alert. In contrast, calves with VTEC-induced diarrhoea, when comparably treated, continue to be dull and rather apathetic in terms of interest in their surroundings or food. The role systemic verotoxin may play in clinical disease in VTEC affected calves is unknown but it is tempting to speculate that there is a neurotoxic effect.

Depending on the severity of the diarrhoea and concomitant dehydration and acidaemia and the size of the calf, 2–10 litres of solution may be required per day during convalescence. Provided this solution supplies sufficient bicarbonate to correct the acidaemia and an adequate amount of sodium at an appropriate ratio to glucose to maximize water absorption and improve extracellular fluid volume, fluid and electrolyte replacement and maintenance will be achieved (Michell *et al.*, 1992). Regardless of whether such an oral electrolyte solution is consumed spontaneously or force-fed (Chapman *et al.*, 1986), the calf should maintain reasonably normal hydration and acid–base balance despite severe ongoing diarrhoea. Occasionally administration by the intravenous, subcutaneous or intraperitoneal route of Ringer's lactate or a commercial solution formulated for parenteral administration to diarrhoeic calves is required because the calves are comatose, severely hypoglycaemic and/or hypothermic, and/or fail to respond within 1 to 2 hours of oral rehydration therapy (Phillips, 1985).

The use of oral antibiotics either alone or in combination with electrolyte replacement therapy for both the treatment and prevention of ETEC-induced NCD has been very controversial. It remains to be seen whether or not antibiotics can be justified in the routine treatment of VTEC-induced disease. The development of antibiotic-resistant strains of enteric bacteria (Tzipori, 1985), depletion of the protective intestinal flora (Shull and Frederick, 1978) and induced intestinal malabsorption (Mero *et al.*, 1985) should prompt veterinarians and stockmen to recognize that the use of oral antibiotics for either ETEC- or VTEC-induced NCD is not without risk. Antiparasympathomimetic drugs have been recommended for the treatment of NCD (Bernschneider and Argenzio, 1982) to address both hypermotility and hypersecretion, although the rationale for this has been described as irrelevant and their use contraindicated (Bywater, 1982).

Prevention

The importance of lacteal immunity and more specifically local immunity within the intestinal lumen relative to protection against ETEC-induced NCD has long been recognized (McEwan *et al.*, 1974). Surprisingly, less than 3–4% of unvaccinated cows possess anti-K99 antibodies (Acres,

1985). The vaccination of pregnant cattle 6 weeks and 2 weeks prior to parturition with whole-cell ETEC bacterins or K99 antigen preparations has been very effective in protecting calves against ETEC infections under experimental conditions (Acres *et al.*, 1982; Tzipori, 1985). Vaccination of the cow late in gestation with a K99 antigen vaccine can ensure high concentrations of anti-K99 colostral antibodies which, when consumed by the calf, act within the intestine to coat the binding sites on the bacterial pili, thus preventing their binding to enterocytes. Unable to bind, these bacteria are then flushed out of the intestine by peristalsis.

Results from field trials have often been less convincing than those in controlled laboratory experiments (Snodgrass *et al.*, 1982; Tzipori, 1985). Moon and Bunn (1993) note that definitive data are not available to assess the efficacy of the commercial vaccines that are in use in the field in the USA. They indicated that health professionals considered that the vaccines were effective, with problems occurring primarily among non-vaccinated animals. As in therapeutic trials conducted under field conditions, mixed infections with ETEC and other enteropathogens tend to confound or at least compromise the results. Furthermore, the issue of the timing of the ingestion of the immune colostrum/milk relative to the ingestion of the pathogenic organism, and virulence and dose of the organism are not under the control of the investigator.

Commercial *E. coli* bacterins contain a variety of pilus antigens depending on the manufacturer (Hjerpe, 1990). All appear to be efficacious provided that they share a pilus antigen in common with the pathogen responsible for the calf diarrhoea problem (Acres, 1985). *E. coli* bacterins in an oil-adjuvant must be given to the pregnant cow once intramuscularly 2–6 months before calving and repeated annually (Collins *et al.*, 1988). It is recommended that non-oil-adjuvanted *E. coli* bacterins be injected 6 weeks and again 3 weeks before the expected calving date and once annually thereafter (Acres, 1985). For the anti-pilus antibody to be protective the calf must ingest an adequate quantity of the immune colostrum very soon after birth. The usual recommendation is the ingestion of an amount of colostrum equal to 10% of the calf's birthweight by 2 hours after birth. If this is not possible or has not occurred then the calf should be force fed such a volume of immune colostrum using an oesophageal feeder.

Commercially produced monoclonal antibody against the K99 antigen of *E. coli* has been developed for the prevention of ETEC-induced NCD (Sherman *et al.*, 1983). This antibody should be administered within 12 hours of birth to prevent mucosal attachment and enterotoxin-induced hypersecretion (Tzipori, 1985). Although its use does not change the incidence of diarrhoea in the herd, severity of clinical signs and mortality are significantly reduced. Accordingly, the prophylactic use of K99 monoclonal antibody is viewed as a sound, economic alternative to annual parenteral immunization of all pregnant cows in herds with either a low or sporadic incidence of this problem. Powdered egg yolk from hens immunized with K-99 pili is protective for calves experimentally challenged with a K99-positive bovine ETEC (Ikemori *et al.*, 1992) and may be an economical alternative source of anti-K99 antibodies.

Other approaches to prevention or treatment of calf diarrhoea due to *E. coli* are under investigation. One approach involves antibiotics which reduce the binding of ETEC to the intestinal epithelium, presumably because they impair pilus synthesis. Thus, subinhibitory concentrations of tiamulin have been reported to reduce the hydrophobicity of the bacterial cell surface and to inhibit binding of K99-positive O101:K30 bovine ETEC strains to red blood cells (Larsen, 1989). Mouricout *et al.* (1990) demonstrated that glycoprotein glycans derived from the non-immunoglobulin fraction of bovine plasma inhibited the binding of K99-positive bovine ETEC to erythrocyte glycoconjugates and protected colostrum-deprived calves from a lethal challenge of 10^{10} ETEC.

Certain mucopolysaccharides, non-digestible carbohydrate structures with galactose residues in the end positions on the molecule can form an effective biomatrix to which enteropathogens can bind. Following experimental infection with an O9:H30:K99 ETEC, the calves were treated with this substance together with electrolyte solution containing glucose and glycine or with the electrolyte solution alone (cited by Verschoor and Christensen, 1990). The combination prevented bodyweight loss up to the eighth day of the experiment and reduced the excretion of ETEC.

In spite of the availability of very effective vaccines for the prevention of ETEC-induced enteric colibacillosis, experience with field outbreaks often on the same farm in consecutive years emphasizes the importance of sound management practices relative to calf housing, feeding and hygiene. Unless these factors and environmental contamination with ETEC and VTEC as well as other enteropathogens are controlled, immunity derived from vaccines may be overcome. Although risk factors for shedding of VTEC by cattle have been investigated (Wilson *et al.*, 1993) no specific recommendations are available for preventing diseases due to VTEC in calves.

Concluding Remarks

This chapter has discussed the roles of ETEC and VTEC in enteric disease in calves. These two types of *E. coli* are certainly the ones that have been most extensively investigated. However, there is evidence that other types of *E. coli* may be involved in enteric disease in calves. There are a number of reports of *E. coli* which are similar to enteropathogenic *E. coli*, in that they cause attaching and effacing lesions in the small intestine, do not produce any known diarrhoeagenic toxins, and are associated with diarrhoea. Also, Espinasse *et al.* (1991) in France have reported their observations on a diarrhoeic syndrome associated with ataxia in 1–2-week-old Charolais calves. The diarrhoea was moderate and did not lead to dehydration. Nervous system signs included depression, hypoaesthesia, and ataxia or paresis. Oedema of the eyelid was observed in some calves. Leucocytosis and neutrophilia were the only significant haematological changes. The strains of *E. coli* recovered from the faeces do not produce verotoxins and the most consistent features are production of antigen CS31A and possession of the Col V plasmid. The authors suggested that the strains colonized the intestine extensively and produced a transient bacteraemia and subacute endotoxaemia. Thus, it is likely that in the future other types of *E. coli* will also be recognized for their importance in calf diarrhoea.

References

Acres, S.D. (1985) Enterotoxigenic *E. coli* infections in newborn calves: a review. *Journal of Dairy Science* 68, 229–256.

Acres, S.D., Saunders, J.R. and Radostits, O.M. (1977) Acute undifferentiated neonatal diarrhea of beef calves: the prevalence of enterotoxigenic *E. coli*, reo-like (rota) virus and other enteropathogens in cow-calf herds. *Canadian Veterinary Journal* 18, 113–121.

Acres, S.D., Forman, A.J. and Kapitany, R.A. (1982) Antigen-extinction profile in pregnant cows, using a K99-containing whole-cell bacterin to induce passive protection against enterotoxigenic colibacillosis of calves. *American Journal of Veterinary Research* 43, 569–575.

Ashkenazi, S., Cleary, T.G., Lopez, E. and Pickering, L.K. (1988) Anticytotoxin-neutralizing antibodies in immune globulin preparations: potential use in hemolytic-uremic syndrome. *Journal of Pediatrics* 113, 1008–1014.

Bernschneider, H.M. and Argenzio, R.A. (1982) A pathophysiological approach to the treatment of infectious diarrhea in the neonatal calf and pig. *Iowa State University Veterinarian* 44, 66–76.

Besser, T.E. and Gay, C.C. (1985) Septicemic colibacillosis and failure of passive transfer of colostral immunoglobulin in calves. *Veterinary Clinics of North America, Food Animal Practice* 1, 445–459.

Beutin, L., Montenegro, M.A., Ørskov, I., Ørskov, F., Prada, J., Zimmerman, S. and Stephan, R. (1989) Close association of verotoxin (Shiga-like toxin) production with enterohemolysin production in strains of *Escherichia coli*. *Journal of Clinical Microbiology* 27, 2559–2564.

Beutin, L., Geier, D., Steinruck, H., Zimmermann, S. and Scheutz, F. (1993) Prevalence and some properties of verotoxin (Shiga-like toxin) producing *Escherichia coli* in seven different species of healthy domestic animals. *Journal of Clinical Microbiology* 31, 2483–2488.

Blanco, J., Gonzalez, E.A., Garcia, S., Blanco, M., Regueiro, B. and Bernardez, I. (1988) Production of toxins by *Escherichia coli* strains isolated from calves with diarrhoea in Galicia (North western Spain). *Veterinary Microbiology* 18, 297–311.

Blanco, M., Blanco, J., Blanco, J.E. and Ramos, J. (1993) Enterotoxigenic, verotoxigenic, and necrotoxigenic *Escherichia coli* isolated from cattle in Spain. *American Journal of Veterinary Research* 54, 1446–1451.

Blood, D.C. and Radostits, O.M. (1989) *Veterinary Medicine*, 7th edn. Baillière Tindall, London. p. 619.

Borman-Eby, H.C., McEwen, S.A., Clarke, R.C., McNab, W.B., Rahn, K. and Valdivieso-Garcia, A. (1993) The seroprevalence of verocytotoxin producing *Escherichia coli* in Ontario dairy cows and associations with production and management. *Preventive Veterinary Medicine* 15, 261–274.

Braaten, B.A. and Myers, L.L. (1977) Biochemical characteristics of enterotoxigenic and nonenterotoxigenic *Escherichia coli* isolated from calves with diarrhoea. *American Journal of Veterinary Research* 38, 1989–1991.

Bulte, M., Montenegro, M.A., Helmuth, R., Trumpf, T. and Reuter, G. (1990) Detection of verotoxin producing *E. coli* (VTEC) in healthy cattle and swine with the DNA colony hybridization method. *Berliner und Münchener Tierärztliche Wochenschrift* 103, 380–384.

Bywater, R.J. (1982) Pathophysiology and treatment of calf diarrhea. *Proceedings of the World Congress on Diseases of Cattle*, Vol. 1. The Netherlands, pp. 291–297.

Chanter, A., Morgan, J.H., Bridger, J.C., Hall, G.A. and Reynolds, D.J. (1984) Dysentery in gnotobiotic calves caused by atypical *Escherichia coli. Veterinary Record* 114, 71.

Chanter, N., Hall, G.A., Bland, A.P., Hayle, A.J. and Parsons, D.R. (1986) Dysentery in calves caused by an atypical strain of *Escherichia coli* (S102–9). *Veterinary Microbiology* 12, 241–253.

Chapman, H.W., Butler, D.G. and Newell, M. (1986) The route of liquids administered to calves by esophageal feeder. *Canadian Journal of Veterinary Research* 50, 84–87.

Cieslak, P.R., Barrett, T.J. and Griffin, P.M. (1993) *Escherichia coli* O157:H7 infection from a manured garden. *Lancet* 342, 367.

Clarke, R.C., Read, S.C., McEwen, S.A., Lynch, J., Schoonderwoerd, M., Lior, H. and Gyles, C.L. (1993) Isolation of verocytotoxin-producing *Escherichia coli* from animals and food products. In: Todd, E. and MacKenzie, J. (eds) *Escherichia coli O157:H7 and Other Verotoxigenic E. coli in Foods*. Polyscience Publications, Ottawa, pp. 121–131.

Collins, N.F., Halbur, T. and Schwenk, W.H. (1988) Duration of immunity and efficacy of an oil emulsion *Escherichia coli* in cattle. *American Journal of Veterinary Research* 49, 674–677.

Dean, A.G., Ching, Y.-C., Williams, R.G. and Harden, L.B. (1972) Test for *Escherichia coli* enterotoxin using infant mice. Application in a study of diarrhea in children in Honolulu. *Journal of Infectious Diseases* 125, 407–411.

Donnenberg, M.S., Tzipori, S., McKee, M.L., O'Brien, A.D., Alroy, J. and Kaper, J.B. (1993) The role of the *eae* gene of enterohemorrhagic *Escherichia coli* in intimate attachment *in vitro* and in a porcine model. *Journal of Clinical Investigation* 92, 1418–1424.

Dorn, C.R., Scotland, S.M., Smith, H.R., Willshaw, G.A. and Rowe, B. (1989)

Properties of Vero cytotoxin producing *Escherichia coli* of human and animal origin belonging to serotypes other than O157 : H7. *Epidemiology and Infection* 103, 83–95.

Ellis, R.P. and Kienholz, J.C. (1977) Heat-labile enterotoxin produced by *Escherichia coli* serogroup O149 isolated from diarrheic calves. *Infection and Immunity* 15, 1002–1003.

Espinasse, J., Navetat, H., Contrepois, M., Baroux, D. and Schelcher, F. (1991) A new diarrhoeic syndrome with ataxia in young Charolais calves: clinical and microbiological studies. *Veterinary Record* 128, 422–425.

Fey, H. (1971) Immunology of the newborn calf: its relationship to colisepticemia. *Annals of the New York Academy of Sciences* 176, 49–63.

Fey, Hans (1972) *Colibacillosis in Calves*. Verlag Hans Huber, Bern, pp. 15–22.

Field, M., Graf, L.H. Jr, Laird, W.J. and Smith, P.L. (1978) Heat-stable enterotoxin of *Escherichia coli, in vitro* effects on guanylate cyclase activity, cyclic GMP concentration, and ion transport in small intestine. *Proceedings of the National Academy of Sciences of the United States of America* 75, 2800–2804.

Gannon, V.P.J., Gyles, C.L. and Friendship, R.W. (1988) Characteristics of verotoxigenic *Escherichia coli* from pigs. *Canadian Journal of Veterinary Research* 52, 331–337.

Gay, C.C. (1965) *Escherichia coli* and neonatal disease in calves. *Bacteriological Reviews* 29, 75–101.

Gianella, R.A. (1976) Suckling mouse model for detection of heat stable *E. coli* enterotoxin: characteristics of the model. *Infection and Immunity* 14, 95–99.

Girardeau, J.P., der Vartanian, M., Ollier, J.L. and Contrepois, M. (1988) CS31A, a new K88-related fimbrial antigen on bovine enterotoxigenic and septicemic *Escherichia coli* strains. *Infection and Immunity* 56, 2180–2188.

Girón, J.A., Ho, S.Y. and Schoolnik, G.K. (1991) An inducible bundle-forming pilus of enteropathogenic *Escherichia coli. Science* 254, 710–713.

Glantz, P.J., Dunne, H.W., Heist, C.E. and Hokanson, J.F. (1959) Bacteriological and serological studies of *Escherichia coli* serotypes associated with calf scours. *Pennsylvania State University Agricultural Experimental Station Bulletin* 654, 1–22.

Gonzalez, E.A. and Blanco, J. (1989) Serotypes and antibiotic resistance of verotoxigenic (VTEC) and necrotizing (NTEC) *Escherichia coli* strains isolated from calves with diarrhoea. *Federation of European Microbiological Societies Microbiology Letters* 60, 31–36.

Gosling, J., McKay, K.A. and Barnum, D.A. (1964) Colibacillosis of calves in Ontario. II. The association of certain serotypes of *Escherichia coli* with calf scours. *Canadian Veterinary Journal* 5, 1205–1209.

Griffin, P.M. and Tauxe, R.V. (1991) The epidemiology of infections caused by *Escherichia coli* O157 : H7, other enterohemorrhagic *E. coli*, and the associated hemolytic uremic syndrome. *Epidemiological Reviews* 13, 60–98.

Groutides, C.P. and Michell, A.R. (1990a) Changes in plasma composition in calves surviving or dying from diarrhoea. *British Veterinary Journal* 146, 205–210.

Groutides, C.P. and Michell, A.R. (1990b) Intravenous solutions for fluid therapy in calf diarrhoea. *Research in Veterinary Science* 49, 292–297.

Gulati, B.R., Sharma, V.K. and Taku, A.K. (1992) Occurrence and enterotoxigenicity of F17 fimbriae bearing *Escherichia coli* from calf diarrhoea. *Veterinary Record* 131, 348–349.

Hadad, J.J. (1980) Factors in the establishment of enteropathogenic *Escherichia coli* in the small intestine of calves. Unpublished PhD Thesis, University of Guelph.

Hadad, J.J. and Gyles, C.L. (1982) Scanning and transmission electron microscope study of the small intestine of colostrum-fed calves infected with selected strains of *Escherichia coli. American Journal of Veterinary Research* 43, 41–49.

Haggard, D.L. (1985) Bovine enteric colibacillosis. In: Hunt, E. (ed.) *Veterinary Clinics of North America: Food Animal Practice*. W.B. Saunders, Philadelphia, pp. 495–508.

Hall, G.A., Reynolds, D.J., Chanter, N., Morgan, J.H., Parsons, K.R., Debney, T.G., Bland, A.P. and Bridger, J.C. (1985) Dysentery caused by *Escherichia coli* (SlO2–9) in calves: natural and experimental disease. *Veterinary Pathology* 22, 156–163.

Hancock, D.D., Besser, T.E., Kinsel, M.L., Tarr, P.I., Rice, D.H. and Paros, M.G. (1994) The prevalence of *Escherichia coli* O157:H7 in dairy and beef cattle. *Epidemiology and infection* (in press).

Hjerpe, C.A. (1990) Bovine vaccines and herd vaccination programs: *Escherichia coli* bacterins. In: Hunt, E. (ed.) *Veterinary Clinics of North America: Food Animal Practice*. W.B. Saunders, Philadelphia, pp. 242–245.

Ikemori, Y., Kuroki, M., Peralta, R.C., Yokoyama, H. and Kodama, Y. (1992) Protection of neonatal calves against fatal enteric colibacillosis by administration of egg yolk powder from hens immunized with K99-piliated enterotoxigenic *Escherichia coli. American Journal of Veterinary Research* 53, 2005–2008.

Isaacson, R.E., Moon, H.W. and Schneider, R.A. (1978) Distribution and virulence of *Escherichia coli* in the small intestines of calves with and without diarrhoea. *American Journal of Veterinary Research* 39, 1750–1755.

Janke, B.H., Francis, D.H., Collins, J.E., Libal, M.C., Zeman, D.H. and Johnson, D.D. (1989) Attaching and effacing *Escherichia coli* infections in calves, pigs, lambs, and dogs. *Journal of Veterinary Diagnostic Investigations* 1, 6–11.

Janke, B.H., Francis, D.H., Collins, J.E., Libal, M.C., Zeman, D.H., Johnson, D.D. and Neiger, R.D. (1990) Attaching and effacing *Escherichia coli* infection as a cause of diarrhoea in young calves. *Journal of the American Veterinary Medical Association* 196, 897–901.

Karmali, M.A. (1989) Infection by verocytotoxin-producing *Escherichia coli. Clinical Microbiological Reviews* 2, 15–38.

Krogh, H.V. (1983) Occurrence of enterotoxigenic *Escherichia coli* in calves with acute neonatal diarrhoea. *Nordisk Veterinary Medicine* 35, 346–352.

Larsen, J.L. (1989) Subinhibitory concentrations of tiamulin. Effects on *Escherichia coli* (K88, K99) adhesion. *Dansk Veterinaertidsskrift* 72, 923–926.

Levine, M. M. (1987) *Escherichia coli* that cause diarrhea: enterotoxigenic, enteropathogenic, enteroinvasive, enterohemorrhagic and enteroadherent. *Journal of Infectious Diseases* 155, 377–389.

Mainil, J.G., Jacquemin, E.R., Kaeckenbeeck, A.E. and Pohl, P.H. (1993) Association between the effacing (eae) gene and the Shiga-like toxin-encoding genes in *Escherichia coli* isolates from cattle. *American Journal of Veterinary Research* 54, 1064–1068.

Marshall, R.F., Wolfe, K.H. and Reed, D.E. (1986) A rapid enzyme-linked immunosorbent assay to detect enterotoxigenic *E. coli* in calves. *Modern Veterinary Practice* 67, 542–544.

McEwan, A.D., Fisher, E.W. and Selman, I.E. (1974) Observations on the immune globulin levels of neonatal calves and their relationship to disease. *Journal of Comparative Pathology* 80, 259–265.

Mero, K.N., Rollin, R.E. and Phillips, R.W. (1985) Malabsorption due to selected oral antibiotics. In: Hunt, E. (ed.) *Veterinary Clinics of North America: Food Animal Practice*. W.B. Saunders, Philadelphia, pp. 581–588.

Michell, A.R., Brooks, H.W., White, D.G. and Wagstaff, A.J. (1992) The comparative effectiveness of three commercial oral solutions in correcting fluid, electrolyte and acid–base disturbances caused by calf diarrhoea. *British Veterinary Journal* 148, 507–522.

Mohammad, A., Peiris, J.S.M., Wijewanta, E.A., Mahalingam, S. and Gunasekara, G. (1985) Role of verocytotoxigenic *Escherichia coli* in cattle and buffalo calf diarrhoea. *Federation of European Microbiological Societies Microbiology Letters* 26, 281–283.

Mohammad, A., Peiris, J.S.M. and Wijewanta, E.A. (1986) Serotypes of verocytotoxigenic *Escherichia coli* isolated from cattle and buffalo calf diarrhoea. *Federation of European Microbiological Societies Microbiology Letters* 35, 261–265.

Moll, T. and Ingalsbe, C.K. (1955) The pathogenicity of certain strains of *Escherichia coli* for young mice. *American Journal of Veterinary Research* 16, 337–341.

Montenegro, M.A., Bulte, M., Trumpf, T., Aleksic, S., Reuter, G., Bulling, E. and Helmuth, R. (1990) Detection and characterization of fecal verotoxin producing *Escherichia coli* from healthy cattle. *Journal of Clinical Microbiology* 28, 1417–1421.

Moon, H.W. and Bunn, T.O. (1993) Vaccines for preventing enterotoxigenic *Escherichia coli* infections in farm animals. *Vaccine* 11, 213–220.

Morris, J.A., Thorns, C.J. and Sojka, W.J. (1980) Evidence for two adhesive antigens on the K99 reference strain *Escherichia coli* B41. *Journal of General Microbiology* 118, 107–113.

Morris, J.A., Thorns, C.J., Scott, A.C., Sojka, W.J. and Wells, G.A. (1982) Adhesion *in vitro* and *in vivo* associated with an adhesive antigen (F41) produced by a K99 mutant of the reference strain *Escherichia coli* B41. *Infection and Immunity* 36, 1146–1153.

Mouricout, M., Petit, J.M., Carias, J.R. and Julien, R. (1990) Glycoprotein glycans that inhibit adhesion of *Escherichia coli* mediated by K99 fimbriae: treatment of experimental colibacillosis. *Infection and Immunity* 58, 98–106.

Moxley, R.A. and Francis, D.H. (1986) Natural and experimental infection with an attaching and effacing strain of *Escherichia coli* in calves. *Infection and Immunity* 53, 339–346.

Myers, L.L. and Guinee, P.A.M. (1976) Occurrence and characteristics of enterotoxigenic *Escherichia coli* isolated from calves with diarrhea. *Infection and Immunity* 13, 1117–1119.

Pearson, G.R. and Logan, E.F. (1979) The pathogenesis of enteric colibacillosis in neonatal unsuckled calves. *Veterinary Record* 105, 159–164.

Pearson, G.R., Watson, C.A., Hall, G.A. and Wray, C. (1989) Natural infections with an attaching and effacing *Escherichia coli* in the small and large intestines of a calf with diarrhoea. *Veterinary Record* 124, 297–299.

Phillips, R.W. (1985) Fluid therapy for diarrheic calves: what, how and how much? *Veterinary Clinics of North America* 1, 541–562.

Read, S.C., Clarke, R.C., Martin, A., McFadden, K., Brouwer, A., Charlebois, R. and Lior, H. (1990) Prevalence of verocytotoxigenic *Escherichia coli* in domestic and imported beef. *Epidemiology and Infection* 105, 11–20.

Saeed, A.M.K., Magnuson, N.S., Gay, C.C. and Greenberg, R.N. (1986) Characterization of heat-stable enterotoxin from a hypertoxigenic *Escherichia coli* strain that is pathogenic for cattle. *Infection and Immunity* 53, 445–447.

Schoonderwoerd, M., Clarke, R.C., Van Dreumel, A.A. and Rawluk, S.A. (1988) Colitis in calves: natural and experimental infection with a verotoxin producing strain of *Escherichia coli* O111:NM. *Canadian Journal of Veterinary Research* 52, 484–487.

Sherman, D.M., Acres, S.D., Sadowski, P.L., Springer, J.A., Bray, B., Raybould, T.J.G. and Muscoplat, C.C. (1983) Protection of calves against fatal enteric colibacillosis by orally administering *E. coli* K99-specific monoclonal antibody. *Infection and Immunity* 42, 653–658.

Sherwood, D., Snodgrass, D.R. and O'Brien, A.D. (1985) Shiga-like toxin production from *Escherichia coli* associated with calf diarrhoea. *Veterinary Record* 116, 217–218.

Shimizu, M., Sakano, T., Yamamoto, J. and Kitajima, K. (1987) Incidence and some characteristics of fimbriae FY and 31A of *Escherichia coli* isolates from calves with diarrhea in Japan. *Microbiology and Immunology* 31, 417–426.

Shull, J.J. and Frederick, H.M. (1978) Adverse effect of oral antibacterial prophylaxis and therapy on incidence of neonatal calf diarrhea. *Veterinary Medicine, Small Animal Clinics* 73, 924–930.

Sivaswamy, G. and Gyles, C.L. (1976) The prevalence of enterotoxigenic *Escherichia coli* in the faeces of calves with diarrhea. *Canadian Journal of Comparative Medicine* 40, 241–246.

Smith, H.W. and Gyles, C.L. (1970) The relationship between two apparently different enterotoxins produced by enteropathogenic strains of *Escherichia coli* of porcine origin. *Journal of Medical Microbiology* 3, 387–401.

Smith, H.W. and Halls, S. (1967a) Studies on *Escherichia coli* enterotoxin. *Journal of Pathology and Bacteriology* 93, 531–543.

Smith, H.W. and Halls, S. (1967b) Observations by the ligated intestinal segment and oral inoculation methods on *Escherichia coli* infections in pigs, calves, lambs and rabbits. *Journal of Pathology and Bacteriology* 93, 499–529.

Smith, H.W. and Huggins, M.B. (1978) Experimental infection of calves, piglets and lambs with mixtures of invasive and enteropathogenic strains of *Escherichia coli*. *Journal of Medical Microbiology* 12, 500–510.

Smith, H.W. and Linggood, M.A. (1971) Further observations on *Escherichia coli* enterotoxins with particular regard to those produced by atypical piglet strains and by calf and lamb strains: the transmissible nature of these enterotoxins and of a K antigen possessed by calf and lamb strains. *Journal of Medical Microbiology* 5, 243–249.

Snodgrass, D.R., Smith, M.L. and Krautil, F.L. (1982) Interaction of rotavirus and enterotoxigenic *Escherichia coli* in conventionally-reared dairy calves. *Veterinary Microbiology* 7, 51–60.

Thorns, C.J., Bell, M.M., Chasey, D., Chesham, J. and Roeder, P.L. (1992) Development of monoclonal antibody ELISA for simultaneous detection of bovine coronavirus, rotavirus serogroup A, and *Escherichia coli* K99 antigen in faeces of calves. *American Journal of Veterinary Research* 53, 36–43.

To, S.C.M. (1984) F41 antigen among porcine enterotoxigenc *Escherichia coli* strains lacking K88, K99, and 987P pili. *Infection and Immunity* 43, 549–554.

Tokhi, A.M., Peiris, J.S.M., Scotland, S.M., Willshaw, G.A., Smith, H.R. and Cheasty, T. (1993) A longitudinal study of vero cytotoxin producing *Escherichia coli* in cattle calves in Sri Lanka. *Epidemiology and Infection* 110, 197–208.

Tzipori, S. (1985) The relative importance of enteric pathogens affecting neonates of domestic animals. In: Cornelius, C.E. and Simpson, C.F. (eds) *Advances in Veterinary Science and Comparative Medicine*, Vol. 29. Academic Press, Toronto, pp.103–206.

Tzipori, S.R., Makin, T.J., Smith, M.L. and Krautil, F.L. (1981) Clinical manifestations of diarrhea in calves infected with rotavirus and enterotoxigenic *Escherichia coli*. *Journal of Clinical Microbiology* 13, 1011–1016.

Tzipori, S., Smith, M., Halpin, C., Makin, T. and Krautil, F. (1983) Intestinal changes associated with rotavirus and enterotoxigenic *Escherichia coli* infection in calves. *Veterinary Microbiology* 8, 35–43.

Ulbrich, F. (1954) Serologische Typendifferenzierung und Prüfung toxischer und immunisierender Eigenschaften von *Escherichi* Colistämmen, die von gesunden und von an Coliruhr arkrankten Jungtieren isoliert wurden. Veterinary Thesis, PhD Berlin. (Cited by Fey, 1972.)

van Zijderveld, P.G., Moerman, A., de Leeuw, P.W., Overdijk, E. and Baanvinger, T. (1982) Epidemiological aspects of enterotoxigenic *E. coli* infections in calves. *Proceedings of the XIIth World Congress on Diseases of Cattle, The Netherlands* I, 258–264.

Verschoor, J and Christensen, C.R. (1990) Fluid therapy with specific mucopolysaccharides. A new approach to diarrhea. In: Hunt, E.D. (ed.) *Veterinary Clinics of North America: Food Animal Practice*. W.B. Saunders, Philadelphia, pp. 69–75.

Wieler, L.H., Bauerfeind, R. and Baljer, G. (1992) Characterization of Shiga-like toxin producing *Escherichia coli* (SLTEC) isolated from calves with and without diarrhoea. *Zentralblatt für Bakteriologie* 276, 243–253.

Wilson, J.B., McEwen, S.A., Clarke, R.C., Leslie, K.E., Wilson, R.A., Waltner-Toews D. and Gyles, C.L. (1992) Distribution and characteristics of verocytotoxigenic *Escherichia coli* isolated from Ontario dairy cattle. *Epidemiology and Infection* 108, 423–439.

Wilson, J.B., McEwen, S.A., Clarke, R.C., Leslie, K.E., Waltner-Toews D. and Gyles, C.L. (1993) Risk factors for bovine infection with verocytotoxigenic *Escherichia coli* in Ontario. *Preventive Veterinary Medicine* 16, 159–170.

Wolk, M., Ohad, E., Shpak, B., Adler, H. and Nahari, N.A. (1992) Survey of enterotoxigenic *Escherichia coli* from calves and lambs in the region of the Western Galilee in Israel during winter 1989–90. *Israel Journal of Veterinary Medicine* 47, 7–10.

Wramby, G. (1948) Investigations into the antigenic structure of *Bact. coli* isolated from calves with special reference to coli septicaemia (white scours). *Appelbergs Bokytryckeriaktiebolag, Uppsala*, 112–153.

Wray, C., McLaren, I. and Pearson, G. R. (1989) Occurrence of 'attaching and effacing' lesions in the small intestine of calves experimentally infected with bovine isolates of verocytotoxic *E. coli. Veterinary Record* 125, 365–368.

Escherichia coli Mastitis

5

A.W. Hill
AFRC Institute for Animal Health, Compton, Newbury, Berkshire RG16 0NN, UK

Introduction

Mastitis can be succinctly defined as an inflammation of the mammary gland, however, the complex interaction between host, pathogen and environment which finally culminates in the clinical disease is poorly understood. As early as 1918 the 'colon bacillus' was known to be capable of causing bovine mastitis (Wall, 1918). It was recognized that an inflammatory response could bring about elimination of bacteria between 3 and 21 days after infection, but infections occurring soon after calving could cause a 'high grade, possibly fatal septic intoxication, accompanied by severe symptoms of fever'. There is little doubt that chance infections of the mammary gland with *E. coli* have always occurred where the environment is contaminated with faecal material, but its incidence was overshadowed by the predominance of new infections caused by contagious Gram-positive pathogens. In recent years, changes in management systems and widespread adoption of postmilking teat disinfection and antibiotic therapy at drying off have dramatically reduced mastitis caused by contagious pathogens. The result has been that mastitis caused by *E. coli* has become one of the most common forms of the disease associated with housed cattle in early lactation.

Clinical Aspects

Mastitis caused by *E. coli* can have the widest possible range of clinical severities from fatal through peracute, acute and recurrent clinical to a subclinical infection, which can only be detected on cultural examination of the milk. The form that any particular infection will take is dependent upon the response of the host and not the infecting bacterium. Although the most severe forms of the disease attract the most attention, because of the financial loss to the farmer, they constitute only a small part of *E. coli* mastitis and an even smaller part of new intramammary infections by the organism (Bushnell, 1974). The distinction between the severities is often arbitrary and the symptoms presented may vary throughout the course of a single infection.

Peracute mastitis

This form of the disease is characterized by its very rapid onset soon after parturition. The animal may appear normal at one milking, but at the next displays pronounced clinical signs including shivering, fever, anorexia, rumen stasis and diarrhoea. In the more severe forms the animal may quickly become recumbent, with marked depression, hypotension, dehydration and a rectal temperature which is often below normal. The condition can soon deteriorate, leading to disseminated intravascular coagulation, circulatory failure, generalized organ malfunction and death within hours of onset of the disease. Some affected quarters may be swollen and hard with teat thickening and oedema and the milk rapidly becoming serous and clotted and, in the very severe cases, bloody. In others, inflammatory signs in the udder may be minimal or not detectable and the milk may appear normal. Irrespective of the appearance of the milk and local clinical signs the animal may develop acute endotoxic shock. In the absence of local signs, the disease can appear very similar to parturient hypocalcaemia (Radostits, 1970; Griel *et al.*, 1975), and even the most experienced clinician may consider a diagnosis other than mastitis.

Should the animal survive, a prolonged illness ensues which does not respond to antibiotic therapy; appetite is poor and there is progressive weight loss and general agalactia. It has been estimated that 10% of cows that develop peracute mastitis die, 70% become agalactic, and 20% return to milk (Bushnell, 1974).

Acute mastitis

This is the most common form of *E. coli* mastitis; both the systemic signs and the inflammatory response are less severe and characteristically of short duration. There may be a transient fever, with the infected quarter becoming swollen and hard. The milk will show varying degrees of abnormality, with discoloration and clots; it will invariably have a very high somatic cell count which will persist for several days despite the elimination of the bacteria. Milk taken at the onset of clinical signs may already be free of bacteria and such samples are thought to account for most of the 20–30%

of mastitic milk samples which fail to reveal causative bacteria (Hill *et al.*, 1978). The recovery of animals with acute symptoms is usually attributed to the intramammary antibiotic therapy which they almost invariably receive, although it has been shown experimentally (Hill *et al.*, 1978) that most of these animals would have recovered at the same rate without therapy. Experimental infections of animals during mid and late lactation show that not only do most animals recover without therapy, but the signs can be so mild and transient that many would be missed even by the most diligent milkers (A.W. Hill, IAH, unpublished observations), and the animal soon returns to the preinfection milk yield.

Chronic or recurrent mastitis

This describes an infection which is of long duration with one or more clinical episodes. In its chronic form, the milk produced during the intervals between exacerbations appears normal, but has a high cell count; in the recurrent form of the disease the milk is normal in every respect. The clinical episodes which display the symptoms and signs of acute mastitis are preceded by an elevation of bacterial numbers in the milk. However, by the time clinical signs are apparent the bacteria may have been eliminated. This type of infection usually ends spontaneously after a clinical episode (Murphy and Hanson, 1943) or inexplicably following several courses of antibiotic therapy (Hill and Shears, 1979).

Subclinical mastitis

This describes the condition of latent infection within the udder. Organisms can be isolated from milk over extended periods in the absence of inflammatory signs. This incongruous and relatively rare situation of pathogenic, toxin-producing bacteria apparently surviving and growing in the udder is well documented (Jasper *et al.*, 1975), but difficult to justify, particularly in light of all experimental data. It appears to be limited to isolated herds in which a large proportion of the animals are infected. The mechanism by which this situation is maintained remains unclear, but continual exposure to the same serological type of organism may have induced an immunological response which restricts the growth of the bacteria and may detoxify the endotoxin.

Characteristics of *E. coli* Involved

Work by Carroll and his colleagues (1973) has shown that the ability of coliform organisms to survive or grow in bovine serum was a prerequisite for growth in the udder and the production of mastitis. They found that intramammary inoculation of high numbers of bacteria ($>10^6$) of strains sensitive to serum could produce a transient mastitis, but this was attributed to the preformed lipopolysaccharide (LPS) in the inoculum. It has been assumed that the complement sensitivity of these organisms was the major factor bringing about their killing within the udder. It is worth noting, however, that both serum-sensitive and serum-resistant organisms are capable of growing in milk which has been freshly drawn from the udder and that haemolytic complement assays have failed to show the presence of complement in normal milk (Mueller *et al.*, 1982). Poutrel and Caffin (1983) did show the presence of complement using a much more sensitive technique, but did not conclusively demonstrate the presence of all complement units. It is possible that a mild inflammatory response follows the infection of the udder, allowing the movement of sufficient serum products to inhibit bacterial growth. It is more likely that existing levels of complement together with the physical conditions within the udder produce a bactericidal environment. Compared with serum susceptibility the ability of a strain to grow in milk or milk whey is not a good indicator of virulence within the mammary gland.

Two surveys (Sanchez-Carlo *et al.*, 1984b; Barrow and Hill, 1989) have examined very large numbers of *E. coli* isolated from cases of bovine mastitis for the presence of a wide range of pathogenic mechanisms and virulence factors commonly associated with other diseases caused by the species. Despite a vast amount of work, both groups concluded that the only consisent characteristic of all the strains was serum resistance.

Linton *et al.* (1979) found 67 different *E. coli* O-serotypes in a survey of 279 isolates from individual cows with clinical mastitis. Similarly, of 141 typeable isolates, Sanchez-Carlo *et al.* (1984a) found 57 O-serotypes represented and concluded that the disease was as a result of non-specific infection.

Influence of Host Defence Mechanisms on Incidence and Severity of Disease

Depending upon the lactational stage of the udder, the host's defence mechanisms have varying success at dealing with serum-resistant *E. coli* once they have passed through the streak canal and into the lumen of the gland. The results can vary from preventing the multiplication of the bacteria in the non-lactating gland to peracute disease, sometimes with fatal consequences in the newly calved animal.

Infection during the dry period

The rates of new infections during the dry period may be as much as four times greater than that during lactation (Smith *et al.*, 1985), but the development of clinical mastitis is a rare event. Experimental challenge of the non-lactating udder with *E. coli* rarely establishes an intramammary infection or produces clinical mastitis, whereas lactating cattle challenged with the same strain invariably developed clinical mastitis (Bramley, 1976). Dry cow secretion shows *in vitro* inhibitory properties to many strains of *E. coli* of mammary origin, but those isolated during the early dry period are more resistant to inhibition (Todhunter *et al.*, 1990). Secretion from the dry gland is high in the iron-binding protein lactoferrin, but low in citrate, whereas in lactating cattle the level of lactoferrin in gland secretion is much reduced and the level of citrate much higher. The inhibition of bacterial growth by dry secretion can be reversed by the addition of iron (Reiter and Bramley, 1975) or citrate (Todhunter *et al.*, 1990). Excess iron can saturate the lactoferrin, citrate can acquire iron from lactoferrin and the iron citrate can be utilized by the organisms. Clearly, the availability of iron in dry secretion is limiting. The citrate/lactoferrin molar ratio has been shown to be more important than the actual concentrations of either component alone. Furthermore, Todhunter *et al.* (1990) observed that the presence of antibody specific to the bacterium increased the inhibitory effect of lactoferrin, but this has not been the conclusion of all workers (Rainard, 1986).

Infection during lactation

E. coli multiply very quickly within the lumen of the lactating gland. Whereas the attachment of slower-growing mammary pathogens to epithelia may allow them to overcome removal from the gland during the milking process and be an important parameter in disease development, there is no indication from data collected *in vitro* (Frost, 1975) or *in vivo* (Frost *et al.*, 1980) that *E. coli* attach to epithelia. The speed of bacterial multiplication ensures that numbers sufficient to produce disease are generated in the udder during an intermilking period.

It is assumed that macrophages, which form the major proportion of resident milk leucocytes, are stimulated either by bacteria or their products to release interleukins such as tumour necrosis factor, interleukin 1 or interleukin 6 (Nathan, 1987). The production of such factors has not been demonstrated in the mammary gland, but these inflammatory intermediates are thought to induce the production of leucocyte adhesion molecules on the surface of local endothelium (Lasky, 1992). The overall effect is the rapid margination and diapedesis of polymorphonuclear leucocytes (PMN), and their appearance within the interstitial connective tissue of the udder. Experimental bacterial challenge has revealed that the PMN move from the tissue into the gland cistern through focal lesions in the epithelium resulting in mounds of PMN (Frost *et al.*, 1980) (Fig. 5.1). In some cases this situation can develop into massive accumulations of PMN, and large areas which are denuded of epithelia.

With the exception of rumen stasis, most clinical aspects of mastitis can be reproduced by intramammary infusions of LPS (Verheijden *et al.*, 1983). However, it is unlikely that the total pathogenesis can be attributed to LPS. Electron microscope studies indicate that low doses of LPS do not produce lesions (although freshly prepared culture filtrate does) and PMN move between the epithelial cells resulting in a lawn of PMN rather than mounds (Fig. 5.2). This may explain the observation of Reiter and Sharpe (1968) that small amounts of purified LPS only induce PMN invasion and

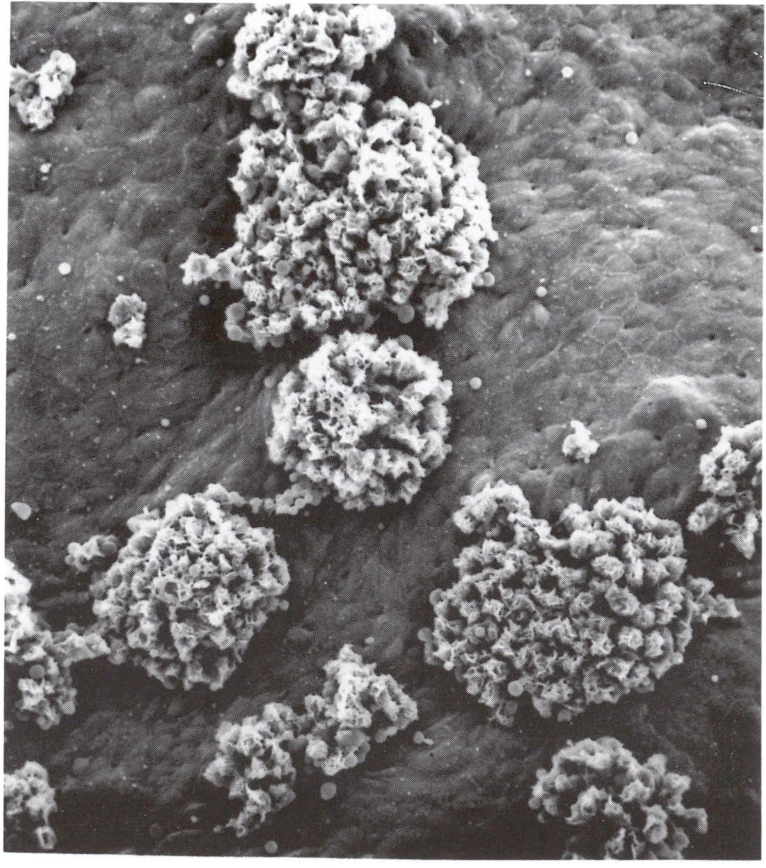

Fig. 5.1. Scanning electron micrograph showing mounds of polymorphonuclear leucocytes on the lactiferous sinus epithelium of the bovine mammary gland during the early pathogenesis of *E. coli* mastitis.

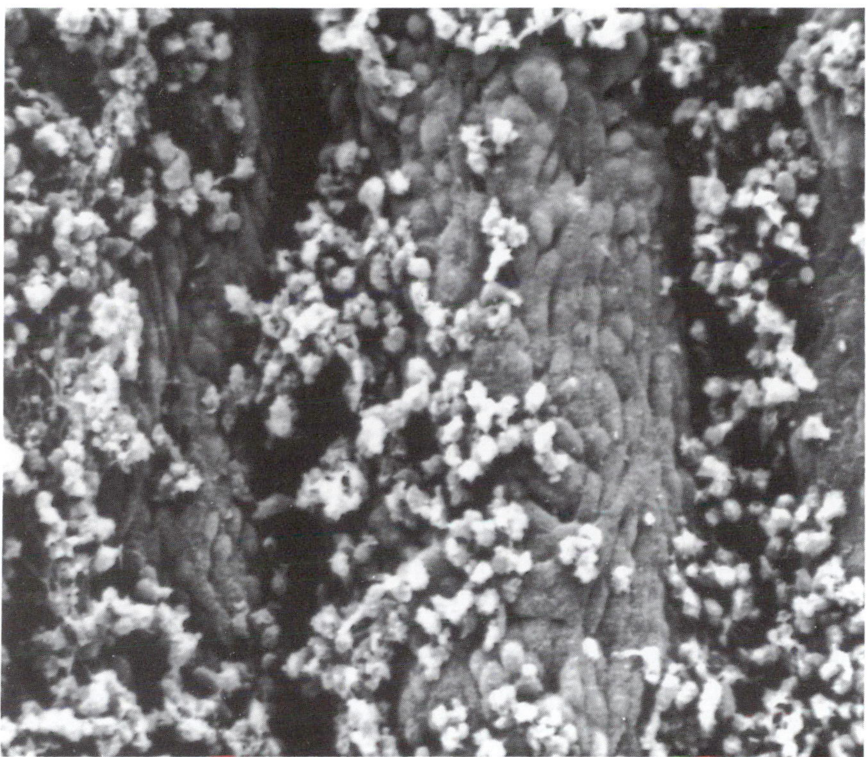

Fig. 5.2. Scanning electron micrograph showing a lawn of polymorphonuclear leucocytes on the teat sinus epithelium of the bovine mammary gland following an infusion of purified endotoxin.

not the leakage of serum proteins. The swift appearance of vast numbers of PMN in the gland sinus, which is sufficient to produce a transient neutropenia in the peripheral circulation, often brings about the elimination of the bacteria from the gland. This elimination can be so rapid and efficient that despite the inflammatory response resulting in the development of clinical mastitis, no bacteria can be cultured from the abnormal milk sample (Hill *et al.*, 1978). In certain laboratories up to 30% of all mastitic milk samples prove to be bacteriologically negative, but the detection of LPS in over 80% of naturally occurring sterile milks (Hill, 1981) proved the involvement of *E. coli* and suggests that the level of new intramammary infection with *E. coli* is much higher than original estimates.

Cells derived from the basal layer of the two-cell-thick epithelium soon form a continuous monolayer covering the exposed basement membrane

(Brooker *et al.*, 1981). This serves to stem the flow of lymph from the lower interstitial tissue, with the result that the milk soon returns to a normal colour and other clinical signs rapidly resolve. PMN numbers in the milk remain high for several days and may not return to normal for up to 2 weeks. The maintenance of this inflammatory response in the absence of bacteria is likely to be due to the activated PMN which have the ability to degranulate, releasing inflammatory lysosomal enzymes (Jain *et al.*, 1972). Although the form of the disease produced by this pathogenesis may at times appear dramatic, the affected animal will not loose body condition and usually returns to preinfection milk yield.

Infection during early lactation

In early lactation the inflammatory response, which results in the PMN infiltration of the gland, can fail or be delayed (Hill *et al.*, 1979) allowing unimpeded bacterial growth. The physiological reasons for this inflammatory deficiency are still to be elucidated. The LPS associated with these high numbers of bacteria cause severe damage to the mammary epithelia and, indirectly, produce the systemic signs of endotoxaemia which together produce the clinical manifestations of peracute and severe acute disease outlined earlier. PMN can subsequently be seen in the mammary secretion, but unlike the prompt PMN infiltration of mid and late lactation, they appear to be unable to sterilize the gland. To establish conditions suitable for eliminating bacteria the ratio of PMN : bacteria must be high; it is possible therefore that the rate of bacterial killing is equal to bacterial multiplication. An alternative theory is that the physical conditions within the udder are not favourable for PMN killing of bacteria, particularly in relationship to oxygen levels. One of the bactericidal systems within the phagolysosomes is oxygen dependent, but the oxygen tension in the gland is much reduced by the preferential aerobic growth of the bacteria (Mayer *et al.*, 1988). Another factor which may influence the elimination of the *E. coli* is that the inflammatory response soon changes into a mononuclear cell infiltration (Hill *et al.*, 1984), which may not have the same ability to kill bacteria. The outcome of some infections during early lactation is that often, despite therapy with an antibiotic of known *in vitro* efficacy, viable bacteria can be isolated from the milk for many days or even weeks. Tissue taken from animals which have been in this condition for a period of time reveals dramatic changes in appearance. The chronic irritation of the bacteria and their toxins induces epithelial hyperplasia in the infected quarter(s) (Fig. 5.3) and involution of the non-infected quarters. It is not known when or if these changes totally resolve.

Histological examination of the mammary gland tissue from animals in the immediate postpartum period which have died as a result of *E. coli* mastitis reveals extensive damage to the ductular and secretory system

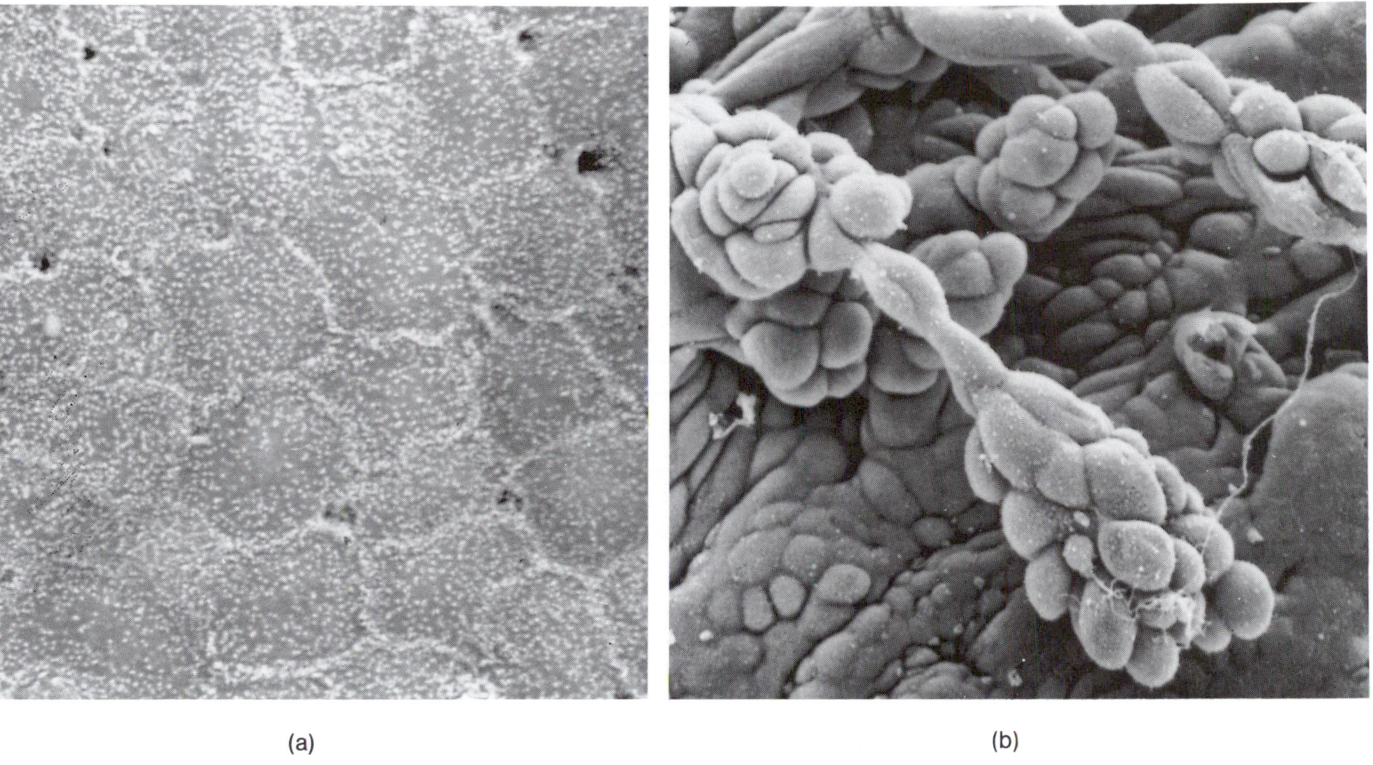

Fig. 5.3. Scanning electron micrographs of epithelia of the bovine lactiferous sinus. (**a**), Normal epithelium showing polygonal cells and microvilli. **(b)** After 14 days of infection with *E. coli*, showing distorted architecture and filiform hyperplastic projections. (From Hill *et al.*, 1984, reproduced by kind permission of *Research in Veterinary Science*.)

involving most areas of the gland (Frost and Brooker, 1986). Epithelia are denuded, particularly in the sinus and ductular regions, and large areas of the interstitial tissue are haemorrhagic. Large numbers of bacteria are seen throughout the gland with evidence of substantial phagocytosis of bacteria by cells of the secretory epithelia, but there is no invasion of the parenchyma. In most cases the udder was totally devoid of PMN. The data suggest that the severe pathogenesis was due to a complete failure of the inflammatory response as predicted from experimental work (Hill *et al.*, 1979). Clearly the speed and magnitude of accumulation of the PMN in the lumen of the infected udder is pivotal for the outcome of an *E. coli* infection. It must be remembered that under most conditions, PMN are only capable of phagocytosing and killing bacteria which are opsonized with antibody. In the non-immune cow IgM appears to be the most important isotype (Williams and Hill, 1982). Opsonic deficiency is not considered to be responsible for the severity of cases of mastitis in early lactation. Early lactation pooled whey (5–10 days postpartum) was found to be opsonic for all strains of *E. coli*, whereas mid-lactation pooled milk whey from cows with no history of mastitis was opsonic only for non-encapsulated strains (Hill *et al.*, 1983a). The milk of mid-lactation animals infected with an encapsulated organism may have insufficient opsonic activity during the early stages of the disease, before inflammation has elevated IgM levels in the milk. Infection of a single mammary quarter with an encapsulated strain stimulates a long-lasting opsonic activity in all quarters not only to the homologous strain but also to others with antigenically similar polysaccharide capsules (Hill *et al.*, 1983b). This induced activity was associated with an increase in the IgM fraction and an appearance of activity in the IgG2 fraction.

Environmental and Management Influences on Disease Incidence

Much of the work which has investigated the influence of the environment on the rate of new intramammary infection refers more generally to coliform organisms, however Bramley (1985) reported that, in a survey of a large UK dairy farm, 77% of this grouping was represented by *E. coli*. The natural flora of the intestine includes a large proportion of *E. coli* and as a result faeces are one of the most important sources of the organism in the environment. There is no indication that herd problems are associated with single strains (Saran-Rosenzuaig and Cohen, 1972). It is assumed, therefore, that *E. coli* is not highly contagious and that new infections are likely to result from environmental contamination. Much of the available data supports this conclusion and indicate that modern intensive farming methods with more confinement and less pasture grazing have tended to exacerbate the situation.

The ability of a particular bedding type to support bacterial numbers has been shown to positively influence the bacterial contamination of teat ends and the ensuing numbers of new cases of mastitis (Bramley, 1985). After pasture, sand was shown to be the most satisfatory, followed by straw, woodshavings, and finally sawdust proving a most unsuitable form of bedding. Although a change to sand bedding can prove an effective method of controlling new infection within a problem herd, its acceptability to the animals and abrasion of hocks can result in welfare problems. If the benefits of availability and cow comfort afforded by sawdust and woodshavings are considered to be important, then daily replacement of the bedding material has been shown to be one of the few effective ways of keeping down bacterial numbers to an acceptable level.

Little information is available on the influence of climate on mastitis incidence, but clearly factors such as humidity, precipitation and ambient temperature (which affect bacterial multiplication in the environment and its ability to adhere to the udder) will have a detrimental effect on disease incidence. As might be predicted, animals grazed in summer and housed in winter show a preponderance of *E. coli* mastitis in the winter months. In contrast, herds which are zero grazed show a higher incidence of disease during the warmer summer months when there is an increased rate of bacterial multiplication in the bedding.

The milking machine has always been implicated as an important factor in udder disease. Three interrelated ways have been identified in which the machine might be involved in increasing the rate of new *E. coli* intramammary infections: induction of teat end erosion and other physical damage allowing the survival of higher populations of organisms; the actual delivery of organisms through the teat canal; and finally their inadequate cleaning allowing the system to serve as a reservoir of organisms. Little information is available on the interaction between the milking machine and *E. coli* mastitis. For the most comprehensive review see the IDF Bulletin No. 215 (1987).

Treatment

At the first signs of clinical mastitis, before an aetiological diagnosis is available, the farmer's initial response is to administer antibiotic therapy. The driving force behind this action is usually a combination of animal welfare and the desire to achieve a rapid clinical cure and a return to the production of milk suitable for sale. At the time when therapy may need to be initiated the milker cannot know if the new infection is due to *E. coli* or whether the defence mechanisms of the animal are being mobilized sufficiently quickly to eliminate the infection. From the discussions of earlier sections of this chapter, it is clear that many cases of mastitis caused by *E. coli* will already be bacteriologically negative when clinical signs appear, and many more will be so within a few hours (Hill *et al.*, 1978). It is under these circumstances that many animals receive unnecessary intramammary antibiotic therapy since evidence suggests that recovery of the udder would have been as quick if therapy had been withheld.

On the other hand, despite early and intensive antibiotic therapy, some intramammary *E. coli* infections will still progress to the acute or peracute forms of the disease, resulting in animals which are fit only for salvage culling once good body condition has been re-established. Many non-antibacterial forms of treatment may offer the same or better prognosis for peracute cases. The old remedy of milking out the affected quarter as often as practical (usually by hand) to continually remove bacteria, toxins and endogenous mediators has many attributes, but is often unrealistic in large modern dairy enterprises with high labour costs. Supportive fluid and corticosteroid therapy often have beneficial results. Large amounts of balanced electrolyte solution will counteract the dehydration caused by diarrhoea and forces diuresis which serves to maintain renal function for the excretion of toxic metabolites. The protective effect of corticosteroids against endotoxic shock has been the basis for their use in the severe form of *E. coli* mastitis. The high doses used would be capable of inducing abortion in late pregnancy, but the severity of mastitis warranting its use are rarely, if ever, seen in later lactation. Similarly, the endotoxaemia associated with severe mastitis can induce abortion. It is worth pointing out that glucocorticoids are pre-eminent anti-inflammatory agents and one of their actions is to modulate PMN margination (Cronstein *et al.*, 1992) and they may therefore enhance microbial infection. It is unlikely however that such observations would negate their use since it is an inflammatory failure which resulted in the condition in the first place.

Hypocalcaemia may also be associated with some cases of peracute and acute mastitis particularly in very early lactation. It has been reported that intravenous calcium can reverse some of the signs induced by intravenous endotoxin (Griel *et al.*, 1975), however this form of treatment should only be used with extreme care since it can cause severe cardiac damage in animals already suffering from toxic shock (Radostits, 1970; Bushnell, 1974).

Prevention

Most available methods for controlling new intramammary infections by *E. coli* have already been alluded to earlier in this chapter. Postmilking teat disinfection with a long-acting germicide effectively reduces new intramammary infections caused by the contagious Gram-positive bacteria such as *Staphylococcus aureus* and *Streptococcus agalactiae* but is totally ineffective against *E. coli*. This failure may be related to the fact that, in contrast to the contagious organisms, *E. coli* often contaminates but does not colonize the teat end prior to penetration of the teat canal and entry into the sinus (Eberhart, 1977).

The most effective preventive measure is to ensure that the udders and particularly the teat ends of the animals are free of faecal and environmental contamination just prior to the attachment of a clean and correctly functioning milking machine. This is best achieved by allowing cattle to spend the intermilking period on pasture. Clearly, in many parts of the world, housing is essential during the winter months and in some cases is preferred as a management system throughout the year. Under these conditions, the washing and drying of teats, the choice of bedding material, the frequency of its replacement (Bramley, 1985) and the space alloted per cow will directly influence the level of *E. coli* contamination of the udder and subsequent rates of new intramammary infections.

In an attempt to improve the control of environmental mammary pathogens, two groups have extended the principle of teat cleansing to include a disinfection step after washing and drying. One group has shown a reduction in *E. coli* infections (Pankey *et al.*, 1987), whereas the other reported limited success, showing a benefit only on individual farms (Shearn *et al.*, 1992). This added step in teat preparation does not appear to guarantee a benefit, furthermore it has been shown that the realistic contact time of the disinfectant in a modern milking parlour is too short to kill the bacteria. The greater attention to udder preparation required by the experimental 'pre-dip' routine may account for any apparent benefits.

There is increasing evidence from field trials that parenteral vaccination of cattle during the dry period with a rough (Rc) mutant of *E. coli* (O111:B4) J5 reduces the rate of clinical coliform mastitis (Gonzalez *et al.*, 1989; Hogan *et al.*, 1992a). However, the same regimen either had no effect (Hill, 1991) or slightly mitigated the clinical signs (Hogan *et al.*, 1992b) following experimental intramammary challenge. The rationale for use of the vaccine is that it induces cross-reacting, neutralizing antibody against the LPS thus reducing the severe systemic and local effects of the toxin. Clearly the benefit of the vaccine seen in the field trials cannot be due to a reduction in the rates of new intramammary infection, and the only explanation which can be offered at present is that it does reduce the severity of a mild infection to a point where it is missed by milking staff. Although this approach does not prevent *E. coli* mastitis or alleviate the severe effects of endotoxin, it may prove not only to be a valuable adjunct to good management but also a harbinger of later generations of vaccines which will be capable of eliminating all the local and systemic effects of the toxin. High titres of cross-reacting antibody together with a pharmacologically manipulated, prompt inflammatory response would minimize the significance of a new intramammary infection.

Conclusions

Mastitis caused by *E. coli* remains one of the most intractable forms of the disease in housed cattle. Its containment requires diligent attention to housing, milking machine maintenance and cleaning and to premilking udder preparation. There is little evidence that antibiotics play any major part in ameliorating the prognosis of an infected animal and a better understanding of the pathogenesis of the disease in the cow has served to emphasize that the outcome is determined by the inflammatory response of the host rather than the virulence of the invading organism.

Rigid compliance with existing 'on farm' guidelines for disease control will continue to be essential. However, pharmacological or immunological intervention may in the future augment the host's own defence mechanisms by ensuring a prompt inflammatory response, particularly in early lactation, and limit toxic shock by the induction of cross-reacting antibodies to lipopolysaccharide, or may even regulate bacterial multiplication within the udder.

References

Barrow, P.A. and Hill, A.W. (1989) The virulence characteristics of strains of *Escherichia coli* isolated from cases of bovine mastitis in England and Wales. *Veterinary Microbiology* 20, 35–48.

Bramley, A.J. (1976) Variation in the susceptibility of lactating and non-lactating bovine udders to infection when infused with *Escherichia coli. Journal of Dairy Research* 43, 205–211.

Bramley, A.J. (1985) The control of coliform mastitis. In: *Proceedings of the 24th Annual Meeting of the National Mastitis Council, Las Vegas*. NMC, Arlington, Virginia, pp. 4–17.

Brooker, B.E., Hill, A.W. and Frost, A.J. (1981) Epithelial regeneration in the bovine mammary gland: the closure of lesions produced by *Escherichia coli. Proceedings of the Royal Society London B* 213, 81–91.

Bushnell, R.B. (1974) Where are we on coliform mastitis? In: *Proceedings of the 13th Annual Meeting of the National Mastitis Council*. NMC, Arlington, Virginia, p. 62.

Carroll, E.J., Jain, N.C., Schalm, O.W. and Lasmanis, J. (1973) Experimentally induced coliform mastitis: inoculation of udders with serum-sensitive and serum-resistant organisms. *American Journal of Veterinary Research* 34, 1143–1146.

Cronstein, B.N., Kimmel, S.C., Levin, R.I., Martiniuk, F. and Weissmann, G. (1992) A mechanism for the antiinflammatory effects of corticosteroids.

Proceedings of the National Academy of Sciences of the United States of America 89, 9991–9995.

Eberhart, R.J. (1977) Coliform mastitis. *Journal of the American Veterinary Medical Association* 170, 1160–1163.

Frost, A.J. (1975) Selective adhesion of microorganisms to the ductular epithelium of the bovine mammary gland. *Infection and Immunity* 12, 1154–1156.

Frost, A.J. and Brooker, B.E. (1986) Hyperacute *Escherichia coli* mastitis of cattle in the immediate post-partum period. *Australian Veterinary Journal* 63, 327–331.

Frost, A.J., Hill, A.W. and Brooker, B.E. (1980) The early pathogenesis of bovine mastitis due to *Escherichia coli. Proceedings of the Royal Society of London B* 209, 431–439.

Gonzalez, R.N., Cullor, J.S., Jasper, D.E., Farver, T.B., Bushnell, R.B. and Oliver, M.N. (1989) Prevention of clinical coliform mastitis in dairy cows by a mutant *Escherichia coli* vaccine. *Canadian Journal of Veterinary Research* 53, 301–305.

Griel, L.C., Zarkower, A. and Eberhart, R.J. (1975) Clinical and clinopathological effects of *Escherichia coli* endotoxin in mature cattle. *Canadian Journal of Comparative Medicine* 39, 1–6.

Hill, A.W. (1981) Factors influencing the outcome of *Escherichia coli* mastitis in the dairy cow. *Research in Veterinary Science* 31, 107–112.

Hill, A.W. (1991) Vaccination of cows with rough *Escherichia coli* mutants fails to protect against experimental intramammary bacterial challenge. *Veterinary Research Communications* 15, 7–16.

Hill, A.W. and Shears, A.L. (1979) Recurrent coliform mastitis in the dairy cow. *Veterinary Record* 105, 229–230.

Hill, A.W., Shears, A.L. and Hibbitt, K.G. (1978) The elimination of serum-resistant *Escherichia coli* from experimentally infected single mammary glands of healthy cattle. *Research in Veterinary Science* 25, 89–93.

Hill, A.W., Shears, A.L. and Hibbitt, K.G. (1979) The pathogenesis of experimental *Escherichia coli* mastitis in newly calved dairy cows. *Research in Dairy Science* 26, 97–101.

Hill, A.W., Heneghan, D.J.S. and Williams, M.R. (1983a) The opsonic activity of bovine milk whey for the phagocytosis and killing by neutrophils of encapsulated and non-encapsulated *Escherichia coli. Veterinary Microbiology* 8, 293–300.

Hill, A.W., Heneghan, D.J.S., Field, T.R. and William, M.R. (1983b) Increase in specific opsonic activity in bovine milk following experimental *Escherichia coli* mastitis. *Research in Veterinary Science* 35, 222–226.

Hill, A.W., Frost, A.J. and Brooker, B.E. (1984) Progressive pathology of severe *Escherichia coli* mastitis in dairy cows. *Research in Veterinary Science* 37, 179–187.

Hogan, J.S., Smith, K.L., Todhunter, D.A. and Schoenberger, P.S. (1992a) Field trial to determine efficacy of an *Escherichia coli* J5 mastitis vaccine. *Journal of Dairy Science* 75, 78–84.

Hogan, J.S., Weiss, W.P., Todhunter, D.A., Smith, K.L. and Schoenberger, P.S. (1992b) Efficacy of an *Escherichia coli* J5 mastitis vaccine in an experimental challenge trial. *Journal of Dairy Science* 75, 415–422.

IDF Bulletin No. 215 (1987) *Machine Milking and Mastitis*. International Dairy Federation, Brussels.

Jain, N.C., Schalm, O.W., Carroll, E.J. and Lasmanis, J. (1972) Leucocyte and tissue factors in the pathogenesis of bovine mastitis. *American Journal of Veterinary Research* 33, 1137–1145.

Jasper, D.E., Dellinger, J.D. and Bushnell, R.B. (1975) Herd studies on coliform mastitis. *Journal of the American Veterinary Medical Association* 166, 778–780.

Lasky, L.A. (1992) Selectins: interpreters of cell-specific carbohydrate information during inflammation. *Science* 258, 964–969.

Linton, A.H., Howe, K., Sojka, W.J. and Wray, C. (1979) A note on the range of *Escherichia coli* O-serotypes causing clinical bovine mastitis and their antibiotic resistance spectra. *Journal of Applied Bacteriology* 46, 585–590.

Mayer, S.J., Waterman, A.E., Keen, P.M., Craven, N. and Bourne, F.J. (1988) Oxygen concentration in milk of healthy and mastitic cows and implications of low oxygen tension for the killing of *Staphylococcus aureus* by bovine neutrophils. *Journal of Dairy Research* 55, 513–519.

Mueller, R., Carroll, E.J. and Panico, L. (1982) Complement C3 levels and haemolytic activity in normal and mastitic whey. *Zentralblatt für Veterinarmedizin B* 29, 99–106.

Murphy, J.M. and Hanson, J.J. (1943) Infection of the bovine udder with coliform bacteria. *Cornell Veterinarian* 33, 61–77.

Nathan, C.F. (1987) Secretory products of macrophages. *Journal of Clinical Investigation* 79, 319–326.

Pankey, J.W., Wildman, E.E., Drechsler, P.A. and Hogan, J.S. (1987) Field trial evaluation of premilking teat disinfection. *Journal of Dairy Science* 70, 867–872.

Poutrel, B. and Caffin, J.P. (1983) A sensitive microassay for the determination of haemolytic complement activity in bovine milk. *Veterinary Immunology and Immunopathology* 5, 177–184.

Radostits, O.M. (1970) The clinical aspects of coliform mastitis in cattle. In: *Proceedings of the IV International Conference on Cattle Diseases*. American Association of Bovine Practitioners, Philadelphia, p. 67.

Rainard, P. (1986) Bacteriostasis of *Escherichia coli* by bovine lactoferrin, transferrin, and immunoglobulins (IgG1, IgG2, IgM) acting alone or in combination. *Veterinary Microbiology* 11, 103–115.

Reiter, B. and Bramley, A.J. (1975) Defence mechanisms of the udder and their relevance to mastitis control. In: Dodd, F.H., Griffen, K. and Kingwill, R.G. (eds) *Proceedings of Seminar on Mastitis Control*. IDF, Brussels, pp. 210–215.

Reiter, B. and Sharpe, M.E. (1968) Inducement of leucocytosis by endotoxin in the bovine udder. In: *Biennial Review of National Institute for Research in Dairying, UK*. University of Reading, UK, p. 61.

Sanchez-Carlo, V., Wilson, R.A., McDonald, J.S. and Packer, R.A. (1984a) Biochemical and serologic properties of *Escherichia coli* isolated from cows with acute mastitis. *American Journal of Veterinary Research* 45, 1771–1774.

Sanchez-Carlo, V., McDonald, J.S. and Packer, R.A. (1984b) Virulence factors of *Escherichia coli* isolated from cows with acute mastitis. *American Journal of Veterinary Research* 45, 1775–1777.

Saran-Rosenzuaig, A. and Cohen, R. (1972) *Escherichia coli* serotypes isolated from cases of acute bovine mastitis in two Israeli dairy herds. *Refuah Veterinarith* 29, 117.

Shearn, M.F.H., Langridge, S., Teverson, R.M., Booth, J.M. and Hillerton, J.E. (1992) Effect of pre-milking teat dipping on clinical mastitis. *Veterinary Record* 131, 488–489.

Smith, K.L., Todhunter, D.A. and Schoenberger, P.S. (1985) Environmental mastitis: cause, prevalence and prevention. *Journal of Dairy Science* 68, 1531–1553.

Todhunter, D., Smith, K.L. and Hogan, J.S. (1990) Growth of Gram-negative bacteria in dry cow secretions. *Journal of Dairy Science* 73, 363–372.

Verheijden, J.H.M., Schotman, A.J.H., Van Miert, A.S.J.P.A.M. and Van Duin, C.T.M. (1983) Pathophysiological aspects of *Escherichia coli* mastitis in ruminants. *Veterinary Research Communications* 7, 229–236.

Wall, S. (1918) Udder-colibacillosis. In: *Mastitis in the Cow* (translated by W.J. Crocker). Lippincott, The Washington Square Press, Philadelphia, pp. 62–70.

Williams, M.R. and Hill, A.W. (1982) A role for IgM in the *in vitro* opsonisation of *Staphylococcus aureus* and *Escherichia coli* by bovine polymorphonuclear leucocytes. *Research in Veterinary Science* 33, 47–53.

6

Diseases Due to *Escherichia coli* in Sheep

J.C. HODGSON
Moredun Research Institute, 408 Gilmerton Road, Edinburgh EH17 7JH, UK

Modern intensive methods of rearing domestic animals create a contaminated environment with a high risk of bacterial infection from ubiquitous *E. coli*. Early information on *E. coli* disease in sheep (Sojka, 1965) emphasized the particular vulnerability of the neonatal lamb (within 2 days of birth) to *E. coli* infection and suggested that predisposing factors were present at birth. Work reviewed here implicates the immature immune status and digestive physiology of the neonatal lamb as two important contributory factors to its disease susceptibility. One of two disease syndromes may develop, depending on the characteristics of the *E. coli* involved (Morris and Sojka, 1985):

1. Enteric colibacillosis, characterized by diarrhoea, with badly affected animals dying within 6–10 days of birth.
2. Systemic colibacillosis, characterized by septicaemia and rapid death, occurring usually within 2–3 days of birth.

The relative prevalence of enteric to systemic colibacillosis in cases investigated by Veterinary Investigation Centres is approximately 2:1 (VIDA (Veterinary Investigation Diagnosis Analysis) data from 1975 to 1993; MAFF, Central Veterinary Laboratory, Addlestone, Surrey, UK). In both syndromes the *E. coli* operate as opportunistic pathogens but the pathogenesis of disease and characteristics of the *E. coli* involved differ markedly (Acres, 1985).

Enteric Disease

History

Uncertainty regarding the role of the common gut commensal *E. coli* in diseases of lambs and other domestic animals prevailed during the first half of this century. The review by Sojka (1965) established the importance of *E. coli* infections in sheep and subsequent work identified fimbrial adhesins (Smith and Linggood, 1972; Ørskov *et al.*, 1975; Smith and Huggins, 1978; Morris *et al.*, 1980a, 1982, 1983) and the ability to produce enterotoxin (Smith and Halls, 1967a, b; Smith and Linggood, 1972) as critical virulence determinants for *E. coli* involved in enteric disease. Strains of *E. coli* which produced colonizing fimbriae and enterotoxin were termed enterotoxigenic *E. coli* (ETEC). Early work, summarized by Sellwood and Lees (1981), indicated that different fimbriae were associated with ETEC from different animal species. The fimbriae detected on ETEC isolated from diarrhoeic lambs and calves were initially called 'common' K antigen (Kco) (Smith and Linggood, 1972) but later designated K99 (Ørskov *et al.*, 1975). This fimbrial antigen is also called F5. The virulence attributes and pathogenic mechanisms of various types of *E. coli* have been the subject of several reviews (Sojka, 1971; Acres, 1985; Wray and Morris, 1985). This section of the present review collates the limited information relating to ETEC scour in lambs, drawing on relevant comparative data from other species as necessary.

Clinical aspects

Neonatal animals are most at risk of developing a profuse diarrhoea resembling cholera in humans (Morris and Sojka, 1985). Lambs are susceptible to *E. coli* scour from birth to about 2 days of age (Smith and Halls, 1967a; Smith and Linggood, 1972; Tzipori *et al.*, 1981; King and Angus, 1991). Scour results from ETEC adhering to intestinal epithelial cells (Gross and Rowe, 1985; Newsome *et al.*, 1987; Mohamed ou Said *et al.*, 1988) and inducing hypersecretion via the release of enterotoxins (Acres, 1985). Animals become dull and weak, reluctant to stand or suck and dehydrate rapidly. The causative *E. coli* are confined to the lumen of the small intestine. Enteritis or bacteraemia are not features of the disease but autolytic changes in the intestinal epithelium and extraintestinal invasion in the terminal stages confounded the interpretation of events before critical aspects of pathogenesis were understood (Smith, 1962). Colibacillary diarrhoea comprised 17% of all diagnoses made in lambs between 1975 and 1980 in England and Wales (Morris and Sojka, 1985). The apparent cause of death is dehydration, acidosis and shock due to fluid and electrolyte loss (Whipp, 1978).

There are no specific postmortem lesions. There are signs of dehydration, the stomach is distended with clotted milk and the intestine with fluid, mucus, gas and particles of digesta. Some parts appear congested, while others are pale, although in most animals examined immediately at death there is no congestion or other sign of inflammation (Smith, 1962).

A constant bacteriological finding is the intense proliferation of certain serotypes of *E. coli* in the small intestine while the numbers of other bacteria in the gut (*Lactobacillus*, *Streptococcus*, *Clostridium*) remain normal (Morris and Sojka, 1985). Numbers of ETEC in the small and large intestine are abnormally high ($>10^8\ g^{-1}$ ileal mucosal scrapings). Bacteria are found postmortem adhering to the brush border of villous enterocytes throughout the lower jejunum and ileum, associated with hyperaemia of mucosal vessels, distension of lacteals and neutrophil infiltration (Tzipori *et al.*, 1981).

Characteristics of ovine ETEC

Strains of ETEC which cause acute infectious scour in lambs belong to O serogroups 8, 9, 20 or 101 (Wray, 1984; Morris and Sojka, 1985) and produce plasmid-encoded virulence determinants – fimbrial adhesion proteins and enterotoxin (Ørskov *et al.*, 1975; Smith and Huggins, 1978; Acres, 1985). Most strains produce the fimbrial adhesin K99 (Acres, 1985), but some produce also, either alone or in combination with K99, another attachment fimbria, F41 (Morris *et al.*, 1982, 1983; Isaacson and Richter, 1984). Both heat labile (LT) and heat stable (STa and STb) forms of enterotoxin have been reported but, in calves and lambs, the enterotoxin produced is of the STa type (Smith and Linggood, 1972; Acres, 1985; Gyles, 1992). Both adhesion and enterotoxic factors must be present for disease to occur (Wray and Morris, 1985).

The same serological OK groups of ETEC are involved in diarrhoea in lambs and calves; the strains are therefore often referred to as calf-lamb strains (Morris and Sojka, 1985; Chapter 4). The polysaccharide of the O and K antigens may enhance colonization (Smith and Huggins, 1978) but detailed information on the role of these antigens is lacking. Similarly, flagellar (H) antigens are uncommon on calf ETEC and their contribution to virulence is undefined. Acquisition of iron may be facilitated by the production of the iron-chelator enterobactin but its role in the virulence of *E. coli* which cause intestinal infections has not been studied (Griffiths, 1991).

Pathogenesis

Pathogenesis of ETEC diarrhoea in lambs is the same as has been described for ETEC in calves (Chapter 4). Adherence to the intestinal epithelium via

K99 or F41 adhesins allows the ETEC to overcome the effects of peristalsis and to colonize the gut (Acres, 1985; Smyth and Smith, 1992). Infecting lambs with an ETEC strain from which the K99 antigen had been eliminated failed to produce disease and inclusion of K88 plasmid from a typical porcine ETEC strain did not restore virulence in the lamb model. Scour was induced only in lambs given $K99^+$ strains (Smith and Linggood, 1972). The K99 antigen was concluded to have a similar function in lambs and calves as K88 in piglets, as an adhesin that allows colonization and growth (Smith and Linggood, 1972). The natural immunity to *E. coli* which develops at about 2 days of age may be linked to maturation of epithelial cells and the loss of adhesin receptors, as gut closure occurs (Acres, 1985; Staley and Bush, 1985).

Early work studied the effects of ETEC enterotoxins on gut epithelium using ligated pig and calf gut segments and measuring the degree of fluid accumulation after exposure to toxin (Smith and Halls, 1967a, b; Smith and Linggood, 1972). Dilatation occurred with typical lamb, calf and piglet enterotoxigenic strains. Enterotoxin production by lamb ETEC strains is transmissible and coded for on Ent plasmids (Smith and Huggins, 1978).

Differential diagnosis

There is no single pathognomonic sign which differentiates enteric colibacillosis from other forms of scour. Diagnosis is based on a combination of clinical and laboratory evidence and elimination of other possible causes, such as lamb dysentery (Sojka, 1971; King and Angus, 1991). The age of the lamb is important. The development of fatal diarrhoea within the first 2 days of life helps differentiate the disease from diarrhoea associated with other common pathogens such as rotavirus and *Cryptosporidium*, which exert their effects later (King and Angus, 1991). Bacterial counts exceeding 10^8 per g of intestinal contents, determined in freshly killed lambs to avoid postmortem proliferation, contribute to a positive diagnosis (Sojka, 1971). The presence of K99 or F41 adhesins may be confirmed by a variety of techniques, including gel diffusion, immunoelectrophoresis, immunofluorescence, and haemagglutination assays. The culture conditions are important, and strains have to be cultured at 37°C to express the fimbriae (Sellwood and Lees, 1981; Tzipori *et al.*, 1981; Morris *et al.*, 1982; King and Angus, 1991).

Production of heat stable enterotoxin STa may be assessed in bioassays (suckling mouse test; ligated gut test) or in immunoassays. Recent trends are towards DNA-based techniques involving hybridization or polymerase chain reaction amplification to detect genes for virulence factors (Cook, 1993; Chapter 21).

Treatment

Lambs showing profuse scour will soon die unless treated quickly with appropriate fluids. Oral rehydration therapy for lambs should include bicarbonate precursors such as citrate to help correct metabolic acidosis and be supplemented with glucose to help prevent hypoglycaemia (Michell, 1989). Antibiotic therapy may assist in elimination of the ETEC in the intestine and should be started during the early stages of disease to be effective.

Prevention

Because of the short interval during which lambs are susceptible to scour due to ETEC, vaccination of the lamb is not feasible. Boosting the maternal antibody levels in colostrum by vaccinating the ewe with a K99 antigen preparation is of benefit only to those lambs which obtain an early and sufficient supply of colostrum. Experimentally, scour was reproduced in lambs by oral infection, within 5–12 hours of birth, with ETEC of serogroups O8, O9, O101, despite high serum antibody levels (Smith and Halls, 1967a). However, colostrum from K99-vaccinated ewes protected lambs against experimental challenge with K99-positive strains of *E. coli* (Sojka *et al.*, 1978; Morris *et al.*, 1980b).

Poor management and inadequate hygiene predispose to disease (Mitchell and Linklater, 1983). Sick lambs should be isolated in clean, disinfected pens with fresh bedding (King and Angus, 1991).

Septicaemic Disease

History

The main consequence of extraintestinal infections due to *E. coli* in young livestock is systemic disease, involving bacteraemia, septicaemia and shock (Morris and Sojka, 1985). In newborn lambs this manifests as watery mouth disease (Hodgson, 1993). Early work on this disease showed that a coli septicaemia was present postmortem (Haig, 1981), but it was considered not to be a causative factor (Gilmour *et al.*, 1985). The role of *E. coli* in the disease remained an enigma until detailed work using gnotobiotic animals monocontaminated with *E. coli* showed watery mouth disease to be a form of endotoxic shock (Hodgson *et al.*, 1989a, b). Infection by *E. coli* may also contribute to mastitis (Jones, 1991) and endometritis in ewes (Sokkar *et al.*, 1980). It is now accepted widely that a major predisposing factor to neonatal disease is colostrum deprivation (Gay, 1984; Contrepois *et al.*, 1986; Hodgson, 1993). This review will expand on these observations and focus on the contribution that the peculiar digestive physiology of the neonate makes to the lamb's vulnerability to disease.

Clinical aspects

Systemic colibacillosis in lambs affects primarily the immunocompromised neonate, commonly 12–48 hours old, reared indoors under intensive conditions (Jensen, 1974; King and Hodgson, 1991). The majority of these lambs become bacteraemic within 12 hours of birth (Hodgson *et al.*, 1992), leading to acute or chronic disease. In the acute form, lambs become ill with little advance warning. High-grade bacteraemia with $>10^5$ colony forming units (c.f.u.) ml^{-1} of blood is present (Hodgson *et al.*, 1989b) and the progress of disease is rapid. Without intensive care death usually occurs within 6–12 hours from onset as a result of endotoxic shock. This is recognized clinically as watery mouth disease and is common in the UK, accounting for about 25% of all neonatal lamb deaths. It is recognized also in Spain and a similar syndrome in goat kids has been reported in France and Canada (Hodgson, 1993). In chronic cases, lambs appear to tolerate low-grade bacteraemia ($<10^4$ c.f.u. ml^{-1} blood) with no clinical signs of disease, but problems such as joint ill or hypopyon develop within 2–3 days after infection as bacteria accumulate at particular anatomical sites.

Signs of disease include excess salivation, lacrimation, dullness, anorexia, abdominal distension, gut stasis and laboured breathing, but scour is not a consistent finding (King and Hodgson, 1991). Body temperature of acutely ill lambs usually falls, consistent with results obtained during experimental endotoxaemia in newborn lambs (Pittman *et al.*, 1973). Detailed clinical biochemistry and physiological monitoring from cases of natural systemic colibacillosis in lambs are not available but experimental reproduction of disease in lambs has shown changes in some key parameters used to define human septicaemia (van Deventer *et al.*, 1988), including lactacidaemia (Hodgson *et al.*, 1989a) and altered blood pressure (O'Brien *et al.*, 1985).

Characteristics of ovine septicaemic E. coli

The serotype of *E. coli* most frequently isolated from cases of systemic colibacillosis is O78:K80 (Sojka, 1971; Wray and Morris, 1985), which is often present as a commensal in the alimentary tract of sheep and cattle (Jensen, 1974). Other virulent serogroups include O15, O26, O35, O86, O115, O117, O119 and O137 (Morris and Sojka, 1985) but the dominant serotype may vary with country of origin (Contrepois *et al.*, 1986).

Plasmid-encoded fimbriae, such as vir (Smith, 1974; Lopez-Alvarez and Gyles, 1980) and CS31A (Contrepois *et al.*, 1986; Girardeau *et al.*, 1988), are characteristic of septicaemic strains. However, only 50% of

E. coli isolated from cases of bovine systemic colibacillosis adhered to enterocytes *in vitro* (Mohamed Ou Said *et al.*, 1988), indicating that the critical attributes of virulent strains relate to the ability to resist serum killing and clearance by the reticuloendothelial system, rather than to the possession of attachment factors. An important indicator of bacterial virulence and survival within host tissues appears to be colicin V production, which occurs in a high proportion of septicaemic *E. coli* (Smith and Huggins, 1976). Colicin V is not a virulence factor, but it indicates the presence of other bacterial factors implicated in virulence such as the iron chelator, aerobactin (see Contrepois *et al.*, 1986).

Pathogenesis

E. coli capable of causing septicaemia in human patients have been extensively investigated (Chapter 13). Although the comparable isolates from animals have not been well characterized, they appear to have similar virulence properties, but to belong to different serological groups (Smith and Huggins, 1976, 1978; Morris and Sojka, 1985; Mohamed Ou Said *et al.*, 1988).

Bacteraemic strains of *E. coli* present in the gut can cause systemic disease if certain conditions affecting bacterial translocation from the gut are met. Three major factors which promote translocation are: (i) bacterial overgrowth; (ii) host immunological deficiencies; (iii) increased permeability of the gut epithelium (Berg, 1992). All three may be present in the colostrum-deprived neonatal lamb.

Bacterial overgrowth

Gastric secretions in the neonatal lamb are neutral (Hill, 1956) and gut motility is reduced during the first 24–48 hours of life (Eales *et al.*, 1985). Both these features are conducive to survival and multiplication of infective bacteria (Sojka, 1971).

Host immunological deficiences

The lamb is born without protective antibodies and relies on an early and adequate intake of colostrum to provide passive protection against infectious disease both at the gut and systemic levels (Hardy, 1970). Colostral antibody may compete with bacteria for attachment sites on the gut epithelium (Staley and Bush, 1985) and reduce, but not prevent, translocation of bacteria from the gut to host tissues (Smith and Halls, 1968; Smith and Huggins, 1979). Activation of the reticuloendothelial system is the main defence mechanism against *E. coli* bacteraemia (Smith and Halls, 1968); systemic antibody activates the classical complement pathway and phagocytosis, thereby increasing the efficiency of bacterial killing (Taylor, 1983).

Failure of passive transfer of colostral immunoglobulins is not uncommon due to mis-mothering, sibling competition, weakness or poor colostrum production. Consequently, a proportion of neonates remains immunocompromized (Gay, 1984; Hodgson, 1993).

Increased permeability of the gut epithelium

The small intestine of the neonatal ruminant is lined with highly adapted intestinal epithelial cells which ingest intact and functional macromolecules by an endocytic mechanism similar to phagocytosis by cells of the reticuloendothelial system (Hill, 1956; Staley and Bush, 1985). These specialized cells may carry receptors for adherent *E. coli* and allow gut bacteria to compete with other macromolecules for translocation into host tissues (Staley and Bush, 1985; Finlay and Falkow, 1988), predisposing the neonatal ruminant to systemic colibacillosis (Murata *et al.*, 1979). However, whether the initial host–bacteria interaction involves receptors is unclear; bacterial uptake seems not to require attachment pili and no host receptors have been identified (Finlay and Falkow, 1988). ETEC and septicaemic *E. coli* strains are equally successful at penetrating gut epithelium (Smith and Halls, 1968) and strains representative of septicaemic, enteropathogenic and non-enteropathogenic *E. coli* can all be isolated from the blood of colostrum-deprived lambs after oral infection (Smith and Huggins, 1979; Contrepois *et al.*, 1986; Hodgson *et al.*, 1989b). Within 24–48 hours of birth and coincident with the lamb's reducing susceptibility to *E. coli* disease, the intestinal epithelium is renewed and the phagocytic capability is lost by all but the epithelial or M cells overlaying Peyer's patches (Staley and Bush, 1985), a process referred to as 'gut closure' (Lecce and Morgan, 1962; Hardy, 1970; Blood and Radostits, 1989).

Disease and death linked with *E. coli* infection in older lambs with a similar pathology have been reported, although *Clostridium perfringens* type D toxin was found in a proportion of affected lambs (Kater *et al.*, 1963). This may have predisposed lambs to *E. coli* infection by increasing epithelial permeability via inflammation and ulceration, suggesting a common aetiology despite a difference in age. Early work (Dalling, 1926) showed that experimental disease was reproduced by feeding mixed cultures of *C. perfringens* and *E. coli* but not by feeding *E. coli* alone.

Differential diagnosis

Clinical signs in *E. coli* septicaemia in lambs are similar to those seen in experimental endotoxic shock in calves (Contrepois *et al.*, 1986; Nagaraja *et al.*, 1979) and in other diseases in which endotoxin is implicated, such as systemic pasteurellosis in sheep (Gilmour, 1980). There are no pathognomonic signs (Contrepois *et al.*, 1986). Thus, diagnosis is based on clinical, pathological and laboratory findings and exclusion of other possible causes. The majority (80%) of field cases occur in lambs aged less than 72 hours (Collins *et al.*, 1985) and less than a third of diseased lambs show signs of scour, although enteritis is the most common pathological observation (Gilmour *et al.*, 1985). Mild interstitial pneumonia is present in some lambs and hepatitis may affect others. Additionally, the abomasum is often full of gas.

Pure cultures of *E. coli* usually can be obtained from most tissues but serotyping of O antigens alone may not be sufficient to differentiate between enteric and systemic strains of *E. coli*. Hodgson *et al.* (1989a) reproduced systemic disease using an *E. coli* serogroup O101 strain, despite this being the same O serogroup as the reference strain for the strictly enteric O101:K99:F41. Differences within a single serogroup are explained by plasmid-controlled factors, the plasmids being preferentially associated with certain serogroups. Septicaemic strains may be differentiated by plasmid-encoded factors which they produce and which correlate with virulence. These include vir, colicin V and CS31A (Lopez-Alvarez and Gyles, 1980; Girardeau *et al.*, 1988; Mohamed Ou Said *et al.*, 1988).

Other diseases which have been confused with colisepticaemia in the past include lamb dysentery, haemorrhagic enterotoxaemia and enterotoxaemia of suckling lambs, caused by *C. perfringens* (Jensen, 1974), which can now be diagnosed by analysis for the relevant beta or epsilon toxin.

Prevention

Systemic colibacillosis is a problem only in colostrum-deprived or colostrum-deficient neonates (Contrepois *et al.*, 1986; Hodgson *et al.*, 1989a). Newborn lambs which receive colostrum before oral infection with *E. coli* are resistant to systemic disease (Smith and Halls, 1967a, 1968; Hodgson *et al.*, 1989a). Prevention of disease is possible, therefore, by ensuring the neonate obtains an early intake of good quality colostrum (Gay, 1984) and by taking steps to avoid the build up of environmental contamination.

Provision of antibodies

Vaccination of the ewe can boost the content of anti-*E. coli* antibodies in the colostrum but the basic problem of ensuring the lamb drinks colostrum remains. The minimum quantity of colostrum required by the newborn lamb to prevent watery mouth disease has been estimated at 50 ml kg^{-1} lamb bodyweight (King and Hodgson, 1991) and should be provided within 6 hours of birth. Alternative sources of colostral antibody may be used to supplement or substitute for ewe colostrum (Hodgson *et al.*, 1992; Hodgson, 1993). Oral antibiotics may be used prophylactically (Hodgson,

1993) as a convenient, quick and relatively cheap option but should be targeted to lambs at risk (e.g. triplet lambs). Indiscriminate dosing may lead to the development of bacterial resistance.

Control of environmental contamination

The incidence of watery mouth disease increases as lambing progresses and as bacterial contamination may be expected to increase. Good husbandry can help control the build up of contamination by ensuring that yards and pens are disinfected and provided regularly with clean bedding, that contaminated fleece from around the ewe's udder is removed and that equipment is sterilized thoroughly.

The umbilicus is another route of infection (Smith and Halls, 1968) and should be cleaned and sterilized (e.g. by dipping in iodine solution) as soon after birth as possible. Early castration of male lambs may reduce their colostrum intake at a critical period and should be delayed until the lambs are 24 hours old.

Treatment

Treatment consists of oral and intramuscular antibiotic combined with feeding glucose/electrolyte solutions and supplementary warming of affected lambs (Eales, 1987). This method is labour intensive and the outcome uncertain. The use of enemas or drugs to restore gut motility has been advocated (Eales, 1987; Scott, 1988) and may have some effect by reducing the overall bacterial numbers in the gut. However, in advanced cases of disease, effective treatment may only be possible by targeting key stages of the cascade of events comprising endotoxic shock. Preliminary work has shown that prophylactic use of human anti-endotoxin serum prevents endotoxaemia and its sequelae in colostrum-deprived newborn lambs (Hodgson *et al.*, 1993) but the effectiveness of antiserum in treating systemic colibacillosis in neonatal ruminants has not been examined.

Mastitis

Mastitis is of increasing concern to sheep farmers (Jones, 1991). Most cases (80%) of mastitis in ewes are due to *Pasteurella haemolytica* and *Staphylococcus aureus*, the remaining 20% to *E. coli* and *Streptococcus* or other *Staphylococcus* species (Jones, 1991). Acute, chronic and subclinical forms are recognized and the acute form can result in rapid death of affected ewes. Approximately 50% of infections occur at or shortly after weaning and the remainder at or near lambing (Ahmed *et al.*, 1992). Treatment with antibiotic is effective but diseased tissue does not recover, highlighting the need to detect disease earlier (Jones, 1991). Attempts at detecting subclinical mastitis in ewes have been described (Maisi *et al.*, 1987).

Serum-resistant bacteria more commonly are the cause of bovine mastitis (Taylor, 1983), in which adhesion to mammary gland epithelial cells may be important for pathogenesis (Amorena *et al.*, 1990). Overproduction of the inflammatory cytokines tumour necrosis factor alpha (TNF-α) and interleukin 1 (IL-1) as an end-event in both Gram-negative and Gram-positive infection (de Bont *et al.*, 1993), may contribute to shock and death in acute mastitis, necessitating treatment directed against these compounds for effective control (Lohuis *et al.*, 1988).

Effective vaccines are not available but improvements in vaccination strategies for cows have been suggested through the inclusion of recombinant cytokines (IL-2 and GM-CSF) (Blecha, 1991) and their benefit in sheep vaccination programmes or manufacture may be an area to develop in the future.

Concluding Remarks

E. coli diseases in sheep are very similar to the diseases in cattle. The colonizing fimbriae and enterotoxin that are produced by ETEC, and the serotypes of *E. coli* that are implicated in both the enteric and the septicaemic disease are identical. Much of the understanding of the disease process in lambs is based on extrapolation from data developed in calves. In the future, it may be useful to use lambs both as a model for the diseases in calves and as a means of obtaining data directly for application to sheep.

References

Acres S.D. (1985) Enterotoxigenic *Escherichia coli* infections in newborn calves: a review. *Journal of Dairy Science* 68, 229–256.

Ahmed G., Timms, L.L., Morrical, D.G. and Brackelsberg, P.O. (1992) Ovine subclinical mastitis: efficacy of dry treatment as a therapeutic and prophylactic measure. *Sheep Research Journal* 8, 30–33.

Amorena B., Baselga, R. and Aguilar, B. (1990) Factors influencing the degree of *in vitro* bacterial adhesion to ovine mammary gland epithelial cells. *Veterinary Microbiology* 24, 43–50.

Berg, R.D. (1992) Bacterial translocation from the gastrointestinal tract. *Journal of Medicine* 23, 217–244.

Blecha, F. (1991) Cytokines: applications in domestic food animals. *Journal of Dairy Science* 74, 328–339.

Blood, D.C. and Radostits, O.M. (1989) *Veterinary Medicine. A textbook of the diseases of cattle, sheep, pigs, goats and horses*, 7th edn. Baillière Tindall, London, pp. 95–121.

Collins, R.O., Eales, F.A. and Small, J. (1985) Observations on watery mouth in newborn lambs. *British Veterinary Journal* 141, 135–140.

Contrepois, M., Dubourguier, H.C., Parodi, A.L., Girardeau, J.P. and Ollier, J.L. (1986) Septicaemic *Escherichia coli* and experimental infection of calves. *Veterinary Microbiology* 12, 109–118.

Cook, G.C. (1993) Diagnostic procedures in the investigation of infectious diarrhoea. *Baillières Clinical Gastroenterology* 7, 421–449.

Dalling, T. (1926) Lamb dysentery. An account of some experimental field work in 1925 and 1926. *Journal of Comparative Pathology and Therapeutics* 39, 148–163.

de Bont, E.S., Martens, A., van Raan, J., Samson, G., Fetter, W.P., Okken A. and de Leij, L.H. (1993) Tumor necrosis factor-alpha, interleukin-1 beta, and interleukin-6 plasma levels in neonatal sepsis. *Pediatric Research* 33, 380–383.

Eales, A. (1987) Watery mouth. *In Practice* 9, 12–17.

Eales, F.A., Small, J., Murray, L. and McBean, A. (1985) Abomasal size and emptying time in healthy lambs and in lambs affected by watery mouth. *Veterinary Record* 117, 332–335.

Finlay, B.B. and Falkow, S. (1988) A comparison of microbial invasion strategies of *Salmonella*, *Shigella* and *Yersinia* species. In: Horwitz, M.A. (ed.) *Bacteria–Host Cell Interactions*. Alan R. Liss, New York, pp. 227–243.

Gay, C.C. (1984) Failure of passive transfer of colostral immunoglobulins and neonatal disease in calves: a review. In: Acres S. (ed.) *Proceedings of the Fourth International Symposium on Neonatal Diarrhea*. Veterinary Infectious Disease Organization, Saskatoon, Saskatchewan, pp. 346–362.

Gilmour, J.S., Donachie, W. and Eales, F.A. (1985) Pathological and microbiological findings in 38 lambs with watery mouth. *Veterinary Record* 117, 335–337.

Gilmour, N.J.L. (1980) *Pasteurella haemolytica* infections in sheep. *Veterinary Quarterly* 2, 191–198.

Girardeau J.P., Der Vartanian, M., Ollier, J.L. and Contrepois, M. (1988) CS31A, a new K88-related fimbrial antigen on bovine enterotoxigenic and septicaemic *Escherichia coli* strains. *Infection and Immunity* 56, 2180–2188.

Griffiths, E. (1991) Iron and bacterial virulence – a brief overview. *Biology of Metals* 4, 7–13.

Gross, R.J. and Rowe, B. (1985) *Escherichia coli* diarrhoea. *Journal of Hygiene* 95, 531–550.

Gyles, C.L. (1992) *Escherichia coli* cytotoxins and enterotoxins. *Canadian Journal of Microbiology* 38, 734–746.

Haig, G. (1981) Lamb survival (Letter). *Veterinary Record* 108, 195.

Hardy, R.N. (1970) Absorption of macromolecules from the intestine of the newborn animal In: Phillipson, A.T. (ed.) *Physiology of Digestion and Metabolism in the Ruminant*. Oriel Press, Newcastle upon Tyne, pp. 150–165.

Hill, K.J. (1956) Gastric development and antibody transference in the lamb, with some observations on the rat and guinea pig. *Journal of Physiology* 41, 421–432.

Hodgson, J.C. (1993) Watery mouth disease in newborn lambs. *Veterinary Annual* 33, 102–106.

Hodgson, J.C., King, T.J., Hay, L.A. and Elston, D.A. (1989a) Biochemical and haematological evidence of endotoxic shock in gnotobiotic lambs with watery mouth disease. *Research in Veterinary Science* 47, 119–124.

Hodgson, J,C., King, T., Moon, G., Donachie, W. and Quirie, M. (1989b) Host responses during infection in newborn lambs. *Federation of European Microbiological Societies Microbiology and Immunology* 47, 311–312.

Hodgson, J.C., Moon, G.M., Hay, L.A. and Quirie, M. (1992) Effectiveness of substitute colostrum in preventing disease in newborn lambs. *British Society of Animal Production, Occasional Publications* 15, 163–165.

Hodgson, J.C., Barclay, G.R., Hay, L.A., Moon, G.M. and Poxton, I.R. (1993) Prevention of endotoxaemia in colostrum-deprived, newborn lambs using human anti-LPS antiserum. (Abstract). *Veterinary Immunology and Immunopathology* 35 (Suppl. PS), 7.5.

Isaacson, R.E. and Richter, P. (1984) Molecular and genetic analysis of K99 plasmids. In: Acres. S. (ed.) *Proceedings, Fourth International Symposium on Neonatal Diarrhea, Saskatchewan*. Veterinary Infectious Disease Organization, Saskatoon, Saskatchewan, pp. 179–190.

Jensen, R. (1974) Colibacillosis in lambs. In: *Diseases of Sheep*. Lea and Febiger, Philadelphia, pp. 76–80.

Jones, J.E.T. (1991) Mastitis. In: Martin, W.B. and Aitken, I.D. (eds) *Diseases of Sheep*, 2nd edn. Blackwell Scientific Publications, Oxford, pp. 75–78.

Kater, J.C., Davis, E.A., Haughey, K.G. and Hartley, W.J. (1963) *Escherichia coli* infection in lambs. *New Zealand Veterinary Journal* 11, 32–38.

King, T. and Hodgson, C. (1991) Watery mouth in lambs. *In Practice* 13, 23–24.

King, T.J. and Angus, K.W. (1991) Neonatal disease. In: Martin, W.B. and Aitken, I.D. (eds) *Diseases of Sheep*, 2nd edn. Blackwell Scientific Publications, Oxford, pp. 12–19.

Leece, J.G. and Morgan, D.O. (1962) Effect of dietary regimen on cessation of intestinal absorption of large molecules (closure) in neonatal pig and lamb. *Journal of Nutrition* 78, 263–268.

Lohuis, J.A., Verheijden, J.H., Burvenich C. and van Miert, A.S. (1988) Pathophysiological effects of endotoxins in ruminants. 1. Changes in body temperature and reticulo-rumen motility, and the effect of repeated administration. *Veterinary Quarterly* 10, 109–116.

Lopez-Alvarez, J. and Gyles, C.L. (1980) Occurrence of the vir plasmid among animal and human strains of invasive *Escherichia coli. American Journal of Veterinary Research* 41, 769–774.

Maisi, P., Junttila, J. and Seppanen, J. (1987) Detection of subclinical mastitis in ewes. *British Veterinary Journal* 143, 402–409.

Michell, A.R. (1989) Oral and parenteral rehydration therapy. *In Practice* 11, 96–99.

Mitchell, G. and Linklater, K. (1983) Differential diagnosis of scouring in lambs. *In Practice* 5, 5–11.

Mohamed Ou Said, A., Contrepois, M.G., Der Vartanian, M. and Girardeau, J.P. (1988) Virulence factors and markers in *Escherichia coli* from calves with bacteremia. *American Journal of Veterinary Research* 49, 1657–1660.

Morris, J.A. and Sojka, W.J. (1985) *Escherichia coli* as a pathogen in animals. In: Sussman, M. (ed.) *The Virulence of* Escherichia coli. *Reviews and Methods*. Academic Press, London, pp. 47–77.

Morris, J.A., Thorns, C.J. and Sojka, W.J. (1980a) Evidence for two adhesive antigens on the K99 reference strain *Escherichia coli* B41. *Journal of General Microbiology* 118, 107–113

Morris, J.A., Wray, C. and Sojka, W.J. (1980b) Passive protection of lambs against enteropathogenic *Escherichia coli*: role of antibodies in serum and colostrum of dams vaccinated with K99 antigen. *Journal of Medical Microbiology* 3, 265–271.

Morris, J.A., Thorns, C., Scott, A.C., Sojka, W.J. and Wells, G.A. (1982) Adhesion *in vitro* and *in vivo* associated with an adhesive antigen (F41) produced by a K99 mutant of the reference strain *Escherichia coli* B41. *Infection and Immunity* 36, 1146–1153.

Morris, J.A., Wells, G.A., Scott, A.C. and Sojka, W.J. (1983) Colonization of the small intestine of lambs by an enterotoxigenic *Escherichia coli* producing F41 fimbriae. *Veterinary Record* 113, 471.

Murata, H., Yaguchi, H. and Namioka, S. (1979) Relationship between the intestinal permeability to macromolecules and invasion of septicemia-inducing *Escherichia coli* in neonatal piglets. *Infection and Immunity* 26, 339–347.

Nagaraja, T.G., Bartley, E.E., Anthony, H.D., Leipold, H.W. and Fina, L.R. (1979) Endotoxin shock in calves from intravenous injection of rumen bacterial endotoxin. *Journal of Animal Science* 49, 567–582.

Newsome, P.M., Burgess, M.N., Burgess, M.R., Coney, K.A., Goddard, M.E. and Morris, J.A. (1987) A model of acute infectious neonatal diarrhoea. *Journal of Medical Microbiology* 23, 19–28.

O'Brien, W.F., Golden, S.M., Davis, S.E. and Bibro, M.C. (1985) Endotoxemia in the neonatal lamb. *American Journal of Obstetrics and Gynecology* 151, 671–674.

Ørskov, I., Ørskov, F., Smith, H.W. and Sojka, W.J. (1975) The establishment of K99, a thermolabile, transmissible *Escherichia coli* K antigen, previously called 'Kco', possessed by calf and lamb enteropathogenic strains. *Acta Pathologica Microbiologica Scandinavica B* 83, 31–36.

Pittman, Q.J., Cooper, K.E., Veale, W.L. and Van Petten, G.R. (1973) Fever in newborn lambs. *Canadian Journal of Physiology and Pharmacology* 51, 868–872.

Scott, P.R. (1988) The possible use of metoclopramide to prevent watery mouth in lambs in commercial flocks. *British Veterinary Journal* 144, 570–572.

Sellwood, R. and Lees, D. (1981) Adhesion of *Escherichia coli* pathogenic in pigs, calves and lambs to intestinal epithelial cell brush-borders. In: de Leeuw, P.W. and Guinee, P.A.M. (eds) *Laboratory Diagnosis in Neonatal Calf and Pig Diarrhoea*. Martinus Nijhoff Publishers, The Hague, pp. 163–174.

Smith, H.W. (1962) Observations on the aetiology of neonatal diarrhoea (scours) in calves. *Journal of Pathology and Bacteriology* 84, 147–168.

Smith, H.W. (1974) A search for transmissible pathogenic characters in invasive strains of *Escherichia coli*: the discovery of a plasmid-controlled toxin and a plasmid-controlled lethal character closely associated, or identical, with colicine V. *Journal of General Microbiology* 83, 95–111.

Smith, H.W. and Halls, S. (1967a) Observations by the ligated intestinal segment and oral inoculation methods on *Escherichia coli* infections in pigs, calves, lambs and rabbits. *Journal of Pathology and Bacteriology* 93, 499–529.

Smith, H.W. and Halls, S. (1967b) Studies on *Escherichia coli* enterotoxin. *Journal of Pathology and Bacteriology* 93, 531–543.

Smith, H.W. and Halls, S. (1968) The experimental infection of calves with bacteraemia-producing strains of *Escherichia coli*: the influence of colostrum. *Journal of Medical Microbiology* 1, 61–78.

Smith, H.W. and Huggins, M.B. (1976) Further observations on the association of the colicine V plasmid of *Escherichia coli* with pathogenicity and with survival in the alimentary tract. *Journal of General Microbiology* 92, 335–350.

Smith, H.W. and Huggins, M.B. (1978) The influence of plasmid-determined and other characteristics of enteropathogenic *Escherichia coli* on their ability to proliferate in the alimentary tracts of piglets, calves and lambs. *Journal of Medical Microbiology* 11, 471–492.

Smith, H.W. and Huggins, M.B. (1979) Experimental infection of calves, piglets and lambs with mixtures of invasive and enteropathogenic strains of *Escherichia coli. Journal of Medical Microbiology* 12, 507–510.

Smith, H.W. and Linggood, M.A. (1972) Further observations on *Escherichia coli* enterotoxins with particular regard to those produced by atypical piglet strains and by calf and lamb strains: the transmissible nature of these enterotoxins and of a K antigen possessed by calf and lamb strains. *Journal of Medical Microbiology* 5, 243–250.

Smyth. C.J. and Smith, S.G.J. (1992) Bacterial fimbriae: variation and regulatory mechanisms. In: Hormaeche, C.E., Penn, C.W. and Smyth, C.J. (eds) *Molecular Biology of Bacterial Infection: Current Status and Future Perspectives*. Cambridge University Press, Cambridge, pp. 267–297.

Sojka, W.J. (1965) *Escherichia coli* infection in sheep. In: Escherichia coli *in Domestic Animals and Poultry*. Commonwealth Agricultural Bureaux, Farnham Royal, UK, pp. 97–103.

Sojka, W.J. (1971) Enteric diseases in new-born piglets, calves and lambs due to *Escherichia coli* infection. *Veterinary Bulletin* 41, 509–522.

Sojka, W.J., Wray, C. and Morris, J.A. (1978) Passive protection of lambs against experimental enteric colibacillosis by colostral transfer of antibodies from K99-vaccinated ewes. *Journal of Medical Microbiology* 11, 493–499.

Sokkar, S.M., Kubba, M.A. and Al-Augaidy, F. (1980) Studies on natural and experimental endometritis in ewes. *Veterinary Pathology* 17, 693–698.

Staley, T.E. and Bush, L.J. (1985) Receptor mechanisms of the neonatal intestine and their relationship to immunoglobulin absorption and disease. *Journal of Dairy Science* 68, 184–205.

Taylor, P.W. (1983) Bactericidal and bacteriolytic activity of serum against gram-negative bacteria. *Microbiological Reviews* 47, 46–83.

Tzipori, S., Sherwood, D., Angus, K.W., Campbell, I. and Gordon, M. (1981) Diarrhea in lambs: experimental infections with enterotoxigenic *Escherichia coli*, rotavirus, and *Cryptosporidium* sp. *Infection and Immunity* 33, 401–406.

van Deventer, S.J., Buller, H.R., ten Cate, J.W., Sturk, A. and Pauw, W. (1988)

Endotoxaemia: an early predictor of septicaemia in febrile patients. *Lancet* i, 605–609.

Whipp, S.C. (1978) Physiology of diarrhea – small intestines. *Journal of the American Veterinary Medical Association* 173, 662–666.

Wray, C. (1984) Enteric diseases in animals caused by *Escherichia coli*: their control and prevention. *Biochemical Society Transactions* 12, 191–193.

Wray, C. and Morris, J.A. (1985) Aspects of colibacillosis in farm animals. *Journal of Hygiene* 95, 577–593.

7

Neonatal Diarrhoea in Pigs

T.J.L. Alexander

Department of Clinical Veterinary Medicine, University of Cambridge, Madingly Road, Cambridge CB3 OES, UK

Diarrhoea is one of the most common diseases of suckled pigs worldwide. Large intensive herds are rarely completely free from it. In a recent US National Swine Survey of preweaning disease, diarrhoea had the highest morbidity and represented 10.8% of preweaning mortality (Tubbs *et al.*, 1993). This survey covered a wide range of herds. In the best managed herds, the morbidity of piglet diarrhoea particularly in newborn piglets is much lower and mortality may be very low indeed. In such herds a target level of mortality from *E. coli* of 0.5% of live births is achievable (M.R. Muirhead, Garth Veterinary Group, Beeford, Driffield, North Humberside, 1993, personal communication).

Piglet diarrhoea, through whatever cause, may occur at any time during suckling but the highest incidence of life-threatening diarrhoea occurs during the first 3–5 days of life with less serious peaks occurring later. In diarrhoea of the newborn piglet (i.e. in the first 3–5 days of life) enterotoxigenic *E. coli* are frequently the primary and sole infectious cause. In diarrhoea that occurs later in the suckling period other agents may also be involved. The term 'neonatal' is sometimes restricted to the very early diarrhoea but in this chapter it will be broadened to cover the whole suckling period (Blood and Studdert, 1988; Fairbrother, 1992).

History

Diarrhoea in suckled piglets has always been a problem but when sows were kept in small numbers and piglets were weaned at 8–12 weeks postfarrowing, it tended to occur at 3–6 weeks of age (Morrison, 1926; Fishwick, 1947; Dunne, 1958). Diarrhoea of the newborn piglet came to be recognized as a serious problem during the late 1950s and 1960s with the emergence of the modern pig industry. *E. coli* was deemed to be involved and 'pathogenic' serotypes were identified initially by the frequency of their isolation from diarrhoeic pigs (Sojka *et al.*, 1960). Dunne (1964), reviewing the studies of a number of research workers, concluded that the most important O serological groups associated with piglet diarrhoea were 08, 0138, 0139 and 0141, of which 0141 appeared most frequently. Colostrum was known to be important in protection. Although lactogenic immunity was recognized in relation to transmissible gastroenteritis (TGE), its importance in preventing *E. coli* diarrhoea was not recognized until around 1970 (Allen and Porter, 1970, 1973; Porter *et al.*, 1970; Porter, 1973b). The virulence factors of pathogenic *E. coli* were not known and precise cause and effect were difficult to prove mainly because of the unreliability of reproducing the disease in naturally reared piglets (Moon *et al.*, 1968; Dunne and Bennett, 1970). Many research workers in different countries applied themselves to the problem and the number of publications expanded accordingly. The use of porcine gut loops (Moon *et al.*, 1966; Gyles and Barnum, 1967; Dunne and Bennett, 1970) and of colostrum-deprived and primary specific pathogen free pigs (Kramer and Nderito, 1967; Kramer, 1969) and later of gnotobiotic pigs (Brandenburg and Wilson, 1972) opened the way for more precise and better-controlled studies. It was shown that 'enteropathogenic' serotypes of *E. coli* adhered to the villous surface of the small intestine (Arbuckle, 1972; Bertschinger and Moon, 1972; Rutter and Jones, 1972) and produced enterotoxins which acted on the enterocytes resulting in diarrhoea (Smith and Halls, 1968; Smith and Gyles, 1970; Brandenburg and Wilson, 1972; Dobrescu and Huygelen, 1972; Pesti and Semjén, 1972). The production of both the adhesins and enterotoxins was found to be governed by transmissible plasmids (Smith and Halls, 1968; Smith and Linggood, 1971).

The terminology used for pathogenic serotypes became confused because different workers applied the terms differently. It is now generally accepted that the term 'enterotoxigenic *E. coli*' (ETEC) refers to *E. coli* which adhere to the villi of the small intestine and produce enterotoxins that act locally on enterocytes. These are the ones predominantly associated with neonatal diarrhoea in piglets. Other terms such as 'enteropathogenic *E. coli*', 'enteroinvasive *E. coli*' and 'enterohaemorrhagic *E. coli*' refer to *E. coli* which produce diarrhoea by other mechanisms (Levine, 1987). Diarrhoea due to these types of *E. coli* is uncommon in the young unweaned piglet.

Clinical Signs

Neonatal diarrhoea may occur sporadically, affecting only one or two pigs in a litter or sometimes whole litters; or it may occur more frequently building up until successive litters are almost all affected. In its most severe acute form it may affect piglets in the first 1–2 hours of life, sometimes so soon after birth that the farrowing house attendants may report that the piglets are scouring at birth. In such severe early acute outbreaks, the morbidity and mortality are often high and may reach alarming numbers unless prompt prophylactic and therapeutic measures are taken. More commonly the onset of diarrhoea is delayed for several hours or days after birth. The disease is then usually less severe. Morbidity is variable and may be high but mortality is usually low if prompt treatment is given. The very first clinical signs in individual pigs may be raised hair and a slight shiver. In pens with minimal bedding often the first signs noted by the attendant are pools of liquid faeces on the solid parts of the farrowing pen floor or on the solid surfaces under perforated pen floors, depending on the pen design. The pools of faeces may be brown and watery, or brightly coloured creamy-white, grey or fawn. When voided by the piglet the liquid faeces tend to dribble down the perineum, staining it and sometimes making it and the tail red and sore. Affected piglets rapidly lose condition, becoming thin, hairy, dehydrated and weak, with discoloured, sometimes dirty skin. In well-bedded farrowing pens dehydration and thinness and possibly even a dead pig may be the first signs noted because the watery faeces are hidden in the bedding and staining of the perineum may be minimal. In outdoor herds, where the farrowing huts are also well bedded but where the air is normally fresh and sweet smelling, the first sign noted is often the distinctive odour of diarrhoeic faeces which may sometimes be detected on the sow's skin when she is outside the hut feeding. As the diarrhoea progresses the eyes become dull and sunken, the emaciation progresses and the ribs, spinal bones and pelvic bones become increasingly prominent. If untreated, severely affected piglets become recumbent, cold, comatose and die. The dams of such piglets and other older pigs in the same room do not develop diarrhoea.

Bacterial Characteristics

The virulence factors of *E. coli* are described in Part III of this book and those of porcine postweaning diarrhoea in Chapter 8. They have also been reviewed by Gyles (1986). All available evidence suggests that the majority of *E. coli* which cause neonatal diarrhoea in piglets are ETEC. In the UK many are haemolytic on sheep blood agar whereas in Australia they tend to be non-haemolytic (D.J. Hampson, Murdoch, Australia, 1993, personal communication). Their important virulence factors are adhesive fimbriae and enterotoxins. There is some evidence that attaching and effacing *E. coli* (AEEC) may also cause diarrhoea in piglets before weaning but this is thought to be rare (G.R. Pearson, School of Veterinary Science, Langford, Bristol, UK; R.J. Higgins, MAFF, Veterinary Investigation Centre, Thirsk, York, UK, 1993, personal communication). There is also at least one report of haemorrhagic diarrhoea in piglets possibly caused by attaching haemorrhagic *E. coli* (AHEC) (Faubert and Drolet, 1992) but clinically obvious haemorrhage in piglet diarrhoea, except for that caused by *Clostridium perfringens* type C, is uncommon. In the UK it seems to be found at postmortem examination more often than it used to be.

The long filamentous fimbriae which radiate from the surface of the ETEC bacteria that cause diarrhoea in piglets possess an antigen that specifically adheres to the surfaces of enterocytes (Gaastra and de Graaf, 1982; Moon, 1990). In the majority of cases this is what was originally called the K88 antigen (K88ab and K88ac) and is now known as fimbrial adhesin 4 (F4). F4 can be regarded as a virulence factor specific to ETEC strains that colonize pigs since it is only found in pigs. It is also the commonest fimbrial adhesin in porcine ETEC. Another adhesin specific to ETEC strains that colonize pigs is F6 (987P). While it seems to be more common now in the UK than it used to be, it is present in only about 2% of isolates (C. Wray, Weybridge, Surrey, UK, 1993, personal communication). In contrast, in the USA, Wilson and Francis (1986) found F6 to be present on 30% of porcine isolates. F5 (K99) and F41, which usually occur together and which are mainly associated with ETEC of calves and sheep, are occasionally found on ETEC from piglets. ETEC which have none of the above adhesins have been shown to adhere to the ileum of weaned pigs but there appear to be no reports of this in sucking piglets (Nagy *et al.*, 1992). ETEC possessing adhesive F antigens may also possess non-adhesive capsular polysaccharide K antigens.

ETEC bacteria which have specific adherent F antigens tend to be associated with a limited array of somatic O serogroups. Thus in the UK at present the commonest serotypes associated with piglet diarrhoea are O8, O138, O147, O149 and O157 (C. Wray, I. McLaren and P.J. Carroll, Central Veterinary Laboratory, Weybridge, UK, 1993, personal communication). Similarly, in North America the commonest were classically serotypes O8, O147, O149 and O157 all with F4 (K88) and producing LT and ST enterotoxin (Wilson and Francis, 1986; Harel *et al.*, 1990). More recently, however, in North America ETEC of other serogroups (e.g. O9, O64 and O101) have been increasingly isolated. These produce fimbrial antigen F5 (K99), F41 or F6 (987P) and STa and/or STb enterotoxin(s) (Fairbrother, 1992). In Australia the most common O groups currently encountered are O9, O20, O101 (Woodward *et al.*, 1993). Many of these isolates lack the adhesins usually associated with porcine strains. It has been hypothesized that these strains may have increased because of the selective effect of widescale vaccination with preparations incorporating pilus antigens. These emerging strains originate from diverse genetic backgrounds, suggesting that pathogenic potential is linked directly or indirectly to their particular somatic antigen type. In contrast to this diversity of strains, a single clonal group of strains of O149 infecting neonatal piglets has apparently predominated in Sweden since the 1960s (Kuhn *et al.*, 1985). This same clonal grouping is present in Indonesia and Australia, where it is related to certain clones of O149 that cause post-weaning diarrhoea (Hampson *et al.*, 1993).

Pathogenesis

The great majority of viable piglets while still *in utero* prior to parturition are microbiologically sterile. From the time of their emergence from the vagina on to the farrowing pen floor pigs are exposed to a massive number and array of bacteria. The sow's faeces, which are likely to be on the floor where the piglet is born, contain several hundred different bacterial species. The great majority of them are non-pathogenic anaerobes but low numbers of potentially pathogenic *E. coli* are frequently present. The air which the little pig breathes also contains faecal and other bacteria which are trapped in its respiratory mucociliary system and swallowed. Within a few minutes of birth the viable piglet makes its way around its dam, often first to her head and then to her teats and in so doing takes in and swallows more bacteria. The pH of the stomach and duodenum is relatively alkaline and the production of digestive enzymes is low. The gastrointestinal tract of the newborn piglet provides a favourable environment throughout its length for the rapid multiplication of bacteria but it is selective and only a limited array of species grow initially. The number of species increases gradually and unevenly over days and weeks but the intestinal flora does not become fully mature until after weaning.

In the first day of life, streptococci and coliform bacteria, including potentially pathogenic *E. coli*, seed down and multiply throughout the tract, but as the pH of the stomach and duodenum falls, due to the secretion of acids both by the stomach and the lactobacilli and streptococci which begin to line it, the population of *E. coli* moves more posteriorly. The multiplication of aerobic bacteria reduces the oxygen tension enabling anaerobic bacteria to multiply. Among the earliest of these is *Clostridium perfringens* followed soon by *Fusobacterium* and *Bacteroides* species. These have a suppressive effect on the multiplication of *E. coli*.

The first few hours of life are highly hazardous for the newborn piglet. One of several reasons for this is because of the rapid multiplication of *E. coli* throughout its small intestine. A proportion of these *E. coli* are likely to be ETEC which are capable of adhering to the enterocytes along the villi, multiplying, producing enterotoxins and hence diarrhoea. The main barrier to attachment is the secretory IgA in the dam's colostrum and milk. If for some reason the intake of this is delayed or its level in the intestine is too low relative to the number of ETEC bacteria then the *E. coli* can attach and multiply.

ETEC strains possessing the K88 antigen which commonly cause diarrhoea in piglets differ from calf strains in that they usually produce a heat labile enterotoxin (LT) in addition to heat stable enterotoxin (ST). LT is a high-molecular-weight protein similar to cholera toxin, and is antigenically constant regardless of the serotype of *E. coli* that produces it. ST refers to low-molecular-weight heat-stable enterotoxin, which may be STa or STb. In a study of the prevalence of enterotoxin genes among *E. coli* isolated from swine, Moon *et al.* (1986) in the USA found that of 874 isolates the most prevalent combination was LT-STb. Woodward *et al.* (1990) reported similar findings in the UK. In US studies, 35% of the ETEC from piglets under 1 week of age with enteric colibacillosis were of the STaP-only genotype whereas 33% of the ETEC from older pigs with enteric colibacillosis were of the STb-only genotype. (STaP is the heat-stable genotype enterotoxin found in ETEC from pigs as distinct from STaH, the heat-stable genotype enterotoxin which is found in ETEC from people.)

The biochemical actions of the enterotoxins have been reviewed recently by Fairbrother (1992) and are discussed in Chapter 14. They bind to different receptors on the surface of the enterocytes and affect the metabolism of the enterocyte in different ways. LT activates adenylate cyclase which stimulates the production of cyclic adenosine monophosphate resulting in increased secretion of Cl, Na, HCO_3 and water. It may also block the absorption of Na by mature enterocytes. STa activates guanylate cyclase which stimulates the production of guanosine monophosphate resulting in reduced absorption of electrolytes and water from the intestine lumen. The action of STb is not well understood but the net effect of all three is secretory and results in ionic imbalance, dehydration, acidosis and raised blood K.

Diagnosis

Since ETEC is the commonest cause of diarrhoea in the first 3–4 days of life, a presumptive diagnosis of primary colibacillosis when moderate levels of diarrhoea are occurring at this age is likely to be right but the probabilities lessen in diarrhoea that occurs after 7 days of age. Under everyday farm conditions therefore, if the neonatal diarrhoea is sporadic and is responding to treatment, farrowing house attendants on the advice of their herd veterinarian tend to take a pragmatic view. They assume that the diarrhoea is colibacillosis and treat piglets individually without recourse to laboratory diagnostic tests. It is only when severe flare-ups of diarrhoea occur, with an increase in mortality and postdiarrhoea debility or if the diarrhoea fails to respond to treatment, that recourse is made to laboratory diagnostic tests.

A simple common approach, particularly if mortality is low, is to take rectal swabs for culture. Dry swabs are often used but as a general rule, particularly if there is to be a delay, it is better to use transport medium. The swabs are cultured overnight, classically on sheep blood agar (on which some strains of ETEC may be haemolytic) and MacConkey or Tergitol-7 agar. The next day suspect *E. coli* colonies are picked off and tested in slide or tube agglutination tests to determine whether they belong to a known ETEC serogroup. If they belong to such a serogroup, their susceptibility to antimicrobial drugs commonly used for piglet diarrhoea may be tested. There is not always a good correlation between the results of such tests and the efficacy of the antibiotics in the field.

This simple approach does not provide a reliable diagnosis. The ETEC serogroup detected in the rectal faeces may not necessarily be the causal agent in the small intestine, although if it is in pure profuse culture it is more likely that it is. The reliability of the diagnosis is greatly improved if one or more untreated live early cases, or, failing that, freshly dead untreated diarrhoeic piglets are made available. Cultures can then be prepared from the surface lining of the ileum. Profuse pure growth of *E. coli* belonging to a known ETEC serogroup is strongly suggestive of colibacillosis.

Laboratories may carry out more extensive procedures routinely or on request to confirm that the isolate is ETEC and to eliminate other causes. Histology of the jejunum and ileum may show bacterial adhesion to intact apparently normal villi supporting the diagnosis of primary colibacillosis. If the villi are abnormal and stunted the cause may be viral or coccidial. To confirm that the isolate is ETEC fimbrial antigens K88, K99 and 987P and toxins LT and STa can be identified by latex agglutination tests and/or ELISAs. In some countries these tests can be purchased in kit form. Some laboratories make impression smears of the ileal surface and carry out fluorescent antibody tests using monoclonal antibodies against K88, K99 and 987P. Mullaney *et al.* (1991) compared seroagglutination (SAT), enzyme-linked immunosorbent assay (ELISA) and indirect fluorescent antibody staining tests (IFAT) for reliability in detecting the pilus antigens K88, K99 and 987P on isolates that had been previously serotyped and characterized for pilus genes by DNA probe. All three tests were found to be specific but the SAT was the least sensitive and the IFAT the most sensitive. In a few laboratories, DNA probes are used to detect LT, STa and STb, but these tests are relatively slow and expensive and are generally only used in conjunction with research projects. (For further information see Chapter 21.)

Differential Diagnosis

Diarrhoea in suckled piglets may be caused by infections other than ETEC. The commonest of these are rotavirus and *Clostridium perfringens* type C, and in some countries or regions transmissible gastroenteritis virus (TGEV), porcine epidemic diarrhoea virus (PEDV) type II (PEDV type I affects only older weaned pigs) and coccidia. The differential diagnosis of these in the laboratory has already been referred to under 'Diagnosis'. This section will deal mainly with key differences in the clinicopathological syndromes.

Clostridium perfringens type C is widespread throughout the world. Its spores are almost ubiquitous, yet many herds remain clinically unaffected. In affected herds it causes diarrhoea or dysentery mainly in piglets under 10 days of age. Whole litters or groups of litters may be affected with a high mortality. In young recently born piglets the dysentery is severe and acute. In unvaccinated herds the faeces are bloody, the piglets rapidly become toxic and depressed, response to antibacterial drugs is poor and most affected piglets soon die. In older piglets (i.e. around 2 weeks of age) the disease may be milder with yellow-brown faeces. Affected piglets of this age that survive are often severely debilitated. Milder sporadic forms of the disease often without dysentery may occur in herds where the sows have been vaccinated but not adequately protected. Gross postmortem examination of the more severely affected piglets is diagnostic. The wall of the jejunum is dark red or purple and the contents are like port wine. The appearance of many large Gram-positive rods in impression smears of the jejunal mucosa and detection by ELISA of toxin (predominantly beta) in the gut contents confirm the diagnosis. In less severely affected older piglets the lesions may be less distinctive, the bacterial flora more mixed and the toxin less easy to demonstrate.

Rotavirus does not cause such dramatic outbreaks but tends to remain endemic in most herds, perpetuated in young weaned pigs subclinically or causing mild diarrhoea. It can cause diarrhoea of varying severity in nursing piglets but rarely under about 7 days of age unless piglets are colostrum deprived. Its clinical occurrence is sporadic affecting individual litters or small groups of litters. Affected pigs may lose condition rapidly, appear depressed, and may stop eating creep feed for a day or two. The faeces are often yellow and watery. Mortality is usually low and recovery takes place gradually after about 5 days and often more quickly if the pigs are weaned early. Bodily condition is helped by oral electrolytes but there is no response to antibacterial drugs. At postmortem examination of unweaned pigs the stomach usually contains clotted milk and the small intestine a creamy liquid. Villous stunting is seen but is less severe than in TGE or PED. Diagnosis is confirmed by electron microscopy or PAGE (polyacrylamide gel electrophoresis) on faeces or sometimes by the fluorescent antibody test (FAT).

There are two simple tests that can be done on the farm to distinguish viral from ETEC diarrhoea. One is to test the pH of the diarrhoeic faeces. If it is alkaline it is likely to be a secretory diarrhoea such as colibacillosis whereas if it is acid it is likely to be a malabsorption diarrhoea and is more likely to be viral. The second test is to examine the gently washed opened mucosal surface of the ileum under saline with a good hand lens or scanning microscope. If villous stunting is severe the cause is likely to be TGE or PED virus, if it is less severe it may be rotavirus, but if no stunting is visible then it is more likely to be ETEC.

TGE occurs in most pig-rearing countries of the world. PED type II is widespread in Europe but is thought to be absent from North America. Both differ from colibacillosis in that they classically cause epizootic outbreaks of acute diarrhoea which spread rapidly between and through susceptible naive herds affecting all age groups including adults. In both, the faeces are very liquid, often highly coloured, with a distinctive odour. It tends to shoot out from the rectum as if from a hosepipe rather than trickle down the perineum and often sticks to the skin all over the piglets' bodies. The diarrhoea in an individual pig lasts about 4–5 days after which most pigs over about 1 week of age recover spontaneously. Mortality from TGE under 10 days of age may approach 100%. Mortality from PED, which is usually less severe, is lower. At postmortem examination, the wall of the gastrointestinal tract appears thin and transluscent. In the lumen, there is often gas and sparse highly coloured liquid. The villi are severely stunted and deformed, a feature which immediately distinguishes it from ETEC. STb produced by some ETEC has been reported to cause villous stunting but the effect is too small to be readily observed in diagnosis (Rose *et al.*, 1987). Specific diagnosis is usually made by FATs on sections of frozen ileum.

The prevalence of coccidiosis due to *Isospora suis* is difficult to assess since histological confirmation on intestinal sections collected from sacrificed acutely diarrhoeic piglets is essential but not always done. Laboratories which make a point of looking for it histologically diagnose it fairly frequently. Its occurrence at 7–10 days of age may be mistaken for colibacillosis or rotavirus diarrhoea. The severity of the diarrhoea varies from transient whitish faecal softening to profuse yellowish watery liquid. Such piglets become thin and hairy and some may remain so for several weeks or recover well particularly when weaned. Littermates of affected piglets may remain clinically unaffected. At postmortem examination the wall of the jejunum and ileum may appear thickened. The contents may be creamy or more liquid. The villi are stunted and there may be very localized points of haemorrhage. A noticeable increase in necrotic enteritis in 7–14-day-old piglets has been associated with more severe forms of *I. suis* enteritis (R.J. Higgins, MAFF Veterinary Investigation Centre, Thirsk, York, UK, 1993, personal communication). Specific diagnosis is made by histology of the jejunum/ileum since most damage to the intestine occurs during the prepatent period when oocysts are not found in faeces.

Other infections have been implicated in piglet diarrhoea but in general their aetiological role has not been well defined or their incidence and importance are not known and are probably low. They include astrovirus, calicivirus (other than vesicular exanthema virus), adenovirus, *Clostridium perfringens* type A, *Campylobacter coli*, *Cryptosporidium* and *Strongyloides*. Further information on them and on the other diarrhoeas discussed above can be found in standard textbooks (e.g. Russell and Eddington, 1985; Taylor, 1986; Pensaert, 1989; Leman *et al.*, 1992).

Piglet diarrhoea is thought to occur as a result of non-infectious primary factors such as changes in the dam's ration, oversupply of sows' milk, stale mouldy creep feed or dirty water supplies. For example, in herds feeding home-mixed waste materials such as milk by-products, waste dog or human biscuits, surplus fats, or lemonade, a sudden increase of an ingredient such as waste fat may appear to trigger off an outbreak of piglet diarrhoea, presumably by altering the nature of the sows' milk. Whether such events are predisposing factors for colibacillosis or are the sole cause of diarrhoea is usually not determined. These events are generally one-time events and the cause and effect are not clearly defined.

Treatment

On a day-to-day basis, when the incidence of neonatal diarrhoea in a herd is low, farrowing house staff generally treat clinical cases on an individual pig or litter basis with an antibacterial preparation that they and their veterinary adviser have found from experience to be effective. Treatment may be by mouth or parenteral injection. A wide range of therapeutic products are available, varying in different countries. Examples of drugs in common use are apramycin, ceftifur sodium, framycetin, gentamicin, neomycin, semisynthetic penicillins, spectinomycin, furizolidone and potentiated sulfa drugs. The use of antisecretory drugs, such as bencetimide or loperamide, with or without antibacterial drugs, has been advocated (Solis *et al.*, 1993).

When a flare-up of acute diarrhoea in newborn piglets occurs a more positive approach may be required. This may involve routine dosing of all piglets soon after birth with an antibacterial drug such as gentamicin by injection or spectinomycin or semisynthetic penicillin by mouth. In severe outbreaks such treatment may be repeated daily or twice daily for several days. Oral electrolytes may also be provided and are particularly helpful in preventing dehydration, ionic imbalance and maintaining body condition when diarrhoea occurs in pigs over 7 days of age. The diarrhoea makes them thirsty and they drink the solutions readily. Oral electrolyte solutions usually contain potassium salts and sodium chloride, glycine, dextrose to provide energy, and sometimes additional compounds. It is important that the solution is made up strictly according to the instructions because if it is hypertonic it will have an adverse effect. In underdeveloped countries where modern antibacterial drugs may not be readily available some herb remedies prepared directly from plants seem to be effective.

In a serious outbreak, booster vaccination of all pregnant females may be instituted and additional booster doses given to sows when they are moved to the farrowing house. Feedback of diarrhoeic faeces from the farrowing house to gilts and sows may be started or stepped up (see also under 'Prevention' below). The sow's colostrum may be supplemented with commercially available gamma globulins given orally to every pig or to smaller or weaker piglets and those which are last to be born in each litter. Some people use goat colostrum for this. It is cheaper and can be stored frozen. Cows' colostrum from animals hyperimmunized against K88 and K99 antigens, which has been pasteurized and deep frozen in small batches, is also a useful adjunct, two doses of 10 ml each being given soon after birth and a few hours later (M.R. Muirhead, Garth Veterinary Group, Beeford, York, 1993, personal communication). Plasma or serum from sows at slaughter has also been used but the results have been disappointing. Furthermore, collecting blood at slaughter houses carries the risk of contamination with other pathogens and feeding it without sterilization to pigs may be illegal in some countries.

It is important also to check the farrowing house management as discussed under 'Prevention' below.

Role of Antibodies

Passively acquired maternal antibodies play a vitally important role in the prevention of neonatal colibacillosis. To be protected against ETEC and other potential infectious pathogens in the farrowing house, the piglet must ingest an adequate quantity of its dam's colostrum as soon after birth as possible. This not only provides a wide spectrum of circulating and mucosally associated antibodies but also energy, physiological homeostasis and warmth. It also satisfies the piglet's hunger drive so that it can rest contentedly in a clean warm protected place for an hour or so until it feeds again.

The role of colostrum and lactogenic immunity in the pig has been reviewed by Roth (1992). Colostrum contains a high level of the gamma globulins IgG, IgM and IgA, in roughly similar proportions to those in the dam's plasma. The intestines of the newborn piglet are immature and lacking in proteolytic enzymes. They are able to absorb the gamma globulins unchanged to reach a level and spectrum in the blood stream comparable to that of the dam's. The piglets' ability to absorb gamma globulins declines over the first 12 hours after birth. It declines more rapidly if the piglet eats or drinks, but more slowly if the piglet is prevented from ingesting liquid or solid food.

The passively acquired circulating antibodies provide a strong defence against systemic infection, including coliform septicaemia, but are not effective against ETEC since these organisms are confined to the intestine. During the time that colostral antibodies are in the intestines, they do provide protection against adherence and proliferation of ETEC. In this setting, the main defence is secretory IgA (SIgA) (Allen and Porter, 1973). Normal sows' milk, postcolostrum, has a low but effective level of SIgA which maintains the protection. Unlike the calf and lamb, it is essential for the piglet to suck its dam every 1–2 hours in order to replenish and sustain this protection.

Ninety per cent of the IgA in sows' milk is produced by primed plasma cells in the subepithelial tissue of the mammary gland. The other 10% is derived from sows' plasma. It is transported through the epithelial cells into the lumen of the acini and small ducts and in so doing picks up a secretory component. This component confers important additional characterisitics on the IgA dimer. It protects against proteolysis by intestinal and bacterial enzymes and also aids in absorption into the mucus which bathes the inner surface of the intestine. Secretory IgA thus provides a barrier against infection. If SIgA has specificity for the fimbrial adhesin, it blocks adhesion of ETEC to the enterocytes. With the aid of complement and lysozyme, it may bring about bacteriolysis. SIgA also neutralizes LT but not ST.

The secretory IgA response of the sows' mammary gland results from specific antigenic stimulation by ETEC of cells of the immune system, mainly in the Peyer's patches of the intestines, with consequent lymphocyte trafficking terminating as specific IgA plasma cells in the mammary tissue. Experimentally it can be brought about by injection of antigen direct into the mammary tissue. Injection into one gland will result in the production of specific secretory IgA in all the glands.

The lactogenic immunity, mediated by secretory IgA, lasts throughout lactation but seems to be most effective in the first week, its effectiveness apparently waning at 10–14 days postpartum. At weaning the provision of this passive protection obviously ceases and the passively acquired mucosally associated antibodies rapidly decline.

First litter gilts are generally less able to provide a fully adequate level of passive immunity than mature sows. Whether this is solely due to lack of intestinal antigenic stimulation or whether the relatively late development of the mammary gland and its immune system plays a role is not known.

Prevention

Although ETEC are necessary primary pathogens in *E. coli* diarrhoea, for practical purposes colibacillosis is best thought of as primarily a husbandry disease since husbandry factors play such an important predisposing role. Management of the dry sow and gilt and of the pigs in the farrowing room is all important in prevention.

Factors that influence the incidence of neonatal diarrhoea include stimulation of the mucosal immune system of the dry sows and gilts by exposure to ETEC antigens naturally or by vaccination, a non-slip surface for the piglets in the first hour or so of life, provision of a warm dry environment for the piglets, a high standard of hygiene in the farrowing rooms, and quiet sow and gilt management to allow uninterrupted farrowing and suckling.

Stimulation of the mucosally associated antibodies by exposure of the dry sows and gilts to ETEC antigens can be brought about and enhanced in a number of ways. If the animals are loose housed in pens or straw yards it may be sufficient to put faeces from the farrowing house in with them on the floor in the feeding area. If the dry sows and gilts are individually housed in stalls, they will have little access to faeces at all and it may be necessary to take more positive measures. Piglet faeces from the farrowing rooms can be mixed in a grinder with water and poured on to the feed of the dry sows and gilts in amounts of about 100–250 ml per animal twice or three times each week from about 4 weeks to about 4 days prior to farrowing. Diarrhoeic faeces can be swabbed up with paper towels and put in the mix. Some veterinarians advise that small amounts of afterbirth be ground up with the mixture to provide a protective vehicle for the ETEC en route through the stomach to the intestines. (This should not be confused with feedback of afterbirth to prevent the SMEDI (still births, mummification, embryonic death and infertility) syndrome.)

Feedback is highly effective in preventing diarrhoea in the first few days of life but it is less effective in diarrhoea in older suckled piglets, possibly because ETEC may then not be the primary or sole cause. Feedback is contraindicated in herds with endemic swine dysentery or clinical cases of erysipelas. It will not prevent piglet dysentery caused by *Clostridium perfringens* and may make it worse.

In some herds feedback is carried out routinely on a continuous basis. In others, it is only adopted when there are flare-ups of colibacillosis. Some pig attendants find it aesthetically displeasing and object to carrying it out at all.

A variety of vaccines are commercially available and are used as an alternative or supplement to feedback. In theory, oral dosing of ETEC antigens should be more effective in stimulating lactogenic immunity than parenteral vaccines. Kohler (1974) showed that piglets could be protected against neonatal enteric colibacillosis with colostrum and milk from sows which had been dosed orally during pregnancy with cultures in milk prepared from the small intestinal contents of piglets with diarrhoea. This method of boosting immunity was adopted by practising veterinarians mainly in the USA to suppress serious outbreaks of piglet diarrhoea. It was effective but with the advent of more sophisticated commercial vaccines has largely fallen out of use. Porter and co-workers (Porter, 1973a; Allen *et al.*, 1982) in the UK developed a commercial feed in which the particles were coated with *E. coli* antigens. It was fed to preparturient sows for the colostral protection of their piglets postpartum (Chidlow and Porter, 1978). This feed is no longer commercially available.

The majority of commercially available vaccines used today are for parenteral injection of pregnant gilts and sows. They consist variously of inactivated whole bacterial cells of selected serogroups and/or purified fimbrial antigens F4, F5, F6 and F41, sometimes with detoxified LT enterotoxin included and usually with an adjuvant. Methods such as recombinant DNA technology have helped to refine such vaccines. They are usually given twice, about 6 and 2 weeks prepartum, during the first pregnancy and once during subsequent ones. In some herds they are given routinely to gilts and sows of all parities, in others only to first pregnancy gilts, and in others they are only used to suppress outbreaks when they occur. In theory they only stimulate a humoral response which would not be likely to provide much intestinal protection. It may be that specific IgG leakage into the intestine occurs because in practice these vaccines are useful as an aid to boosting immunity but do not result in solid protection and are not usually as effective as oral dosing.

The presence of high levels of protective antibodies in colostrum and milk are no use unless the newborn piglet can suck the sow's teats soon after birth and frequently thereafter. A delay in taking the first drink of colostrum allows colonization of the intestine and adhesion to the villi by ETEC. Such a delay can be brought about by wet slippery floors particularly if the newborn piglet has a tendency to splaylegs, or by maternal problems such as swollen sore mammary glands, mastitis, agalactia or piglet-savaging by gilts. A quiet calm farrowing room environment is also helpful because frequent disturbances interrupt farrowing and suckling.

A constantly warm and dry environment for the piglet is important for several reasons. The young piglet has limited control over its body temperature and is quickly chilled. This reduces its energy and hunger drive and lowers its already fragile immunity, predisposing it to colibacillosis. Dampness and draughts exacerbate this downward spiral. Worn wet farrowing house floors, poor drainage, and too rapid turn-around of pens which have not had time to dry, are likely to lead to colibacillosis.

A high standard of hygiene in the farrowing house is also important. The maternally derived colostral and lactogenic immunity is finite and can be overwhelmed by high oral doses of ETEC. Each successive litter that is born builds up the concentration of *E. coli* in the farrowing room. To break this cycle all-in all-out farrowing room systems can be adopted with a thorough clean-up, disinfection and drying between each batch. This is relatively easy to organize in large herds, particularly if the farrowing rooms are small, but may be difficult in smaller herds. Whether all-in all-out farrowing is used, it is important that the water and creep feed available to the piglet is clean, fresh, and not contaminated by faeces, and that there is no dirty water lying in pools which the piglet may drink. Bedding, if used, should be clean and adequate. Prompt and thorough treatment of piglets when they develop diarrhoea is also helpful in slowing the build-up of virulent strains.

The ration fed to the sow and the feeding regime before farrowing and during the suckling period has a bearing on piglet diarrhoea but the detailed mechanisms involved are imprecise. Ready availability of clean water for the sow is also important. Some sows are reluctant to rise to drink before and just after farrowing, they become dehydrated which may then lead to poor milk flow. Oedema of the udder which may result from a poor feeding and watering regime, may also inhibit milk flow.

The overall aim of the farrowing room attendants should be to ensure that the delicate balance between ETEC and maternally derived immunity is always weighted in favour of the latter.

An additional approach to prevention has been suggested, namely to breed pigs for hereditary resistance to ETEC adhesive antigen (Sellwood *et al.*, 1975). It has been shown that within pig populations some individual pigs lack the enterocyte receptor for the F4 (K88) fimbrial antigen. This trait however is mediated by a recessive gene. Thus three genotypes exist. Homozygous dominant (SS) and heterozygous piglets (Ss) possess the receptor and are susceptible; homozygous recessive (ss) piglets do not possess the receptor and are resistant.

Litters born to SS or Ss sows in a herd in which virulent F4 bearing ETEC are in high numbers are protected by specific antibodies in colostrum and milk. Litters born to ss sows by an ss boar are also protected because the F4 antigen cannot adhere. But litters born to ss sows by Ss or SS boars are highly susceptible to F4-ETEC because they possess receptors but their dams provide insufficient specific lactogenic antibodies, presumably because of lack of multiplication of F4-ETEC in their intestines. Consequently, although some attempts have been made to breed pure ss lines they have not been adopted on any scale. Two additional reasons for not breeding pure ss lines are that this would reduce the selection pressure on other more economically desirable traits and no protection would be offered against ETEC strains which produce adhesins other than F4.

Combinations of *E. coli* and Other Agents

Other non-infectious factors, mostly associated with poor management (as outlined in 'Prevention' above), predispose to piglet colibacillosis but unlike diarrhoea in the calf, the majority of cases of diarrhoea caused by ETEC in piglets up to about 5 days of age appear to have a single aetiology and other infectious agents are rarely implicated at the same time. The recent exception to this is porcine reproductive and respiratory syndrome (PRRS) virus. Virulent strains of PRRS virus entering a naive herd for the first time may trigger off severe neonatal colibacillosis. Sometimes ETEC can be cultured from faeces of piglets with TGE but it seems unlikely that they play any role since the villi are badly damaged and antibacterial therapy has no effect. Detailed investigation of diarrhoea in the older suckled piglet may reveal other *E. coli* serotypes, rotavirus and/or coccidia and other viruses as well as ETEC (Wilson and Francis, 1986) but it is not known whether there is any interplay among them.

Concluding Remarks

Substantial developments in understanding characteristics of ETEC implicated in neonatal diarrhoea in pigs began in the early 1960s. These observations have led to improvements in our ability to detect ETEC in the laboratory, to carry out epidemiological studies, to prevent disease and to treat affected piglets. Vaccination of pregnant sows to protect nursing piglets against ETEC diarrhoea is now common practice, which appears to have resulted in a reduction in incidence and severity of disease. However, the fact that the major virulence attributes of ETEC are plasmid borne and that *E. coli* is highly adaptable suggest that a vigilant watch needs to be maintained for the appearance of new types of porcine ETEC.

Acknowledgements

The author is grateful for information and advice freely given by P.W. Blackburn, W.T. Christianson, J. Connor, D.J. Hampson, R.J. Higgins, J. Hunter, M.A. Jones, M.A. Holmes, T. Loula, M.R. Muirhead and C. Wray and for the help of H. Lindsay in the preparation of the script and references.

References

Allen, W.D. and Porter, P. (1970) The demonstration of immunoglobulins in porcine intestinal tissue by immunofluorescence with observations on the effect of fixation. *Immunology* 18, 799–806.

Allen, W.D. and Porter, P. (1973) Localization by immunofluorescence of secretory component and IgA in the intesinal mucosa of the young pig. *Immunology* 24, 365–374.

Allen, W.D., Lingwood, M., Blades, J.A. and Porter, P. (1982) Novel mucosal antimicrobial functions associated with 'in-feed' vaccination using Intagen (Unifeeds Ltd). A review of international trials evaluating environmental and production parameters in sows and piglets. In: *Proceedings of the Seventh International Pig Veterinary Society Congress, Mexico*. IPVS, p. 17.

Arbuckle, J.B.R. (1972) The attachment of some intestinal pathogenic bacteria to small intestinal villi of pigs. In: *Proceedings of the Second International Pig Veterinary Society Congress, Hannover*. IPVS, p. 15.

Bertschinger, H.U. and Moon, H.W. (1972) Localisation of enteropathogenic *Escherichia coli* in ligated intestinal loops of piglets. In: *Proceedings of the Second International Pig Veterinary Society Congress, Hannover*. IPVS, p. 24.

Blood, D.C. and Studdert, V.P. (1988) *Baillières Comprehensive Veterinary Dictionary*. Chaucer Press, London, p. 614.

Brandenburg, A.C. and Wilson, M.R. (1972) IgG immunoglobulin in passive immunity to colibacillosis in pigs. In: *Proceedings of the Second International Pig Veterinary Society Congress, Hannover*. IPVS, p. 47.

Chidlow, J.W. and Porter, P. (1978) The role of oral immunisation in stimulating *Escherichia coli* antibody of the IgM class in porcine colostrum. *Research in Veterinary Science* 24, 254–257.

Dobrescu, L. and Huygelen, C. (1972) Comparative studies of *E. coli* enterotoxins in pigs and in laboratory animals. In: *Proceedings of the Second International Pig Veterinary Society Congress, Hannover*. IPVS, p. 47.

Dunne, H.W. (1958) Streptococcosis and colibacillosis. In: Dunne, H.W. (ed.) *Diseases of Swine*. Iowa State University Press, Ames, Iowa, pp. 371–376.

Dunne, H.W. (1964) Streptococcosis, colibacillosis and bordetellosis. In: Dunne, H.W. (ed.) *Diseases of Swine*. Iowa State University Press, Ames, Iowa, pp. 462–467.

Dunne, H.W. and Bennett, P.C. (1970) Colibacillosis and edema disease. In: Dunne, H.W. (ed.) *Diseases of Swine*, 3rd edn. Iowa State University Press, Ames, Iowa, pp. 597–616.

Fairbrother, J.M. (1992) Enteric colibacillosis. In: Leman, A.D., Straw, B.E., Mengeling, W.L., D'Allaire, S. and Taylor, D.J. (eds) *Diseases of Swine*, 7th edn. Iowa State University Press, Ames, Iowa, pp. 489–497.

Faubert, C. and Drolet, R. (1992) Hemorrhagic gastroenteritis caused by *Escherichia coli* in piglets: clinical, pathological and microbiological findings. *Canadian Veterinary Journal* 33, 251–256.

Fishwick, V.C. (1947) *Pigs; Their Breeding, Feeding, and Management*. Crosby Lockwood and Son Ltd, London.

Gaastra, W. and de Graaf, F.K. (1982) Host-specific fimbrial adhesins of non-invasive enterotoxigenic *Escherichia coli* strains. *Microbiological Reviews* 46, 129–161.

Gyles, C.L. (1986) *Escherichia coli*. In: Gyles, C.L. and Thoen, C.O. (eds) *Pathogenesis of Bacterial Infections in Animals*. Iowa State University Press, Ames, Iowa, pp. 114–131.

Gyles, C.L. and Barnum, D.A. (1967) *Escherichia coli* in ligated segments of pig intestine. *Journal of Pathology and Bacteriology* 94, 189–194.

Hampson, D.J., Woodward, J.M. and Connaughton, I.D. (1993) Genetic analysis of *Escherichia coli* from porcine postweaning diarrhoea. *Epidemiology and Infection* 110, 575–581.

Harel, J., LaPointe, H., Fallara, A., Lortie, L.A., Bigras-Poulin, M., Larivière, S. and Fairbrother, J.M. (1990) Detection of genes for fimbrial antigens and enterotoxins associated with *Escherichia coli* serogroups isolated from pigs with diarrhoea. *Journal of Clinical Microbiology* 29, 745–752.

Kohler, E.M. (1974) Protection of pigs against neonatal enteric colibacillosis with colostrum and milk from orally infected sows. *American Journal of Veterinary Research* 35, 331–338.

Kramer, T. (1969) Effects of various *E. coli* strains on pathogen free 1-day old fasting pigs. In: *Proceedings of the First International Pig Veterinary Society Congress, Cambridge*. IPVS, p. 26.

Kramer, T.T. and Nderito, P.C. (1967) Experimental *Escherichia coli* diarrhoea in hysterectomy-derived, one day old, fasting pigs. *American Journal of Veterinary Research* 28, 959–964.

Kuhn, I., Franklin, A., Soderlind, O. and Mollby, R. (1985) Phenotypic variations among enterotoxigenic *Escherichia coli* from Swedish piglets with diarrhoea. *Medical Microbiology and Immunology* 174, 119–130.

Leman, A.D., Straw, B.E., Mengeling, W.L., D'Allaire, S. and Taylor, D.J. (eds) (1992) *Diseases of Swine*, 7th edn. Iowa State University Press, Ames, Iowa.

Levine, M.M. (1987) *Escherichia coli* that cause diarrhoea: enterotoxigenic, enteropathogenic, enteroinvasive, enterohemorrhagic and enteroadherent. *Journal of Infectious Diseases* 155, 377–389.

Moon, H.W. (1990) Colonization factor antigens of enterotoxigenic *Escherichia coli* in animals. *Current Topics in Microbiology and Immunology* 151, 147–165.

Moon, H.W., Sorensen, D.K. and Sautter, J.M. (1966) *Escherichia coli* infection of the ligated intestinal loop of the newborn pig. *American Journal of Veterinary Research* 27, 1317–1325.

Moon, H.W., Sorensen, D.K. and Sautter, J.M. (1968) Experimental enteric colibacillosis in piglets. *Canadian Journal of Comparative Medicine* 32, 493–497.

Moon, H.W., Schneider, R.A. and Moseley, S.L. (1986) Comparative prevalence of four enterotoxin genes among *Escherichia cloi* isolated from swine. *American Journal of Veterinary Research* 47, 210–212.

Morrison, R. (1926) *The Individuality of the Pig*. John Murray, London, p. 325.

Mullaney, C.D., Francis, D.M. and Willgohs, J.A. (1991) Comparison of seroagglutination, ELISA, and indirect fluorescent antibody staining for the detection of K99, K88, and 987P pilus antigens of *Escherichia coli*. *Journal of Veterinary Diagnostic Investigation* 3, 115–118.

Nagy, B., Arp, L.H., Moon, H.W. and Casey, T.A. (1992) Colonization of the small intestine of weaned pigs by enterotoxigenic *Escherichia coli* that lack known colonization factors. *Veterinary Pathology* 29, 239–246.

Pensaert, M.B. (ed.) (1989) *Virus Infections of Porcines*. Elsevier Science, Amsterdam.

Pesti, L. and Semjén, G. (1972) Studies on heat stable and heat-labile enterotoxins of swine-enteropathogenic *E. coli* strains isolated from Hungary. In: *Proceedings of the Second International Pig Veterinary Society Congress*. IPVS, p. 127.

Porter, P. (1973a) An 'in-feed' *Escherichia coli* vaccine for oral immunisation in the young pig. *Veterinary Annual* 13, 65–68.

Porter, P. (1973b) Intestinal defence in the young pig – a review of the secretory antibody systems and their possible role in oral immunisation. *Veterinary Record* 92, 658–664.

Porter, P., Noakes, D.E. and Allen, W.D. (1970) Secretory IgA and antibodies to *Escherichia coli* in porcine colostrum and milk and their significance in the alimentary tract of the young pig. *Immunology* 18, 245–257.

Rose, R., Whipp, S.C. and Moon, H.W. (1987) Effects of *Escherichia coli* heat stable enterotoxin b on small intestinal villi in pigs, rabbits and lambs. *Veterinary Pathology* 24, 71–79.

Roth, J.A. (1992) Immune system. In: Leman, A.D., Straw, B.E., Mengeling, W.L., D'Allaire, S. and Taylor, D.J. (eds), *Diseases of Swine*, 7th edn. Iowa State University Press, Ames, Iowa, pp. 21–39.

Russell, P.H. and Eddington, N. (1985) *Veterinary Viruses*. Burlington Press, Cambridge.

Rutter, J.M. and Jones, G.W. (1972) The role of the K88 antigen of *Escherichia coli* in neonatal diarrhoea of piglets. In: *Proceedings of the Second International Pig Veterinary Society Congress, Hannover*. IPVS, p. 141.

Sellwood, R., Gibbons, R.A., Jones, G.W. and Rutter, J.M. (1975) Adhesion of enteropathogenic *Escherichia coli* to pig intestinal brush border: The existence of two pig phenotypes. *Journal of Medical Microbiology* 8, 405–411.

Smith, H.W. and Gyles, C.L. (1970) The relationship between two apparently different enterotoxins produced by enteropathogenic strains of *Escherichia coli* of porcine origin. *Journal of Medical Microbiology* 3, 387–401.

Smith, H.W. and Halls, S. (1968) The transmissible nature of the genetic factor in *Escherichia coli* that controls enterotoxin production. *Journal of General Microbiology* 52, 319–334.

Smith, H.W. and Linggood, M.A. (1971) Observations on the pathogenic properties of the K88, Hly and Ent plasmids of *Escherichia coli* with particular reference to porcine diarrhoea. *Journal of Medical Microbiology* 4, 467–485.

Sojka, W.J., Lloyd, M.K. and Sweeney, E.J. (1960) *Escherichia coli* serotypes associated with certain pig diseases. *Research in Veterinary Science* 1, 17–27.

Solis, Ch.A., Sumano, L.H. and Marin, H.H.A. (1993) Treatment of *Escherichia coli* induced diarrhoea in piglets with antisecretory drugs alone or combined with antibacterials. *Pig Veterinary Journal* 30, 83–88.

Taylor, D.J. (1986) *Pig Diseases*, 4th edn. Burlington Press, Cambridge.

Tubbs, R.C., Hurd, H.S., Dargatz, N. and Hill, G. (1993) Preweaning morbidity and mortality in the United States swine herd. *Swine Health and Production* 1, 21–28.

Wilson, R.A. and Francis, D.H. (1986) Fimbriae and enterotoxins associated with *Escherichia coli* serogroups isolated from pigs with colibacillosis. *American Journal of Veterinary Research* 47, 213–217.

Woodward, J.M., Connaughton, I.D., Fahy, V.A., Lymbery, A.J. and Hampson, D.J. (1993) Clonal analysis of *Escherichia coli* of serogroups O9, O20, and O101 isolated from Australian pigs with neonatal diarrhoea. *Journal of Clinical Microbiology* 31, 1185–1188.

Woodward, M.J., Kearsley, R., Wray, C. and Roeder, P.L. (1990) DNA probes for the detection of toxin genes in *Escherichia coli* isolated from diarrhoeal disease in cattle and pigs. *Veterinary Microbiology* 22, 277–290.

8

Postweaning *Escherichia coli* Diarrhoea in Pigs

D.J. Hampson
School of Veterinary Studies, Murdoch University, Murdoch, Western Australia 6150

History and Significance

It is common for piglets to develop a diarrhoea which starts 3–10 days after weaning. This condition, which has been called porcine postweaning diarrhoea (PWD), was first clearly described in Canada by Richards and Fraser (1961), who associated it with a proliferation of beta-haemolytic *E. coli* in the proximal small intestines of affected pigs. Previously, throughout the 1950s, there had been numerous reports of the role that specific serotypes of haemolytic *E. coli* played in the aetiology of oedema disease (see Sojka, 1965). Oedema disease is essentially a toxaemia of weaned pigs, although it is sometimes accompanied by diarrhoea (Smith and Halls, 1968). Other less common toxaemic conditions associated with haemolytic *E. coli* are the 'shock in weaner syndrome' and 'haemorrhagic enteritis' (reviewed by Morris and Sojka, 1985). This chapter is restricted to a consideration of PWD.

Throughout the 1960s, as the pig industry in Europe and the USA became more intensively managed, PWD was recognized as being widespread. Numerous attempts were made to elucidate its pathogenesis (Gregory, 1962; Kenworthy and Crabbe, 1963; Smith and Jones, 1963; Palmer and Hulland 1965; Kenworthy and Allen, 1966; Smith and Halls, 1968). Much of the experimental work at this time was on pigs weaned at 3–4 weeks of age, even though it was then more usual to wean pigs commercially at 6–8 weeks. Most piggeries now wean at 3–4 weeks, and it has been suggested that this trend towards early weaning may have been responsible for a parallel increase in the occurrence of PWD in the intervening years (Blood and Radostits, 1989).

Postweaning colibacillosis is still a major cause of economic loss to the pig industry from both mortality and reduced growth rates (van Beers-Schreurs *et al.*, 1992), and is the most common cause of postweaning mortality on many farms, killing 1.5–2.0% of pigs weaned. In Australia, for example, loss of production on typically affected piggeries, excluding expenditure on antimicrobial drugs, has been estimated to cost around $80 per year for every sow (Cutler and Gardner, 1988).

Although specific serotypes of *E. coli* have a central role in the aetiology of PWD, the condition is complex and multifactorial. Even in the absence of diarrhoea, early-weaned pigs usually show a reduction in growth rate in the fortnight after weaning (Leece *et al.*, 1979; Armstrong and Clawson, 1980; Hampson, 1983). This poor performance is not surprising given the nutritional, physiological, psychological and often environmental stresses that are imposed on early-weaned pigs. These factors may also predispose to the development of PWD (see below).

Clinical Aspects of *E. coli* PWD

The principal sign in PWD is a fluid, yellowish or grey diarrhoea, lasting for a week or more and causing progressive emaciation (Richards and Fraser, 1961). Affected pigs appear depressed, their appetite is reduced, they develop a rough hair coat, become pot-bellied and may shiver. Sometimes one or more pigs in good condition may die suddenly at the outset of the disease. Signs of diarrhoea usually start within 3–5 days of weaning, and, over a 2–3 day period, most of the pigs in a group become affected to a greater or lesser extent. The group mortality rate can reach 25% in the absence of adequate medication.

Pigs which have died are usually in poor condition and are dehydrated. Their small intestines are hyperaemic, dilated, thin walled and contain varying amounts of fluid contents and accumulations of gas. The stomach is often full, and the contents of the large intestine may be semifluid. Heavy growths of haemolytic *E. coli* can be recovered from sites throughout the intestinal tract (Svendsen, 1974; Svendsen *et al.*, 1977).

According to Fahy *et al.* (1987), a second form of disease is seen on some farms. This starts at around 10 days after weaning, and, whilst there is often chronic diarrhoea, variable neurological signs may also be seen. This syndrome would appear to be a form of oedema disease rather than typical PWD.

Characteristics of *E. coli* Involved in PWD

Origin

When pigs are weaned, at whatever age and regardless of whether PWD occurs or not, it is usual for there to be a sudden increase in numbers of haemolytic *E. coli* throughout the small and large intestines (Kenworthy and Crabbe, 1963; Hinton *et al.*, 1985). It is uncommon to detect these bacteria in the gastrointestinal tract of sucking pigs, or in mature animals. They are presumably present however, since investigation into the source of these bacteria in weaned pigs has demonstrated that they can be carried into a new unused weaner house by healthy sucking pigs (Hampson *et al.*, 1987). Colonization of weaners can also occur following their exposure to the contaminated environment of weaner houses that have contained pigs (Hampson *et al.*, 1987).

Haemolysin

Haemolytic strains of *E. coli* appear to have some selective advantage that allows them to proliferate and to dominate the intestinal *E. coli* flora of newly weaned pigs. Many of these haemolytic strains have the potential to induce PWD, although occasionally non-haemolytic strains may be associated with the condition (Hoblet *et al.*, 1986a). Smith and Linggood (1971) investigated the role of the *E. coli* haemolysin as a virulence determinant by undertaking curing experiments to remove the Hly plasmid that codes for the haemolysin. The resulting non-haemolytic cured strain was still capable of colonizing and inducing diarrhoea after experimental challenge. This demonstrated that the haemolysin is not an essential virulence factor. It does not exclude the likelihood that, under natural conditions, the strains possessing the haemolysin are best adapted to colonize the intestines of recently weaned pigs.

Serotypes

Strains of *E. coli* that cause PWD are of a limited range of serotypes. Some of these serotypes may also be isolated from cases of neonatal diarrhoea, although not all neonatal strains cause PWD (Svendsen, 1974). Some of the more common serotypes reported from cases of PWD are shown in Table 8.1. The studies referred to in the table varied in a number of respects, including size and methodology, but generally it can be seen that the main O groups involved in various parts of the world have been O8, O138, O139, O141, O147, O149 and O157. Of these, O8, O141 and O149 are most commonly reported worldwide. O149 is particularly interesting since it only emerged as an important serogroup in the late

Table 8.1 Some serogroups[a] of *E. coli* reported from cases of porcine postweaning diarrhoea.

Serogroup	Authors[b]/location/period										
	1 UK 1961	2 — 1968	3 Ontario 1967–70	4 Denmark 1971	5 Denmark 1970–75	6 Switzerland 1977	7 USA 1980–82	8 Japan 1981–84	9 Sweden 1983–84	10 Hungary 1980s?	11 Canada 1979–89
O8:K87				+	+			+	+	+	+
O8:K87:K88	+	+	+[c]				+		+	+	+
O45:'E65',K88			+								+
O116:'V17':K88			+[c]								
O138:K81			+	+	+	+				+	+
O139:K82				+		+				+	+
O141:K85a,b / O141:K85a,c	+	+		+	+	+[c]		+	+	+	+
O141:K87		+									
O141:K85a,c:K88a,b	+	+									
O147:K87		+	+		+					+	+
O149:K91				+[c]	+[c]			+[c]	+[c]	+	+
O149:K91:K88						+[c]	+[c]	+	+[c]	+[c]	+
O157						+	+	+[c]		+	+

[a] Other serogroups less commonly encountered: O9; O10; O20; O26; O35; O64; O98; O101; O115; O119 (Fahy *et al.*, 1987; Soderlind *et al.*, 1988; Harel *et al.*, 1991); K antigens not always specified.
[b] Authors: 1, Sojka, 1965; 2, Nielsen *et al.*, 1968; 3, Gyles *et al.*, 1971; 4, Dam and Knox, 1974; 5, Larsen, 1976; 6, Bertschinger *et al.*, 1979a; 7, Wilson and Francis, 1986; 8, Nakazawa *et al.*, 1987; 9, Soderlind *et al.*, 1988; 10, Nagy *et al.*, 1990; 11, Harel *et al.*, 1991.
[c] Predominant serotype(s) in that study.

1960s and early 1970s (Dam and Knox, 1974). O157 also appears to have been more frequently encountered in the late 1970s and 1980s than it was previously. Regional differences also seem to occur, with, for example, O45 only being frequently reported from Canada. It is generally assumed that the disease induced by these different serotypes is identical.

The question of why only a limited range of serotypes cause PWD is not fully answered. It might be predicted that *E. coli* which cause PWD consist of a few clonal groups that have become widely disseminated throughout the world. These would possess specific virulence determinants or other selective advantages that would allow them to proliferate in the intestines of weaned pigs, and thence to cause PWD. This does not seem to be the case, however, since the genetic diversity amongst serotypes from pigs with PWD is in the same order as that seen for the whole species (Hampson *et al.*, 1993). This implies that something specifically associated with or linked to these particular somatic antigen types facilitates their ability to establish and proliferate in the newly weaned pig intestine, independent of their overall genetic background.

Adhesive factors

Where PWD occurs, viable counts of haemolytic *E. coli* in the anterior jejunum are 10^3–10^5 higher than in healthy weaners (Svendsen *et al.*, 1977). These bacteria are closely associated with the intestinal mucosa, and possess specific adhesive factors which prevent them from being dislodged (Smith and Linggood, 1971). The best characterized of these factors in porcine *E. coli* is the K88 pilus or fimbria (Jones and Rutter, 1972). This has been renamed F4, and may be found associated with all the main PWD serogroups, but particularly with O149 (Tzipori, 1985). These fimbriae can exist as antigenic variants, K88ab, K88ac and K88ad, all of which allow adhesion to villous enterocytes throughout the small intestine. Other pili on porcine *E. coli* include K99 (F5), 987P (F6) and F41, but these are not commonly associated with PWD strains (Nakazawa *et al.*, 1987; Nagy *et al.*, 1990).

The absence of the four major pili on many PWD strains led to a search for other adhesive factors. A new fimbria called F107 has been demonstrated on an oedema-disease strain of the O139 serogroup (Bertschinger *et al.*, 1990), whilst other fimbriae have been recorded on PWD strains of the O141 serogroup (Kennan and Monckton, 1990), and on O141 and O157 serogroups (Nagy *et al.*, 1992). Isolates bearing such 'fine pili', called 2134P, apparently preferentially colonize villi over Peyer's patches (Nagy *et al.*, 1992). Another colonization factor called '8813' has also recently been found on PWD strains of serogroups O25, O108, O138, O141, O147 and O157 (Salajka *et al.*, 1992). It is not clear how this colonization factor relates to the 'fine pili' of Nagy *et al.* (1992), but colonization factors of this sort may ultimately be found to be common to many PWD strains. Since susceptibility of the porcine intestine to adhesion by the new pili described by Nagy *et al.* (1992) apparently increases over the first 3 weeks of life, this may offer an explanation of why these strains are only prevalent in weaned pigs.

Interestingly, it has been suggested that isolates bearing the K88 pilus are more likely to cause diarrhoea around 4 days after weaning, whilst isolates that lack K88 tend to cause diarrhoea 7–10 days postweaning (Fahy *et al.*, 1987). This difference may be associated with changes that occur in the small intestinal mucosa and associated epithelial receptors in the period immediately after weaning. In experiments conducted in one piggery it was shown that haemolytic isolates of serogroup 0138 usually predominated after weaning, but that a strain of serogroup 0139 could be induced to proliferate later, either following movement of weaner pigs, or if pigs were weaned, returned to the sow, and then weaned again (Hampson *et al.*, 1988a).

Toxins

E. coli isolates from PWD are mostly enterotoxigenic (ETEC strains), producing either heat stable toxin ‘a’ (STa), heat stable toxin ‘b’ (STb), heat labile toxin (LT), or combinations of these (Morris and Sojka, 1985). Enterotoxins induce a secretory diarrhoea, generally without inducing histological changes, although STb may cause shortening of villi (Rose *et al.*, 1987). The small intestine apparently becomes more susceptible to enterotoxins immediately after weaning (Stevens *et al.*, 1972). STa for example only causes fluid accumulation in the intestines of piglets less than 2 weeks of age (Burgess *et al.*, 1978), or in those that have just been weaned (Mezoff *et al.*, 1991). The genes encoding the enterotoxins, like those for most of the fimbriae, are located on transmissible plasmids (Smith and Huggins, 1978).

Some PWD isolates produce another toxin, called verotoxin 2e (VT2e), or Shiga-like toxin type-II variant (SLT-IIv). Isolates produce VT2 either with or without the production of enterotoxins (Smith *et al.*, 1983; Nagy *et al.*, 1990). SLT-IIv is mainly produced by classical oedema disease serotypes (O138, O139 and O141), although not exclusively (Smith *et al.*, 1983; Gannon *et al.*, 1988). It has been suggested that SLT-IIv could play a role in PWD (Gannon *et al.*, 1988; Harel *et al.*, 1991), but this has not been established experimentally. Certain other strains of serotype O45:K‘E65’ do not possess known toxins or adhesins, but may produce attaching-effacing lesions on the brush border of enterocytes in the small and large intestine (Hélie *et al.*, 1991). It has been suggested that this could be a mechanism in the development of some forms of PWD (Harel *et al.*, 1991). Recently *E. coli* strains lacking any recognized enterotoxin, cytotoxin, invasion or effacement traits have been shown to cause fluid diarrhoea in rabbit models following intestinal colonization (Schlager *et al.*, 1990). The significance of this finding is not known in relation to the aetiology of PWD in pigs, but it may be important. In one study in Japan, for example, almost 50% of *E. coli* strains isolated from cases of PWD produced neither LT nor STa, although assays for other toxins, including STb, were not conducted (Nakazawa *et al.*, 1987).

Predisposition to PWD

Background

Although there is a strong association between colonization of the small intestine of recently weaned pigs by haemolytic ETEC and the occurrence of diarrhoea, oral dosing with these bacteria often fails to induce disease (Smith and Jones, 1963; Kenworthy and Allen, 1966; Armstrong and Cline, 1977). Furthermore, haemolytic strains proliferate in the intestinal tracts of healthy pigs after weaning, although to lower numbers than in littermates that develop diarrhoea (Kenworthy and Crabb, 1963; Svendsen *et al.*, 1977). In some cases poor colonization may be linked to an absence of appropriate receptors for K88 fimbriae on the brush borders of small intestinal enterocytes (Sarmiento *et al.*, 1988). Resistance to colonization is not common, since the presence of the receptor is controlled by an autosomal dominant gene (Gibbons *et al.*, 1977). Other genetic factors influencing susceptibility probably also operate. Smith and Halls (1968) used an enterotoxigenic strain of O141:K85ac, which lacked K88, to reproduce diarrhoea and oedema disease in weaned pigs. This strain colonized pigs from nine different farms, but disease was only reproduced in animals from one of the sources. The inoculated strain was present in the faeces of pigs from this farm at about two to three logs higher than it was in the animals from the other piggeries. This increased susceptibility could have been due to the presence of receptors for other adhesins possessed by that strain, for example, the recently described F107 adhesin (Stamm and Bertschinger, 1992).

Loss of sows' milk

Although diarrhoea can be induced in unweaned pigs of weaning age by dosing them orally with ETEC (Sarmiento *et al.*, 1988), PWD, by definition, only naturally occurs in newly weaned pigs. Its occurrence is always preceded by the recent withdrawal of sows' milk, and this material has a number of specific and non-specific protective effects. Therefore, the withdrawal of a regular supply of this protective material at weaning increases the opportunity for enteropathogens to proliferate, provided that they possess selective growth advantages over other components of the intestinal flora. The protective influence of milk in weaners has been experimentally demonstrated by supplementing their diet with sows' milk, and thereby inhibiting the normal postweaning proliferation of haemolytic *E. coli* (Deprez *et al.*, 1986).

Physiological factors

Recently weaned pigs appear to be predisposed to develop PWD by a number of physiological changes that occur following weaning. Generally these developmental changes are exacerbated by management practices whereby piglets are weaned at an early age.

Gastric acidity

It has been suggested that the pH of the gastric contents increases to non-bactericidal levels after weaning, and that these changes allow ingested ETEC to survive and gain access to the small intestine (Schulman, 1973). This effect could be important in the spread of infection throughout a pen of pigs. However, Hampson *et al.* (1985) found that weaned pigs tended to have both more acidic gastric contents and fewer viable coliform organisms in the stomach than did unweaned pigs. Initiation of disease is most likely to result from an increase in numbers of bacteria that have already colonized the intestines of piglets before weaning.

Small intestinal structure and function

Piglets develop a series of changes in small intestinal structure and enterocyte brush border enzyme activities immediately after weaning (Kenworthy, 1976; Smith, 1984; Hampson, 1986a; Hampson and Kidder, 1986; Miller *et al.*, 1986). The height of villi can be reduced by 25% within 24 hours of weaning, whilst crypt depth normally increases steadily over an 11-day period after weaning. Other changes occur concomitant with these alterations in architecture of the villi, and with increases in rates of both crypt cell production and shedding of villous enterocytes. For example, brush border lactase activity declines, sucrase declines to a minimum by 5 days after weaning, then increases, the maltases increase, whilst alkaline phosphatase is largely unaffected. Sodium-dependent alanine transport and capacity for xylose absorption are reduced. The net effect is a temporary reduction in intestinal digestive and absorptive function after weaning.

There are probably different components to these changes, and their causes are still disputed (Hampson, 1987a). They have been suggested to be the result of hypersensitivity to dietary antigens (Miller *et al.*, 1984), to the action of viruses (Lecce *et al.*, 1983), to a lack of dietary intake (Kelly *et al.*, 1984) or to be normal adaptive changes that are exaggerated by early weaning (Hampson, 1983; Kelly *et al.*, 1991a). Whatever the exact causes, these changes could predispose to PWD. A reduction in digestive and absorptive function of the small intestine would encourage the development of an osmotic diarrhoea, whilst unabsorbed dietary material might act as a substrate for ETEC in the gastrointestinal tract. Furthermore, changes in villous enterocyte populations might expose new receptors, for example for the ETEC strains that do not possess K88 (Nagy *et al.*, 1992).

Fermentation in the large intestine

Unweaned pigs have small, underdeveloped large intestines, which rapidly increase in size and content following weaning at 3 weeks of age (Hampson, 1987b). The large intestine is a major site of water and electrolyte absorption in the weaned pig (Hamilton and Roe, 1977), and this activity is facilitated by absorption of volatile fatty acids (VFAs) (Argenzio, 1982). It has been suggested that newly weaned pigs are predisposed to develop diarrhoea because their large intestinal microflora is incompletely developed. Fermentation is therefore limited, so that water and electrolyte movement associated with absorption of VFAs may also be diminished (Hampson, 1987b). Conversely, it has been argued that consumption of poorly digestible diets by weaner pigs results in increased bacterial fermentation, with an increased VFA production, which in turn causes an osmotic diarrhoea (Etheridge *et al.*, 1984).

Nutritional factors

Many aspects of nutrition have been investigated in relation to the development of PWD and reductions in growth rate. A review of the influence of diet on the development of PWD has been published elsewhere (Hampson, 1987a).

Dietary intake and composition

There are conflicting views about the interaction between dietary intake, both before and after weaning, and the occurrence of PWD. For example, it has been argued that consumption of small amounts of creep food before weaning may 'prime' intestinal hypersensitivity reactions to dietary antigens after weaning, and exacerbate PWD (Miller *et al.*, 1984). Most workers have not been able to substantiate this suggestion (Hampson and Smith, 1986; Hampson *et al.*, 1988b; Kelly *et al.*, 1990a, b; Sarmiento *et al.*, 1990), although there is good evidence that soyabean meal in the diet may be capable of inducing immunological responses that damage the intestine (Dunsford *et al.*, 1989; Li *et al.*, 1990, 1991). Intake of creep feed is probably mainly important in increasing bodyweight at weaning, which in turn reduces the risk of developing PWD (Madec and Josse, 1983).

Restriction of dietary intake after weaning, alone or in combination with an increased fibre content of the diet, reduces both the proliferation of haemolytic *E. coli* and the occurrence of PWD (Smith and Halls, 1968; Bertschinger *et al.*, 1979b). It is generally presumed that this manipulation reduces the amount of substrate available in the intestinal tract, which would otherwise be selectively utilized by haemolytic *E. coli*. Lecce *et al.* (1983) found that a high postweaning nutrient intake fed three times a day produced more prolonged diarrhoea and a greater colonization by haemolytic *E. coli* than did the same diet fed in 24 equal hourly increments per day. Hampson and Smith (1986) also found a direct positive relationship between the amount of weaner diet consumed, the duration of faecal excretion of haemolytic *E. coli*, and the occurrence of PWD. This was not however found in a subsequent experiment (Hampson *et al.*, 1988b). Some workers have noted that high concentrations of fish meal or sugars in the weaner ration predispose to PWD, again presumably by supplying substrate for bacterial proliferation (Smith and Halls, 1968; Vasenius, 1969). Weaned pigs may be particularly susceptible to this effect because they normally develop a 'malabsorption syndrome' after weaning (Kenworthy and Allen, 1966). Their reduced digestive and absorptive capacity may not, however, be as limiting as once thought, since weaned pigs actually have considerable 'spare' digestive capacity for cereal-based weaner diets (Kelly *et al.*, 1991b).

Physical form of the diet

There is some evidence to suggest that feeding liquid weaner diets can reduce the number of coliform bacteria in the intestinal tract (Decuypere and Van der Heyde, 1972), and prevent both postweaning growth reduction (Lecce *et al.*, 1979) and PWD (Tzipori *et al.*, 1984). This is most evident for regularly fed milk-based diets (Deprez *et al.*, 1986), where a direct antibacterial effect can be postulated, but may also occur with other ingredients. In some cases, this protective effect may be associated with other changes in the intestinal tract after weaning. For example, the reductions that normally occur in height of villi, crypt cell production rates and brush border enzyme activities after weaning are apparently triggered by exposure to dry pelleted meal at weaning (Hall and Byrne, 1989). This is supported by the observations that the extent of these morphological changes is reduced if the weaner diet consists of a liquid sow milk replacer (Hampson 1986b), if it is fed as a liquid slurry (Deprez *et al.*, 1987), or if it consists of regular 2-hourly feeds of ewes' milk (Pluske *et al.*, 1991). Whether or not PWD occurs in susceptible pigs in any one situation is therefore likely to be governed by a very complex series of interactions between morphological and functional changes in the intestine, the amount and composition of the dietary ingredients, and the extent of proliferation of haemolytic *E. coli*.

Environmental temperature

Exposing weaned pigs to cold temperatures or to temperature fluctuations predisposes them to PWD (Kelley, 1982). For example, English (1981) found that a sudden drop in temperature could precipitate PWD, even in pigs on an optimal diet. In studies of risk factors associated with the occurrence of PWD, Madec and Josse (1983) identified large temperature fluctuations as conferring a high risk of developing PWD. Under experimental conditions, Wathes *et al.* (1989) also showed that moderate cold stress (15 °C) increased susceptibility to PWD, although restriction of food intake at the same time compensated for this effect.

The mechanism whereby inadequate thermal environments predispose to PWD is not well defined. In experiments by Armstrong and Cline (1977), chilling did cause increased PWD in one group of pigs, but numbers of haemolytic *E. coli* in the intestine were not elevated above the control group. In the experiments of Wathes *et al.* (1989), chilled pigs with PWD did have elevated numbers of haemolytic *E. coli* in their faeces. Chilling increases the rate of passage of ingesta through the intestinal tract (Pouteaux *et al.*, 1982), encourages increased food consumption (Le Dividich *et al.*, 1977), and reduces antibody-mediated immune responses (Blecha and Kelley, 1981). Any or all of these effects could interact in the predisposition to PWD.

Rotavirus infections

Infection with rotavirus has been implicated in some outbreaks of PWD (Lecce and King, 1978). Experimentally, sequential infection of gnotobiotic piglets with rotavirus and haemolytic *E. coli* has been shown to produce a more severe diarrhoea than that resulting from infection with each agent separately (Tzipori *et al.*, 1980). It has been suggested that rotavirus infection at weaning damages the intestine and causes villous atrophy which provides an environment that favours subsequent colonization and growth of haemolytic *E. coli* (Lecce *et al.*, 1982). However, atrophy induced experimentally with transmissible gastroenteritis virus has actually been shown to cause both a marked decrease in intestinal response to *E. coli* heat stable toxins (Whipp *et al.*, 1985), and a diminished susceptibility of villous enterocytes to adhesion with K88ac$^+$ *E. coli* (Cox *et al.*, 1988). Furthermore, damage induced by rotavirus infection at weaning is only short-lived (Hall *et al.*, 1989). These findings cast some doubts on the potential role of rotaviruses in the aetiology of PWD, particularly as rotavirus, with or without haemolytic *E. coli*, can often be recovered from healthy weaned pigs (Hampson *et al.*, 1985; Fu and Hampson, 1987). Moreover, at least one commercially available porcine-origin rotavirus vaccine has been found to be ineffective against PWD (Hoblet *et al.*, 1986b). However, this is not conclusive evidence, since there are a number of groups and serotypes of rotaviruses, and up to five different electrophoretypes of the virus may be found on some piggeries (Fu *et al.*, 1989). Age at weaning may also be important, since piglets weaned at 2 weeks of age have a much higher prevalence of rotavirus excretion than do those weaned at 4–5 weeks (Svensmark, 1983). It remains likely that rotavirus infections can predispose to some outbreaks of PWD.

Diagnosis

Diagnosis of PWD is relatively straightforward, being based on the findings of diarrhoea in groups of weaned pigs, with minimal gross changes in the intestinal mucosa, and recovery of profuse pure growths of haemolytic *E. coli* from the small intestine. Furthermore, the disease is often endemic in many piggeries. The *E. coli* isolates can be further identified by serotyping, and/or examining for specific virulence determinants (colonization factors and toxins). These may be detected using a variety of techniques that are appropriate for each determinant, including immunological assays (e.g. agglutination and coagglutination), biological assays (e.g. CHO cells and Y1 adrenal cells), and methods for identification of specific DNA sequences (polymerase chain reaction and nucleic acid probes). These techniques are described in detail in Chapter 21. Although sophisticated methods for detecting the presence of virulent strains of *E. coli* are now available, some care must be exercised in interpretation since these bacteria may also be found in healthy pigs.

PWD is unlikely to be confused with other diseases, except perhaps intestinal spirochaetosis/colitis, swine dysentery or salmonellosis. These diseases are unlikely to remain confined to newly weaned pigs, usually result in more mucoid diarrhoea or dysentery, and generally cause obvious gross and histological lesions in the mucosa of the large intestines of affected pigs.

Treatment

Affected pigs require antimicrobials and electrolyte replacement therapy. Initially drugs should be given orally or parenterally, and then provided in the water (preferably), or through the feed. Sensitivity testing should be undertaken where possible, since multiple antimicrobial drug resistance is common in strains of *E. coli* from weaned pigs (Gannon *et al.*, 1988). In the first instance, the potentiated sulfonamides or neomycin are recommended. It is also important to reduce predisposing factors, particularly cold and fluctuating environmental temperatures, and to restrict the amount of food available for 2–3 days. A good supply of palatable water should also be available.

Prevention

There are two broad approaches to the prevention of PWD. The first attempts to minimize factors that predispose to PWD, whilst the second is more specifically directed at the *E. coli*. Management factors that predispose to PWD should be addressed wherever practical. Increasing the age at weaning, or preferably weaning on weight (e.g. >6 kg), is helpful, provided there is sufficient space to keep piglets in the farrowing house longer. The temperature in the weaner house at weaning should start in the range 28–32°C, with minimal temperature fluctuations, and no drafts. Stressors such as mixing pigs should be minimized, for example by multiple suckling. A good quality fresh creep feed should be made available, particularly to pigs that are to be weaned at more than 3 weeks of age. The weaner diet can initially consist of the creep feed, but weaner diets in general should be highly digestible and should not contain high concentrations of soyabean meal. A liquid diet based on milk protein is probably ideal, but is neither practical nor economical in most situations. Sometimes it may be necessary to restrict dietary intake in the first few days after weaning, and provide fibre in the diet. Wherever possible, the pigs should not be overstocked, and should have an adequate slatted dunging area. Good hygiene should be maintained, with dung removed daily, and pens thoroughly cleaned and disinfected between groups of pigs.

There are a number of strategies available that are aimed directly at reducing the build-up of numbers of haemolytic *E. coli* in the intestine after weaning. Prophylactic antimicrobials are used in many piggeries, but this is not an ideal situation. Their routine use encourages development of drug resistance, and, indeed, the spectrum of resistance in many PWD strains of *E. coli* is alarming. Addition of organic acids to the water supply or weaner diets is thought to reduce gastric acidity and minimize survival of ingested *E. coli* (Thomlinson and Lawrence, 1981). Again, this procedure has variable results, and may delay onset of PWD rather than prevent it completely. Other workers have supplemented feed with cultures of *Lactobacillus* spp., *Streptococcus faecium* or *Bacillus cereus* to compete for colonization sites for *E. coli*. Generally, the use of these 'probiotics' in weaned pigs has not been particularly helpful (De Cupere *et al.*, 1992). Other approaches include dosing with microencapsulated protease preparations, which are believed to remove receptor sites for K88 (Chandler and Luke, 1987), the addition of non-absorbed antibacterial polymers to the drinking water, or zinc oxide to the feed, the feeding of cows' milk or egg yolk containing specific antibodies against *E. coli* adhesins (Yokoyama *et al.*, 1992), or breeding pigs that are resistant to adhesion by the bacteria (Chandler and Luke, 1987; Stamm and Bertschinger, 1992).

Vaccination has not been widely used as a means of prophylaxis. Bertschinger *et al.* (1979a) demonstrated that administration of live cultures of *E. coli* before weaning offered subsequent protection against PWD, provided that the procedure was combined with low energy diets. Unfortunately this manipulation resulted in depressed growth rates. In Australia, Fahy *et al.* (1987) have had success in controlling PWD using live oral autogenous *E. coli* given before weaning. Although there is little published evidence on the efficacy of killed whole cell bacterins as a means of controlling PWD, personal experience with one of these products in Australia has suggested that they can be helpful in reducing the severity of the disease. With the recognition of new colonization factors, and their likely incorporation into future vaccines, vaccination will probably become the major means of controlling PWD.

References

Argenzio, R.A. (1982) Volatile fatty acid production and absorption from the large intestine of the pig. In: LapLace, J.P., Corring, T. and Rerat, A. (eds) *Digestive Physiology in the Pig*. Institut National de la Recherche Agronomique, Paris, pp. 207–216.

Armstrong, W.D. and Clawson, A.J. (1980) Nutrition and management of early-weaned pigs: effect of increased nutrient concentrations and (or) supplemental liquid feeding. *Journal of Animal Science* 50, 377–384.

Armstrong, W.D. and Cline, T.R. (1977) Effect of various nutrient levels and environmental temperatures on the incidence of colibacillary diarrhea in pigs: intestinal fistulation and titration studies. *Journal of Animal Science* 45, 1042–1050.

Bertschinger, H.U., Tucker, H. and Pfirter, H.P. (1979a) Control of *Escherichia coli* infection in weaned pigs by use of oral immunization combined with a diet low in nutrients. *Fortschritte der Veterinaermedizin* 29, 73–81.

Bertschinger, H.U., Eggenberger, E., Tucker, H. and Pfirter, H.P. (1979b) Evaluation of low nutrient, high fibre diets for the prevention of porcine *Escherichia coli* enterotoxaemia. *Veterinary Microbiology* 3, 281–290.

Bertschinger, H.U., Bachmann, M., Mettler, C., Pospischil, A., Schraner, E.M., Stamm, M., Sydler, T. and Wild, P. (1990) Adhesive fimbriae produced *in vivo* by *Escherichia coli* O139:K12(B):H1 associated with enterotoxaemia in pigs. *Veterinary Microbiology* 25, 267–281.

Blecha, F. and Kelley, K.W. (1981) The effect of cold and weaner stressors on the antibody-mediated immune response of pigs. *Journal of Animal Science* 53, 439–447.

Blood, D.C. and Radostits, O.M. (1989) *Veterinary Medicine*, 7th edn. Baillière Tindall, London, pp. 639–642.

Burgess, M.N., Bywater, R.J., Cowley, J.M., Mullen, N.A. and Newsome, P.M. (1978) Biological evaluation of a methanol soluble, heat-stable *Escherichia coli* enterotoxin in infant mice, pigs, rabbits and calves. *Infection and Immunity* 21, 526–531.

Chandler, D.S. and Luke, R.K.J. (1987) Alternative approaches to treatment of postweaning scours. In: Australasian Pig Science Association Committee (eds) *Manipulating Pig Production*. Australasian Pig Science Association, Werribee, Victoria, Australia, pp. 215–229.

Cox, E., Cools, V., Thoonen, H., Hoorens, J. and Houvenaghel, A. (1988) Effect of experimentally-induced villous atrophy on adhesion of K88ac-positive *Escherichia coli* associated with enteritis and enterotoxaemia in just weaned piglets. *Veterinary Microbiology* 17, 159–169.

Cutler, R. and Gardner, I. (1988) *A Blue Print for Pig Health Research*. Australian Pig Research Council, Canberra, Australia, pp. 39–40.

Dam, A. and Knox, B. (1974) Haemolytic *Escherichia coli* associated with enteritis and enterotoxaemia in pigs in Denmark, with particular reference to the rapid spread of serogroup O149:K91. *Nordisk Veterinaermedicin* 26, 219–225.

De Cupere, F., Deprez, P., Demeulenaere, D. and Muylle, E. (1992) Evaluation of the effect of 3 probiotics on experimental *Escherichia coli* enterotoxaemia in weaned pigs. *Journal of Veterinary Medicine B* 39, 277–284.

Decuypere, J. and Van der Heyde, H. (1972) Study of the gastrointestinal microflora of suckling piglets and early-weaned piglets reared using different feeding systems. *Zentralblatt für Bakteriologie, Mikrobiologie und Hygiene A* 221, 492–510.

Deprez, P., Van Den Hende, C., Muylle, E. and Oyaert, W. (1986) The influence of the administration of sow's milk on the postweaning excretion of haemolytic *Escherichia coli* in the pig. *Veterinary Research Communications* 10, 469–478.

Deprez, P., Deroose, P., Van Den Hende, C., Muylle, E. and Oyaert, W. (1987) Liquid versus dry feeding in weaned piglets: the influence on small intestinal morphology. *Journal of Veterinary Medicine* 34, 254–259.

Dunsford, B.R., Knabe, D.A. and Haensly, W.E. (1989) Effect of dietary soybean meal on the microscopic anatomy of the small intestine in the early-weaned pig. *Journal of Animal Science* 67, 1855–1863.

English, P.R. (1981) Establishing the early weaned pig. *The Pig Veterinary Society Proceedings* 7, 29–37.

Etheridge, R.D., Seerley, R.W. and Huber, T.L. (1984) The effect of diet on fecal moisture, osmolarity of fecal extracts, products of bacterial fermentation and loss of minerals in feces of weaned pigs. *Journal of Animal Science* 58, 1403–1411.

Fahy, V.A., Connaughton, I.D., Driesen, S.J. and Spicer, E.M. (1987) Postweaning colibacillosis. In: Australasian Pig Science Association Committee (eds)

Manipulating Pig Production. Australasian Pig Science Association, Werribee, Victoria, pp. 189–201.

Fu, Z.F. and Hampson, D.J. (1987) Group A rotavirus excretion patterns in naturally infected pigs. *Research in Veterinary Science* 43, 297–300.

Fu, Z.F., Blackmore, D.K., Hampson, D.J. and Wilks, C.R. (1989) Epidemiology of typical and atypical rotavirus infections in New Zealand pigs. *New Zealand Veterinary Journal* 37, 102–106.

Gannon, V.P.J., Gyles, C.L. and Friendship, R.W. (1988) Characteristics of verotoxigenic *Escherichia coli* from pigs. *Canadian Journal of Veterinary Research* 52, 331–337.

Gibbons, R.A., Sellwood, R., Burrows, M. and Hunter, P.A. (1977) Inheritance of resistance to neonatal *E. coli* diarrhoea in the pig. Examination of the genetic system. *Theoretical and Applied Genetics* 51, 65–70.

Gregory, D.W. (1962) Hemolytic *Escherichia coli* enteritis of weanling pigs. *Journal of the American Veterinary Medicine Association* 141, 947–949.

Gyles, C.L., Stevens, J.B. and Craven, J.A. (1971) A study of *Escherichia coli* strains isolated from pigs with gastro-intestinal disease. *Canadian Journal of Comparative Medicine* 35, 258–266.

Hall, G.A. and Byrne, T.F. (1989) Effects of age and diet on small intestinal structure and function in gnotobiotic piglets. *Research in Veterinary Science* 47, 387–392.

Hall, G.A., Parsons, K.R., Waxler, G.L., Bunch, K.J. and Batt, R.M. (1989) Effects of dietary change and rotavirus infection on small intestinal structure and function in gnotobiotic piglets. *Research in Veterinary Science* 47, 219–224.

Hamilton, D.L. and Roe, W.E. (1977) Electrolyte levels and net fluid and electrolyte movements in the gastrointestinal tract of weanling swine. *Canadian Journal of Comparative Medicine* 41, 241–250.

Hampson, D.J. (1983) Postweaning changes in the piglet small intestine in relation to growth checks and diarrhoea. PhD thesis, University of Bristol.

Hampson, D.J. (1986a) Alterations in piglet small intestine structure at weaning. *Research in Veterinary Science* 40, 32–40.

Hampson, D.J. (1986b) Attempts to modify changes in the piglet small intestine after weaning. *Research in Veterinary Science* 40, 313–317.

Hampson, D.J. (1987a) Dietary influences on porcine postweaning diarrhoea. In: Australasian Pig Science Association Committee (eds) *Manipulating Pig Production*. Australasian Pig Science Association, Werribee, Victoria, Australia, pp. 202–214.

Hampson, D.J. (1987b) The osmolality of caecal contents in piglets following weaning. *New Zealand Veterinary Journal* 35, 35–36.

Hampson, D.J. and Kidder, D.E. (1986) Influence of creep feeding and weaning on brush-border enzyme activities in the piglet small intestine. *Research in Veterinary Science* 40, 24–31.

Hampson, D.J. and Smith, W.C. (1986) Influence of creep feeding and dietary intake after weaning on malabsorption and occurrence of diarrhoea in the newly weaned pig. *Research in Veterinary Science* 41, 63–69.

Hampson, D.J., Hinton, M. and Kidder, D.E. (1985) Coliform numbers in the stomach and small intestine of healthy pigs following weaning at three weeks of age. *Journal of Comparative Pathology* 95, 353–362.

Hampson, D.J., Fu, Z.F. and Robertson, I.D. (1987) Investigation of the source of haemolytic *Escherichia coli* infecting weaned pigs. *Epidemiology and Infection* 99, 149–153.

Hampson, D.J., Fu, Z.F., Bettleheim, K.A. and Wilson, M.W. (1988a) Managemental influences on the selective proliferation of two strains of haemolytic *Escherichia coli* in weaned pigs. *Epidemiology and Infection* 100, 213–220.

Hampson, D.J., Fu, Z.F. and Smith, W.C. (1988b) Pre-weaning supplementary feed and porcine post weaning diarrhoea. *Research in Veterinary Science* 44, 309–314.

Hampson, D.J., Woodward, J.M. and Connaughton, I.D. (1993) Genetic analysis of *Escherichia coli* from porcine postweaning diarrhoea. *Epidemiology and Infection* 110, 575–581.

Harel, J., Lapointe, H., Fallara, A., Lorfie, L.A., Bigras-Poulin, M., Larivière, S. and Fairbrother, J.M. (1991) Detection of genes for fimbrial antigens and enterotoxins associated with *Escherichia coli* serogroups isolated from pigs with diarrhoea. *Journal of Clinical Microbiology* 29, 745–752.

Heliè, P., Morin, M., Jacques, M. and Fairbrother, J.M. (1991) Experimental infection of newborn pigs with attaching and effacing *Escherichia coli* O45 : KE65 strain. *Infection and Immunity* 59, 814–821.

Hinton, M., Hampson, D.J., Hampson, E. and Linton, A.H. (1985) A comparison of the ecology of *Escherichia coli* in the intestines of healthy unweaned pigs and pigs after weaning. *Journal of Applied Bacteriology* 58, 471–478.

Hoblet, K.H., Kohler, E.M., Saif, L.J., Theil, K.W. and Ingalls, W.l. (1986a) Study of porcine postweaning diarrhoea involving K88(-) hemolytic *Escherichia coli. American Journal of Veterinary Research* 47, 1910–1912.

Hoblet, K.H., Saif, L.J., Kohler, E.M., Theil, K.W., Bech-Nielsen, S. and Stitzlein, G.A. (1986b) Efficacy of an orally administered modified-live porcine-origin rotavirus vaccine against postweaning diarrhoea in pigs. *American Journal of Veterinary Research* 47, 1697–1703.

Jones, G.W. and Rutter, J.M. (1972) Role of the K88 antigen in the pathogenesis of neonatal diarrhoea cause by *Escherichia coli* in piglets. *Infection and Immunity* 6, 918–927.

Kelley, K.W. (1982) Environmental effects on the immune system of pigs. *Pig News and Information* 3, 395–400.

Kelly, D., Greene, J., O'Brien, J.J. and McCracken, K.J. (1984) Gavage feeding of early-weaned pigs to study the effect of diet on digestive development and changes in intestinal microflora. In: *Proceedings of the 8th International Pig Veterinary Society Congress, Ghent*. IPVS, p. 317.

Kelly, D., O'Brien, J.J. and McCracken, K.J. (1990a) Effect of creep feeding on the incidence, duration and severity of post-weaning diarrhoea in pigs. *Research in Veterinary Science* 49, 223–228.

Kelly, D., Smyth, J.A. and McCracken, D.J. (1990b) Effect of creep feeding on structural and functional changes of the gut of early weaned pigs. *Research in Veterinary Science* 48, 350–356.

Kelly, D., Smyth, J.A. and McCracken, K.J. (1991a) Digestive development of the early-weaned pig. 1. Effect of continuous nutrient supply on the development of the digestive tract and on changes in digestive enzyme activity during the first week post-weaning. *British Journal of Nutrition* 65, 169–180.

Kelly, D., Smyth, J.A. and McCracken, K.J. (1991b) Digestive development of the early-weaned pig. 2. Effect of level of food intake on digestive enzyme activity during the immediate post-weaning period. *British Journal of Nutrition* 65, 181–188.

Kennan, R.M. and Monckton, R.P. (1990) Adhesive fimbriae associated with porcine enterotoxigenic *Escherichia coli* of the O141 serotype. *Journal of Clinical Microbiology* 28, 2006–2011.

Kenworthy, R. (1976) Observations of the effects of weaning in the young pig. Clinical and histopathological studies of intestinal function and morphology. *Research in Veterinary Science* 21, 69–75.

Kenworthy, R. and Allen, W.D. (1966) The significance of *Escherichia coli* to the young pig. *Journal of Comparative Pathology* 76, 31–44.

Kenworthy, R. and Crabb, W.E. (1963) The intestinal flora of young pigs, with reference to early weaning, *Escherichia coli* and scours. *Journal of Comparative Pathology* 73, 215–228.

Larsen, J.T. (1976) Differences between enteropathogenic *Escherichia coli* strains isolated from neonatal *E. coli* diarrhoea (N.C.D.) and post weaning diarrhoea (P.W.D.) in pigs. *Nordisk Veterinaermedicin* 28, 417–429.

Lecce, J.G. and King, M.W. (1978) Role of rotavirus (Reo-like) in weanling diarrhea of pigs. *Journal of Clinical Microbiology* 8, 454–458.

Lecce, J.G., Armstrong, W.D., Crawford, P.C. and Ducharme, G.A. (1979) Nutrition and management of early-weaned pigs: liquid vs dry feeding. *Journal of Animal Science* 48, 1007–1014.

Lecce, J.G., Balsbaugh, R.K., Clare, D.A. and King, M.W. (1982) Rotavirus and hemolytic enterpathogenic *Escherichia coli* in weanling diarrhea of pigs. *Journal of Clinical Microbiology* 16, 715–723.

Lecce, J.G., Clare, D.A., Balsbaugh, R.K. and Collier, D.N. (1983) Effect of dietary regimen on rotavirus – *Escherichia coli* weanling diarrhea of piglets. *Journal of Clinical Microbiology* 17, 689–695.

Le Dividich, J., Aumaitre, A. and Berbigier, P. (1977) Influence of air temperature and velocity on performance of pigs weaned at 3 weeks. *Annales de Zootechnie* 26, 465.

Li, D.F., Nelssen, J.L., Reddy, P.G., Blecha, F., Hancock, J.D., Allee, G.L., Goodband, R.D. and Klemm, R.D. (1990) Transient hypersensitivity to soybean meal in the early-weaned pig. *Journal of Animal Science* 68, 1790–1799.

Li, D.F., Nelssen, J.L., Reddy, P.G., Blecha, F., Klemm, R. and Goodband, R.D. (1991) Interrelationship between hypersensitivity to soybean proteins and growth performance in early-weaned pigs. *Journal of Animal Science* 69, 4062–4069.

Madec, F. and Josse, J. (1983) Influence of environmental factors on the onset of digestive disorders of the weaned piglet. *Annales de Recherches Veterinaire* 14, 456–462.

Mezoff, A.G., Jensen, N.J. and Cohen, M.B. (1991) Mechanisms of increased susceptibility of immature and weaned pigs to *Escherichia coli* heat-stable enterotoxin. *Pediatrics Research* 29, 424–428.

Miller, B.G., Newby, T.G., Stokes, C.R. and Bourne, F.J. (1984) Influence of diet on postweaning malabsorption and diarrhoea in the pig. *Research in Veterinary Science* 36, 187–193.

Miller, B.G., James, P.S., Smith, M.W. and Bourne, F.J. (1986) Effects of weaning on the capacity of pig intestinal villi to digest and absorb nutrients. *Journal of Agricultural Science* 107, 579–589.

Morris, J.A. and Sojka, W.J. (1985). *Escherichia coli* as a pathogen in animals. In: Sussman, M. (ed.) *The Virulence of Escherichia coli*. Academic Press, London, pp. 47–77.

Nagy, B., Casey, T.A. and Moon, H.W. (1990) Phenotype and genotype of *Escherichia coli* isolated from pigs with postweaning diarrhea in Hungary. *Journal of Clinical Microbiology* 28, 651–653.

Nagy, B., Casey, T.A., Whipp, S.C. and Moon, H.W. (1992) Susceptibility of porcine intestine to pilus-mediated adhesion by some isolates of piliated enterotoxigenic *Escherichia coli* increases with age. *Infection and Immunity* 60, 1285–1294.

Nakazawa, M., Sugimoto, C., Isayama, Y. and Kashiwazaki, M. (1987) Virulence factors in *Escherichia coli* isolated from piglets with neonatal and post-weaning diarrhoea in Japan. *Veterinary Microbiology* 13, 291–300.

Nielsen, N.O., Moon, H.W. and Roe, W.E. (1968) Enteric colibacillosis in swine. *Journal of the American Veterinary Medicine Association* 153, 1590–1606.

Palmer, N.C. and Hulland, T.J. (1965) Factors predisposing to the development of coliform gastroenteritis in weaned pigs. *Canadian Veterinary Journal* 6, 310–316.

Pluske, J.R., Williams, I.H. and Aherne, F.X. (1991) Maintained of villous height and crypt depth in the small intestine of weaned piglets. In: Batterham, E.S. (ed.) *Manipulating Pig Production III*. Australasian Pig Science Association. Werribee, Victoria, p. 143.

Pouteaux, V.A., Christison, G.I. and Rhodes, C.S. (1982) The involvement of dietary protein source and chilling in the etiology of diarrhea in newly weaned pigs. *Canadian Journal of Animal Science* 62, 1199–1209.

Richards, W.P.C. and Fraser, C.M. (1961) Coliform enteritis of weaned pigs. A description of the disease and its association with haemolytic *Escherichia coli*. *Cornell Veterinarian* 51, 245–257.

Rose, R., Whipp, S.C. and Moon, H.W. (1987) Effects of *Escherichia coli* heat stable enterotoxin b on small intestinal villi in pigs, rabbits and lambs. *Veterinary Pathology* 24, 71–79.

Salajka, E., Salajkova, Z., Alexa, P. and Hornich, M. (1992) Colonization factor different from K88, K99, F41 and 987P in enterotoxigenic *Escherichia coli* strains isolated from postweaning diarrhoea in pigs. *Veterinary Microbiology* 32, 163–175.

Sarmiento, J.I., Dean, E.A. and Moon, H.W. (1988) Effects of weaning on diarrhea caused by enterotoxigenic *Escherichia coli* in three-week-old pigs. *American Journal of Veterinary Research* 49, 2030–2033.

Sarmiento, J.I., Runnels, P.L. and Moon, H.W. (1990) Effects of preweaning exposure to a starter diet on enterotoxigenic *Escherichia coli*-induced postweaning diarrhea in swine. *American Journal of Veterinary Research* 51, 1180–1183.

Schlager, T.A., Wanke, C.A. and Guerrant, R.L. (1990) Net fluid secretion and impaired villous function induced by colonization of the small intestine by nontoxigenic colonizing *Escherichia coli. Infection and Immunity* 58, 1337–1343.

Schulman, A. (1973) Effect of weaning on the pH changes of the contents of the piglet stomach and duodenum. *Nordisk Veterinaermedicin* 25, 220–225.

Smith, M.W. (1984) Effect of postnatal development and weaning upon the capacity of pig intestinal villi to transport alanine. *Journal of Agricultural Science* 102, 625–633.

Smith, H.W. and Halls, S. (1968) The production of oedema disease and diarrhoea in weaned pigs by the oral administration of *Escherichia coli*: factors that influence the course of the experimental disease. *Journal of Medical Microbiology* 1, 45–59.

Smith, H.W. and Huggins, M.B. (1978) The influence of plasmid-determined and other characteristics of enteropathogenic *Escherichia coli* on their ability to proliferate in the alimentary tracts of piglets, calves and lambs. *Journal of Medical Microbiology* 11, 471–492.

Smith, H.W. and Jones, J.E.T. (1963) Observations on the alimentary tract and its bacterial flora in healthy and diseased pigs. *Journal of Pathology and Bacteriology* 86, 387–412.

Smith, H.W. and Linggood, M.A. (1971) Observations on the pathogenic properties of the K88, Hly and Ent plasmids of *Escherichia coli* with particular reference to porcine diarrhoea. *Journal of Medical Microbiology* 4, 467–485.

Smith, H.W., Green, P. and Potsell, Z. (1987) Vero cell toxins in *Escherichia coli* and related species: transfer by phage and conjugation and toxic action in laboratory animals, chickens and pigs. *Journal of General Microbiology* 129, 3121–3137.

Soderlind, O., Thafvelin, B. and Mollby, R. (1988) Virulence factors in *Escherichia coli* strains isolated from Swedish piglets with diarrhea. *Journal of Clinical Microbiology* 26, 879–884.

Sojka, W.J. (1985) Escherichia coli *in Domestic Animals and Poultry*. Commonwealth Agricultural Bureaux, Farnham Royal, UK.

Stamm, M. and Bertschinger, H.U. (1992) Identification of pigs genetically resistant to oedema disease by testing adhesion of *E. coli* expressing fimbriae 107 to intestinal epithelial cells. In *Proceedings of the 12th International Pig Veterinary Society Congress*, The Hague, The Netherlands, p. 242.

Stevens, J.B., Gyles, C.L. and Barnum, D.A. (1972) Production of diarrhea in pigs in response to *Escherichia coli* enterotoxin. *American Journal of Veterinary Research* 33, 2511–2526.

Svendsen, J. (1974) Enteric *Escherichia coli* diseases in weaned pigs. *Nordisk Veterinaermedicin* 26, 226–238.

Svendsen, J., Riising, H.J. and Christensen, S. (1977) Studies on the pathogenesis of enteric *Escherichia coli* in weaned pigs: bacteriological and immunofluorescence studies. *Nordisk Veterinaermedicin* 29, 212–220.

Svensmark, B. (1983) Prevalence rate of porcine rotavirus in Danish swine herds. *Annales de Recherche Veterinaire* 14, 433–436.

Thomlinson, J.R. and Lawrence, T.L.J. (1981) Dietary manipulation of gastric pH in the prophylaxis of enteric disease in weaned pigs: some field observations. *Veterinary Research* 109, 120–122.

Tzipori, S. (1985) The relative importance of enteric pathogens affecting neonates of domestic animals. *Advances in Veterinary Science and Comparative Medicine* 29, 103–206.

Tzipori, S., Chandler, D., Makin, T. and Smith, M. (1980) *Escherichia coli* and rotavirus infections in four-week-old gnotobiotic piglets fed milk or dry food. *Australian Veterinary Journal* 56, 279–284.

Tzipori, S., McCartney, E., Chang, H.S. and Dunkin, A. (1984) Postweaning diarrhoea in pigs: an interaction between change to dry food and colibacillosis. *Federation of European Microbiological Societies Microbiology Letters* 24, 313–317.

van Beers-Schreurs, H.M.G., Vellenga, L., Wensing, Th. and Breukink, H.J. (1992) The pathogenesis of the post-weaning syndrome in weaned piglets; a review. *Veterinary Quarterly* 14, 29–34.

Vasenuis, H. (1969) The influence of dietary carbohydrate on the multiplication and colonisation of inoculated *Escherichia coli* strains in pig's intestine. II Investigations in pigs at weaning age. *Nordisk Veterinaermedicin* 21, 535–544.

Wathes, C.M., Miller, B.G. and Bourne, F.J. (1989) Cold stress and post-weaning diarrhoea in piglets inoculated orally or by aerosol. *Animal Production* 49, 483–496.

Whipp, S.C., Moon, H.W., Kemeny, L.J. and Argenzio, R.A. (1985) Effect of virus-induced destruction of villous epithelium on intestinal secretion induced by heat-stable *Escherichia coli* enterotoxins and prostaglandin E_1 in swine. *American Journal of Veterinary Research* 46, 637–642.

Wilson, R.A. and Francis, D.H. (1986) Fimbriae and enterotoxins associated with *Escherichia coli* serogroups isolated from pigs with colibacillosis. *American Journal of Veterinary Research* 47, 213–217.

Yokoyama, H., Perahta, R.C., Diaz, R., Sendo, S., Ikemori, Y. and Kodama, Y. (1992) Passive protective effect of chicken egg yolk immunoglobulins against experimental enterotoxigenic *Escherichia coli* infection in neonatal pigs. *Infection and Immunity* 60, 998–1007.

Oedema Disease of Pigs

9

H.U. Bertschinger[1] and C.L. Gyles[2]

[1]*Institut für Veterinärbakteriologie der Universität Zürich, Winterthurerstrasse 270, 8057 Zürich, Switzerland and*
[2]*Department of Veterinary Microbiology and Immunology, University of Guelph, Guelph, Ontario Canada N1G 2W1*

History

The first clinical description of what is now known as oedema disease came from Ireland, when Shanks (1938) reported an 'unusual condition affecting the digestive organs of the pig'. He proposed no specific name, but speculated that the condition might be an enterotoxaemia, and that the introduction of more concentrated feeds might be an important factor. The association with nutritious feed led to the long-held concept of a protein intoxication (Eiweissvergiftung) or a disease due to overeating.

Intensive research on oedema disease occurred in two periods, in the 1950s and in the last decade. The research of the early period was driven by a phenomenally high incidence of oedema disease in the 1940s and has been reviewed in detail by Sojka (1965). The resurgence of interest in the disease stems from discoveries about the oedema disease toxin and the *E. coli* adhesin that is involved in colonization of the intestine.

Timoney (1950) was the first author to report reproduction of the disease by intravenous injection of extracts prepared from intestinal contents of affected pigs. The observation that haemolytic *E. coli* are associated with the disease was made independently by Schofield and Davis (1955) and by Gregory (1955). The general concept of an enterotoxaemia was consolidated when Erskine *et al.* (1957) described reproduction of oedema disease by intravenous injection of freeze–thaw extracts from cultures of six strains of haemolytic *E. coli* recovered from oedema disease. However, at that time, it was not possible to reproduce the syndrome by oral administration of bacterial cultures.

A new era began when Konowalchuk *et al.* (1977) discovered that certain strains of *E. coli* of human origin and one oedema disease strain produced a toxin (verotoxin) that was lethal for Vero cells. Soon thereafter, researchers provided evidence that verotoxin and oedema disease toxin were the same (Blanco *et al.*, 1983; Dobrescu, 1983; Smith *et al.*, 1983) and it was possible to replace weaned pigs with tissue culture to assay oedema disease toxin. The new tool, combined with molecular genetics, led to purification and characterization of the toxin which turned out to be a classical bacterial exotoxin (MacLeod and Gyles, 1990) highly toxic to the pig (MacLeod *et al.*, 1991).

Colonization of the intestine by oedema disease strains of *E. coli* was first addressed by Smith and Halls (1968), who induced oedema disease by oral administration of an oedema disease *E. coli* isolate to weaned pigs from a specific farm. They demonstrated that failure to produce the disease in pigs from other farms was associated with failure of the organism to colonize the intestine of these pigs. They concluded, from differential viable counts, that, in susceptible pigs, the inoculated bacteria were present in larger numbers in mucosal scrapings compared with contents of the anterior small intestine. However, the mechanism by which the mucosa became colonized remained unidentified for over two decades before Bertschinger *et al.* (1990) reported their discovery of a new type of adhesive fimbriae which was shown to occur in most *E. coli* strains harbouring the genes coding for the toxin causing oedema disease (Imberechts *et al.*, 1992a; Imberechts *et al.*, 1994).

Clinical Aspects

Epidemiology

Oedema disease is most often seen as sporadic cases or small outbreaks limited to a certain age group. Outbreaks do not conform to the usual pattern associated with outbreaks of highly transmissible diseases, but tend to occur in a herd indiscriminately and at intervals in a haphazard fashion (Timoney, 1950). On premises where the disease occurs, the *E. coli* responsible are detected only in affected pigs, or their in-contact penmates (Sojka *et al.*, 1957). Four weeks after an outbreak the organism cannot be isolated any more.

Oedema disease is chiefly a disease of recently weaned pigs, occurring most often 7–10 days after weaning, or after transfer to fattening premises. However, sporadic cases and solitary outbreaks are seen in suckling pigs 2 weeks of age and older. According to Timoney (1950), decreased susceptibility with age is suggestive of development of immunity. Oedema disease in brood sows and boars is not rare in Switzerland (Bürgi *et al.*, 1992). The disease takes a more protracted course than in younger pigs, and outbreaks may extend over longer periods.

A salient feature of the vast majority of outbreaks of oedema disease is the sudden onset of illness affecting several pigs in rapid succession followed by abrupt termination of the outbreak (Timoney, 1950). Death losses usually cease within 4–5 days from the first appearance of the disease and, as a general rule, no further cases appear in the lot of pigs. The frequent recurrences at varying intervals on the same premises suggest persistence of the organism. Isolates of the same serotype from one farm show a high degree of homogeneity (Tschäpe *et al.*, 1992). In summary, oedema disease has many characteristics of an endemic transmissible disease.

In a study based on 19 herds and 1970 pigs at risk, a morbidity of 16%, and a case mortality rate of 64% were observed (Kernkamp *et al.*, 1965). The average duration of outbreaks was 8 (4–15) days.

Clinical signs

The precise observations reported by Timoney (1950) in natural outbreaks give an illustrative picture of oedema disease. Pigs are frequently found dead without previous signs of illness. Pigs with early symptoms move with a staggering gait towards the feeding trough, where they may eat sparingly or only place their noses in the feed. The symptoms progress to a marked staggering gait followed by loss of control of either the hind or the fore limbs. Within a few hours the paralysis is complete, and the pig is unable to rise. Generalized fine muscle tremors are frequently seen in this stage. In other cases, recumbency is accompanied by attacks of convulsive running movements. Swelling of the eyelids, frequently combined with slight reddening of the skin, may develop at different stages of the disease and may be the chief symptom in pigs affected with a mild form of oedema disease, from which they recover. The ears may be inclined to droop (Fig. 9.1). A peculiar squeal attributable to laryngeal oedema is sometimes noted. Forced respiratory movements through the wide open mouth, sometimes associated with a snoring sound, are in most cases recognized shortly before death. The rectal temperature is normal with few exceptions. Constipation is a marked feature of most cases, but in outbreaks due to strains of *E. coli* which produce one or more than one enterotoxin, diarrhoea may precede the symptoms of oedema disease. In a small number of cases, diarrhoea is a terminal event and is sometimes haemorrhagic. Most affected animals die within 24 hours, but occasional animals linger on for 48–72 hours. This is especially the case in older pigs (Bürgi *et al.*, 1992).

Haemograms of affected and of moribund pigs are usually within normal limits (Kurtz *et al.*, 1969). A glycosuria is present in a minority of cases (Timoney, 1950).

In certain outbreaks, pigs may survive and develop chronic disease characterized by slower growth with or without signs of a focal encephalopathy (Bertschinger and Pohlenz, 1974; Kausche *et al.*, 1992). The

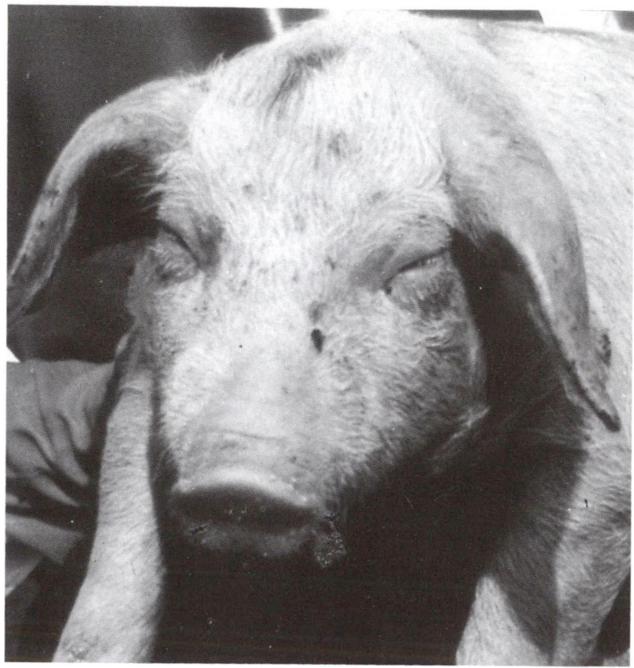

Fig. 9.1. Severe oedema of the eyelids, frontal area and ears in a pig infected with an *E. coli* strain of serogroup O139.

condition had been called cerebrospinal angiopathy, before its identity with chronic oedema disease was recognized.

Gross lesions

Excellent descriptions of the lesions detected at postmortem have been provided by Luke and Gordon (1950), Timoney (1950) and Barker and van Dreumel (1985). The lesions may be present in various combinations, and the severity of the changes shows enormous variation. In typical acute cases, the pigs are in good condition and subcutaneous oedema is seen in the eyelids, in the frontal area, over the nasal bone, in the groin and over the belly. Subcutaneous lymph nodes are oedematous with a reddish mottled cut surface.

Serous effusions with occasional or numerous white fibrinous strands can be found in the serous cavities. Occasional petechiae may be detected on the heart. Variable oedema is present in the lungs and in the wall of the gall bladder.

The stomach is often full of unusually dry and fresh looking crumbly feed. The mucosa is pale. Submucosal oedema of variable thickness can be detected in the cardiac region (Fig. 9.2). The small intestine may be almost completely empty, whereas the colon usually contains a moderate amount of solid faeces. Submucosal oedema is occasionally detected in the wall of the caecum or the colon. The mesentery of the spiral coil of the colon and of the terminal colon is commonly oedematous (Fig. 9.3), whereas the mesentery of the small intestine is often simply moist. The mesenteric lymph nodes may be oedematous and swollen and a circumscribed dark red discoloration of the periphery is frequently seen.

In exceptional peracute cases characterized by terminal diarrhoea, there is sometimes extensive haemorrhage associated with oedematous lesions in the stomach and the large intestine. The mucosa in the terminal portion of the small intestine and, more rarely, the caecum and the upper colon is roughened and covered by fibrin and by clotted fresh blood (Fig. 9.4) (Timoney, 1950; Bertschinger and Pohlenz, 1983). These changes are rare in subacute or chronic cases, where malacia confined to the brain stem (Kurtz *et al.*, 1969) may exceptionally be grossly detectable.

Distribution Among Countries

Oedema disease has been reported from a great number of countries (Sojka, 1965). In 1957, Lloyd observed that Australia was the only continent

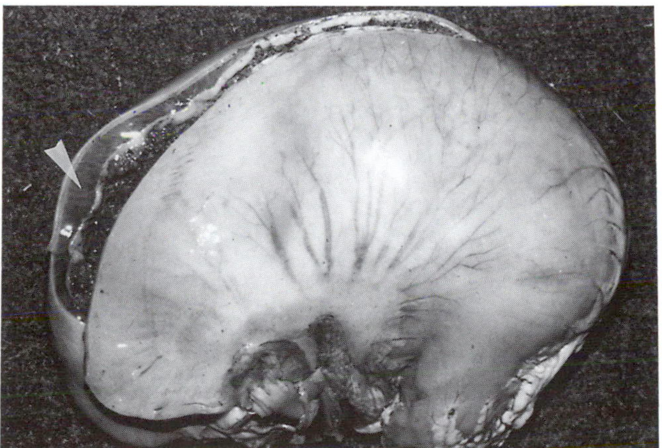

Fig. 9.2. Marked oedema of the stomach wall in the submucosa of the cardiac region (arrow).

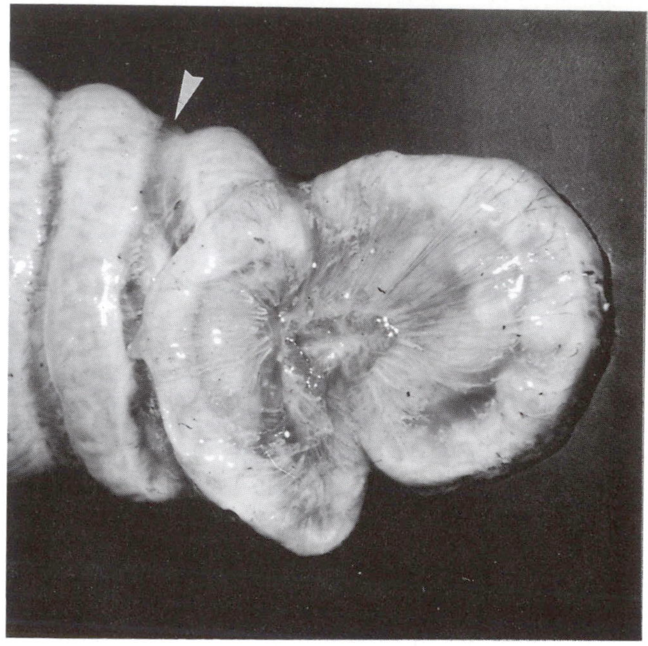

Fig. 9.3. Colonic coil with severe oedema of the mesentery (arrow).

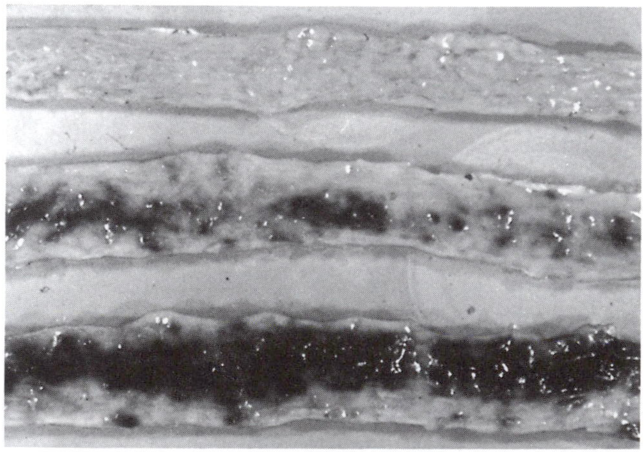

Fig. 9.4. Small intestinal segments from a case of oedema disease with terminal bloody diarrhoea. Circumscribed mucosal haemorrhage occurs preferentially over Peyer's patches. The upper jejunum is free of haemorrhage.

which did not have cases of this disease, but oedema disease was recently reported from Australia (Fahey *et al.*, 1990).

It is difficult to obtain good estimates of the incidence of oedema disease. This can be explained by the failure of some reports to distinguish between diarrhoea and oedema disease among weaned pigs with *E. coli* diseases, and the use of confusing terminology in other cases. Sometimes the terms enterotoxicosis or enterotoxaemia are used for both oedema disease and postweaning *E. coli* diarrhoea. In a German study, total *E. coli* mortality of weaned pigs amounted to 1.8% (Jahn and Uecker, 1987). This figure may also apply to Switzerland, where in a retrospective analysis of postmortem examinations oedema disease and postweaning *E. coli* diarrhoea were regarded as the cause of death in 22% and 33%, respectively, of the cases between 4 and 12 weeks of age (Häni *et al.*, 1976).

The incidence of oedema disease is subject to great variation relating to time and geographic region. Barker and Van Dreumel (1985) state that oedema disease and postweaning *E. coli* diarrhoea have apparently declined in prevalence in many parts of North America. Change of disease incidence over time is possibly associated with change of dominating serotypes. The latter has been followed by Wittig and Fabricius (1992) in Saxony over the last 28 years. Serogroup O139:K82, the main or only type causing oedema disease in that region, was prevalent until 1973, and again from 1986 on. Between 1973 and 1986 this serogroup was replaced by serogroup O149:K91:F4. A given serotype may be equipped with different toxins in different regions. Isolates of serogroup 0139 from Switzerland harbour no enterotoxin genes (Boss *et al.*, 1992, Imberechts *et al.*, 1994) whereas a significant proportion of German and Canadian isolates produces enterotoxin (Truszczynski *et al.*, 1985, Gannon *et al.*, 1988).

Characteristics of *E. coli* Involved

Production of oedema disease toxin (Shiga-like toxin)

Timoney (1950) demonstrated that intravenous injection of pigs with supernatant from centrifuged intestinal contents of pigs that had succumbed to oedema disease induced the characteristic signs and lesions of oedema disease. The toxic factor was heat labile and induced neutralizing antibody (Timoney, 1957). However, further characterization of the toxic factor was delayed for over three decades, due to the cumbersome assay in pigs, and because it was not possible to obtain pure preparations of the factor. The toxic factor was given names such as oedema disease toxin, oedema disease principle, neurotoxin, angiotoxin and vasotoxin. The term neurotoxin was proposed by Gregory (1960), who recognized similarities between the oedema disease toxin and the neurotoxin of *Shigella dysenteriae*, also called Shiga toxin.

A cytotoxic effect of culture supernatants of oedema disease strains of *E. coli* on Vero cells was first reported by Konowalchuk *et al.* (1977) and later confirmed by Kashiwazaki *et al.* (1981), Dobrescu (1983) and Smith *et al.* (1983) as well as others. Similar cytotoxic substances were detected in pathogenic *E. coli* from other animal species and humans (Gyles, 1992; Imberechts *et al.*, 1992b). The cytotoxins were first called verotoxins (VTs) because of their lethality for cultured Vero cells, but later called Shiga-like toxins (SLTs) because of their close relationship to Shiga toxin (see Chapter 15 for greater detail). The toxin produced by *E. coli* isolates from pigs with oedema disease was compared by Marques *et al.* (1987) with SLT-I and SLT-II, produced by *E. coli* from humans. They concluded that the toxic factor was a variant of SLT-II, which led to the designation SLT-IIv. *E. coli* strains containing genetic information for SLT-IIv production can be identified with accuracy by application of polymerase chain reaction (PCR) amplification procedures (Gyles *et al.*, 1988; Imberechts *et al.*, 1992a).

A single antigenic type of the toxin is found within a wide range of isolates and serogroups (Gannon and Gyles, 1990). Contrasting with other SLTs, SLT-IIv is weakly enterotoxigenic and is approximately 1% as active in causing fluid accumulation in ligated intestinal loops in rabbits. The toxin exerts a direct dose-related cytotoxic effect on cultured porcine vascular endothelial cells (Gyles, 1992). SLTs other than SLT-IIv are rarely detected in porcine isolates not implicated in oedema disease (Gannon and Gyles, 1990). Intravenous injection of highly purified SLT-IIv in pigs induced the clinical signs and postmortem lesions of oedema disease (MacLeod *et al.*, 1991). The LD_{50} of the preparation was 3 ng per kg of bodyweight.

Some oedema disease strains of *E. coli* produce not only SLT-IIv but also enterotoxins such as STIa, STII and LTp (Konowalchuk *et al.*, 1977; Blanco *et al.*, 1983; Gannon *et al.*, 1988; Nagy *et al.*, 1990; Boss *et al.*, 1992; Imberechts *et al.*, 1994). Pigs infected with strains producing SLT-IIv and LT usually die from diarrhoea and dehydration (Boss *et al.*, 1992), whereas those infected with strains producing SLT-IIv and STIa and/or STII may die with signs of either diarrhoea, sudden death or oedema disease (Gannon *et al.*, 1988).

Production of haemolysin

Cultures on blood-containing agar media demonstrated that *E. coli* strains associated with outbreaks of oedema disease were markedly haemolytic and this provided a valuable marker in the early period for the differentiation of *E. coli* implicated in oedema disease from other *E. coli* (Gregory, 1955; Schofield and Davis, 1955). The haemolysin is detectable in the cell-free supernatant of broth cultures and is designated alpha-haemolysin (Smith, 1963). Production of alpha-haemolysin is common among verotoxigenic porcine isolates with only occasional exceptions (Gannon *et al.*, 1988). However, haemolytic activity is of only limited value for the recognition of oedema disease strains of *E. coli*, since non-typable haemolytic *E. coli* are common in the faeces of healthy weaned pigs. Smith (1963) isolated haemolytic *E. coli* from 59% of 200 faecal samples from healthy pigs. Such strains may occur in high numbers in the faeces of weaned pigs without doing any harm (unpublished observations of the authors).

There is no evidence that alpha-haemolysin contributes to virulence in oedema disease. Variants of a strain with and without haemolysin were administered orally to experimental pigs. Both variants induced diarrhoea and oedema disease of equal severity and with comparable mortality (Smith and Linggood, 1971).

Belonging to a limited number of serotypes

Shortly after it became evident that haemolytic *E. coli* were regularly associated with outbreaks of oedema disease, Sojka *et al.* (1957) reported that the great majority of the isolates could be assigned to two serotypes. They described type strains E57 and E4, later assigned the international antigen formulae O138:K81(B):H14 and O139:K82(B):H1, respectively (Ewing *et al.*, 1958). The capsular antigen K82 was later found to be closely related to K12 and therefore dropped (Semjen *et al.*, 1977). A third type strain, E68II (O141:K85a, b[B]:H4), was described by Lloyd (1957). Capsular antigens of this serotype undergo an a,b → a,c variation (Ørskov *et al.*, 1961). A total of not more than four serotypes comprises the great majority of isolates from outbreaks of oedema disease reported all over the world. A variable but high proportion of isolates assigned to these four serotypes produces the oedema disease toxin (Schimmelpfennig, 1970; Smith *et al.*, 1983; Gonzales and Blanco, 1985; Linggood and Thompson, 1987; Gannon *et al.*, 1988). Production of verotoxin has been reported for isolates of serogroups O149:K91, O157:K'V17', O2, O45, O120 and O121, but these are only occasionally implicated in oedema disease (Gannon *et al.*, 1988; Salajka *et al.*, 1992).

There is some controversy regarding toxin production by strains of the four common serogroups isolated from healthy pigs. Linggood and Thompson (1987) found that British isolates of oedema disease serotypes recovered from pigs with oedema disease produced Shiga-like toxin but those from healthy pigs did not produce Shiga-like toxin. In contrast, Gannon *et al.* (1988) isolated verotoxigenic strains of these serotypes with similar frequency from healthy weaned pigs and weaned pigs with enteric disease in Canada.

Wittig and Fabricius (1992) published a retrospective analysis of serotypes of isolates from 16,064 pigs with postweaning enteric *E. coli* infections through 28 years. They found an impressive but rather slow change in the prevalence of some serotypes.

Adhesive fimbriae

No fimbriae were detected on oedema disease strains of *E. coli* grown on artificial media, and the mechanism of intestinal colonization remained a mystery until a richly fimbriated variant of a field strain of serotype O139:K12(B):H1 was described by Bertschinger *et al.* (1990). The fimbriae were provisionally designated F107. An antiserum prepared against these fimbriae reacted strongly with bacteria of a field strain in the intestinal environment. In an experiment with a different field strain, fimbriae with the morphology of F107 could be visualized on bacteria colonizing the intestine. Binding of anti-F107 fimbrial antibody to these fimbriae was shown by immunoelectron microscopy (Bertschinger *et al.*, 1990).

Fimbriae F107 are present on bacteria in variable, but often high numbers. They are long, slender and flexible with a diameter of about 4.6 nm (Fig. 9.5). They are not expressed at 18 °C, and do not agglutinate human or animal red blood cells. There is no antigenic relationship to fimbriae F4, F5, F6 or F41 of porcine enterotoxigenic *E. coli*. Bacteria with fimbriae F107 strongly adhere to brush border fragments of small intestinal enterocytes (Bertschinger *et al.*, 1990). The prevalence of fimbriae F107 was examined in an indirect immunofluorescence test involving smears from the small intestinal mucosa of pigs representing 90 outbreaks of oedema disease and/or postweaning diarrhoea (Stamm *et al.*, 1990). Four-fifths of the cases that yielded massive growth of *E. coli* of serogroups O139:K12 or O141:K85a,b showed strong fluorescence. Negative or inconclusive preparations resulted from pigs infected with *E. coli* of serogroup O149:K91:K88.

Three research teams independently reported new fimbriae on certain *E. coli* isolated from postweaning diarrhoea (Kennan and Monckton, 1990; Nagy *et al.*, 1992a; Salajka *et al.*, 1992). Comparison of these fimbriae with fimbriae F107 revealed that they are closely related in morphology, antigenicity and genetic organization (H. Imberechts, Brussels, 1992, personal communication). So far, two antigenic variants have been defined with a common antigenic factor designated a and two specific factors called b and c (Nagy *et al.*, 1992b; H. Imberechts, Brussels, 1992, personal communication; H.U. Bertschinger, 1990, unpublished results).

A large collection of *E. coli* isolated from weaned pigs in Saxony was examined for expression of fimbriae under specially developed cultural conditions (Wittig *et al.*, 1994). Fimbriae F107 were serologically identified in nearly all isolates, which belong to 11 serogroups. In some serogroups, both antigenic variants, 107a,b and 107a,c, were represented.

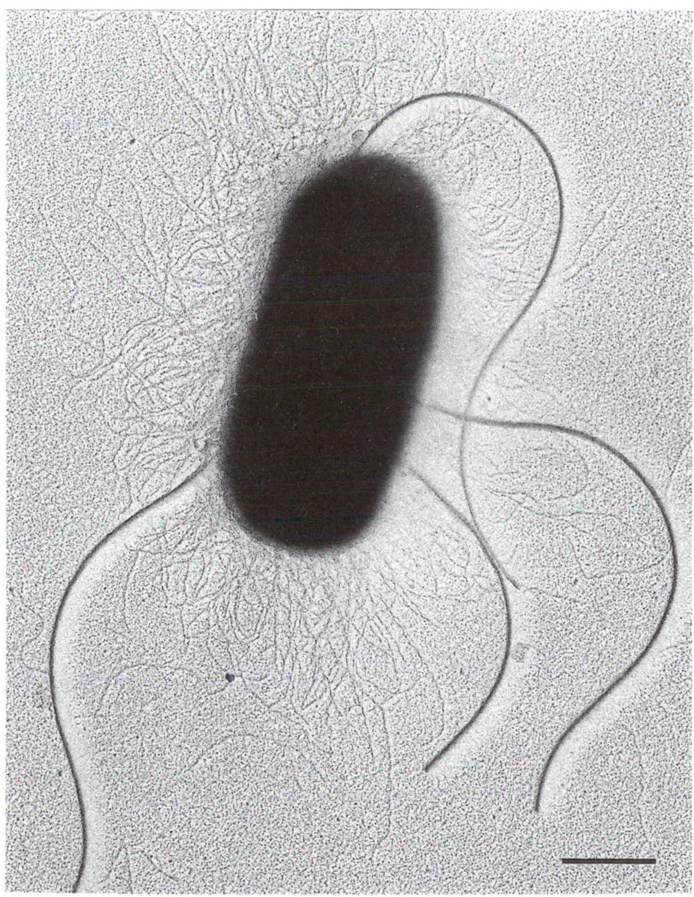

Fig. 9.5. *E. coli* strain 107/86 grown aerobically on Isonsensitest agar (Oxoid) at 37 °C, showing numerous long slender fimbriae. Platinum shadowing. Scale bar = 0.5 μm. (Laboratory of P. Wild, University of Zurich.)

A PCR amplification procedure developed by Imberechts *et al.* (1992a) recognized strains of *E. coli* with both antigenic variants of fimbriae F107 (H. Imberechts, Brussels, 1993, personal communication).

Other characteristics

Production of verotoxin by oedema disease strains of *E. coli* was not associated with production of colicin, haemolysin or any of 23 biochemical characteristics examined by Gannon *et al.* (1988).

Pathogenesis

Colonization of the intestine

Large numbers of *E. coli* are typically found in the small intestines of pigs examined early in the disease (Smith and Jones, 1963). Viable counts may reach 10^9 c.f.u. cm^{-1} of intestine (wall and contents) (Bertschinger and Pohlenz, 1983; Bertschinger *et al.*, 1990). This proliferation of *E. coli* is not associated with a disturbance of other components of the gastro-intestinal flora. Quantitative studies of the latter failed to show significant deviations (Smith and Jones, 1963; Schulze, 1977). In some pigs with oedema disease, the viable counts of *E. coli* are highest in the more anterior regions of the small intestine (Smith and Halls, 1968), whereas in others the counts are maximal in the terminal ileum (Timoney, 1957; Bertschinger *et al.*, 1990).

In frozen sections and in scanning electron micrographs, the surface of small intestinal villi from infected pigs is covered by the bacteria either as continuous layers or in a patchy way with irregularly arranged micro-colonies of various sizes (Fig. 9.6) (Bertschinger and Pohlenz, 1983). In ultrathin sections, the bacteria are visible along the brush border (Methiyapun *et al.*, 1984; Bertschinger *et al.*, 1990). Most of the adherent bacteria are surrounded by a translucent zone preventing the bacterial outer membranes from direct contact with each other as well as with the microvilli. In well-preserved sites, thick layers of bacteria sticking together are present. Such bacterial aggregates are also seen in smears from the mucosal surface examined by light microscopy.

The morphology of the enterocytes including the microvilli is not changed, and the large intestine is not involved (Methiyapun *et al.*, 1984). All other SLT-producing *E. coli* implicated in diseases in other host species preferentially colonize parts of the large intestine and induce an 'attaching and effacing' lesion.

Adhesion of *E. coli* causing oedema disease is mediated in most, if not all, cases by fimbriae of the type F107. This was proven in microscopic adhesion tests where identical strains with and without the fimbriae were compared (Bertschinger *et al.*, 1990; Imberechts *et al.*, 1992a).

Toxin production and kinetics

From early experiments with intestinal contents as for example those of Timoney (1957), it can be concluded that only a small proportion of the toxin present in the intestinal lumen reaches the vascular system. Further details such as the amounts of SLT-IIv produced *in vivo*, permeation of the intestinal barrier, concentrations of toxin in body fluids, and final

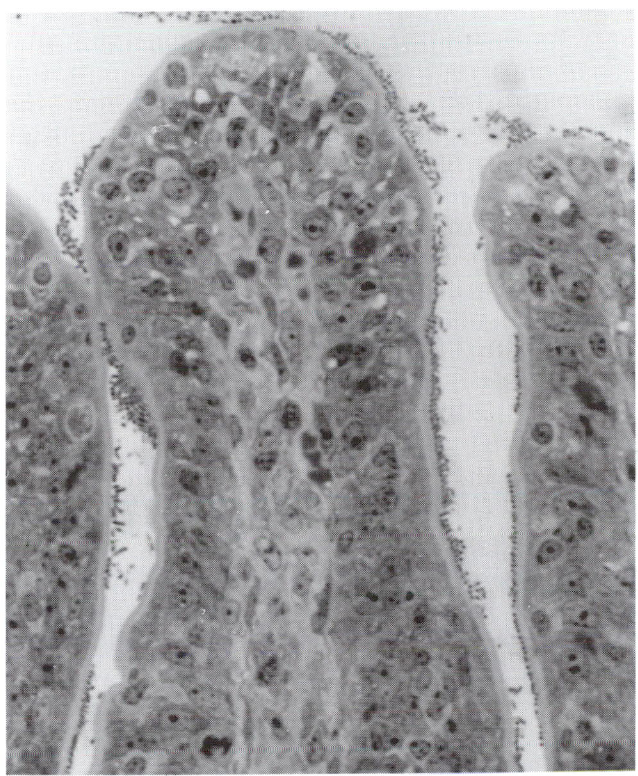

Fig. 9.6. Small intestinal villi colonized with *E. coli* serotype O139:K12(B):H1:F107 without alteration of the enterocyte or brush border morphology. Semithin section stained with toluidine blue. (Laboratory of P. Wild, University of Zurich.)

disposition of the toxin are not known. The long delay between colonization of the intestine and appearance of signs of illness in the experimental disease (Smith and Halls, 1968) may be the result of the slow rate of passage of toxin from the intestine to the blood and tissues. The presence of the toxin in the vascular compartment is deduced from successful reproduction of oedema disease by intravenous injection of toxin preparations.

Effects of the toxin

Shiga-like toxins are composed of one A subunit and five B subunits. The A subunit has RNA glycosidase activity, which removes an adenine residue from the 28S subunit of eukaryotic ribosomal RNA, thereby inhibiting protein synthesis of the animal cell (Saxena *et al.*, 1989). The B subunit determines the binding specificity. SLT-IIv binds to certain glycolipids (primarily globotetraosyl ceramide) in vascular endothelium. The distribution of receptors in porcine tissues appears to coincide with the tissues that show abnormalities in oedema disease (Boyd *et al.*, 1993). Differences in receptor specificities and in tissue distribution of receptors help to explain differences in the disease syndromes associated with the various SLTs (Samuel *et al.*, 1990).

Intravenous injection of purified SLT-IIv induces principally the same signs as seen in the natural disease (MacLeod *et al.*, 1991). Speed of onset and severity of clinical signs and gross pathological lesions are related to the dose of the toxin. Intervals between injection and onset of disease vary from 7 to 28 hours, the mean times to death from 24 to 42 hours. The microscopic changes of blood vessels include perivascular oedema, haemorrhage and vascular necrosis. The latter is characterized by amorphous hyaline changes in the walls of small arteries and arterioles. Haemorrhage is seen in the cerebellum, the stomach and the caecum. These haemorrhages, as well as superficial mucosal erosions in the colon and the caecum, are not usually found in the natural disease. Coagulative haemorrhagic necrosis may be caused by ischaemia, and is more subtle in pigs receiving lower doses of the toxin. Ultrastructural examination of the central nervous system of pigs injected with a semipurified preparation of SLT-IIv did not reveal a clear-cut morphological basis for the neurological symptoms (Clugston *et al.*, 1974).

Reproduction of disease by oral inoculation of pigs with E. coli

Many researchers who have attempted to reproduce oedema disease by oral inoculation of pigs with *E. coli* cultures have failed repeatedly (Lloyd, 1957; Smith and Jones, 1963; C.L. Gyles, 1991, unpublished). Smith and Halls (1968) were the first to reproduce the disease. They found that pigs from one farm only were suitable for this type of experiment, whereas pigs procured from other farms were refractory, suggesting that only pigs from some sources were genetically susceptible. Failure to induce experimental disease was associated with failure of colonization of the intestine by the *E. coli* that were administered.

Within 3–6 days after administration of strains producing enterotoxin as well as SLT-IIv, pigs suffered from diarrhoea for 1 or 2 days and ate very little (Smith and Halls, 1968). During the diarrhoeic phase very high numbers of the *E. coli* strain administered were found in the anterior regions of the small intestine. Clinical signs of oedema disease developed 7–9 days after inoculation. At that time, diarrhoea was no longer present in most pigs and signs of nervous system involvement were apparent. By this time bacterial numbers were much lower.

In pigs exposed to a strain producing SLT-IIv only, anorexia was not seen before 5 days postinoculation (Bertschinger *et al.*, 1978). The proportion of pigs which developed the characteristic syndrome was variable, and in one experiment, several pigs exhibited the haemorrhagic type of the disease (Bertschinger and Pohlenz, 1983). In the experiments reported by Kausche *et al.* (1992), a minority of pigs suffered from typical oedema disease, whereas nearly all developed vascular lesions within 2 weeks. Surviving pigs sometimes showed reduced growth with or without neurological signs.

Host Factors

Genetic resistance

Genetic resistance to disease which was suggested by earlier researchers (Lloyd, 1957; Smith and Halls, 1968) was placed on a scientific basis by studies involving the fimbriae F107 produced by oedema disease strains of *E. coli*. Retrospective analysis of a field experiment with oedema disease revealed a highly significant influence of the boar on intestinal colonization by the causative bacteria and on mortality (Bertschinger *et al.*, 1986), suggesting the existence of genetic resistance against colonization by *E. coli* causing oedema disease. Subsequently, it was concluded from an experiment aimed at breeding resistant pigs that resistance against colonization is controlled by one locus, and that susceptibility dominates resistance against colonization (Bertschinger *et al.*, 1993). It is now evident that genetic resistance is a consequence of the absence of receptors for the fimbriae F107 from the enterocyte membrane. Resistant pigs can be identified by microscopic adhesion tests (Stamm and Bertschinger, 1992). An identical mode of inheritance was reported previously for resistance of pigs to colonization by enterotoxigenic *E. coli* bearing fimbriae F4 (Gibbons *et al.*, 1977).

Investigation of a number of blood factors for use as genetic markers allowed localization of the locus for the receptor for fimbriae F107 on chromosome 6, the chromosome harbouring the porcine stress syndrome gene. Absence of receptor is frequently associated, however, with stress susceptibility (Vögeli *et al.*, 1992).

Immunity

Salajka *et al.* (1975) demonstrated that the milk of sows contained antibody against O and K antigens of *E. coli* serotypes associated with oedema disease. Specific antiserum, but not normal serum, given to weaned pigs in the drinking water, prevented the pathogenic serotype from becoming dominant. These observations support the view that weaning favours intestinal colonization by withdrawal of antibody. Deprez *et al.* (1986) showed that late lactation sows' milk fed to weaned pigs almost completely inhibited the proliferation of haemolytic *E. coli* and concluded that the inhibitory effect was likely to be due to specific and/or non-specific antimicrobial factors. They demonstrated that cows' milk did not possess this inhibitory effect.

It appears that anti-oedema disease toxin antibody is not prevalent in the blood of pigs. In early studies normal pig serum failed to neutralize the toxic effects of preparations which contained oedema disease toxin (Timoney, 1957). In recent studies, MacLeod *et al.* (1991) reported that young pigs were uniformly susceptible to the toxin administered by the intravenous route and Gannon *et al.* (1988) found that antibodies against SLT-IIv were not detectable in sera from neonatal and from weaned pigs (Gannon *et al.*, 1988).

Antitoxic antibodies can protect pigs against oedema disease. Smith and Linggood (1971) investigated the effects on experimental oedema disease of subcutaneous administration of antisera prepared in pigs against cultures of an oedema disease strain of *E. coli*. They found evidence for protective antitoxic immunity: several of the passively immunized pigs that were challenged showed colonization of the intestine and developed diarrhoea but failed to develop oedema disease.

Intestinal colonization induces immunity against subsequent colonization. Oral reinoculation 15–18 days after initial inoculation of recovered pigs with the same or a different strain does not re-induce infection (Smith and Halls, 1968). Interestingly, antihaemolysin and bactericidal, but not anti-O or anti-K antibodies, increased in the serum of challenged pigs which died or recovered after oral administration of an oedema disease isolate of *E. coli*. Awad-Masalmeh *et al.* (1989) reported that a glutaraldehyde-inactivated crude oedema disease toxin preparation was highly effective in stimulating protective immunity in pigs. Of 56 vaccinated pigs that were challenged, one died due to oedema disease; of 49 control pigs, 23 died of oedema disease. Surviving vaccinated animals were reported to have shed the challenge strain of *E. coli* for 2–3 days, in contrast to 2–6 days for survivors from the control group. This observation suggests that the vaccine also stimulated some anticolonization effects, which may have been induced by fimbrial or other surface antigens. MacLeod and Gyles (1991) used purified SLT-IIv inactivated with glutaraldehyde to protect passively and actively immunized pigs against challenge with the toxin.

Live cultures of oedema disease strains of *E. coli* may be used as an effective vaccine. Pigs protected by a diet low in protein and high in fibre may be immunized by oral administration of a virulent culture of a strain of *E. coli* O139:K12(B):H1 (Bertschinger *et al.*, 1981). Optimal protection against rechallenge is not achieved until 12 days after initial exposure. In this type of experiment, the diet slows down bacterial proliferation, and protection depends on the quantity of antigen administered. A total dose of up to 1×10^9 c.f.u. is ineffective, whereas maximal protection is seen with doses of 6×10^{11} c.f.u. or more (Bertschinger *et al.*, 1984).

Feed and feeding

Surveys of feeds on premises where oedema disease occurred resulted in a miscellaneous list with considerable farm-to-farm variation. It was not possible to correlate outbreaks of oedema disease with any particular type of meal (Luke and Gordon, 1950; Timoney, 1950). However, it was noteworthy that outbreaks were often associated with a high level of nutrition and that the fastest-growing animals appeared to be highly susceptible.

Smith and Halls (1968) compared the effects of six dietary regimens on susceptibility of pigs to experimental oedema disease. Three diets, one composed of barley meal alone, a second composed of barley meal plus 10% fish meal, and a third composed of barley meal plus 20% fish meal represented highly nutritious rations. Three diets, one of barley meal plus 10% fish meal administered at one-third the normal daily intake, a second composed of sweetened barley fibre, and a third consisting of barley fibre plus 10% fish meal constituted poorly nutritious rations. All pigs except those restricted to one-third the normal intake were allowed free access to feed. Smith and Halls (1968) found that much lower numbers of the inoculated *E. coli* O141:K85a,c were found in rectal contents of the pigs fed the poorly nutritious diets and that no clinical disease or deaths developed in challenged pigs on those diets. Oedema disease developed at similarly high frequencies in pigs on all three highly nutritious diets, suggesting that protein content was not a significant factor. The authors suggested that the physiological state of the intestine played a role in determining whether or not bacteria adhered to the intestinal epithelium. Certainly, whether receptor molecules for fimbriae are largely adherent to epithelial cells or are shed into the overlying mucus can determine whether or not colonization takes place.

The findings of Smith and Halls (1968) were confirmed by Bertschinger *et al.* (1978) working with larger numbers of pigs, and with an *E. coli* strain O139:K12(B):H1 producing no enterotoxin. These authors tested the usefulness of such poor diets for prevention of oedema disease and determined that, in order to be effective, diets had to be so low in nutrients that growth of the pigs was seriously retarded. The effect of the diet on bacterial proliferation was abolished by supplementation with fish meal, but not with starch or fat. Such diets may be of practical use for protection of weaned pigs for a limited period during the course of active immunization.

Diagnosis

Oedema disease is easily identified when it occurs in a typical outbreak. However, sporadic cases, especially those affecting atypical age groups, require differentiation from other conditions characterized by a short course and by neurological signs, such as pseudorabies, enteroviral polioencephalomyelitis, swine fever, bacterial meningoencephalitis caused by *Streptococcus suis* or *Haemophilus parasuis*, otitis media or water deprivation.

Characteristic gross lesions may be missing especially in cases where severe diarrhoea precedes development of oedema disease, and in protracted forms. Microscopic lesions are often missed in acute cases. Single vessels only may be affected and are most easily detected in the brain, where they may occur in every area, but more often in the brain stem (Kurtz *et al.*, 1969). Histological lesions in small arteries and arterioles consist of pyknosis and karyorrhexis of nuclei in the tunica media, swelling of endothelial nuclei, necrosis of smooth muscle cells followed by fibrinoid changes. Globules of eosinophilic material are often scattered around affected brain vessels (Fig. 9.7).

Bacteriology is of limited diagnostic value. The high numbers of colonizing bacteria may have disappeared in protracted cases, where the haemolytic strain may be detected as part of a mixed large intestinal flora

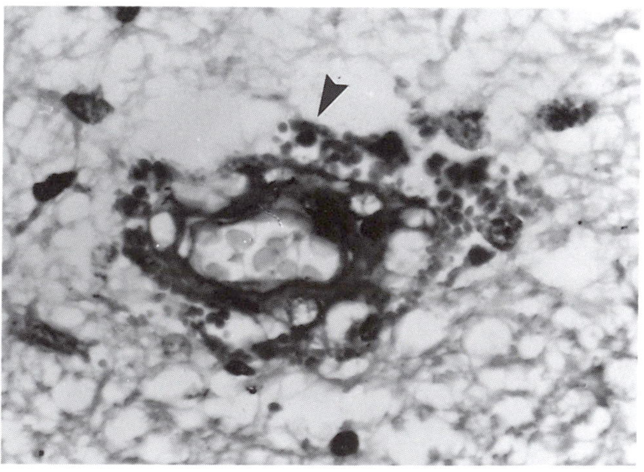

Fig. 9.7. Degenerative arteriopathy in the brain stem of a pig 4 weeks after oral administration of *E. coli* O139:K12(B):H1:F107. The pig was killed because of poor growth, depression, and a slight twisting of the head. Perivascular plasma droplets (arrow) and exudation in the vascular wall are evident. PAS reaction. (Laboratory of A. Pospischil, University of Zurich.)

not distinct from findings in pigs living in pen-contact with affected pigs. Simplified serotyping limited to slide agglutination of fresh cultures in OK-sera is strongly recommended, because haemolysis is not a reliable criterion. Preceding sections of this chapter and Chapter 21 may be consulted for methods for detection of the virulence determinants SLT-IIv and fimbriae F107.

Treatment

The unpredictable course of outbreaks has seriously hampered the evaluation of therapeutic measures and none of the many substances proposed through the years has found a definitive place in the veterinarian's armament. Some animals die before signs of illness are observed and others are in advanced stages of illness when they are first seen to be affected. As a rule, pigs that show neurological signs have a poor prognosis. The most effective response is to attempt to protect unaffected pigs. Withholding the feed is thought to impair colonization of the gut and is a valuable measure still recommended to the owners of pigs on a farm on which an outbreak has been recognized. Antimicrobials are also administered in the feed with this objective in mind.

Prevention

Prevention of oedema disease is highly desirable, since there is no reliable therapy. Most published methods of prevention, however, have only been tested under field conditions, and without adequate controls.

Diet

In most problem herds either diets with reduced nutrient contents (Smith and Halls, 1968; Bertschinger *et al.*, 1978) or limited amounts of conventional diets (Smith and Halls, 1968) may be offered for the first 2–3 weeks after weaning or after introduction of new batches of pigs into fattening establishments. Where limited feeding is practised, sufficient creep space must be available.

Chemoprophylaxis

Antibacterial substances are frequently added to the feed in problem herds despite two serious drawbacks. The first is that prophylactic medication may interfere with active immunization, thereby allowing clinical signs and mortality to develop after withdrawal of the antimicrobial drugs from the feed. This shortcoming is observed in varying degrees even within different weaner batches on the same premises. Variation may be due to uneven time and level of exposure to infection, variable feed intake and variable interaction of the drug with the carrier feed. The second problem is associated with the ease with which antimicrobial resistance develops in *E. coli* subjected to the selection pressure of antimicrobials in the feed. The frequencies of resistance against various drugs vary in different regions (Table 9.1), mostly as a consequence of the different patterns of use of antibacterial drugs. The number of resistance determinants per isolate continues to increase. Even the polymyxins (including colistin) may decrease in efficacy. Susceptibility testing by the agar diffusion method does not allow detection of this type of resistance.

Probiotics

Probiotics are preparations of selected bacteria that have been suggested as an alternative to antibiotics. These microorganisms are thought to have an inhibitory effect on proliferation of *E. coli* in the intestine but they have not been shown to be protective in rigorous tests of their effectiveness. De Cupere *et al.* (1992) evaluated three probiotics (*Streptococcus faecium*, *Lactobacillus* sp. and *Bacillus cereus* [toyoi]) in an experimental model for enterotoxaemia. Supplementation with each of the bacteria did not prevent clinical symptoms and mortality.

Table 9.1. Prevalence of resistance against antimicrobials among porcine *E. coli* isolates of the O groups 138, 139 and 141 in Canada (Gannon *et al.*, 1988) and in Belgium (Pohl *et al.*, 1991).

	Resistant isolates (%)	
Antimicrobial agent	Canada 1970–86 (n = 39)	Belgium 1986–90 (n = 153)
Ampicillin	69	30
Chloramphenicol	28	32
Tetracycline	85	60
Streptomycin	87	57
Neomycin/kanamycin	15	9
Gentamicin	0	0
Enrofloxacin	Not tested	0
Sulfonamide	67	52
Trimethoprim	Not tested	22
Sulfamethoxazole plus trimethoprim	0	Not tested

Immunoprophylaxis

Long before purified toxin was available it was shown that antiserum produced against toxic bowel supernatants from pigs with oedema disease neutralized the effect of such supernatants (Timoney, 1957). MacLeod and Gyles (1991) demonstrated that toxoid from purified SLT-IIv induces protection against the toxin. Protection can be passively transferred with serum from immunized pigs. An SLT-IIv toxoid vaccine produced from less purified material protected against the disease and shortened the period of intestinal colonization (Awad-Masalmeh *et al.*, 1989). There have been some problems associated with incomplete detoxification of protein toxins by formaldehyde treatment, but glutaraldehyde appears to effect complete inactivation. No toxoid vaccine is marketed at present. An enzymatic mutant of the toxin which is free of detectable cytotoxic activity and is immunogenic has been constructed by Gordon *et al.* (1992).

The vaccine strain evaluated by Bertschinger *et al.* (1984) as an oral antigen turned out to be not sufficiently stable under conditions of mass application. A commercial vaccine is not available.

As outlined above, genetic resistance may be the most economical method in the long range. However, at present a practical method to identify breeding stock without the intestinal receptor for fimbriae F107 is unavailable.

Concluding Comments

Important advances in knowledge on pathogenesis of oedema disease have been made in the past 10 years. These have filled in some of the gaps in the earlier literature, and have also served to highlight both the remarkable insight and impeccable experiments and meticulous field observations made by the researchers of the 1950s and 1960s. The early studies established that:

1. Haemolytic *E. coli* belonging to three or four serotypes were responsible for oedema disease.
2. The disease process involved colonization of the small intestine by the *E. coli*.
3. Colonization depended on changes in the intestinal environment at weaning, and on the diet of the pigs.
4. Some pigs were susceptible and others were refractory to infection.
5. Toxin produced by the *E. coli* in the intestine had to be absorbed into the circulation.
6. The toxin was heat labile and neutralizable by specific antiserum.

As early as 1960, both Timoney and Gregory recognized that oedema disease toxin had several similarities to the Shiga neurotoxin of *S. dysenteriae*. Recent advances include purification and characterization of the oedema disease toxin, identification and characterization of the fimbriae that are involved in colonization, and elucidation of the genetic basis of resistance of pigs to colonization by oedema disease strains of *E. coli*. Remaining gaps in our understanding of the disease process include identification of the receptor for the F107 fimbriae, determining the physiological factors associated with weaning that affect colonization and absorption of toxin, and identifying how diet affects colonization of the intestine.

References

Awad-Masalmeh, M., Schuh, M., Köfer, J. and Quakyi, E. (1989) Ueberprüfung der Schutzwirkung eines Toxoidimpfstoffes gegen die Oedemkrankheit des Absetzferkels im Infektionsmodell. *Deutsche tierärztliche Wochenschrift* 96, 419–421.

Barker, I.K. and Van Dreumel, A.A. (1985) The alimentary system. In: Jubb, K.V.F., Kennedy, P.C. and Palmer, N. (eds) *Pathology of Domestic Animals*, 3rd edn. Academic Press, Orlando, pp. 130–132.

Bertschinger, H.U. and Pohlenz, J. (1974) Cerebrospinale Angiopathie bei Ferkeln mit experimenteller Coli-Enterotoxämie. *Schweizer Archiv für Tierheilkunde* 116, 543–554.

Bertschinger, H.U. and Pohlenz, J. (1983) Bacterial colonization and morphology of the intestine in porcine *Escherichia coli* enterotoxemia (edema disease). *Veterinary Pathology* 20, 99–110.

Bertschinger, H.U., Eggenberger, E., Jucker, H. and Pfirter, H.P. (1978) Evaluation of low nutrient, high fibre diets for the prevention of porcine *Escherichia coli* enterotoxaemia. *Veterinary Microbiology* 3, 281–290.

Bertschinger, H.U., Jucker, H., Halter, H.M. and Pfirter, H.P. (1981) Zur Prophylaxe der Colienterotoxämie des Schweines: Dauer der oralen Immunisierung mit virulenten Erregern unter dem Schutz eines Diätfutters. *Schweizer Archiv für Tierheilkunde* 123, 61–68.

Bertschinger, H.U., Jucker H. and Pfirter, H.P. (1984) Orale Vakzination von Ferkeln gegen Colienterotoxämie mit einer Streptomycin-Dependenz-Revertante von *Escherichia coli*. *Schweizer Archiv für Tierheilkunde* 126, 497–509.

Bertschinger, H.U., Munz-Müller, M., Pfirter, H.P. and Schneider, A. (1986) Vererbte Resistenz gegen Colienterotoxämie beim Schwein. *Zeitschrift für Tierzüchtung und Züchtungsbiologie* 103, 255–264.

Bertschinger, H.U., Bachmann, M., Mettler, C., Pospischil, A., Schraner, E.M., Stamm, M., Sydler, T. and Wild, P. (1990) Adhesive fimbriae produced *in vivo* by *Escherichia coli* O139:K12(B):H1 associated with enterotoxaemia in pigs. *Veterinary Microbiology* 25, 267–281.

Bertschinger, H.U., Stamm, M. and Vögeli, P. (1993) Inheritance of resistance to oedema disease in the pig: experiments with an *Escherichia coli* strain expressing fimbriae 107. *Veterinary Microbiology* 35, 79–89.

Blanco, J., Gonzalez, E.A., Bernardez, I. and Regueiro, B. (1983) Differentiated biological activity of Vero cytotoxins (VT) released by human and porcine *Escherichia coli* strains. *Federation of European Microbiological Societies Microbiology Letters* 20, 167–170.

Boss, P., Monckton, R.P., Nicolet, J. and Burnens, A.P. (1992) Nachweis von Toxingenen verschiedener *E. coli* Pathotypen beim Schwein mit nichtradioaktiv markierten Sonden. *Schweizer Archiv für Tierheilkunde* 134, 31–37.

Boyd, B., Tyrrell, G., Maloney, M., Gyles, C., Brunton, J. and Lingwood, C. (1993) Alteration of the glycolipid binding specificity of the pig edema toxin from globotetraosyl ceramide alters *in vivo* tissue targetting and results in a verotoxin 1-like disease in pigs. *Journal of Experimental Medicine* 177, 1745–1753.

Bürgi, E., Sydler, T., Bertschinger, H.U. and Pospischil, A. (1992) Mitteilung über das Vorkommen von Oedemkrankheit bei Zuchtschweinen. *Tierärztliche Umschau* 47, 582–588.

Clugston, R.E., Nielsen, N.O. and Smith, D.L.T. (1974) Experimental edema disease of swine (*E. coli* enterotoxemia). III. Pathology and pathogenesis. *Canadian Journal of Comparative Medicine* 38, 34–43.

De Cupere, F., Deprez, P., Demeulenaere, D. and Muylle, E. (1992) Evaluation of the effect of 3 probiotics on experimental *Escherichia coli* enterotoxaemia in weaned piglets. *Journal of Veterinary Medicine B* 39, 277–284.

Deprez, P., Van den Hende, C., Muylle, E. and Oyaert, W. (1986) The influence of the administration of sow's milk on the postweaning excretion of hemolytic *E. coli* in the pig. *Veterinary Research Communications* 10, 469–478.

Dobrescu, L. (1983) New biological effect of edema disease principle (*Escherichia coli* – neurotoxin) and its use as an *in vitro* assay for this toxin. *American Journal of Veterinary Research* 44, 31–34.

Erskine, R.G., Sojka, W.J. and Lloyd, M.K. (1957) The experimental reproduction of a syndrome indistinguishable from oedema disease. *Veterinary Record* 69, 301–303.

Ewing, H.W., Tatum, H.W. and Davis, B.R. (1958) *Escherichia coli* serotypes associated with edema disease of swine. *Cornell Veterinarian* 48, 201–206.

Fahey, V.A., Cutler, R.S. and Spicer, E.M. (1990) Diseases of weaned pigs. In: Gardner, J.A.A., Dunkin, A.C. and Lloyd, L.C. (eds) *Pig Production in Australia*. Butterworths, Sidney, pp. 169–170.

Gannon, V.P.J. and Gyles, C.L. (1990) Characteristics of the Shiga-like toxin produced by *Escherichia coli* associated with porcine edema disease. *Veterinary Microbiology* 24, 89–100.

Gannon, V.P.J., Gyles, C.L. and Friendship, R.W. (1988) Characteristics of verotoxigenic *Escherichia coli* from pigs. *Canadian Journal of Veterinary Research* 52, 331–337.

Gibbons, R.A., Sellwood, R., Burrows, M. and Hunter, P.A. (1977) Inheritance of resistance to neonatal *E. coli* diarrhoea in the pig: examination of the genetic system. *Theoretical and Applied Genetics* 51, 65–70.

Gonzalez, E.A. and Blanco, J. (1985) Production of cytotoxin VT in enteropathogenic and non-enteropathogenic *Escherichia coli* strains of porcine origin. *Federation of European Microbiological Societies Microbiology Letters* 26, 127–130.

Gordon, V.M., Whipp, S.C., Moon, H.W., O'Brien, A.D. and Samuel, J.E. (1992) An enzymatic mutant of Shiga-like toxin II variant is a vaccine candidate for edema disease of swine. *Infection and Immunity* 60, 485–490.

Gregory, D.W. (1955) Role of beta hemolytic coliform organisms in edema disease of swine. *Veterinary Medicine* 50, 609–610.

Gregory, D.W. (1960) The neuro-oedema toxin of haemolytic *Escherichia coli. Veterinary Record* 72, 1208–1209.

Gyles, C.L. (1992) *Escherichia coli* cytotoxins and enterotoxins. *Canadian Journal of Microbiology* 38, 734–746.

Gyles, C.L., De Grandis, S.A., MacKenzie, C. and Brunton, J.L. (1988) Cloning and nucleotide sequence analysis of the genes determining verocytotoxin production in a porcine edema disease isolate of *Escherichia coli. Microbial Pathogenesis* 5, 419–426.

Häni, H., Brändli, A., Nicolet, J., von Roll, P., Luginbühl, H. and Hörning, B. (1976) Vorkommen und Bedeutung von Schweinekrankheiten: Analyse eines Sektionsguts (1971–1973). III. Pathologie des Digestionstraktes. *Schweizer Archiv für Tierheilkunde* 118, 13–29.

Imberechts, H., De Greve, H., Schlicker, Ch., Bouchet, H., Pohl, P., Charlier, G., Bertschinger, H., Wild, P., Vandekerckhove, J., Van Damme, J., Van Montagu, M. and Lintermans, P. (1992a) Characterization of F107 fimbriae of *Escherichia coli* 107/86, which causes edema disease in pigs, and nucleotide sequence of the F107 major fimbrial subunit gene, *fedA. Infection and Immunity* 60, 1963–1971.

Imberechts, H., De Greve, H. and Lintermans, P. (1992b) The pathogenesis of edema disease in pigs. *Veterinary Microbiology* 31, 221–233.

Imberechts, H., Bertschinger, H.U., Stamm, M., Sydler, T., Pohl, P. De Greve, H., Hernalsteens, J.-P., Van Montagu, M. and Lintermans, P. (1994) Prevalence of F107 fimbriae on *Escherichia coli* isolated from pigs with oedema disease or postweaning diarrhoea. *Veterinary Microbiology* 40, 219–230.

Jahn, S. und Uecker, E. (1987) Oekonomische Untersuchungen zur Kolienterotoxämie des Schweines. *Monatshefte für Veterinärmedizin* 42, 769–771.

Kashiwazaki, M., Ogawa, T., Nakamura, K., Isayama, Y., Tamura, K. and Sakazaki, R. (1981) Vero cytotoxin produced by *Escherichia coli* strains of animal origin. *National Institute of Animal Health Quarterly (Japan)* 21, 68–72.

Kausche, F.M., Dean, E.A., Arp, L.H., Samuel, J.E. and Moon, H.W. (1992) An experimental model for subclinical edema disease (*Escherichia coli* enterotoxemia) manifest as vascular necrosis in pigs. *American Journal of Veterinary Research* 53, 281–287.

Kennan, R.M. and Monckton, R.P. (1990) Adhesive fimbriae associated with porcine enterotoxigenic *Escherichia coli* of the O141 serotype. *Journal of Clinical Microbiology* 28, 2006–2011.

Kernkamp, H.C.H., Sorensen, D.K., Hanson, L.J. and Nielsen, N.O. (1965) Epizootiology of edema disease in swine. *Journal of the American Veterinary Medical Association* 146, 353–357.

Konowalchuk, J., Speirs, J.I. and Stavric, S. (1977) Vero response to a cytotoxin of *Escherichia coli. Infection and Immunity* 18, 775–779.

Kurtz, H.J., Bergeland, M.E. and Barnes, D.M. (1969) Pathologic changes in edema disease of swine. *American Journal of Veterinary Research* 30, 791–806.

Linggood, M.A. and Thompson, J.M. (1987) Verotoxin production among porcine strains of *Escherichia coli* and its association with oedema disease. *Journal of Medical Microbiology* 25, 359–362.

Lloyd, M.K. (1957) Oedema disease in swine. Discussion of paper given by J.F. Timoney. *Veterinary Record* 69, 1160–1175.

Luke, D. and Gordon, W.A.M. (1950) Observations on some pig diseases. *Veterinary Record* 62, 179–185.

MacLeod, D.L. and Gyles, C.L. (1990) Purification and characterization of an *Escherichia coli* Shiga-like toxin II variant. *Infection and Immunity* 58, 1232–1239.

MacLeod, D.L. and Gyles, C.L. (1991) Immunization of pigs with a purified Shiga-like toxin II variant toxoid. *Veterinary Microbiology* 29, 309–318.

MacLeod, D.L., Gyles, C.L. and Wilcock, B.P. (1991) Reproduction of edema disease of swine with purified Shiga-like toxin-II variant. *Veterinary Pathology* 28, 66–73.

Marques, L.R.M., Peiris, J.S.M., Cryz, S.J. and O'Brien, A.D. (1987) *Escherichia coli* strains isolated from pigs with edema disease produce a variant of Shiga-like toxin II. *Federation of European Microbiological Societies Microbiology Letters* 44, 33–38.

Methiyapun, S., Pohlenz, J.F.L. and Bertschinger, H.U. (1984) Ultrastructure of the intestinal mucosa in pigs experimentally inoculated with an edema disease-producing strain of *Escherichia coli* (O139:K12:H1). *Veterinary Pathology* 21, 516–520.

Nagy, B., Casey, T.A. and Moon, H.W. (1990) Phenotype and genotype of *Escherichia coli* isolated from pigs with postweaning diarrhoea in Hungary. *Journal of Clinical Microbiology* 28, 651–653.

Nagy, B., Casey, T.A., Whipp, S.C. and Moon, H.W. (1992a) Susceptibility of porcine intestine to pilus-mediated adhesion by some isolates of piliated enterotoxigenic *Escherichia coli* increases with age. *Infection and Immunity* 60, 1285–1294.

Nagy, B., Casey, T.A., Whipp, S.C., Moon, H.W. and Dean-Nystrom, E.A. (1992b) Pili and adhesiveness of porcine post weaning enterotoxigenic and verotoxigenic *Escherichia coli*. In: *Proceedings 12th International Pig Veterinary Society Congress, The Hague*. Royal Netherlands Veterinary Association, ORBIT, GAIB b.v., 's-Hertogenbosch, The Netherlands, p. 240.

Ørskov, I., Ørskov, F., Sojka, W.J. and Leach, J.M. (1961) Simultaneous occurrence of *E. coli* B and L antigen in strains from diseased swine. *Acta pathologica et microbiologica Scandinavica* 53, 404–422.

Pohl, P., Verlinden, M., Lintermans, P., Van Robaeys, G. and Stockmans, F. (1991) Antibiogrammes des entérobactéries pathogènes pour les animaux d'élevage et les pigeons, isolées en Belgique de 1986 à 1990. *Annales de Médecine Vétérinaire* 135, 101–108.

Salajka, E., Cernohous, J. and Sarmanova, Z. (1975) Association of the colonization of the intestine by pathogenic strains of haemolytic *E. coli* in weaned piglets with withdrawal of antibody contained in the dams' milk. *Documenta veterinaria, Brno* 8, 43–55.

Salajka, E., Salajkova, Z., Alexa, P. and Hornich, M. (1992) Colonization factor different from K88, K99, F41 and 987P in enterotoxigenic *Escherichia coli* strains isolated from postweaning diarrhoea in pigs. *Veterinary Microbiology* 32, 163–175.

Samuel, J.E., Perera, L.P., Ward, S., O'Brien, A.D., Ginsburg, V. and Krivan, H.C. (1990) Comparison of the glycolipid receptor specificities of Shiga-like toxin type II and Shiga-like toxin type II variants. *Infection and Immunity* 58, 611–618.

Saxena, S.K., O'Brien, A.D. and Ackerman, E.J. (1989) Shiga toxin, Shiga-like toxin II variant, and ricin are all single-site RNA N-glycosidases of 28 S RNA when microinjected into *Xenopus* oocytes. *Journal of Biological Chemistry* 264, 596–601.

Schimmelpfennig, H.H. (1970) Untersuchungen zur Aetiologie der Oedemkrankheit des Schweines. *Beiheft 13 zum Zentralblatt für Veterinärmedizin*. Verlag Paul Parey, Berlin.

Schofield, F.W. and Davis, D. (1955) Oedema disease (entero-toxaemia) in swine. – II. Experiments conducted in a susceptible herd. *Canadian Journal of Comparative Medicine* 19, 242–245.

Schulze, F. (1977) Quantitative Magen-Darm-Flora-Analysen beim Ferkel vor und nach dem Absetzen unter Berücksichtigung der Pathogenese der Kolienterotoxämie. *Archiv für Experimentelle Veterinärmedizin* 31, 299–316.

Semjen, G., Ørskov, I. and Ørskov, F. (1977) K antigen determination of *Escherichia coli* by counter-current immunoelectrophoresis (CIE). *Acta pathologica microbiologica Scandinavica Sect B.* 85, 103–107.

Shanks, P.L. (1938) An unusual condition affecting the digestive organs of the pig. *Veterinary Record* 50, 356–358.

Smith, H.W. (1963) The haemolysins of *Escherichia coli*. *Journal of Pathology and Bacteriology* 85, 197–211.

Smith, H.W. and Halls S. (1968) The production of oedema disease and diarrhoea in weaned pigs by the oral administration of *Escherichia coli*: factors that influence the course of the experimental disease. *Journal of Medical Microbiology* 1, 45–59.

Smith, H.W. and Jones, J.E.T. (1963) Observations on the alimentary tract and its bacterial flora in healthy and diseased pigs. *Journal of Pathology and Bacteriology* 86, 387–412.

Smith, H.W. and Linggood, M.A. (1971) Observations on the pathogenic properties of the K88, Hly and ent plasmids of *Escherichia coli* with particular reference to porcine diarrhoea. *Journal of Medical Microbiology* 4, 467–485.

Smith, H.W., Green, P. and Parsell, Z. (1983) Vero cell toxins in *Escherichia coli* and related bacteria. Transfer by phage and conjugation and toxic action in laboratory animals, chickens and pigs. *Journal of General Microbiology* 129, 3121–3137.

Sojka, W.J. (1965) *Escherichia coli in Domestic Animals and Poultry*. Commonwealth Agricultural Bureaux, Farnham Royal, UK.

Sojka, W.J., Erskine, R.G. and Lloyd M.K. (1957) Haemolytic *Escherichia coli* and 'oedema disease' of pigs. *Veterinary Record* 69, 293–301.

Stamm, M. and Bertschinger, H.U. (1992) Identification of pigs genetically resistant to oedema disease by testing adhesion of *E. coli* expressing fimbriae 107 to intestinal epithelial cells. In: *Proceedings of the 12th International Pig*

Veterinary Society Congress, The Hague. Royal Netherlands Veterinary Association, ORBIT, GAIB b.v., 's-Hertogenbosch, The Netherlands, p. 242.

Stamm, M., Bertschinger, H.U. and Sydler, T. (1990) Prevalence of fimbriae 107 in the intestine of pigs with oedema disease or postweaning *E. coli* diarrhoea. In: *Proceedings of the 11th International Pig Veterinary Society Congress, Lausanne*. IPVS, Lausanne, p. 142.

Timoney, J.F. (1950) Oedema disease of swine. *Veterinary Record* 62, 748–755.

Timoney, J.F. (1957) Oedema disease in swine. *Veterinary Record* 69, 1160–1175.

Timoney, J.F. (1960) An alternative method to repeated freezing and thawing for the preparation of an extract from a strain of haemolytic *Escherichia coli* which on intravenous injection in pigs mimics the syndrome of oedema disease. *Veterinary Record* 72, 1252.

Truszczynski, M., Ciosek, D. and Wittig, W. (1985) Die Bedeutung der O- und K-Antigene sowie der Enterotoxine als Indikatoren der Pathogenität der *Escherichia-coli*-Stämme vom Schwein. *Archiv für Experimentelle Veterinärmedizin* 39, 470–491.

Tschäpe, H., Bender, L., Ott, M., Wittig, W. and Hacker, J. (1992) Restriction fragment length polymorphism and virulence pattern of the veterinary pathogen *Escherichia coli* O139:K82:H1. *Zentralblatt für Bakteriologie* 276, 264–272.

Vögeli, P., Delacretaz, A.S., Kuhn, B., Stamm, M., Bertschinger, H.U. and Stranzinger, G. (1992) Associations between the H blood group system and the GPI red cell enzyme system and the locus specifying receptors of an *Escherichia coli* strain expressing fimbriae 107 in the pig. *Animal Genetics* 23 (Suppl. 1), 93.

Wittig, W. and Fabricius, Ch. (1992) *Escherichia coli* types isolated from porcine *E. coli* infections in Saxony from 1963 to 1990. *Zentralblatt für Bakteriologie* 277, 389–402.

Wittig, W., Prager, R., Stamm, M., Streckel, W. and Tschäpe, H. (1994) Expression and plasmid transfer for the frimbrial antigen F107 in porcine *Escherichia coli* strains. *Zentralblatt für Bakteriologie* 281, 130–139.

10

Extraintestinal *Escherichia coli* Infections in Pigs

J.M. Fairbrother and M. Ngeleka

Swine Infectious Disease Research Group (Groupe de Recherche sur les Maladies Infectieuses du Porc: GREMIP), Faculty of Veterinary Medicine, University of Montreal, CP5000, St-Hyacinthe, Quebec, Canada J2S 7C6

Septicaemia or Systemic Colibacillosis

Introduction

E. coli may induce extraintestinal infections such as septicaemia, polyserositis, meningitis, arthritis, mastitis and urogenital tract infections (Morris and Sojka, 1985; Fairbrother *et al.*, 1989; Bertschinger *et al.*, 1992). Septicaemia must be distinguished from bacteraemia in which a small number of microorganisms enter the circulatory system over a very short time and are removed by the non-specific mechanisms of host defence (i.e. complement and phagocytic system) without causing symptoms. This bacterial invasion may result in a localized infection manifested as meningitis and/or arthritis. In septicaemia, the microorganisms enter the system, persist in the blood and colonize extraintestinal organs (e.g. lung, liver, kidney, spleen) usually over a period of time. Nevertheless, septicaemia is preceded by a bacteraemic phase in which bacteria enter the system from different sites of infection, especially from the intestinal and respiratory tracts. Septicaemia due to *E. coli* may be primary, occurring predominantly in newborn to 4-day-old pigs, or secondary, when associated with diarrhoea or other compromising diseases in young pigs.

Clinical aspects and gross lesions

Primary septicaemia frequently occurs in neonatal piglets, and is observed less frequently in suckling piglets and rarely in piglets more than 80 days of age (Nielson *et al.*, 1975b; Murata *et al.*, 1979). Clinical signs of infection include depression, lameness, reluctance to move, anorexia, rough haircoat and laboured respiration. The affected piglets may show sternal recumbency and the abdomen may be somewhat distended. Sometimes piglets become unconscious with convulsions and paddling movements; they may be in good bodily condition but cyanosis of the extremities may be observed. Some piglets are found dead whereas others are comatose without any sign of diarrhoea. These clinical signs may develop in the first 12 hours after birth and piglets may die within 48 hours (Taylor, 1989). In older piglets, the clinical signs can include periodical scouring or other ailments which precede the onset of acute septicaemia with symptoms resembling those in the newborn pigs.

In acute primary septicaemia, there may be no gross lesions but congestion of the intestine, the mesenteric lymph nodes and the extraintestinal organs may be observed. In subacute cases, subserous or submucosal haemorrhages and fibrinous polyserositis with gross signs of pneumonia are usually observed, and fibrinopurulent arthritis and meningitis may accompany these lesions (Waxler and Britt, 1972; Morris and Sojka, 1985). In secondary septicaemia resulting from enteric colibacillosis, icterus, petechial haemorrhages in the serosal membranes, and splenomegaly accompanied by severe diarrhoea and dehydration may be observed in some cases (Bertschinger *et al.*, 1992).

In a 4-year study (from 1989 to 1992) of 2266 cases from which *E. coli* were isolated in our laboratory, 318 cases (14%) involved *E. coli* septicaemia with bacteria isolated from the intestine and from more than one extraintestinal organ. Among these cases, 49 (15.4%) were associated with primary septicaemia which included polyserositis, pericarditis and meningitis from which *E. coli* were isolated from extraintestinal organs, and 269 cases (84.6%) were associated with sudden death of piglets due either to primary or secondary septicaemia and from which *E. coli* were isolated in significant numbers from the intestine or extraintestinal organs. In confirmed primary septicaemia, 94% of cases occurred in suckling piglets whereas 6% of cases occurred in piglets more than 2 months of age. In cases of sudden death of piglets, 79% of cases were found in neonatal and suckling piglets, and 21% in piglets more than 2 months of age.

In experimental reproduction of septicaemia in colostrum-deprived newborn piglets, most piglets became depressed and weak, and died within 12–48 hours after intragastric inoculation (Fairbrother *et al.*, 1989; Ngeleka *et al.*, 1993; Table 10.1; personal observations). Fever was observed in some piglets but most of them developed hypothermia as they became moribund. Mucoid diarrhoea was observed sporadically. Lesions of fibrinous polyserositis were observed in many pigs, particularly those which survived more than 24 hours. The thoracic, pericardial, peritoneal and certain limb joint cavities contained small to moderate quantities of yellow fluid. A layer of fibrin adhered to the visceral pleura and peritoneum.

Serotypes

A relatively small number of serogroups have been reported in natural cases of septicaemia. Serogroups O6, O8, O9, O11, O15, O17, O18, O20, O45, O60, O78, O83, O93, O101, O112, O115 and O116 have most commonly been identified in isolates associated with the infection (Nielson *et al.*, 1975a; Morris and Sojka, 1985; Gyles, 1986; Fairbrother *et al.*, 1989). In addition to *E. coli*, other Gram-negative bacteria such as *Klebsiella* spp. and *Pseudomonas* spp. have been reported to be associated with systemic infections in pigs (Bertschinger *et al.*, 1992)

In our 4-year study, the most commonly observed serogroups in isolates from cases of primary septicaemia were O9 (10%) and O20 (18%). Serogroups O1, O18, O60, O78, O101, O141 and O147 were isolated in relatively lower numbers (2–4% of each), but 49% of isolates were non-typable. In cases of sudden death of piglets, serogroups O8 (13%), O141 (3%), O149 (11%) and O157 (5%), often associated with enterotoxigenic isolates, were most commonly isolated, and serogroups O9, O20 and O101 (3% for each) were also isolated. Serogroups O2, O7, O10, O15, O21, O26, O45, O54, O64, O71, O78, O83, O108, O114, O115, O119, O128, O131, O137, O139 and O147 (1–2% for each) were isolated to a lesser extent. However, 42% of isolates from these cases were non-typable.

Not all *E. coli* isolates are able to cause septicaemia in colostrum-deprived piglets (Meyer *et al.*, 1971; Murata *et al.*, 1979; Table 10.1). For instance, we found that certain O115 isolates, and all three O101 isolates that were tested failed to cause septicaemia. Isolates of certain serogroups (O78:K80, O9:K30, O11:K"F12",and O137:K79) appeared to cause septicaemia more rapidly than isolates of other serogroups that were tested.

Characteristics of E. coli *involved*

Septicaemia-inducing strains may express virulence determinants which include fimbriae, polysaccharide capsule and O-antigen capsule, lipopolysaccharide (LPS or O-antigen), the aerobactin system, haemolysin and other cytotoxins (Ngeleka *et al.*, 1993). Fimbrial adhesins play a crucial role in development of many bacterial diseases. Typically, these adhesins are able to mediate attachment of bacteria to erythrocytes of various species *in vitro* (haemagglutination: HA) and to other eukaryotic cells. Pathogenic bacteria may produce one or more of the different serotypes of fimbriae classified as mannose sensitive (MS) (i.e. the attachment mediated by these fimbriae to eukaryotic cells is inhibited by D-mannoside) or mannose-resistant (MR) fimbriae. The MS F1 (type 1) or common fimbriae are encoded by the *pil* or *fim* operon and are produced by most of the pathogenic and non-pathogenic Gram-negative bacteria (Hacker, 1992; Ørskov and Ørskov, 1992).

Table 10.1. Ability of porcine and bovine *E. coli* isolates to cause septicaemia in experimentally inoculated colostrum-deprived piglets.

	Isolates which caused septicaemia/ isolates tested[a]		
Serogroup	Porcine	Bovine	Time of onset of clinical signs (hours)
O9:K28	6/6	1/1	20–72
O9:K30	1/2	3/3	16–48
O11:K"F12"	0/0	1/1	48
O15:K"RVC383"	0/0	1/2	48–72
O20:K"X367"	0/0	1/1	20–43
O78:K80	2/2	0/0	18–24
O101:K30	0/0	0/2	NA
O101:K32	0/1	0/0	NA
O115:K"V165"	5/10	0/0	40–48
O137:K79	0/0	1/1	16
O141:K85ab	1/1	0/1	48

[a] At least two piglets inoculated per isolate.
NA, not applicable.

Among the MR fimbriae, fimbriae of the P family, represented by Pap (pyelonephritis associated pili) encoded by the *pap* operon, are expressed by strains from urinary tract infections in humans. These fimbriae bind to the alpha-D-galactopyranosyl-(1–4)-β-D-galactopyranoside (Gal-α-(1–4)-β-Gal) moiety present in the globoseries of glycolipids on cells lining the urinary tract. Prs (P-related sequence) adhesins are encoded by the *prs* operon and adhere to the galactose-*N*-acetyl-α-(1–3)-galactose-*N*-acetyl (GalNac-GalNac) moiety of the Forssman antigen located on the surface of sheep erythrocytes (Hacker, 1992). The S fimbrial adhesins (Sfa) encoded by the *sfa* operon are related to the F1C non-haemagglutinating fimbriae and are closely associated with *E. coli* causing septicaemia or newborn meningitis in humans. These adhesins recognize α-sialyl-(2–3)-β-galactose containing glycoprotein receptors. The adherence factor termed afimbrial adhesin (Afa) is encoded by the *afa* operon and is expressed by strains from urinary tract infections in humans, in the absence of any fimbrial structures (Hacker, 1992).

The F165 fimbrial complex has been found on *E. coli* isolates from piglets and calves with septicaemia and/or diarrhoea (Fairbrother *et al.*, 1986; Contrepois *et al.*, 1989). These isolates belong principally to serogroups O8, O9, O78 and O115 and biotypes 1 and 2, but isolates belonging to serogroups O15, O101 and O141 and biotypes 10, 12, 14 and 16 have also been reported (Harel *et al.*, 1993). The purified F165 fimbrial complex possesses at least two separate major protein subunits of 19 kDa and 17.5 kDa (Fairbrother *et al.*, 1988) which we have subsequently designated $F165_1$ and $F165_2$, respectively. The $F165_1$ fimbrial component encoded by *f165₁*, a *prs*-like operon, recognizes the GalNAc-GalNAc moiety, and haemagglutinates sheep and porcine erythrocytes (Harel *et al.*, 1992). The $F165_2$ fimbrial component is similar, but not identical, to fimbrial component F1C (Dubreuil and Fairbrother, 1992).

In our 4-year study, 6% of isolates from cases of primary septicaemia were F165 positive as determined by immunofluorescence; F165 was most frequently found in isolates of serogroups O9 (20%). Four per cent of isolates from cases of sudden death of piglets were F165 positive. F165 was most commonly observed in serogroups O8 (8%), O78 (100%) and O141 (43%). Sixteen per cent of isolates from cases of sudden death of piglets expressed fimbrial antigen F4 (K88) associated with enterotoxigenic *E. coli*, especially isolates of serogroups O8 (3%), O20 (1%), O149 (84%) and O157 (54%).

F165-positive porcine isolates, with the exception of those belonging to serogroup O101, induced septicaemia in newborn colostrum-deprived pigs (Fairbrother *et al.*, 1989; Table 10.1; personal observations). They possessed the *pap*, *pap* + *sfa*, or *pap* + *afa* fimbrial operons (Fairbrother *et al.*, 1989, 1993). *pap*-positive strains agglutinated human OP_1, A_1P_1 and bovine erythrocytes whereas *pap* + *sfa*-positive and *pap* + *afa*-positive isolates agglutinated human A_1P_1 and sheep erythrocytes, or human OP_1 and bovine erythrocytes, respectively. Some of these isolates recognized the Gal-α-(1–4)-β-Gal or the GalNac-GalNac moiety (Fairbrother *et al.*, 1993; Harel *et al.*, 1993). These results indicate that adhesins with receptor specificity different from that of $F165_1$ and $F165_2$ are also present on these isolates.

The characteristics of 14 porcine isolates inducing septicaemia in newborn colostrum-deprived pigs and four isolates from primary septicaemia in pigs were studied (Fairbrother *et al.*, 1989; Harel *et al.*, 1993; personal observations). Both F165-positive and F165-negative isolates were represented in this group. Most isolates caused MRHA of erythrocytes from at least two animal species, indicating that fimbriae other than $F165_1$ and $F165_2$ may be associated with septicaemia in pigs. Six of 11 isolates that were tested produced colicin V, 11 of 12 isolates produced the siderophore aerobactin and eight of eight isolates were serum resistant. One of 10 isolates from cases of primary septicaemia produced cytotoxic necrotizing factor 1 (CNF1), whereas four of 65 isolates from cases of sudden death or diarrhoea of piglets produced this toxin (E. Oswald, Maryland, 1992, personal communication). None of the 75 isolates that were examined produced toxin cytotoxic necrotizing factor 2 (CNF2).

Pathogenesis

Neonatal septicaemia occurs in piglets lacking immunity, either due to an absence of ingested colostrum or to ingestion of colostrum lacking specific antibody. The disease may develop after bacterial invasion of the respiratory or the gastrointestinal tract in the non-immune host. Contamination of the umbilicus after birth may also lead to colisepticaemia. However, the intestine is considered to be a major route of *E. coli* invasion since the disease may be experimentally induced by oral or intragastric administration of the organisms (Ngeleka *et al.*, 1993).

Secondary septicaemia may develop after invasion of the host by enterotoxigenic *E. coli* but in most cases development of primary neonatal septicaemia is associated with intestinal permeability to macromolecules (IPM), to some defect of the immune system (e.g. low levels of maternal colostrum), to low birthweight or to sublethal malformations (Murata *et al.*, 1979; Gyles, 1986; Bertschinger *et al.*, 1992).

Bacteria may pass through the mucosa of the alimentary tract, probably by endocytic uptake into intestinal epithelial cells or through the intercellular spaces formed by lateral plasma membranes of adjacent epithelial cells, to locate in the mesenteric lymph nodes before entering the blood stream (Ngeleka *et al.*, 1993). This bacterial invasion may result in a generalized infection (septicaemia, polyserositis) with bacteria disseminated in different extraintestinal organs such as the lung, liver, spleen, kidney, brain and heart blood, or in a localized infection (meningitis or arthritis) (Morris and Sojka, 1985). In the sow, a perpueral sepsis may be induced by an enteric *E. coli* soon after farrowing (Sojka, 1965).

Septicaemia may be produced experimentally in colostrum-deprived piglets by intragastric inoculation with isolates of porcine origin (Ngeleka *et al.*, 1993; Table 10.1). However, the disease can also be reproduced in piglets with isolates from other animals, including cats, poultry and calves (Meyer *et al.*, 1971; Murata *et al.*, 1979; Table 10.1). After intragastric inoculation, the incubation period is very short and may vary from 12 hours to 5 days depending on the strain and the quantity of inoculum used. The inoculated animals survive from 1 to 8 days. The animals may develop fever, anorexia, diarrhoea, dyspnoea or nervous signs. These symptoms may be due in part to the effect of bacterial endotoxin or cytotoxins or to the effects of inflammatory cytokines, such as tumour necrosis factor (TNF) and interleukin 1 (Il-1) induced by these bacterial products (Nakajima *et al.*, 1991; Jesmok *et al.*, 1992).

The role of some of the virulence determinants associated with *E. coli*-inducing septicaemia are only partially understood. Certain LPS, K capsules and O-antigen capsules, and production of siderophores such as aerobactin are thought to allow the bacteria to invade the host and escape its defence mechanisms. These determinants increase bacterial resistance to the bactericidal effect of complement and to phagocytosis, and allow bacterial growth in body fluids with low concentrations of free iron (Crosa, 1989; Ngeleka *et al.*, 1992, 1993).

In an experimental infection of colostrum-deprived newborn gnotobiotic piglets, a serum-resistant *E. coli* strain of O115 serogroup expressing F165 fimbriae, the K"V165" O-antigen capsule, and possessing the aerobactin system and Col V plasmid, induced clinical signs of septicaemia (Ngeleka *et al.*, 1992, 1993). Bacteria were associated with the intestinal goblet cells and the mucous layer more than with the intestinal cells (Fig. 10.1). Experimental inoculation of gnotobiotic piglets with Tn*phoA* and spontaneous mutants of this strain demonstrated that the presence of the $F165_1$ fimbriae and of the K"V165" O-antigen capsule did not seem to play a role in intestinal colonization or passage through the intestinal wall, but was strongly associated with bacterial survival in the extra-intestinal organs and in the blood stream of infected piglets and with pathogenicity for piglets. Fimbrial antigen $F165_1$ promotes adherence of bacteria to porcine polymorphonuclear leucocytes *in vitro*, but enhances resistance to phagocytosis (Ngeleka *et al.*, 1994). O-antigen capsule K"V165" is required for resistance to the bactericidal effects of serum and for resistance to phagocytosis by porcine polymorphonuclear leucocytes *in vitro* (Ngeleka *et al.*, 1992, 1994).

Differential diagnosis

Systemic colibacillosis is generally suspected on the basis of clinical signs (Bertschinger *et al.*, 1992). However, in cases of polyserositis *Mycoplasma hyorhinis* and *Haemophilus suis* need to be considered as possible causes of the disease. The former infection tends to be slower in developing and gross lesions can be detected more than 6 days after infection; the mortality rate is lower than in *E. coli* infection. In infection due to *H. suis* the exudate may be serofibrinous or fibrinous, whereas in polyserositis due to *E. coli*, the exudate encountered in piglets may be serofibrinous or fibrinopurulent to purulent (Waxler and Britt, 1972). Furthermore, infection due to *H. suis* is rarely seen in the early suckling period but usually in piglets of 2–3 months of age. However, a differential diagnosis can be established after isolation of the organism that is involved. In most cases some pigs will die and samples taken at postmortem examination will yield the bacterium in pure culture.

Prevention and treatment

Inadequate hygiene and poor environmental temperature control increase the likelihood of infection (Bertschinger *et al.*, 1992). Thus, prevention of infection should concentrate on reduction or elimination of significant

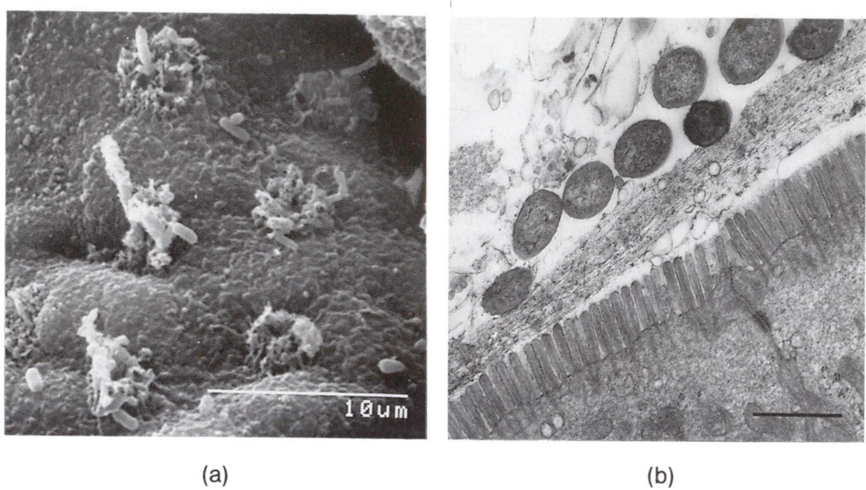

(a) (b)

Fig. 10.1. Colonization of the porcine intestinal mucosa by an O115:K″V165″:F165 strain which caused septicaemia. Scanning (a) and transmission (b) electron micrographs of bacterial cells in association with goblet cells (a) or the mucous layer (b) in the colon of a pig inoculated with a septicaemia-inducing *E. coli*. Scale bar = 1 μm.

pathogenic *E. coli* populations in the environmental area of the piglets, and in providing sufficient colostrum at birth. Good hygiene practices, especially washing and disinfection of the farrowing pens, would greatly contribute to reduction of the infection. Young piglets should be maintained at an even temperature of 35 °C for the first week of life. They must be kept dry and warm in clean surroundings. In small outbreaks, careful monitoring of the causative serogroup(s) and immunization of the pregnant sows with an autogenous vaccine may be useful.

Treatment may be attempted after diagnostic confirmation of *E. coli* infection and antibiotic sensitivity testing. Meanwhile, parenteral or oral administration of a broad-spectrum antibiotic to affected piglets can be suggested. This treatment may be useful in subacute cases of infection but is mostly ineffective after appearance of clinical signs. However, the remaining piglets in the litter and affected piglets in adjacent litters should be treated.

Urogenital Tract Infection

Urinary tract infection (UTI) is an important cause of death in adult pigs (Bertschinger *et al.*, 1992). This infection may be manifested as bacteriuria without apparent clinical signs or as acute infection including cystitis and pyelonephritis. Pyelonephritis is the major cause of death in adult female pigs in certain countries (D'Allaire *et al.*, 1991). The presence of bacteria may increase the risk of subsequently developing mastitis-metritis agalactia (MMA). *Eubacterium suis* has been isolated at a high prevalence in sows with severe urinary tract disease, and may be considered as a specific cause of this disease (Berstchinger *et al.*, 1992). Other bacteria such as *Klebsiella* spp., *Pseudomonas* spp., *Aeromonas* spp., *Staphylococcus* spp., *Enterococcus* spp. and *Bacteroides* spp. are considered as causes of non-specific UTI. *E. coli* is also associated with non-specific UTI (Bertschinger *et al.*, 1992; Carr and Walton, 1992a). In most of these cases no clinical signs are observed and bacteriuria may be associated with low litter size and frequency. Cystitis leads to abnormal urination and possibly vulval discharge in sows. Pyelonephritis often occurs during the first 2 weeks postpartum and typically results in a low rectal temperature, high heart rate, polypnoea, cyanosis and ataxia.

E. coli has been associated with endometritis in sows immediately after parturition (Berner, 1984) and with abortions in swine (Pohl *et al.*, 1993) and has been isolated in pure culture from organs of aborted fetuses (personal observations). Clinical signs of endometritis range from mild (with no fever and some fluid, seromucous exudate) to severe (with fever, abundant exudate) hypogalactia and signs of septicaemia or toxaemia.

The characteristics of *E. coli* associated with UTI in humans have been well studied (reviewed by Johnson, 1991; Ørskov and Ørskov, 1992). These isolates often produce P fimbrial adhesins, especially in cases of pyelonephritis, or Afa, Nfa, Sfa and F1A (type 1) adhesins. They most commonly belong to serogroups O1, O4, O6, O16, and O18, and produce haemolysin, CNF1 and aerobactin. The *E. coli* isolates from porcine UTI have not been well characterized. In one study (Carr and Walton, 1992a), all 52 isolates from the urinary tract of sows with bacteriuria or cystitis and pyelonephritis, and from the genital tract of sows with a vulval discharge, were non-haemolytic and non-typable using antisera against known porcine *E. coli* serogroups, but these isolates were not tested against serogroups commonly associated with UTI infections in other species. Only one isolate appeared to produce P fimbriae. However, one potential virulence determinant was the production of F1A (type 1) fimbriae in 41% of these isolates. P fimbrial adhesins mediate attachment of *E. coli* to the urinary tract epithelium in humans. They permit the bacteria to ascend to and colonize the upper urinary tract and induce pyelonephritis. The role of Prs adhesins, which have been found on *E. coli* isolates associated with septicaemia in pigs, has not been studied in urinary tract isolates from the same species.

The *E. coli* isolates from porcine genital tract infections have not been well characterized. Pohl *et al.* (1993) demonstrated the production of CNF1, but not CNF2, in three of three isolates from aborted fetuses and in two of two isolates from the semen of boars. We have found that most

(14/17) isolates from aborted fetuses are non-typable with antisera against the serogroups most commonly associated with systemic colibacillosis in humans and animals. One isolate belonged to O2 and two belonged to O8 serogroup.

Infection of the upper urinary tract is favoured by the short, wide urethra of the sow; relaxation of the sphincter muscle in late pregnancy; trauma to the urethra and bladder at coitus and parturition; abnormal bacterial colonization of the sinus urogenitales and the genital organs; incomplete closure of the vulva; and catheterization of the bladder (Bertschinger *et al.*, 1992). Chronic *E. coli* infection of the urinary tract appears to predispose sows to ascending infection of the uterus in the first day after parturition (Berner, 1984). Release of high levels of endotoxin from the uterus may result in clinical symptoms resembling toxaemia.

UTI is often non-specific (non-contagious disease of endogenous origin), involving *E. coli* or other bacterial species (Bertschinger *et al.*, 1992), and should be suspected when bacteriological examination of the urine reveals more than 10^4 c.f.u. ml^{-1}. A colony count of more than 10^5 c.f.u. ml^{-1} is indicative of an infection. A count of less then 10^4 c.f.u. ml^{-1} would reflect the normal flora colonizing the vagina and the distal part of the urethra.

In most cases of non-specific UTI the clinical signs were inapparent (Carr and Walton, 1992b). In sows with cystitis and pyelonephritis, biochemical changes of the plasma included azotaemia, hyperkalaemia and raised plasma concentrations of calcium, magnesium and phosphate. Sodium and chloride concentrations of the urine were increased. The blood concentration of urea and creatinine was very high. Examination of the urine may reveal pyuria, haematuria, renal granular casts and bacteriuria.

Treatment of urogenital *E. coli* infections usually consists of antimicrobial therapy to eliminate the bacteria. However, variability in susceptibility of the *E. coli* isolates to different agents, and a high level of resistance to certain antimicrobials such as tetracyclines, streptomycin and ampicillin complicates this task (Bertschinger *et al.*, 1992; Carr and Walton, 1992b). Prolonged parenteral treatment with broad-spectrum or combined antimicrobials has been recommended, although subclinical UTI often persists after treatment. To reduce the incidence of the infection, it has been recommended that sows be checked for UTI and treated if necessary with specific antimicrobial agents before parturition (Bertschinger *et al.*, 1992). A reduction of environmental exposure to faecal drainage and an improvement in housing conditions would also contribute to reduce the infection. Vaccination has not been considered as an alternative for prevention of disease.

Mastitis

Mastitis induced by *E. coli* is often referred to as coliform mastitis, although this term includes mastitis caused by *Klebsiella* spp., *Enterobacter* spp. and *Citrobacter* spp. (Armstrong *et al.*, 1968; Jones, 1968; Ross *et al.*, 1975; Bertschinger *et al.*, 1992). The disease is also termed more descriptively, according to the clinical signs, milk fever, farrowing fever, lactation failure, hypogalactia and agalactia or mastitis-metritis-agalactia (MMA), agalactia postpartum syndrome, agalactia toxaemia, puerperal toxaemia and puerperal mastitis (Pederson *et al.*, 1984; for review, see Bertschinger *et al.*, 1992).

Coliform mastitis (CM) has been described all over the world and may have an incidence of up to 50% in individual herds. Economic losses are due to mortality of piglets resulting from increased farrowing time, starvation and impaired immunity following low uptake of colostral immunoglobulins. Low milk yield of affected sows leads to low weight gain of piglets. *E. coli* has been the organism most often isolated from milk or infected tissues of cases of coliform mastitis (Armstrong *et al.*, 1968; Ross *et al.*, 1975; Wegman and Berstchinger, 1984). Most clinical descriptions of this disease refer to coliform mastitis and not specifically to *E. coli* mastitis, the clinical features being the same for all the coliform organisms.

Clinical signs may range from a very mild to a highly acute form in which the mammary tissue is greatly inflammed and oedematous, the inguinal lymph nodes are swollen, and agalactia or diminished lactation, fever, lethargy, anorexia and weakness are observed (Bertschinger *et al.*, 1992; Smith *et al.*, 1992). The signs are usually manifested 1–2 days after farrowing and last for several days. An initial leucopenia is observed, usually followed by a leucocytosis. Mammary secretions may be serous to purulent, and may contain large quantities of fibrin or blood.

The characteristics of *E. coli* associated with mastitis in sows have not been extensively studied. It does not appear that any serotypes predominate among the isolates from diseased mammary glands, but that multiple serotypes may be found within a herd and even within different glands of one sow (Bertschinger *et al.*, 1992). In one study of *E. coli* isolates from milk samples from agalactic and clinically healthy sows within 48 hours after parturition (Pedersen *et al.*, 1984), 47% of isolates grown in nutrient broth demonstrated mannose-resistant haemagglutination (MRHA) of guinea-pig erythrocytes. In addition 17% of isolates showed both mannose-sensitive haemagglutination (MSHA) and MRHA. However, no correlation was observed between haemagglutination of isolates and clinical findings. Thus, it is not clear if fimbrial adherence is involved in colonization of the porcine mammary gland by *E. coli*.

It is probable that *E. coli* causing mastitis originate from contamination of the nipples by the intestinal flora and the environment. For instance,

Awad-Masalmeh *et al.* (1990) found identical *E. coli* isolates in mammary secretions and faeces of about 25% of sows with mastitis. Invasion of the mammary gland by *E. coli* probably occurs prior to parturition or up to 2 days postpartum (Bertschinger *et al.*, 1992). Bacteria may be found in the inguinal lymph nodes, but systemic invasion is rare (Armstrong *et al.*, 1968; Ross *et al.*, 1983). Bacteria are rapidly eliminated from the mammary gland within 6 days postpartum (Wegmann and Bertschinger, 1984). Certain sows appear to be more susceptible to mastitis induced experimentally by *E. coli* (Ross *et al.*, 1983).

The agalactia and septicaemic effects observed in cases of *E. coli* mastitis are probably due to bacterial release of endotoxin into the circulation. Endotoxaemia was observed more often in sows with mastitis than in healthy control sows (Morkoc *et al.*, 1983). Exposure of sows to endotoxin resulted in hypogalactia (Ferguson *et al.*, 1984) and a decrease in prolactin plasma levels (Smith and Wagner, 1984). Intravenous inoculation of endotoxin in sows also resulted in fever, depression and anorexia (De Ruijter *et al.*, 1988). However, fever was also observed after inoculation of small doses of endotoxin into the mammary glands of sows made tolerant to endotoxin by its repeated intravenous administration. These results suggest that host inflammatory mediators, produced in the mammary gland in response to endotoxin stimulation, are absorbed into the circulation and result in the systemic effects associated with *E. coli* mastitis.

Mastitis due to *E. coli* may be differentiated from that caused by other Gram-negative bacteria of the genera *Klebsiella*, *Enterobacter* and *Citrobacter*, or by Gram-positive bacteria of the genera *Streptococcus* and *Staphylococcus* (Smith *et al.*, 1992). This may be accomplished by bacteriological culture. In lactation insufficiency, non-infectious causes such as malformation, ergot toxicity, psychogenic agalactia, mammary oedema, poor management and nutritional disorders should be considered.

Treatment of *E. coli* mastitis consists of either oral or parenteral administration of appropriate antimicrobial agents and may be supplemented by administration of a glucocorticosteroid or oxytocin (Bertschinger *et al.*, 1992). Prevention of *E. coli* mastitis is aimed at decreasing bacterial contamination of the teats, especially by improving farrowing accommodation. Chemoprophylaxis prior to farrowing has also reduced the severity and morbidity of CM. Use of autologous *E. coli* bacterins has not been successful.

Concluding Remarks

Until recently, there was little information on characteristics of porcine septicaemic strains of *E. coli* and potential virulence factors associated with them. Studies on F165 fimbriae and the K"V165" O-antigen capsule have contributed to our understanding of some of these factors but there is much that is still not understood about this group of organisms. Further characterization of the high percentage of untypeable isolates from septicaemia might determine whether they represent a highly heterogeneous group or include a small number of important O groups that have not previously been serotyped. There is even less known about characteristics of *E. coli* which cause UTIs in pigs, but it is likely that they represent organisms that are particularly adapted to the urinary tract. There is a similar lack of information on features of isolates from mastitis, but evidence from bovine mastitis suggests that these are simply opportunistic agents with no particular virulence properties. Future work should probably concentrate on potential virulence factors of porcine septicaemic strains of *E. coli*, because of the high mortality associated with the condition. It would be interesting to clarify if pigs require specific antibody for protection or can be protected simply by having a sufficiently high level of serum immunoglobulin, as is the case with calves (Chapter 3).

References

Armstrong, C.H., Hooper, B.E. and Martin, C.E. (1968) Microflora associated with agalactia syndrome of sows. *American Journal of Veterinary Research* 29, 1401–1407.

Awad-Masalmeh, M., Baumgartner, W., Passernig, A., Silber, R. and Hinterdorfer, F. (1990) Bakteriologisch Untersuchungen bei an puerperaler mastitis (MMA Syndrom) erkrankten Sauen verschiendener tier bestände oesterreichs. *Tieraerztliche Umschau* 45, 521–535.

Berner, H. (1984) Bacteriological and clinical investigations in pathogenesis of puerperal endometritis in the sows. In: *Proceedings of the 8th Congress of the International Pig Veterinary Society, Gent*. Belgium Section of the International Pig Veterinary Society, Gent, Belgium, p. 284.

Bertschinger, H.U., Fairbrother, J.M., Nielsen, N.O. and Pohlenz, J.F. (1992) *Escherichia coli* infections. In: Leman, A.D., Straw, B.E., Mengeling, W.L., D'Allaire, S. and Taylor, D.J. (eds) *Diseases of Swine*. Iowa State University Press, Ames, pp. 487–521.

Carr, J. and Walton, J.R.W. (1992a) The characterization of *Escherichia coli* isolates from the porcine urogenital tract. In: *Proceedings of the 12th Congress of the International Pig Veterinary Society, The Hague*. Royal Netherlands Veterinary Association, ORBIT, GAIB b.v., 's-Hertogenbosch, The Netherlands, p. 262.

Carr, J. and Walton, J.R.W. (1992b) Characteristics of plasma and urine from normal adult swine and changes found in sows with either asymptomatic bacteriuria or cystitis and pyelonephritis. In: *Proceeding of the 12th Congress of the International Pig Veterinary Society, The Hague*. Royal Netherlands Veterinary Association, ORBIT, GAIB b.v., 's-Hertogenbosch, The Netherlands, p. 263.

Contrepois, M., Fairbrother, J.M., Kaura, Y.K. and Giradeau, J.P. (1989) Prevalence of CS31A and F165 surface antigens in *Escherichia coli* isolates from animals in France, Canada, and India. *Federation of European Microbiological Societies Microbiological Letters* 59, 319–324.

Crosa, J.H. (1989) Genetics and molecular biology of siderophore-mediated iron transport in bacteria. *Microbiology Reviews* 53, 517–530.

D'Allaire S., Drolet, R. and Chagnon, M. (1991) The causes of sows mortality: a retrospective study. *Canadian Veterinary Journal* 32, 241–243.

De Ruijter, K., Verheijden, J.H.M., Pijpers, A. and Berends, J. (1988) The role of endotoxin in the pathogenesis of coliform mastitis in sows. *Veterinary Quarterly* 10, 186–190.

Dubreuil, J.D. and Fairbrother, J.M. (1992) Biochemical and serological characterization of *Escherichia coli* fimbrial antigen $F165_2$. *Federation of European Microbiological Societies Microbiological Letters* 95, 219–224.

Fairbrother, J.M., Lariviére, S. and Lallier, R. (1986) New fimbrial antigen F165 on *Escherichia coli* serogroup O115 strains isolated from piglets with diarrhea. *Infection and Immunity* 51, 10–15.

Fairbrother, J.M., Lallier, R., Leblanc, L., Jacques, M. and Larivière, S. (1988). Production and purification of *Escherichia coli* fimbrial antigen F165. *Federation of European Microbiological Societies Microbiological Letters* 45, 247–252.

Fairbrother, J.M., Broes, A., Jacques, M. and Larivière, S. (1989) Pathogenicity of *Escherichia coli* O115:K"V165" strains isolated from pigs with diarrhoea. *American Journal of Veterinary Research* 50, 1029–1036.

Fairbrother, J.M., Harel, J., Forget, C., Desautels, C. and Moore, J. (1993) Receptor binding specifity and pathogenicity of *Escherichia coli* F165-positive strains isolated from piglets and calves and possessing *pap* related sequences. *Canadian Journal of Veterinary Research* 57, 53–55.

Ferguson, F.G., Confer, F., Pinto, A., Weber, J., Stout, T. and Kensinger, M. (1984) Long-term endotoxin exposure in the sow and neonatal piglet a model for MMA. In: *Proceedings of the 8th Congress of the International Pig Veterinary Society, Gent*. Belgium Section of the International Pig Veterinary Society, Gent, Belgium, p. 289.

Gyles, C.L. (1986) *Escherichia coli*. In: Gyles, C.L. and Thoen, C.O. (eds) *Pathogenesis of Bacterial Infections in Animals*. Iowa State University Press, Ames, Iowa, pp. 114–131.

Hacker, J. (1992) Role of fimbrial adhesins in the pathogenesis of *Escherichia coli* infections. *Canadian Journal of Microbiology* 38, 720–727.

Harel, J., Forget, C., Saint-Amand, J., Daigle, F., Dubreuil, D., Jacques, M. and Fairbrother, J.M. (1992) Molecular cloning of a determinant coding for fimbrial antigen $F165_1$, a Prs-like fimbrial antigen from porcine septicaemic *Escherichia coli*. *Journal of General Microbiology* 138, 1495–1502.

Harel, J., Fairbrother, J.M., Forget, C., Desautels, C. and Moore, J. (1993) Virulence factors associated with F165-positive *Escherichia coli* strains isolated from piglets and calves. *Veterinary Microbiology* 38, 139–155.

Jesmok, G., Lindsey, C., Duerr, M., Fournel, M. and Emerson, T. Jr (1992) Efficacy of monoclonal antibody against human recombinant tumor necrosis factor in *E. coli*-challenged swine. *American Journal of Pathology* 141, 1197–1207.

Johnson, J.R. (1991) Virulence factors in *Escherichia coli* urinary tract infection. *Clinical Microbiology Reviews* 4, 80–128.

Jones, J.E.T. (1968) The cause of death in sows. A one year survey of 106 herds in Essex. *British Veterinary Journal* 124, 45–55.

Meyer, R.C., Saxena, S.P. and Rhoades, H.E. (1971) Polyserositis induced by *Escherichia coli* in gnotobiotic swine. *Infection and Immunity* 3, 41–44.

Morkoc, A., Backstrom, L., Lund, L. and Smith, A.R. (1983) Bacterial endotoxin in blood of dysgalactic sows in relation to microbial status of uterus, milk, and intestine. *Journal of American Veterinary Medical Association* 183, 786–789.

Morris, J.A. and Sojka, W.J. (1985) *Escherichia coli* as a pathogen in animals. In: Sussman, M. (ed.) *The Virulence of* Escherichia coli: *Reviews and Methods*. Academic Press, London, pp. 47–77.

Murata, H., Yaguchi, H. and Namioka, S. (1979) Relationship between the intestinal permeability to macromolecules and invasion of septicemia-inducing *Escherichia coli* in neonatal piglets. *Infection and Immunity* 26, 339–347.

Nakajima, Y., Ishikawa, Y., Momotani, E., Takahashi, K., Madarame, H., Ito, A., Ueda, H., Wada, M. and Takahashi, H. (1991) A comparison of central nervous lesions directly induced by *Escherichia coli* lipopolysaccharide in piglets, calves, rabbits and mice. *Journal of Comparative Pathology* 104, 57–64.

Ngeleka, M., Harel, J., Jacques, M. and Fairbrother, J.M. (1992) Characterization of a non acidic polysaccharide capsular antigen of septicemic *Escherichia coli* O115:K"V165":F165 and evaluation of its role in pathogenicity. *Infection and Immunity* 60, 5048–5056.

Ngeleka, M., Jacques, M., Martineau-Doizé, B., Harel, J. and Fairbrother, J.M. (1993) Pathogenicity of an *Escherichia coli* O115:K"V165" mutant negative for $F165_1$ fimbriae in septicemia of gnotobiotic pigs. *Infection and Immunity* 61, 836–843.

Ngeleka, M., Martineau-Doizé, B. and Fairbrother, J.M. (1994) Septicemia-inducing *Escherichia coli* O115:K"V165" resist killing by porcine polymorphonuclear leukocytes *in vitro*: role of $F165_1$ fimbriae and K"V165" O-antigen capsule. *Infection and Immunity* 62, 398–404.

Nielsen, N.C., Bille, N., Riising, H.J. and Dam, A. (1975a) Polyserositis in pigs due to generalized *Escherichia coli* infection. *Canadian Journal of Comparative Medicine* 39, 421–426.

Nielsen, N.C., Riising, H.J., Larsen, J.L., Bille, N. and Svendsen, J. (1975b) Preweaning mortality in pigs. Acute septicaemias. *Nordisk Veterinary Medicine* 27, 129–139.

Ørskov, F. and Ørskov, I. (1992) *Escherichia coli* serotyping and disease in man and animals. *Canadian Journal of Microbiology* 38, 699–704.

Pederson, A., Krovacec K. and Ekwall H. (1984) Virulence factors in strains of *Escherichia coli* isolated from mastitic milk from agalactic sows. In: *Proceedings of the 8th Congress of the International Pig Veterinary Society, Gent*. Belgium Section of the International Pig Veterinary Society, Gent, Belgium, p. 286.

Pohl, P., Oswald, E., Vanmuylem, K., Jacquemin, E., Lintermans, P. and Mainil, J. (1993) *Escherichia coli* producing CNF1 and CNF2 cytotoxins in animals with different disorders. *Veterinary Research* 24, 311–315.

Ross, R.F., Zimmerman, B.J., Wagner, W.C. and Cox, D.F. (1975) A field study of coliform mastitis in sows. *Journal of American Veterinary Medicine Association* 167, 231–235.

Ross, R.F., Harmon, R.L., Zimmerman, B.J. and Young, T.F. (1983) Susceptibility of sows to experimentally induced *Escherichia coli* mastitis. *American Journal of Veterinary Research* 44, 949–954.

Smith, B.B. and Wagner, W.C. (1984) Suppression of prolactin in pigs by *Escherichia coli* endotoxin. *Science* 224, 605–607.

Smith, B.B., Martineau, G. and Bisaillon, A. (1992) Mammary glands and lactation problems. In: Leman, A.D., Straw, B.E., Mengeling, W.L., D'Allaire, S. and Taylor, D.J. (eds) *Diseases of Swine*. Iowa State University Press, Ames, Iowa, pp. 40–61.

Sojka, W.J. (1965) *Escherichia coli* infections in pigs. In: Sojka, W.J. (ed.) Escherichia coli *in Animals*. Commonwealth Agriculture Bureaux, Farnham Royal, UK, pp. 104–156.

Taylor, D.J. (1989) Bacterial diseases. In: Taylor, D.J. (ed.) *Pig Diseases*. Burlington Press (Cambridge), Foxton, pp. 71–172.

Waxler, G.L. and Britt, A.L. (1972) Polyserositis and arthritis due to *Escherichia coli* in gnotobiotic pigs. *Canadian Journal of Comparative Medicine* 36, 226–233.

Wegmann, P. and Bertschinger, H.V. (1984) Sequential cytological and bacteriological examination of the secretions from sucked and unsucked mammary gland with and without mastitis. In: *Proceedings of the 8th International Pig Veterinary Society, Gent*. Belgium Section of the International Pig Veterinary Society, Gent, Belgium, p. 287.

11

Diseases Due to *Escherichia coli* in Poultry

W.G. Gross
1509 Lark Lane, Blacksburg, Virginia 24060, USA

Among the first reports of infections in poultry caused by coliform organisms were those of David (1938) and Twisselman (1939). Later, Wasserman *et al*. (1954) and Fahey (1955) reported the isolation of *E. coli* from 'air sac disease'. Pathogenic serogroups of *E. coli* are common in the environments in which poultry are raised and may cause air sacculitis, pericarditis, peritonitis, salpingitis, synovitis, osteomyelitis, cellulitis or yolk sac infection. Collectively, these diseases constitute a major economic loss. Except for cellulitis and yolk sac infection, these conditions represent different manifestations of infection with the same *E. coli* implicated in avian septicaemic colibacillosis. Except for yolk sac infections, all of these diseases require a predisposing factor, and losses can be low if the predisposing factors are controlled. Most serogroups isolated from poultry are not pathogenic for other animals, and although serogroup O78:K80 has been associated with enteric disease in humans, and septicaemic disease in calves, sheep and pig, it is likely that there is species specificity in infection by organisms of this serogroup.

Environmental Distribution

The most important reservoir of *E. coli* is the intestinal tract of animals, including poultry. *E. coli* is one of the dominant aerobic organisms in the intestine but is outnumbered 100- to 1000-fold by anaerobic Gram-negative rods. In chickens, there are about 10^9 colony forming units of bacteria per gram of faeces. Of these, 10^6 are *E. coli*, 10–15% of which are pathogenic serogroups (Harry and Helmsley, 1965a). The bacterial flora of the gut has many ecological niches which are filled by the most adapted strains and bacteria which enter from the outside may or may not be able to fill an existing niche. At times, coliforms may be transmitted between poultry and humans (Ojeniyi, 1989), but this is not a human health problem, because poultry do not appear to carry strains that cause disease in humans.

Faeces and dust in the poultry house are important sources of pathogenic *E. coli*. The dust found in poultry houses can contain as many as 10^6 bacteria g^{-1} and there is a positive relationship between serogroups in the dust and those found in septicaemia (Carlson and Whenham, 1968). However, serogroups isolated from systemic infections of chickens are not necessarily the same as those found in their intestinal tracts (Harry and Helmsley, 1965b). Dry dust tends to preserve the bacteria and the level of contamination is reduced with increasing moisture levels. Following fogging, there can be a 85–95% reduction within 7 days (Harry, 1964). Rodent faeces may contain pathogenic serogroups for many months. When coliforms of faecal origin are in dry litter, they tend to be preserved but they do not survive well in wet litter. Feed ingredients are sometimes contaminated with pathogenic serogroups, which are destroyed by hot pelleting. Coliforms are stable in feed at normal 5–10% moisture levels, but tend to die when the moisture levels reach 15–20%. Contaminated drinking water is also a potential source which can be controlled by chlorination (Nagi and Raggi, 1972; Boado *et al.*, 1988).

Disease Syndromes

Yolk sac infection

Yolk sac infections result primarily from faecal contamination of the surface of eggs, usually from dirty nests. *E. coli* penetration of the shell and shell membranes is more frequent if there is visible faecal contamination, the shell is cracked or of poor quality, the eggs are warm, and/or the surface is wet. Other possible minor sources of contamination are salpingitis and ovarian infection.

The incidence of yolk sac infection is greatest when egg shell contamination occurs late in incubation and many affected embryos will die. As few as 10 bacteria of virulent O1:K1 organisms may result in death of all embryos, following inoculation into the yolk sac (Siccardi, 1966). Typically, losses continue during hatching and for an additional 3 weeks. The infected yolk sac is retained and has an abnormal consistency although the yolk sacs of some infected birds appear to be normal. Omphalitis is a frequent finding. Chicks which live longer than 4 days also tend to have pericarditis while some chicks seem to be able to control the infection.

Some serogroups of *E. coli* are of low virulence. Yolk sac infection with

E. coli of serogroup O103 resulted in a 20% decrease in bodyweight with no mortality or decreased hatchability. The only lesion was a small (up to 15 mm) retained caseous yolk sac which persisted for several months (Gross, 1964).

Characteristically, the outer wall of the infected yolk sac is oedematous, and the adjacent zones contain many heterophils and macrophages followed by a layer of giant cells. In the cavity there are masses of necrotic heterophils and bacteria.

Diagnosis is made by isolating *E. coli* from the retained yolk sacs. Isolates can be tested for pathogenicity by dipping embryonating eggs in a broth culture during the week before hatching. Other bacteria, such as *Proteus* spp., *Bacillus* spp. and enterococci are sometimes isolated from yolk sacs (Harry, 1957).

Yolk sac infections are prevented by using clean nests and disinfecting the egg surfaces within 1 hour of laying. Disinfection with formaldehyde or other chemicals seems to reduce the incidence of penetration of the eggs by bacteria. Venting hatchers outside the building reduces spread to other birds. Brooding at below normal temperatures increases the severity and incidence of the clinical diseases. Infected birds benefit greatly from increased brooding temperature. Affected chicks may be treated with nitrofurans or other antimicrobial agents but this might not be cost effective, because survivors may be stunted.

Respiratory tract infection (air sac disease)

Respiratory disease complex, involving a secondary infection by *E. coli* (Gross, 1956), usually occurs between 2 and 12 weeks of age, with most losses occurring between 4 and 9 weeks. This is one of the most common poultry diseases with losses at times being over 20%. Economic loss results from reduced growth and feed efficiency, increased mortality and increased condemnation at processing.

Poultry frequently inhale pathogenic *E. coli* in dust derived from faeces, but the normal host defence prevents respiratory tract infection. However, following infection with respiratory tract agents such as Newcastle disease virus (NDV), infectious bronchitis virus (IBV) and *Mycoplasma gallisepticum* alone or in combination, certain *E. coli* are able to establish in the respiratory tract (Gross, 1961a). Vaccine viruses (NDV and IBV) are as important as the more virulent field strains (Gross, 1961b).

Respiratory infections which predispose to *E. coli* disease are affected by a variety of factors. *M. gallisepticum* can be passed through the egg and disseminated in the hatcher and during brooding. Infection becomes more severe following brooding at temperatures higher or lower than normal. High levels of environmental stress also increase the severity of the respiratory infection (Gross and Siegel, 1965). The severity of the infection is reduced when the birds are socialized to their human associates (Gross and Siegel, 1982). Chickens which were selectively bred for a high antibody (HA) response to sheep erythrocytes were more resistant to respiratory infections than those selected for a low (LA) antibody response (Gross *et al.*, 1980a).

Several host and environmental factors influence susceptibility of chicks to *E. coli*. Resistance to *E. coli* was greatest in LA chickens (Gross *et al.*, 1980a). Resistance to *E. coli* increased as the level of environmental stress increased until protection was close to complete. Further increases in the severity of environmental stress resulted in increased susceptibility (Gross, 1984a). Under very low levels of stress, birds became extremely susceptible. Socialization also resulted in increased resistance (Gross and Siegel, 1982). Exposure to ammonia and dust resulted in deciliation of the epithelium of the respiratory tract which allowed coliforms to invade (Oyetunde *et al.*, 1978; Nagaraga *et al.*, 1984).

While the concentration of respiratory disease agents was greatest during the early stages of infection, susceptibility to inhaled *E. coli* often occurred much later. Susceptibility following *M. gallisepticum* infection first occurred between 12 and 16 days and lasted for at least 30 days. Following exposure to a vaccine strain of NDV, susceptibility to *E. coli* began in about 3 days while maximum susceptibility began at about 8 days and lasted for over 30 days. Losses tend to be more severe and longer lasting under poor management and following mixed respiratory infections (Ibragimov *et al.*, 1983; Smith *et al.*, 1985).

During the first 3 days of respiratory agent infection, both lymphoid cells and heterophils are present in the respiratory tract lesions. The pseudostratified columnar epithelium of the trachea is replaced with 3–8 layers of immature non-ciliated cells (Ficken *et al.*, 1987). As infection progresses, the number of lymphocytes increases while the number of heterophils decreases. Susceptibility to inhaled *E. coli* is associated with a successful overspecialized lymphoid defence against the respiratory tract infections. These lesions contain very few heterophils, which are the initial defenders against *E. coli*. Susceptible chickens can then be infected with small numbers of inhaled *E. coli*. While chickens infected with respiratory tract viruses or mycoplasma are more susceptible to inhaled *E. coli* than are uninfected controls, the stress response to the respiratory infection renders the infected birds more resistant to intravenous challenge than the controls (Gross, 1990).

In normal chickens, a successful defence against *E. coli* inoculated into an air sac can occur within 60 minutes with very little cellular response. Four hours after the feeding of a diet containing 40 mg corticosterone kg^{-1} for a period of 30 minutes, chickens became resistant to *E. coli* air sac challenge. One hour later, susceptibility returned (Gross, 1992).

Resistance to *E. coli* infection was reduced when resources needed for defence were not available. This may occur following fasting or water deprivation. Resistance was increased if the birds were under the influence of chemicals which blocked the stress response (Gross and Chickering, 1987). In another example, when broiler breeders were fed a restricted diet in an effort to control bodyweight, their resistance to *E. coli* was increased because restricted feeding was stressful. Following the return of feeding *ad libitum*, both feed efficiency and growth rate increased. Resistance to *E. coli* was greatly reduced because resources needed for defence were utilized for increased growth (Doa-Ponser *et al.*, 1991). Increased genetic pressure by broiler breeders has resulted in increased resource allocation for feed efficiency and growth rate and fewer resources for antibody production and phagocytic defence. Thus broilers are more susceptible to *E. coli* than layers.

Poultry which are infected with *E. coli* are depressed and often have yellowish or greenish watery droppings. Body temperature is usually increased from a normal of 40°C to 42°C. Just before death, body temperature may reach 44°C.

Air sacs of infected birds are thickened and often have a caseous exudate on the respiratory surface. The earliest microscopic change is oedema followed by heterophil infiltration. Within 12 hours, there is infiltration with mononuclear phagocytes. Later, mononuclear phagocytes become more common. Giant cells line necrotic areas which contain heterophil debris in a caseous mass (Gross, 1957a). The lesions of the predisposing respiratory disease are also present. They consist of lymphoid follicles, and epithelium-lined air passages.

A diagnosis of *E. coli* infection is suggested by the presence of air sacculitis, sometimes associated with pericarditis, although a similar picture may be observed with chlamydia infection. Recovery of *E. coli* from the lesions is confirmatory. The predisposing respiratory disease agents may no longer be present in late stages of the disease, but their association with the syndrome may be determined by demonstration of antibodies in serum and by pathological changes.

Control of the disease by preventing the predisposing respiratory infections has been much more successful than treatment of the secondary *E. coli* infection. *M. gallisepticum* has been eradicated from all commercial breeding stocks and is seldom seen under good management conditions. Most respiratory viruses now resemble the vaccine strains (Alexander *et al.*, 1987) and the severity of these viral infections can be reduced by raising birds under a relatively low level of environmental stress and/or by socializing the birds to their handlers. Eliminating the use of live virus vaccines and preventing the introduction of respiratory viruses eliminates air sac infection.

In some birds, respiratory tract infection is not controlled and the *E. coli* infection becomes bacteraemic.

Bacteraemia

Following oral inoculation of turkeys and chickens with avian adenovirus group 2 (haemorrhagic enteritis (HE) virus), the spleen becomes infected. At first, infection is confined to the spleen. On the sixth day, viraemia is followed by intestinal bleeding and on the seventh day, viraemia disappears and recovery is rapid. At this time, *E. coli* bacteraemia (possibly from an intestinal source) may become a clinical problem. A strong defence against HE renders the bird susceptible to *E. coli*. Factors which favour resistance to HE favour susceptibility to *E. coli* and vice versa. For example, an optimal level of dietary corticosterone or environmental stress results in increased resistance to *E. coli* and increased susceptibility to HE virus. Chickens which are genetically resistant to HE virus are susceptible to *E. coli* and vice versa (Gross and Domermuth, 1988). The successful largely mononuclear defence against HE virus renders the chicken susceptible to intravenous inoculation of small numbers of *E. coli* resulting in severe bacteraemia.

Coliform infection is indicated by the presence of hepatitis in turkeys and pericarditis in chickens, from which *E. coli* can be isolated. The lesions of the predisposing HE infection are usually absent and diagnosis is by history and serology.

Turkeys are often vaccinated against HE, with a virus of low virulence, at about 5 weeks of age in an attempt to prevent secondary *E. coli* infection. Turkeys which are infected with *Bordetella avium* have increased susceptibility to *E. coli* (Alsine and Arp, 1987).

Dhillon (1986) reported increased susceptibility to *E. coli* infection following infection of chickens with infectious bursal disease virus. However, increased susceptibility to *E. coli* is not a common sequel to infectious bursal disease.

Some birds are able to control bacteraemia. In most bacteraemic birds, infection spreads to the myocardium and later to the pericardial sac. Myocardial infection results in changes in the electrical conductivity of the myocardium resulting in major changes in the electrocardiogram (Gross, 1966). This leads to reduced cardiac efficiency resulting in systolic arterial pressure falling from a normal level of 150 mmHg to 40 mmHg just before death. Reduced blood pressure often results in a fibrinous perihepatitis. Bacteraemia by most pathogenic strains of *E. coli* results in a fibrinous pericarditis, which is also a feature of chlamydiosis.

Myocardial infiltration with macrophages occurs before there are macroscopic lesions of pericarditis. Plasma cells may appear after 7 days.

A unilateral panophthalmitis, associated with hypopyon and blindness, sometimes occurs in bacteraemic birds. Many birds die shortly after the onset, while some recover. There is infiltration of the anterior chamber and choroid with heterophils, monocytes and bacteria; giant cells surround areas of necrosis. The choroid is greatly thickened and the retina is destroyed (Gross, 1957b). Panophthalmitis is also seen in *Salmonella* infections.

Some serogroups, for example O15, tend to result in joint infections most frequently of the femorotibular joint. Lesions tend to heal spontaneously in 3–4 weeks (Gross, 1961c). Joint infection may also be caused by other organisms, including staphylococci, salmonella, *Streptobacillus moniliformis* and mycoplasma.

Acute septicaemia of chickens and turkeys

Acute *E. coli* septicaemia is an infection of mature chickens and turkeys, characterized by a firm dark or greenish liver and congested pectoral muscles. Sometimes small necrotic foci can be seen on the liver. The crops are usually full and the birds are in good flesh. In some cases pericarditis and peritonitis are also present. The experimental production of these lesions has not been reported. Currently this infection is not frequently seen in chickens but is seen to a moderate extent in turkeys. When chickens with very poor resistance are challenged with *E. coli*, there may be death with few lesions. Similar liver lesions are more frequently seen in other infections such as those due to fowl typhoid, pasteurellae and streptococci.

Coliform septicaemia in ducks

Coliform septicaemia of ducks is characterized by pericarditis and a moist curd-like exudate on the thoracic and abdominal viscera as well as the surfaces of the air sacs. Typically, postmortem examination reveals a swollen, dark and bile-stained liver and a swollen and dark spleen. *E. coli* serogroup O78:K80 can usually be isolated from the liver, spleen and blood. A characteristic odour can often be noted. All ages of ducklings are susceptible, and losses, which seem to be associated with individual farms rather than hatcheries, are most frequent in autumn and winter. An effective formalin-killed bacterin has been prepared from O78:K80 *E. coli* (Sandu and Layton, 1985).

Pasteurella anatipestifer is another cause of pericarditis in ducks, but infections with this organism usually have less involvement of the air sacs. Thick exudate may be found in the nasal sinuses, trachea, lungs and oviduct and meningitis is often evident.

Salpingitis

Infection of the left greater abdominal air sac allows *E. coli* to reach the oviduct via the attached mesosalpinx. The oviduct becomes greatly enlarged and infected birds never lay eggs (Gross, 1956). Salpingitis can be reproduced in some chickens by injecting large numbers (10^9) of bacteria into the uterus or may occur following artificial insemination in turkeys. Stilboesterol implants result in increased susceptibility. Within the thin-walled oviduct is a large caseous mass consisting of large numbers of necrotic heterophils and fibrin. The lesions in the oviduct wall are mild and consist of a narrow zone of heterophils just under the epithelium (Gross, 1957b). Salpingitis is a frequent cause of loss in many avian species.

Peritonitis

Peritonitis causes a sudden sporadic mortality among laying hens. At the end of a clutch of eggs, there is a genetic tendency for failure of the infundibulum to engulf the ovum which falls into the peritoneal cavity. The yolk is usually absorbed within a few hours. At times, small numbers of *E. coli* reach the peritoneal cavity through the oviduct. This invasion is usually easily controlled. If both events occur at the same time, coliform infection of the yolk results in a severe peritonitis (Gross and Siegel, 1959). Peritonitis due to *E. coli* occurs in many avian species, but the incidence in commercial layers has been reduced by selective breeding.

Swollen head syndrome

Swollen head syndrome (SHS) is characterized by an oedematous swelling, containing a diffuse cellulitis, over the eye of broilers, broiler breeders and in commercial layers. *E. coli* can be isolated from the lesions (O'Brien, 1985). Disease appears to require previous infection with a previously unknown coronavirus, and infection could be reproduced following a combined *E. coli*–coronavirus infection. Broilers were protected from clinical infection following vaccination with attenuated coronavirus. Lesions do not affect the infraorbital sinuses which are affected in infections with *Haemophilus paragallinarum* (Morley and Thomson, 1984). Other viral agents including IBV, NDV, IBD and turkey rhinotracheitis virus (TRTV) have been proposed to predispose to *E. coli* infection and result in SHS (Zellen, 1988). However, a recent study has rejected the association of TRTV with SHS (Shirai *et al.*, 1993).

The lesion consists of gelatinous oedema involving the facial skin and periorbital tissues, and caseous exudate in the conjunctival sac, facial subcutaneous tissues and lacrymal gland (Pattison *et al.*, 1989; Nunoya *et al.*, 1991). Antibacterial medication and an attenuated live-virus vaccine have been reported to control the disease (Morley and Thomson, 1984; Zellen, 1988).

Cellulitis

Cellulitis (sometimes called necrotic dermatitis) of the lower abdomen below the vent and the thighs of broilers does not result in mortality or clinical signs, but the presence of fibrinous plaques under the skin results in substantial losses through condemnation or downgrading of carcasses (Randall *et al.*, 1984; Vaillancourt *et al.*, 1992). In the USA total annual losses due to cellulitis were estimated at $18–20 million (Morris, 1991). *E. coli* is always the predominant bacterium but other bacteria are sometimes recovered as well. O78 : K80 was the serogroup most frequently involved in cellulitis but *E. coli* of serogroups O1 and O2 are also among the most consistently isolated organisms from the subcutaneous lesions (Glunder, 1990; Messier *et al.*, 1993; Peighambari *et al.*, 1993). The condition was reproduced by introducing an O78 : K80 *E. coli* isolate into feather follicles (Glunder, 1990). Valentine and Willsch (1987) isolated *E. coli* of serogroup O1 : K1 from typical lesions and reproduced the condition following inoculation of the isolated bacteria.

Enteritis

A few reports have suggested that *E. coli* may be a cause of enteritis in poultry. The almost universal presence of pathogenic serogroups of *E. coli* in the intestinal tracts of poultry is not associated with any disease. Poultry with severe septicaemic infections often have watery, yellowish droppings. These seem to be associated with rapid reductions in bodyweight. Outbreaks of diarrhoeal disease associated with enterotoxigenic *E. coli* occur rarely and have been reported from the Philippines (Joya *et al.*, 1990). A heat-labile enterotoxin (LT) similar to LT from human enterotoxigenic *E. coli* has been recovered from poultry strains (Tsuji *et al.*, 1988). A small percentage of strains also produced heat-stable enterotoxin (STa). Interestingly, some enterotoxigenic strains have been recovered from outbreaks belonging to O groups 8 and 149, O groups frequently implicated in *E. coli* diarrhoea in pigs.

A severe haemorrhagic typhlitis results from the oral inoculation of *E. coli* into *Eimeria burnetti*-infected chickens (Nagi and Mathey, 1972). Dual infection with *E. coli* and *Eimeria tenella* has been reported by Nakamura *et al.* (1990).

Characteristics of Avian Pathogenic *E. coli*

Serogroups

Many investigators throughout the world have determined the serogroups of *E. coli* involved in disease outbreaks in poultry. Siccardi (1966) found that 74/154 (48%) of the then known serogroups were pathogenic for chicks, embryonating eggs or both. Among the O serogroups that have been reported to be pathogenic for poultry are: 1, 2, 3, 6, 8, 15, 18, 35, 71, 74, 78, 87, 88, 95, 103 and 109. On a worldwide basis, O serogroups 1, 2 and 78 are by far the most common (Sojka and Carnaghan, 1961; Heller and Drabkin, 1977), but many pathogenic isolates do not belong to any of the established O groups and are designated 'untypeable'. These serogroups are not common among isolates from healthy chickens.

Virulence-related factors

E. coli strains that cause avian colibacillosis clearly belong to the class of pathogenic *E. coli* which invade the blood stream from an epithelial surface. In this respect, they are similar to strains of *E. coli* which cause extra-intestinal infections in humans (Chapter 13). It is not surprising, therefore, that several potential virulence factors are common to both types of bacteria. These include pili, resistance to complement (serum resistance), the aerobactin iron scavenging system, and production of the K1 capsule (Rosenburger *et al.*, 1985; Bree *et al.*, 1989; Ellis *et al.*, 1989; Dozois *et al.*, 1992; Wooley *et al.*, 1992; Valvano, 1992). Bree *et al.* (1989) showed that an O2:K1:H7 strain of *E. coli* isolated from respiratory disease in a chicken had the genes for aerobactin production, adhered *in vitro* to chicken pharyngeal cells, and was virulent in axenic and specific pathogen-free chickens. An O2:K1:H$^-$ isolate from the faeces of a healthy chicken lacked all these properties. Interestingly, alpha-haemolysin, which is implicated in virulence of human uropathogenic *E. coli*, is rarely produced by *E. coli* implicated in avian colibacillosis.

Pili

There is good evidence that ability of *E. coli* to adhere to the epithelium of the respiratory tract of chickens is an important virulence attribute of avian colibacillosis strains of the organism. Pili are commonly associated with adhesins in *E. coli* and there have been several studies to identify pili which might bear adhesins that are important in the virulence of avian pathogenic *E. coli*. Naveh *et al.* (1984) demonstrated that three strains of *E. coli* (O2, O78 and O88) from colisepticaemia in poultry produced pili when grown at 37°C but not at 18°C. They showed that piliated strains adhered both *in vitro* and *in vivo* to ciliated tracheal epithelial cells and that inoculation of chickens with piliated strains resulted in a significantly higher occurrence of disease compared with birds inoculated with non-piliated bacteria.

Type 1 pili or genes for type 1 pili have been demonstrated on avian pathogenic *E. coli*. Suwanichkul and Panigrahy (1986) examined pilus production among strains of avian *E. coli* of O groups 1, 2 and 78. They found that O78 strains produced type 1 pili but that pili of strains of the other serogroups were different. Ike and co-workers (1990) reported that 87 of 151 *E. coli* strains recovery from broiler chickens with coli-septicaemia produce type 1 pili. Wooley *et al.* (1992) found that all 40 avian septicaemic isolates of *E. coli* had type 1 pili as indicated by mannose-sensitive haemagglutination, but that only 23 of 40 intestinal isolates had this property.

Adherence to chicken tracheal epithelium is mediated by pili on avian septicaemic strains of O groups 1, 2 and 78 (Dho and Lafont, 1984; Gyimah and Panigrahy, 1988). Gyimah and Panigrahy (1988) blocked adherence with specific anti-pilus antibody, and by D-mannose and certain derivatives of this sugar. Type 1 or type 1-like fimbriae have been detected on O78 strains by Suwanichkul and Panigrahy (1986) and on O2 and O78 strains by Dho-Moulin *et al.* (1990). Chanteloup *et al.* (1991) used immunoblotting techniques with a monoclonal antibody specific for the adhesin of type 1 fimbriae and showed that the adhesin on type 1-like and type 1A fimbriae of avian septicaemic *E. coli* was the same as that on type 1 fimbriae. They also demonstrated that the adhesin was carried at the tips or at both tip and sides of the fimbriae.

Yerushalmi *et al.* (1990) reported that avian O78 : K80 *E. coli* produce pili called AC/I (avian *E. coli* I), which do not agglutinate red blood cells, have subunits of molecular weight of approximately 18 kDa, and are important for adherence *in vitro* and *in vivo*. They used monoclonal antibodies against the pilus subunit to inhibit adherence. Interestingly, strains of O78 : K80 are implicated in diarrhoeal disease in humans and in septicaemia in sheep, cattle and pigs (Dassouli-Mrani-Belkebir *et al.*, 1988). The human ETEC strains possess CFA/I pili and CS31A pili have been identified on bovine strains. Yerushalmi *et al.* (1990) showed that the AC/I pili mediated preferential binding to avian epithelium compared with human epithelium.

Dozois *et al.* (1992) investigated the occurrence among *E. coli* isolates from septicaemic and healthy chickens and turkeys from Quebec of nucleotide sequences which hybridized with *pap* and *pil* probes. They observed that pap + isolates from chickens were associated with septicaemia and all lacked the P adhesin. Four of nine pap + isolates from turkeys expressed P adhesin.

Serum resistance

Resistance to killing by complement in serum is mediated by surface structures such as capsule, lipopolysaccharide or outer membrane protein and is often associated with avian septicaemic strains of *E. coli*. Ellis *et al.* (1988) determined serum resistance of 25 *E. coli* isolates from turkeys and virulence of the strains for 3-week-old turkeys. Eighteen of the strains were either serum resistant and virulent or serum sensitive and avirulent; five strains were serum resistant but avirulent and two strains were serum sensitive and virulent. In a study of 40 *E. coli* isolates from the intestines of normal chickens and 40 isolates from colisepticaemic chickens, Wooley *et al.* (1992) determined that complement resistance was highly associated with the septicaemic isolates. Nolan *et al.* (1992) showed that complement resistance was highly correlated with lethality for chickens and moderately correlated with chick embryo lethality. In an attempt to determine the role of complement resistance in virulence of an avian *E. coli* isolate, Nolan *et al.* (1992) used transposon mutagenesis to produce mutants that had reduced complement resistance. When they tested the virulence of parent and mutant organisms in the chick embryo they found that one of four mutants was reduced in virulence.

Production of aerobactin

The adverse effects on bacterial growth associated with the low levels of free iron in the body of animals are well established (Payne, 1988; Martinez *et al.*, 1990). However, some bacteria possess high affinity iron acquisition systems which can compete with transferrins and thereby satisfy the iron requirements of the bacteria. Bolin and Jensen (1987) demonstrated the relationship between availability of iron and virulence of *E. coli* in septicaemia in turkeys. They showed that there was a hypoferraemia following infection of the air sacs of turkeys with *E. coli* and that both mortality and severity of disease were increased when iron was administered to the infected birds.

Several studies have shown that the majority of avian pathogenic strains of *E. coli* possess the aerobactin iron scavenging system (Chapter 19) which can be used to obtain iron in the low iron environment of the host. Linggood *et al.* (1987) identified aerobactin production in 89% of 61 avian septicaemic *E. coli* isolates that were examined, compared with 11% of 27 isolates from healthy chickens. Emery *et al.* (1992) examined 420 *E. coli* isolates from colisepticaemic turkeys and 80 from colisepticaemic chickens and found that 74% of the chicken isolates and 80% of the turkey isolates produced aerobactin. Dozois *et al.* (1992) reported that 98% of *E. coli* from septicaemic chickens and 73% from septicaemic turkeys had the aerobactin system.

Dho and Lafont (1984) showed that ability of avian *E. coli* strains to grow under iron-limiting conditions was highly correlated with lethality for 1-day-old chickens. Later, Lafont *et al.* (1987) showed that genes which encode the aerobactin iron transport system were present in all of the most virulent avian *E. coli* isolates but absent from all but one avirulent isolate.

The aerobactin iron uptake system is typically carried by Col V plasmids, but other virulence-related properties have been shown on only a limited number of Col V plasmids (Waters and Crosa, 1991). Valvano (1992) showed that 13 of 13 avian septicaemic *E. coli* isolates possessed the aerobactin iron transport system and that the genes for this system were always carried on a Col V-type plasmid. Vidotto *et al.* (1990) also showed that aerobactin production was associated with avian septicaemic *E. coli* and they identified a single transferable, 100-MDa plasmid which carried genes for the aerobactin system, drug resistance and colicin production. Ike *et al.* (1992) examined 115 avian septicaemic *E. coli* recovered from chickens and showed that aerobactin-mediated iron uptake and serum resistance were the most common virulence-associated properties of these strains. However, they noted that there were some strains which were virulent for chickens but lacked both factors. They demonstrated that a virulent O2 strain carried a 100-MDa conjugative plasmid with genes for serum resistance and the aerobactin iron uptake system and that loss of the plasmid resulted in a reduction in virulence and reintroduction of the plasmid restored virulence. Some avian septicaemic strains produce aerobactin but do not produce colicin V (Dassouli-Mrani-Belkebir *et al.*, 1988).

The aerobactin receptor and other iron-regulated proteins are detectable in outer membrane preparations of certain *E. coli* grown under iron limitation. Bolin and Jensen (1987) passively immunized 18-day-old turkeys with antiserum prepared in rabbits against iron-regulated outer membrane proteins of *E. coli*. They challenged the immunized turkeys and control groups with an O78:K80 *E. coli* isolate and showed that the immunized turkeys were protected.

K1 antigen

Most strains of avian septicaemic *E. coli* belong to a limited number of O:K groups. The predominant O groups are 1, 2 and 78, and the most common K antigens are K1 and K80. The K1 antigen is also associated with extraintestinal infections in humans and has been shown to be anticomplementary as well as poorly immunogenic. It is usually associated with O group 1 or 2 and Bree *et al.* (1989) identified the production of K1 polysaccharide capsule as a virulence determinant in avian pathogenic strains of serogroup O2.

Congo Red binding

The ability to bind the dye Congo Red (CR) in agar media has been proposed as a marker for avian pathogenic *E. coli* (Berkhoff and Vinal, 1986; Corbett *et al.*, 1987). Berkhoff and Vinal (1986) demonstrated a CR-positive phenotype for all 144 *E. coli* isolated from lesions of diseased birds in contrast to less than 50% of 170 control isolates obtained from the trachea and cloaca of normal birds and from poultry houses. Corbett *et al.* (1987) later evaluated the association of CR-positive *E. coli* and colisepticaemia in chickens and concluded that CR positivity identified a virulent form of *E. coli* implicated in colisepticaemia in poultry. Yoder *et al.* (1989) provided evidence that, for some strains at least, CR binding may be directly related to virulence; they showed that a CR-positive isolate was consistently more pathogenic for chickens than the CR-negative counterpart of the isolate. It is not known whether the strains were isogenic except for ability to bind CR. Similarly, Gjessing and Berkhoff (1989) reported that a mortality rate of 4.11% and a morbidity rate of 13.4% were obtained when day-old chicks were exposed to an aerosol of a CR-positive *E. coli* strain but no mortality or morbidity was obtained with CR-negative derivatives of the strain.

A number of workers have reported that CR binding did not correlate well with pathogenicity. Yoder (1989) found that if bile salts were added to the test medium, as recommended, then almost all cultures of *E. coli* formed red colonies. If bile salts were not added, then most *E. coli* isolates, including avian pathogens, rarely bound the dye. Panigrahy and Yushen (1990) investigated 21 *E. coli* isolates from chickens and turkeys for their CR-binding properties and their pathogenicity in 1-week-old chicks. They found that 15 strains were pathogenic, that eight of the 15 were CR positive, that all isolates of O group 78 were CR positive and all isolates of O group 2 were CR negative. The finding that all O78 isolates were CR positive is consistent with the findings of Corbett *et al.* (1987), and it appears that CR binding identifies a subset of avian colisepticaemic *E. coli* but is not a marker for pathogenicity. Gjessing and Berkhoff (1989) suggested that some strains of CR-positive *E. coli* should be considered potential primary pathogens, because air sacculitis and septicaemia could be reproduced experimentally by aerosol administration of these strains in the absence of any predisposing factors.

Diagnosis of *E. coli* Infections of Poultry

The clinical picture and/or postmortem lesions often suggest an *E. coli* infection, but isolation of *E. coli* from characteristic lesions is the means by which diagnoses are confirmed. Cultures should be taken from affected tissue such as the liver, spleen, pericardial sac and marrow, taking great care to avoid contamination with intestinal contents. Material should be streaked on Tergitol 7 agar, MacConkey's agar or eosin methylene blue (EMB) agar.

A presumptive diagnosis can be made if the colonies have the characteristic yellow colour on Tergitol 7 agar, the bright pink colour on MacConkey's agar or the metallic sheen on EMB agar. At times, lactose fermentation can be late. During recovery from infection, birds may have characteristic lesions from which bacteria cannot be isolated.

The diagnosis can be strengthened if the isolated cultures belong to a known pathogenic serogroup, such as O1, O2 or O78:K80. Serotyping is expensive and available at only a few specialized centres, but it is possible for a laboratory to obtain antisera against the common serogroups implicated in poultry diseases and to carry out simple agglutination tests. For routine diagnostic work, serotyping is not necessary, but it is of great value when conducting epidemiological studies.

Treatment

Some strains of *E. coli* are susceptible to drugs such as ampicillin, chloramphenicol, chlortetracycline, oxytetracycline, neomycin, gentamicin, nitrofurans, nalidixic acid, trimethoprim-sulfadimethoxine, polymixin B and sulfonamides, but isolates of *E. coli* from poultry are frequently resistant to these drugs (Gross, 1961d; Cloud *et al.*, 1985). Because of great variations in resistance patterns, isolates should be tested for antibiotic resistance so that ineffective treatments may be avoided. Residual lesions of successfully treated birds may result in condemnation at processing.

Treatment with ascorbic acid, which increases the effectiveness of phagocytes, is very effective and is not affected by drug resistance of the bacteria. The optimal dose of ascorbic acid is 100 mg kg^{-1} of feed. Higher or lower doses are much less effective. The actual dose should be determined for local stocks and environments. As the bird's stress level increases, the optimal dose increases and effectiveness decreases (Gross *et al.*, 1988). Optimal doses of corticosterone and deoxycorticosterone also result in increased effectiveness of phagocytes. The effects of increasing effectiveness of phagocytes and the actions of antibiotics are additive (Gross *et al.*, 1980b; Gross and Siegel, 1981; Gross, 1984b).

Vaccination

If birds can survive *E. coli* infection for about 5 days, antibody becomes an important component of host defence. An ELISA test was found to be more efficient than an indirect haemagglutination test in detecting antibodies associated with challenge survival (Leitner *et al.*, 1990). In some very severe infections, detectable levels of antibody may not be produced.

The inoculation of optimal numbers of live bacteria, usually via the intravenous route, results in strong immunity. If infection is too severe, clinical disease results.

Poultry do not naturally develop immunity to the pathogenic serotypes of *E. coli* which are part of their gut flora. The continual inhalation of pathogenic serotypes found in poultry house dust also does not result in immunity.

Various vaccines have employed killed bacteria. Killed bacteria with capsules of the B type of the K antigen, such as the relatively common 078:K80 serogroup, are very effective and are often used to protect ducks. Vaccines consisting of the somatic 'O' antigens result in high antibody titres which do not result in immunity. Most pathogenic serogroups have the L form of the K antigen. Vaccines containing adjuvants and large amounts of bacteria made from these strains are stressful to birds, resulting in non-specific resistance to bacteria for several weeks.

Vaccination of breeders with vaccines containing sonicated bacteria resulted in detectable titres for 160 days. Passive immunity of their chicks was completely protective for 2 weeks. Some protection was present for 45 days (Odagiri *et al.*, 1987; Heller *et al.*, 1990). Passive immunity results in increased clearance of bacteria from the blood, spleen, liver and lungs (Arp, 1982; Myers and Arp, 1987).

Pili increase pathogenicity by mediating adherence of the bacteria to the respiratory tract epithelium (Naveh *et al.*, 1984). Highly purified pilus vaccines containing 180 μg of protein per dose were very effective against bacteria containing the source pilus (Gyimah *et al.*, 1986; Suwanichkul *et al.*, 1987). Six pilus types were identified and type 1 pilus was present on 54% of pathogenic cultures (Suwanichkul and Panigrahy, 1988).

Vaccines against *E. coli* are not widely employed, perhaps because of the large number of serogroups involved in field outbreaks. The cost of vaccination may also be an important factor.

Control of Pathogenic Serogroups in the Intestinal Tract

The most direct method for controlling environmental contamination with pathogenic serotypes would be to control intestinal contamination. As chickens age, the number of *E. coli* belonging to pathogenic serotypes in the intestine tends to decrease. In some flocks, pathogens are not present. Weinack *et al.* (1981) found that pathogenic serotypes could be competitively excluded from the intestinal tract by seeding newly hatched chicks with the intestinal flora of resistant chickens.

Conclusions

Under most situations, *E. coli* is an environmental opportunist. At a given time, only a portion of a population is susceptible. In poultry, interactions between genetic and environmental factors are usually required to produce susceptibility to *E. coli* or to a predisposing infection. Infection with *E. coli* sometimes follows a strong defence effort against another disease-producing organism which elicits a defence response which is different from that required for defence against *E. coli*. Most infections in poultry can be controlled by good husbandry.

A successful defence against *E. coli* is characterized by a rapid response with highly efficient heterophils. This defence requires the expenditure of scarce resources and maximum efficiency is not normally maintained. Defence is weakened if nutritional and/or other resources are not available or have been diverted for other purposes.

Several virulence-associated factors of avian septicaemic *E. coli* have been identified. One of these, pili which mediate adherence to tracheal epithelial cells, is a potential target for vaccine-induced antibodies. However, more needs to be learnt about the range of target antigens on strains of the major serotypes of these *E. coli*.

References

Alexander, D.J., Manvell, R.J., Kemp, P.A., Parsons, G., Collins, M.S., Brockman, S., Russell, P.H. and Lister, S.A. (1987) Use of monoclonal antibodies in the characterization of avian paramyxovirus type 1 (Newcastle disease virus) isolates submitted to an international reference laboratory. *Avian Pathology* 16, 553–565.

Alsine, W.G. and Arp, L.H. (1987) Influence of *Bordetella avium* on association of *Escherichia coli* with turkey trachea. *American Journal of Veterinary Research* 48, 1574–1576.

Arp, L.H. (1982) Effect of passive immunization on phagocytosis in blood borne *Escherichia coli* in spleen and liver of turkeys. *American Journal of Veterinary Research* 43, 1034–1040.

Berkhoff, H.A. and Vinal, A.C. (1986) Congo red medium to distinguish between invasive and noninvasive *Escherichia coli* for poultry. *Avian Diseases* 30, 117–121.

Boado, E., Gonzaliz, A., Masdeu, V., Fonesca, C., Viamontes, O. and Canejo, V.J. (1988) Chloracion del agua de beber contra la coliseptacemia. *Revista Agricultura* 32, 45–58.

Bolin, C.A. and Jensen, A.E. (1987) Passive immunization with antibodies against iron-regulated outer membrane proteins protects turkeys from *Escherichia coli* septicemia. *Infection and Immunity* 55, 1239–1242.

Bree, A., Dho, M. and Lafont, J.P. (1989) Comparative infectivity for axenic and specific-pathogen-free chickens of O2 *E. coli* strains with or without virulence factors. *Avian Diseases* 33, 134–139.

Carlson, H.C. and Whenham, G.R. (1968) Coliform bacteria in chicken broiler house dust and their possible relationship to coli-septacemia. *Avian Diseases* 12, 297–302.

Chanteloup, N.K., Dho-Moulin, M., Esnault, E., Bree, A. and Lafont, J.P. (1991)

Serological conservation and location of the adhesin of avian *Escherichia coli* type 1 fimbriae. *Microbial Pathogenesis* 10, 271–280.

Cloud, S.S., Rosenberger, J.K., Fries, P.A., Wilson, R.A. and Odor, E.M. (1985) *In vitro* and *in vivo* characterization of avian *Escherichia coli*. 1 Serotypes, metabolic activity, and antibiotic sensitivity. *Avian Diseases* 29, 1084–1093.

Corbett, W.T., Berkhoff, H.A. and Vinal, A.C. (1987) Epidemiological study of the relationship between Congo red binding *Escherichia coli* and avian colisepticemia. *Canadian Journal of Veterinary Research* 51, 312–315.

Dassouli-Mrani-Belkebir, A., Contrepois, M., Girardeau, J.P. and Der Vartanian, M. (1988) Characters of *Escherichia coli* O78 isolated from septicaemic animals. *Veterinary Microbiology* 17, 345–356.

David, C.T. (1938) Colibacillosis in young chicks. *Journal of the American Veterinary Medical Association* 92, 518–522.

Dhillon, A.S. (1986) Pathology of avian adenovirus serotypes in the presence of *Escherichia coli* in infectious bursal-disease-virus infected specific-pathogen-free chickens. *Avian Diseases* 30, 81–86.

Dho, M. and Lafont, J.P. (1984) Adhesive properties and iron uptake ability in *Escherichia coli* lethal and nonlethal for chicks. *Avian Diseases* 26, 787–797.

Dho-Moulin, M., van den Bosch, J.F., Girardeau, J.P., Bree, A., Barat, T. and Lafont, J.P. (1990) Surface antigens from *Escherichia coli* O2 and O78 strains. *Infection and Immunity* 58, 740–745.

Doa-Ponser, K., O'Sullivan, N.P., Gross, W.B., Dunnington, E.A. and Siegel, P.B. (1991) Genotype-feeding regimen and diet interactions in meat chicks. III. General fitness. *Poultry Science* 70, 697–701.

Dozois, C.M., Fairbrother, J.M., Harel, J. and Bosse, M. (1992). Pap and pil-related DNA sequences and other virulence determinants associated with *Escherichia coli* isolated from septicemic chickens and turkeys. *Infection and Immunity* 60, 2648–2656.

Ellis, M.G., Arp, L.H. and Lamont, S.J. (1988). Serum resistance and virulence of *E. coli* isolated from turkeys. *American Journal of Veterinary Research* 46, 2034–2037.

Ellis, M.G., Arp, L.H. and Lamont, S.J. (1989) Interaction of turkey complement with *Escherichia coli* isolated from turkeys. *American Journal of Veterinary Research* 50, 1285–1288.

Emery, D.A., Nagaraja, K.V., Shaw, D.P., Newman, J.A. and White, D.J. (1992) Virulence factors of *E. coli* associated with colisepticemia in chickens and turkeys. *Avian Diseases* 36, 504–511.

Fahey, J.E. (1955) Some observations on 'air sac' infection in chickens. *Poultry Science* 34, 582–594.

Ficken, M.D., Edwards, J.F., Lay, J.C. and Tveter, D.E. (1987) Tracheal mucous transport rate and bacterial clearance in turkeys exposed by aerosol to La Sota strain of Newcastle disease virus. *Avian Diseases* 31, 241–248.

Gjessing, K.M. and Berkhoff, H.A. (1989). Experimental reproduction of airsacculitis and septicemia by aerosol exposure of 1-day-old chicks using Congo-red-positive *E. coli*. *Avian Diseases* 33, 473–478.

Glunder, G. (1990) Dermatitis in broilers caused by *Escherichia coli*: isolation of *Escherichia coli*, reproduction of the disease with *Escherichia coli* 078 : K80 and conclusions under consideration. *Journal of Veterinary Medicine Series B* 37, 383–391.

Gross, W.B. (1956) *Escherichia coli* as a complicating factor in chronic respiratory disease in chickens and infectious sinusitis in turkeys. *Poultry Science* 35, 765–771.

Gross, W.B. (1957a) Pathological changes of an *Escherichia coli* infection in chickens and turkeys. *American Journal of Veterinary Research* 18, 724–730.

Gross, W.B. (1957b) *Escherichia coli* infection of the chicken eye. *Avian Diseases* 1, 37–41.

Gross, W.B. (1961a) The development of 'Air sac disease'. *Avian Diseases* 5, 431–439.

Gross, W.B. (1961b) *Escherichia coli* as a complicating factor in Newcastle disease vaccination. *Avian Diseases* 5, 132–134.

Gross, W.B. (1961c) A synovitis caused by a strain of *Escherichia coli. Avian Diseases* 5, 218–220.

Gross, W.B. (1961d) The effect of chlortetracycline, erythromycin and nitrofurans as treatments for experimental 'Air sac disease'. *Poultry Science* 40, 833–841.

Gross, W.B. (1964) Retained caseous yolk sacs caused by *Escherichia coli. Avian Diseases* 8, 438–441.

Gross, W.B. (1966) Electrocardiographic changes in *Escherichia coli* infected birds. *American Journal of Veterinary Research* 27, 1427–1436.

Gross, W.B. (1984a) Combined effects of deoxycorticosterone and furaltadone on *Escherichia coli. American Journal of Veterinary Research* 45, 963–966.

Gross, W.B. (1984b) Effect of a range of social stress severity on *Escherichia coli* challenge infection. *American Journal of Veterinary Research* 45, 2074–2076.

Gross, W.B. (1990) Factors affecting the development of respiratory disease complex in chickens. *Avian Diseases* 34, 607–610.

Gross, W.B. (1992) Effect of short-term exposure of chickens to corticosterone on resistance to challenge exposure with *Escherichia coli* and antibody response to sheep erythrocytes. *American Journal of Veterinary Research* 53, 291–293.

Gross, W.B. and Chickering, W. (1987) Effects of fasting, water deprivation and adrenal-blocking chemicals on resistance to *Escherichia coli* challenge. *Poultry Science* 66, 270–272.

Gross, W.B. and Domermuth, C.H. (1988) Factors influencing the severity of *Escherichia coli* and avian adenovirus type 11 infection in chickens. *Avian Diseases* 17, 767–774.

Gross, W.B. and Siegel, P.B. (1959) Coliform peritonitis of chickens. *Avian Diseases* 3, 370–373.

Gross, W.B. and Siegel, H.S. (1965) Social groupings, stress on resistance to coliform infection in cockerels. *Poultry Science* 44, 1530–1536.

Gross, W.B. and Siegel, P.B. (1981) Some effects of feeding deoxycorticosterone to chickens. *Poultry Science* 60, 2232–2239.

Gross, W.B. and Siegel, P.B. (1982) Socialization as a factor in resistance to infection, feed efficiency and response to antigens in chickens. *American Journal of Veterinary Research* 43, 2010–2012.

Gross, W.B., Siegel, P.B., Domermuth, C.H. and DuBose, T.T. (1980a) Production and persistence of antibodies. 2. Resistance to infectious diseases. *Poultry Science* 59, 205–210.

Gross, W.B., Siegel, P.B. and DuBose, R.T. (1980b) Some effects of feeding corticosterone to chickens. *Poultry Science* 59, 516–522.

Gross, W.B., Jones, D. and Cherry, J. (1988) Effect of ascorbic acid on the disease caused by *Escherichia coli* challenge infection. *Avian Diseases* 32, 407–409.

Gyimah, J.E. and Panigrahy, B. (1988) Adhesin-receptor interactions mediating the attachment of pathogenic *Escherichia coli* to chicken tracheal epithelium. *Avian Diseases* 32, 74–78.

Gyimah, J.E., Panigrahy, B. and Williams, J.D. (1986) Immunogenicity of an *Escherichia coli* multivalent pilus vaccine in chickens. *Avian Diseases* 30, 687–689.

Harry, E.G. (1957) The effect on embryonic and chick mortality of yolk contamination with bacteria from the hen. *Veterinary Record* 69, 1433–1440.

Harry, E.G. (1964) The survival of *E. coli* in the dust of poultry houses. *Veterinary Record* 76, 466–470.

Harry, E.G. and Hemsley, L.A. (1965a) The association between the presence of septicaemic strains of *Escherichia coli* in the respiratory and intestinal tracts of chickens and the occurrence of coli septicaemia. *Veterinary Record* 77, 35–40.

Harry, E.G. and Hemsley, L.A. (1965b) The relationship between environmental contamination with septicaemic strains of *Escherichia coli* and their incidence in chickens. *Veterinary Record* 77, 241–245.

Heller, E.D. and Drabkin, N. (1977) Some characteristics of pathogenic *E. coli* strains. *British Veterinary Journal* 133, 572–578.

Heller, E.D., Leintner, G., Darabken, N. and Melamed, D. (1990) Passive immunization of chicks against *Escherichia coli. Animal Pathology* 19, 345–354.

Ibragimov, A.A., Oskolpov, V.S. and Golod, Y.R. (1983) Pathogenesis and diagnosis of mixed respiratory infections in fowls. *Veterinarya (Moscow)* 12, 33–36.

Ike, K., Kawahara, K., Danbara, H. and Kume, K. (1990) Serum resistance and aerobactin iron uptake in avian *E. coli* mediated by conjugative 100-megadalton plasmid. *Journal of Veterinary Medical Science* 54, 1091–1098.

Joya, J.E., Tsuji, T., Jacaline, A.V., Arita, M., Tsukamoto, T., Honda, T. and Miwatani, T. (1990) Demonstration of enterotoxigenic *Escherichia coli* in diarrheic broiler chicks. *European Journal of Epidemiology* 6, 88–90.

Lafont, J. P., Dho, M., D'hauteville, H.M., Bree, A. and Sansonetti, P.J. (1987) Presence and expression of aerobactin genes in virulent avian strains of *E. coli. Infection and Immunity* 55, 193–197.

Leitner, G., Melamed, D., Drabkin, N. and Heller, E.D. (1990) An enzyme-linked immunoabsorbent assay for detection of antibodies against *Escherichia coli*: association between indirect haemagglutination test and survival. *Avian Diseases* 34, 58–62.

Linggood, M.A., Roberts, M., Ford, S., Parry, H. and Williams, P.H. (1987) Incidence of the aerobactin iron uptake system among *E. coli* isolates from infections of farm animals. *Journal of General Microbiology* 133, 835–842.

Martinez, J. L., D-Iribarren, A. and Baquero, F. (1990) Mechanisms of iron acquisition and bacterial virulence. *Federation of European Microbiological Societies Microbiology Reviews* 75, 45–56.

Messier, S., Quessy, S., Robinson, Y., Devriese, L.A., Hommez, J. and Fairbrother, J.M. (1993) Focal dermatitis and cellulitis in broiler chickens:

bacteriological and pathological findings. *Avian Diseases* 37, 839–844.

Morley, A.J. and Thomson, D.K. (1984) Swollen head syndrome in broiler chickens. *Avian Diseases* 28, 238–243.

Morris, M. P. (1991) Cellulitis in broilers. *Broiler Industry* September, 32–40.

Myers, R.K. and Arp, L.H. (1987) Pulmonary clearance and lesions of lung and air sac in passively immunized and unimmunized turkeys following exposure to aerosolized *Escherichia coli. Avian Diseases* 31, 622–628.

Nagaraja, K.V., Emery, D.A., Jordan, K.A., Sivanandan, V., Newman, J.A. and Pomeroy, B.S. (1984) Effect of ammonia on the quantitative clearance of *Escherichia coli* from lungs, air sacs, and livers of turkeys aerosol vaccinated against *Escherichia coli. American Journal of Veterinary Research* 45, 392–395.

Nagi, M.S. and Mathey, W.J. (1972) Interaction of *Escherichia coli* and *Eimeria burnetti* in chickens. *Avian Diseases* 16, 864–873.

Nagi, M.S. and Raggi, L.G. (1972) Importance to 'airsac' disease of water contaminated with pathogenic *Escherichia coli. Avian Diseases* 16, 718–723.

Nakamura, K., Osobe, T. and Narita, M. (1990) Dual infection of *Eimeria tenella* and *Escherichia coli* in chickens. *Research in Veterinary Science* 49, 125–126.

Naveh, M.W., Zusman, T., Sketulsky, E. and Ron, E.Z. (1984) Adherence pili in avian strains of *Escherichia coli*: effect on pathogenicity. *Avian Diseases* 28, 651–661.

Nolan, L.K., Wooley, R.E. and Cooper, R.K. (1992) Transposon mutagenesis used to study the role of complement resistance in the virulence of an avian *Escherichia coli* isolate. *Avian Diseases* 36, 398–402.

Nunoya, T., Tajima, M., Izuchi, T., Takahashi, K., Otaki, T., Nagasawa, Y. and Hakogi, E. (1991) Pathology of a broiler disease characterized by the swollen head. *Journal of Veterinary Medical Science* 53, 347–349.

O'Brien (1985) Swollen head syndrome. *The Veterinary Record* 117, 619–620.

Odagiri, Y., Jensen, A.E. and Cheville, N.T. (1987) Immunity of chicks against colibacillosis by vaccination of parent breeders. *Bulletin of University of Osaka Prefecture B* 40, 37–44.

Ojeniyi, A.A. (1989) Direct transmission of *Escherichia coli* from poultry to humans. *Epidemiology and Infection* 103, 513–522.

Oyetunde, O.O.F., Thomson, R.G. and Carlson, H.C. (1978) Aerosol exposure of ammonia, dust and *Escherichia coli* in broiler chickens. *Canadian Veterinary Journal* 19, 187–193.

Panigrahy, B. and Yushen, L. (1990) Differentiation of pathogenic and non-pathogenic *E. coli* isolated from poultry. *Avian Diseases* 34, 941–943.

Pattison, M., Chettle, N., Randall, C.J. and Wyeth, P.J. (1989) Observations on swollen head syndrome in broiler and broiler breeder chickens. *Veterinary Record* 125, 229–231.

Payne, S.M. 1988. Iron and virulence in the family Enterobacteriaceae. *CRC Critical Reviews in Microbiology* 16, 81–111.

Peighambari, M., Vaillancourt, J.P., Wilson, R.A. and Gyles, C.L. (1993) Characteristics of *Escherichia coli* isolates from avian cellulitis. In: *Proceedings of the 74th Conference of Research Workers in Animal Diseases*. CRWAD, Chicago.

Randall, C.J., Meakins, P.A., Harris, M.P. and Watt, D.J. (1984) A new skin disease in broilers? *Veterinary Record* 114, 246.

Rosenburger, J.K., Fries, P.A., Cloud, S.S. and Wilson, R.A. (1985) *In vitro* and *in vivo* studies of *Escherichia coli*. 11. Factors associated with pathogenicity. *Avian Diseases* 29, 1094–1107.

Sandu, T.S. and Layton, H.W. (1985) Laboratory and field trials with formalin-inactivated *Escherichia coli* (078)-*Pasteurella anatipestifer* bacterin in White Pekin Ducks. *Avian Diseases* 29, 128–135.

Shirai, J., Maeda, M., Fujii, M. and Kuniyoshi, S. (1993) Swollen head syndrome is not associated with turkey rhinotracheitis virus. *Veterinary Record* 132, 41–42.

Siccardi, F.J. (1966) Identification and disease producing ability of *Escherichia coli* associated with *E. coli* infection of chickens and turkeys. MSc Thesis, University of Minnesota.

Smith, H.W., Cook, J.K.A. and Parcell, Z.E. (1985) The experimental infection of chickens with infectious bronchitis and *Escherichia coli. Journal of General Virology* 66, 777–786.

Sojka, W.J. and Carnaghan, R.B.A. (1961) *Escherichia coli* infection in poultry. *Research in Veterinary Science* 2, 340–352.

Suwanichkul, A. and Panigrahy, B. (1986) Biological and immunological characterization of pili of *E. coli* serotypes O1, O2, and O78 pathogenic to poultry. *Avian Diseases* 30, 781–787.

Suwanichkul, A. and Panigrahy, B. (1988) Diversity of pillus subunits of *Escherichia coli* isolated from avian species. *Avian Diseases* 32, 822–825.

Suwanichkul, A., Panigrahy, B. and Wagner, R.M. (1987) Antigenic relatedness and partial amino acid sequences of pili of *Escherichia coli* serotypes O1, O2 and O78 pathogenic for poultry. *Avian Diseases* 31, 809–813.

Tsuji, T., Joya, J.E., Yao, S., Honda, T. and Miwatani, T. (1988) Purification and characterization of heat-labile enterotoxin isolated from chicken enterotoxigenic *E. coli. Federation of European Microbiological Societies Microbiology Letters* 52, 79–84.

Twisselmann, N.M. (1939) An acute infectious disease of pullets apparently caused by *E. coli* communis. *Journal of the American Veterinary Medical Association* 94, 235–236.

Vaillancourt, J.P., Elfadil, A. and Bisaillon, J.R. 1992. Cellulitis in poultry. *Canada Poultryman* 79, 34–37.

Valantine, A. and Willsch, K. (1987) Unterschungen zur atiologie und pathogense der tiefen dermatitis bei schlacht broilern. *Monatshefte fur Veterinar Medizin* 42, 708–711.

Valvano, M.A. (1992) Diphenylamine increases cloacon DF13 sensitivity in avian septicemic strains of *Escherichia coli. Veterinary Microbiology* 32, 149–161.

Vidotto, M.C., Muller, E.E., de Freitas, J.C., Alfieri, A.A., Guimaraes, I.G. and Santos, D.S. (1990) Virulence factors of avian *E. coli. Avian Diseases* 34, 531–538.

Wasserman, B., Yates, J. and Fry, D.E. (1954) On so called air sac infection. *Poultry Science* 33, 622–623.

Waters, V.L. and Crosa, J.H. (1991) Colicin V virulence plasmids. *Microbiological Reviews* 55, 437–450.

Weinack, O.M., Snoyenbos, G.H., Smyzer, C.F. and Soerjadi, A.S. (1981)

Competitive exclusion of intestinal colonization of *Escherichia coli* in chicks. *Avian Diseases* 25, 696–705.

Wooley, R.E., Spears, K.R., Brown, J., Nolan, L.K. and Fletcher, O.J. (1992) Relationship of complement resistance and selected virulence factors in pathogenic avian *Escherichia coli. Avian Diseases* 36, 679–684.

Yerushalmi, Z., Smorodinsky, N.I., Naveh, M.W. and Ron, E.Z. (1990) Adherence pili of avian strains of *E. coli* O78. *Infection and Immunity* 58, 1129–1131.

Yoder, Jr, H. W. (1989) Congo red binding by *Escherichia coli* isolates from chickens. *Avian Diseases* 33, 502–505.

Yoder, H.W., Jr, Beard, C.W. and Mitchell, B.W. (1989) Pathogenicity of *Escherichia coli* in aerosols for young chickens. *Avian Diseases* 33, 676–683.

Zellen, G. (1988) Swollen head syndrome in broiler chickens. *Canadian Veterinary Journal* 29, 298.

12

Escherichia coli Infections in Rabbits, Cats, Dogs, Goats and Horses

J.E. PEETERS
National Instituut voor Diergeneeskundig Onderzoek, Department of Small Stock Pathology and Parasitology, Groeselenberg 99, B 1180 Brussels, Belgium

Previous chapters have discussed *E. coli* infections in cattle, sheep and pigs, the animal species in which most extensive investigations have been conducted. However, *E. coli* is an important agent of disease in several other animal species and, as methodologies for identification of pathogenic *E. coli* become more readily available, more information is being obtained about the significance of *E. coli* in other animal species. This chapter will discuss *E. coli* diseases in rabbits, dogs, cats, goats and horses. Most emphasis will be placed on the disease in rabbits, because there is considerable information on the role of enteropathogenic *E. coli* in diarrhoeal diseases in rabbits.

E. coli Infections in Rabbits

Enteropathogenic *E. coli* (EPEC) are the only class of pathogenic *E. coli* of importance in rabbits. These organisms constitute one of the main infectious agents in diarrhoeic rabbits and are responsible for 25–40% of the losses (Fig. 12.1). Often different agents are simultaneously involved.

History

Only low levels of *E. coli* are present in the gut of healthy weaned rabbits, because of the inhibitory influence of the caecal volatile fatty acids (VFA) (Prohaszka, 1980). During the 1970s, researchers recognized that diarrhoea in rabbits was often accompanied by a dramatic increase in the numbers of *E. coli* in the intestine. In 1977, Cantey and Blake demonstrated that *E. coli* were implicated in diarrhoea in rabbits and suggested that the

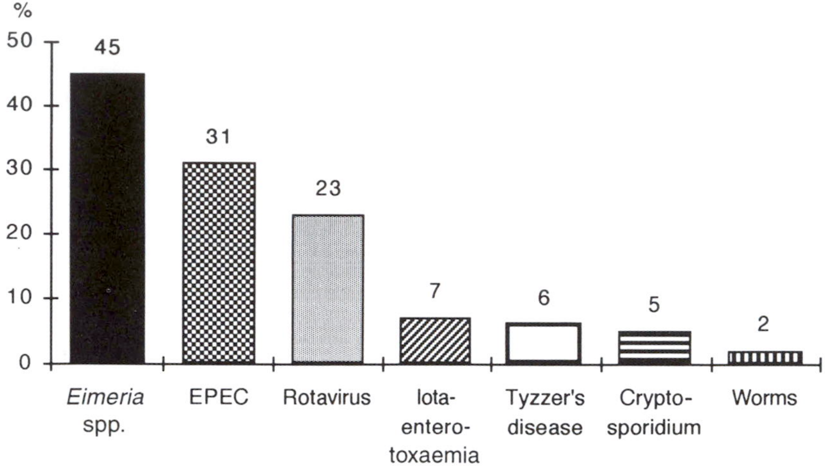

Fig. 12.1. Occurrence of pathogenic agents in commercial diarrhoeic rabbits in Belgium.

mechanism by which they caused disease was distinctly different from that associated with enterotoxigenic *E. coli* (ETEC). They isolated an O15 *E. coli* from diarrhoeal disease in rabbits and called the strain rabbit diarrhoeal *E. coli* 1 (RDEC-1). They showed that experimental infection with as few as 1.5×10^2 cells of *E. coli* strain RDEC-1 caused liquid diarrhoea and high mortality in rabbits. Subsequently, other researchers established the existence of pathogenic *E. coli* strains in rabbits and confirmed the characteristics of these strains.

Characteristics of E. coli *involved*

E. coli which cause intestinal disease in rabbits possess the attributes characteristic of EPEC of human origin. They attach to intestinal epithelial cells and efface microvilli; they do not produce known thermostable or thermolabile enterotoxins and are not enteroinvasive (Cantey and Blake, 1977; Peeters *et al.*, 1984b). Toxigenic types of *E. coli* are rarely identified among rabbit *E. coli* isolates. Pohl *et al.* (1993) examined a collection of 40 rabbit strains of *E. coli* and detected one O26/4+ strain which reacted with an SLT-I probe. One O128/2+ strain has been identified as a producer of cytolethal distending toxin (CLDT) (J.M. Fairbrother and W.M. Johnson, Québec, Canada, 1988, personal communication). Both these strains produced light to moderate diarrhoea after experimental infection.

Rabbit EPEC may be differentiated into sero/biotypes with different tissue tropisms and degrees of pathogenicity (Table 12.1). Some serotypes are mainly pathogenic for suckling rabbits (less than 3 weeks old) and others are associated predominantly with disease in weaned rabbits (Peeters *et al.*, 1984a, 1988b). It appears that specific clones are involved because rabbit EPEC can be divided into several pathotypes characterized by biotype (Table 12.2). The relationships between biotype, serotype, pathogenicity and tropism are outlined in Table 12.1. The occurrence of different serogroups of rabbit EPEC in various countries is shown in Table 12.3. Certain O serogroups, notably O2, O15, O103, O128 and O132, have a wide distribution.

There is conflicting information on the adherence of rabbit EPEC to HEp-2 cells. Reynaud and Federighi (1991) reported that all 20 rhamnose-negative O103 *E. coli* from weaned rabbits with diarrhoea showed localized adhesion to HEp-2 cells, but Pohl *et al.* (1993) found that rabbit EPEC did not have the genes responsible for diffuse, localized or aggregative forms of adherence to HEp-2 cells. There is some information on adhesins that may be involved in mediating attachment of rabbit EPEC to intestinal epithelial cells. Attachment of strain RDEC-1 to enterocytes is mediated by fimbriae called AF/R1 (adherence fimbriae, rabbit 1), but these fimbriae have not been detected on O15 EPEC strains involved in field infections in Belgium and Holland. Also, neither AF/R1 pili nor DNA sequences recognized by an AF/R1-specific DNA probe were detected in a collection of 40 rabbit EPEC of various serotypes. Thus, AF/R1 pili do not seem to constitute the main factor involved with adherence of rabbit EPEC and other bacterial surface proteins must be involved. Milon *et al.* (1990a) identified a 32-kDa adhesin on the surface of O103/8+ and O128/2+ rabbit EPEC strains, but not on O26/4+ strains. Antibodies raised against this adhesin inhibited diffuse adherence to HeLa cells and adherence to 8-day-old rabbit villi *in vitro*. A DNA sequence which hybridizes with an *eae* gene probe was the only common factor of 40 rabbit EPEC tested by Pohl *et al.* (1993). The *eae* gene codes for a 94-kDa outer membrane protein (intimin) involved with intimate attachment of the human EPEC strain E2348/69 to the epithelial cell membrane and with the induction of filamentous actin accumulation in HEp-2 cells. The finding that four out of five rabbit EPEC (O15, O26 and O103) reacted positively with FITC-phalloidin in the FAS (fluorescent actin staining) test confirms the similarity of at least some rabbit EPEC with EPEC of human origin. The basis of this test is discussed in Chapter 20.

Host factors that influence disease

Diets have a profound influence on colibacillosis in rabbits. Caecal *E. coli* numbers are moderated by VFA and pH: at a pH of 6.5 and a VFA

Table 12.1. Characteristics of EPEC pathogenic for neonatal and weanling rabbits.

	Neonatal rabbits	Weanling rabbits
Highly pathogenic strains		
Mortality (%)	100	50–100
Colonization of entire small and large intestine	biotype 1+, O109:K−:H2	biotype 8+, O103:K−:H2
Patchy colonization of ileum, caecum and colon		biotype 3−, 015:K−:H− biotype 4+, O26:K−, H11
Moderately pathogenic strains		
Mortality (%)	0–30	0–30
Patchy colonization of ileum, caecum and colon	biotype 1−, O8:K?:H? biotype 3+, O2:K1:H6 biotype 3−, O15:K−:H− biotype 8+, O103:K−:H2	biotype 1+, O20:K−:H7 biotype 1+, O109:K−:H7 biotype 1+, O153:K−:H7 biotype 2+, O128:K−:H2 biotype 2+, O132:K−:H2 biotype 3+, O2:K1:H6

Table 12.2. Biotypes of enteropathogenic *E. coli* in rabbits.

Biotype	Motility	Ornithine decarboxylase	Dulcitol	Raffinose	Rhamnose	Sorbose
1+	+	+ (97 %)	−	+	+	−
1−	−	+ (97 %)	−	+	+	−
2+	+	+ (98 %)	+	+	+	−
2−	−	+ (98 %)	+	+	+	−
3+	+	+ (96 %)	+	+	+	+
3−	−	+ (100 %)	+	+	+	+
4+	+	+ (100 %)	−	+	−	+
5+	+	− (0 %)	−	−	−	−
6+	+	+ (100 %)	+	−	+	−
6−	−	− (0 %)	+	−	+	−
7+	+	+ 100 %)	+	−	+	+
7−	−	+ (100 %)	+	−	+	+
8+	+	+ (100 %)	+	+	−	−
13+	+	−/+ (40 %)	−	+	+	+
18+	+	+ (100 %)	+	+	−	+
19+	+	−/+ (50 %)	−	−	−	+
19−	−	−/+ (50 %)	−	−	+	+
20+	+	− (0 %)	−	−	+	−
20−	−	− (0 %)	−	−	+	−

Figures in parentheses are percentage of strains positive.

Table 12.3. Serogroups of enteropathogenic *E. coli* in rabbits from different countries.

	O serogroup													
Country	2	7	8	15	18	20	26	49	85	103	109	128	132	153
Belgium	X		X	X		X	X			X	X	X	X	X
France	X			X			X	X	X	X		X	X	
Germany[a]	X		X		X				X	X		X		
Holland				X						X	X	X	X	
Hungary	X	X						X		X		X	X	
Italy	X		X		X			X		X				
Spain							X			X				
UK														X
USA				X										

[a] Strains of O groups 44, 55, 101 and 119 have also been reported from Germany.

concentration of 70 mmol kg^{-1}, proliferation of *E. coli* is impaired (Prohaszka, 1980). At lower pH values lower VFA levels are effective (Fig. 12.2). Thus, any factor which increases caecal pH and/or decreases caecal VFA favours colibacillosis. Feed composition, rate of intestinal transit and feeding method are the main factors that determine caecal pH and VFA levels. Dietary fibre protects weanling rabbits from diarrhoea. High protein diets (>18%) lead to excess levels of undigested protein in the caecum and to an increase in caecal ammonia and pH, which favour not only the proliferation of *E. coli*, but also of *Clostridium spiroforme*. Also, diets low in starch and rich in fibre (>17%) promote diarrhoea (Morisse *et al.*, 1985). Such diets result in a low caecal VFA production and a higher caecal pH by increasing retention of ammonia. Similar events occur when starch is replaced by fat in isoenergetic rations (Peeters *et al.*, 1993).

All factors, such as stress, cold, lack of drinking water and respiratory disease, that lead to reduced feed intake will result in decreased caecal VFA production, increased pH and *E. coli* proliferation. A combination of feed restriction (lower VFA production) and rotavirus infection (increased caecal ammonia concentration as a consequence of tissue destruction) provokes an increase in numbers of *E. coli* in the caecum (Fig. 12.3). Coccidiosis is yet another condition which favours colibacillosis in rabbits. As only higher infection levels result in clinical disease these factors are particularly pertinent in the case of moderately pathogenic EPEC. Such levels can only be reached in continuously occupied rabbit houses, in cases of unsatisfactory hygiene, an inadequate anticoccidiosis programme, or where there is immunosuppression. Moreover, 4- to 5-week-old rabbits are more susceptible to colibacillosis than are older rabbits.

Pathogenesis

Attachment of EPEC is followed by effacement of the epithelial brush borders, destruction of absorptive cells and villous atrophy (Cantey and Blake, 1977). The reduction in the digestive and resorptive capacities of the gut result in diarrhoea, poor feed conversion, weight loss and mortality. Also caecal sodium and chloride resorption is impaired, while ileal permeability for proteins is increased. Infection is associated with the excretion of up to 10^9 EPEC per gram of faeces for 14 days, contributing to the persistence of the infection (Fig. 12.4).

Clinical signs and gross lesions

Suckling rabbits

During a first outbreak of colibacillosis due to O109/1+ *E. coli*, 4–30% of the litters show yellow diarrhoea with soiling of the hind quarters.

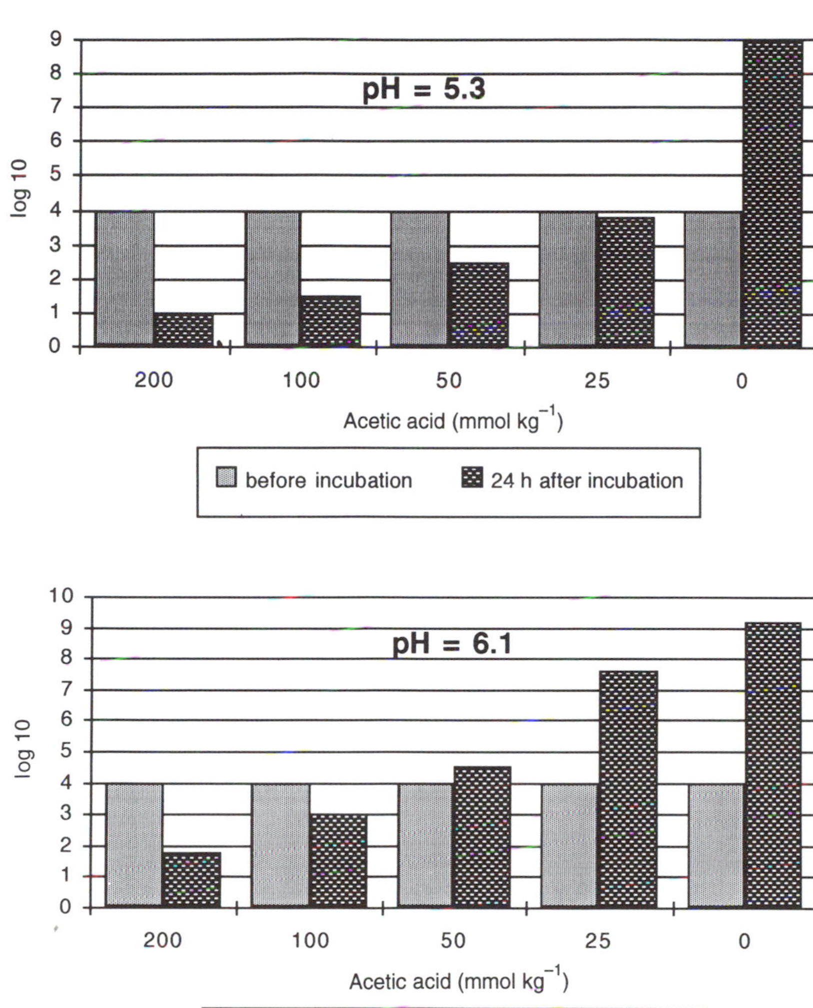

Fig. 12.2. Influence of acetic acid on *E. coli* numbers following incubation *in vitro* at pH 5.3 and 6.1.

Rabbits 3–12 days of age are the main ones that are affected and mortality within a litter reaches 100% in 24–48 hours. Two successive litters are rarely affected. Other sero/biotypes may cause disease, but, typically, half of the littermates will survive. Necropsy shows a congested small intestine and yellowish, liquid to pasty caecal contents. The stomach is filled with

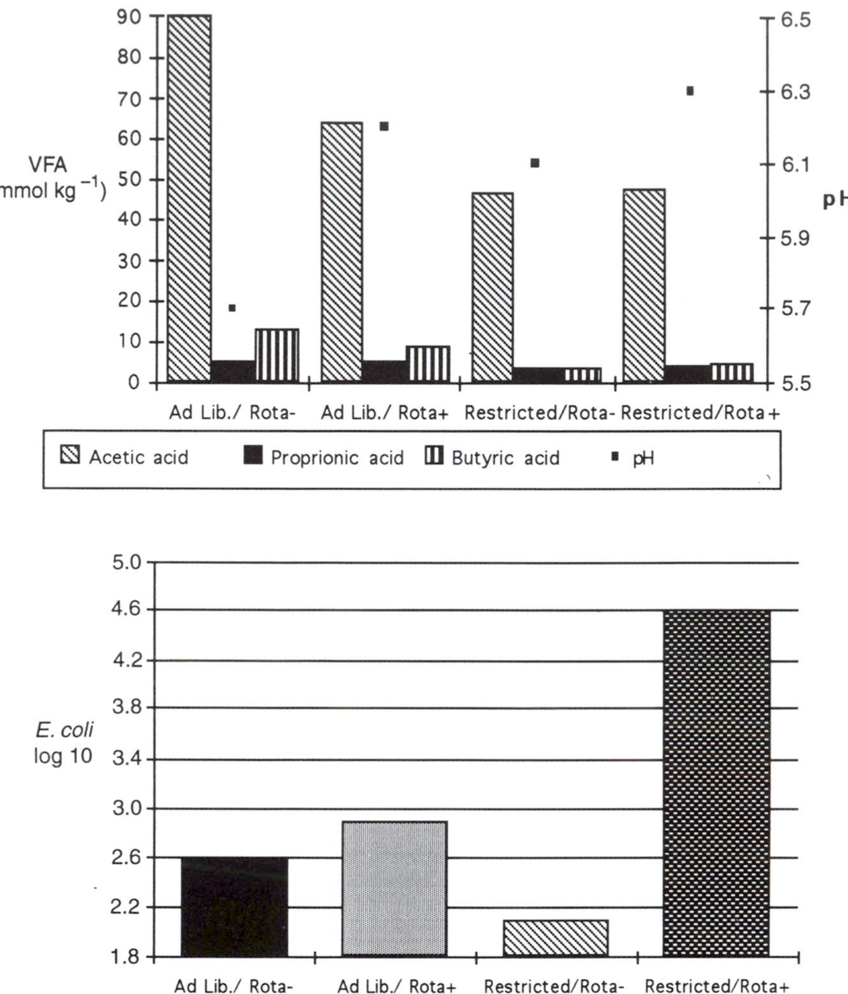

Fig. 12.3. Influence of feed restriction and rotavirus infection on caecal volatile fatty acid concentrations, pH and *E. coli* numbers 14 days after weaning.

curdled milk, indicating the rapid progression of the disease (Okerman *et al.*, 1982).

Weanling rabbits

Diarrhoea occurs 4–10 days after experimental infection with 2×10^6 bacteria. In the field, the first clinical signs appear 5–14 days after weaning. Rabbits older than 3 months are rarely affected. Diarrhoea persists for a

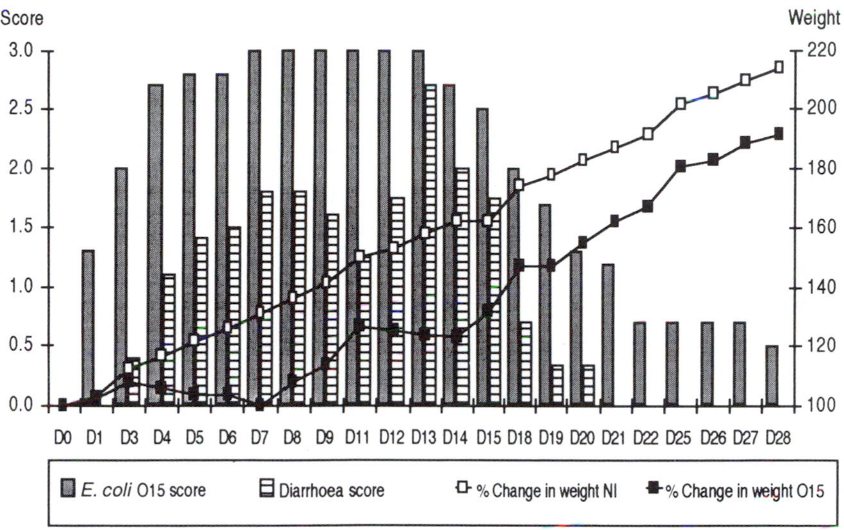

Fig. 12.4. Change in weight, diarrhoea and *E. coli* O15 output after experimental infection with EPEC O15/3−.

mean of 4 days and affected animals stop drinking and eating. Faeces are watery, occasionally mucoid and do not contain blood. Mortality is mostly between 5% and 20% in the case of moderately pathogenic strains, but may reach 50% and more when highly virulent strains are involved. Some animals remain completely cachectic 7–14 days postinfection, while animals which recuperate show a growth retardation of 5–7 days. Infection by low numbers of moderately pathogenic sero/biotypes is followed by poor feed conversion but no overt signs of disease.

At necropsy, lesions are limited to the terminal small intestine, caecum and colon. Mesenteric lymph nodes and Peyer's patches are markedly swollen. Often only foul-smelling, watery and brown caecal content is found. In infections by highly pathogenic strains moderate to severe caecal oedema may be observed, sometimes associated with paintbrush haemorrhage on the caecal serosa in cases of complication with *Clostridium spiroforme* iota-enterotoxaemia.

Microscopic lesions

EPEC may be observed adhering to intestinal epithelial cells. In suckling rabbits the EPEC colonize the full length of the small and large intestine and cause severe villous atrophy. In weaned rabbits sero/biotype O15/3− attaches first to the Peyer's patches from 4 to 12 hours postinfection. By

3 days after infection, small patches of adherent bacteria can be found in the ileum, caecum and colon, and by 6–10 days postinfection large numbers are found attached to these segments and diarrhoea occurs. The caecum is most heavily involved. Sero/biotype O103/8+ also colonizes the proximal small intestine. In both suckling and weanling rabbits the lamina propria is infiltrated by polymorphonuclear cells beneath colonized sites. Electron microscopy shows loss of the microvillous border and bacteria intimately adherent on pedestal-like structures on the epithelial surface (Cantey, 1984).

Immune response

Protection provided by previous colonization is complete. Specific anti-EPEC IgG and IgM, but not IgA, appear in the serum by 4 days postinfection, with a peak 7–15 days post-diarrhoea. Specific secretory anti-EPEC IgA is the only immunoglobulin detected in ileal contents by 7–13 days postinfection and continues to rise as long as 50–55 days postdiarrhoea (O'Hanley and Cantey, 1981). Bile is a major source of specific IgA. We observed similar kinetics after experimental infection of rabbits with EPEC O15/3− and O103/8+ (Fig. 12.5). The progressively increasing synthesis and secretion of IgA in the gut reflects a continuous antigenic stimulation by reingestion of organisms during caecotrophy or by recolonization of the

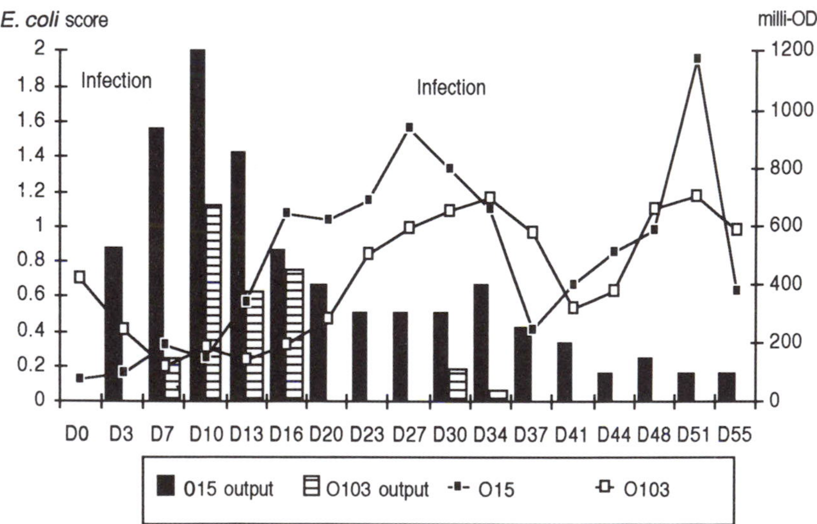

Fig. 12.5. Kinetics of faecal *E. coli* output and specific faecal anti-LPS IgA (ELISA) after experimental infection with EPEC O15/3− and O103/8+.

intestinal tract by hidden foci of organisms in healthy carriers. Although faecal excretion of EPEC does not increase after reinfection, local IgA will rise further.

As the mammary gland and the gut form part of a common mucosal immune system, prolonged antigenic stimulation explains why only one litter of the same doe is usually affected by neonatal colibacillosis. Orogastric administration of live EPEC is followed by large amounts of specific IgA in the milk (Cantey, 1984; Milon and Camguilhem, 1989). Immune IgA purified from rabbit milk and given orally to rabbits prior to and several days after experimental infection prevented attachment and clinical signs (O'Hanley and Cantey, 1981). However, persistence of organisms in the intestinal lumen is not inhibited (McQueen *et al.*, 1992).

Diagnosis

Histology reveals *E. coli* adherent to the intestinal mucosa. Colibacillosis may also be screened by semiquantitative evaluation of *E. coli* numbers in the gut since *E. coli* is present in low numbers in healthy weaned rabbits. There is a 89% correlation between histological confirmation and confluent growth of *E. coli* from samples taken from the mid small intestine. A simple combination of serogrouping and biotyping allows quick diagnosis of highly pathogenic EPEC. A selective Simmons' citrate sorbose medium was developed for screening EPEC of biotypes 3 and 4 (Peeters *et al.*, 1988a). Rabbitries may be screened serologically by ELISA, using LPS as antigen.

Differential diagnosis

In suckling rabbits, rotaviruses and *Cryptosporidium parvum* cause similar clinical signs and gross lesions, although mortality seldom surpasses 50%. Enteritis problems in weaned rabbits are often multifactorial. Therefore differential diagnosis should involve coccidiosis, *Clostridium spiroforme* iota-enterotoxaemia, Tyzzers' disease (*Bacillus piliformis*) and rotavirus infection.

Treatment

Suckling rabbits

Antibiotic treatment of all littermates for 5 days from the first appearance of diarrhoea is highly effective. Treatment of does will not cure their young and impairs development of maternal immunity.

Weanling rabbits

As other pathogenic agents enhance the pathological effects of colibacillosis, all agents involved should be identified correctly. Antibacterial treatment should always be accompanied by appropriate anticoccidial measures. Moderately pathogenic EPEC are easily controlled by administration of any of a number of appropriate antibiotics. Highly pathogenic strains of EPEC, on the contrary, are difficult to control on a long-term basis. Typically, only enrofloxacin, neomycin and, to a lesser extent, chloramphenicol show sufficient activity; sulfonamides, tetracycline, furaltodone, flumequine and colistin are usually ineffective regardless of the *in vitro* sensitivity. Antibiotic resistance is widespread among rabbit EPEC. Treatment should be continued for 7–10 days. Often, prolonged medication, especially with neomycin, is followed by *Clostridium spiroforme* iota-enterotoxaemia. This can be prevented by simultaneous administration of imidazoles or bacitracin. A total of 3–7% of animals remain carriers after treatment. Therefore, an eradication programme should be considered in commercial rabbitries in order to prevent repeated outbreaks in cases of sero/biotypes O15/3− and O103/8+. This was done successfully by screening and eliminating carriers after rectal swabbing and replacing eliminated animals by certified EPEC-free reproduction stock.

Prevention

Vaccination

Oral and intradermal vaccination of does during gestation protects sucklings from neonatal colibacillosis. Parenteral vaccination of weanlings with an O103/8+ strain was not followed by protection. Vaccination of mothers does not protect their offspring after weaning either (Milon and Camguilhem, 1989). However, protection against challenge was reported after administration of formalized vaccines by the drinking water during four consecutive days after weaning (Camguilhem and Milon, 1990). Under field conditions, immunity has to be boosted 3 weeks after the initial vaccination to avoid mortality at the end of the fattening period. Even after booster vaccination, protection is incomplete and EPEC excretion in the faeces is only partly inhibited. Thus, vaccination will not eradicate the disease.

Infection with one sero/biotype may induce cross-protection against other sero/biotypes. In this respect, Milon *et al.* (1990b) obtained good protection after oral vaccination with a live non-pathogenic O103 strain and after vaccination with an O128 strain that expressed the same adhesins as the virulent O103/8+ strain. Nevertheless, vaccination with the first did not completely protect against challenge, while vaccination with the latter was not completely harmless.

Other means of prevention

Before introducing new reproduction stock, the rabbitry of origin should be checked for highly pathogenic EPEC strains (O15/3−, O26/4+, O103/8+). Postponing weaning until the age of 35–38 days limits the susceptibility of weanlings to colibacillosis. Also modification of feed composition in rabbitries at risk is useful: energy content (2200–2300 kcal kg^{-1}) and crude protein level (<16%) should be reduced and a level of ±18% of starch should be maintained. Besides, hygienic measures, which reduce the infection pressure, and a good anticoccidiosis programme will limit the extent of disease.

E. coli Infections in Dogs

ETEC, EPEC, uropathogenic and cytotoxic necrotizing factor (CNF^+) *E. coli* have all been recovered from dogs, but only a few strains have been studied in detail. Although most reports deal with ETEC, the finding of ETEC does not always imply an aetiological role as in most clinical cases additional aetiological agents were established. Possibly, intestinal *E. coli* infections are the result of a concurrent intestinal environment.

Characteristics of E. coli *involved*

ETEC

E. coli strains from dogs which produce the heat-stable enterotoxin STa were first described in 1980 by Josse *et al*. Later, several other reports were published (reviewed by Broes, 1993). The occurrence of ETEC in diarrhoeic dogs varied between 2.7% and 29.5%. Most strains produced STa enterotoxin and LT-producing strains were rarely detected. Most strains belonged to serogroups O4, O6, O8 or O42, but also to serogroups O5, O17, O20, O23, O25, O70 or O105. They often express fimbriae which do not react with anti-CFA1, CFA2, K88 or 987P antiserum. K99 fimbriae were detected in four O42:H37 ETEC strains by Wasteson *et al*. (1988). In these strains, the genes coding for ST were located on a 98-MDa plasmid. Similar strains were shown to carry *hly* plasmids encoding alpha-haemolysin sequences. Mainil *et al*. (1991) used DNA probes for STa1, STa2, STb and LT toxins and for K99, K88, F41 and 987P fimbriae to test 710 strains isolated from 276 dogs. Positive strains showed the following pathotypes:

$STa1^+$ (18), $STa1^+$ STb^+ (70), $STa1^+ + K99^+$ (2) and $STa1^+$ $K99^+$ $F41^+$ (4).

EPEC

EPEC were detected by electron microscopic examination of the intestine of an 8-week-old puppy (Broes *et al.*, 1988). The strain belonged to serotype O49:H10, was not invasive and did not produce any of the known enterotoxins or verotoxins, nor any of the known fimbrial antigens.

Uropathogenic E. coli

E. coli is the most common organism recovered from the urine of dogs with urinary tract infection (UTI) (Van der Stock *et al.*, 1981; Meier *et al.*, 1983; Senior, 1985; Zschock *et al.*, 1988; Schwarz, 1991). These infections include cystitis, endometritis, pyelonephritis and prostatitis. Studies of the numbers of bacteria recovered from urine samples of dogs show that, as in humans, there is a bimodal distribution and a level of 10^5 organisms or more per millilitre of urine is a good basis for distinguishing significant bacteriuria from contamination.

Canine uropathogenic *E. coli* share several attributes of their more extensively studied counterparts from human infections. They belong to a small number of O serogroups, possess fimbrial adhesins which bind to epithelial cells of the urogenital system, are often haemolytic, and sometimes produce aerobactin. Serogroups have been determined in only a limited number of studies, but strains of O groups 2, 4 and 6 appear to be most common (Westerlund *et al.*, 1987; Garcia *et al.*, 1988a; Wilson *et al.*, 1988).

Several researchers have investigated the association of fimbriae with canine uropathogenic *E. coli*. Type 1 (F1) fimbriae which possess mannose-sensitive haemagglutinating activity are often present. Westerlund *et al.* (1987) found that 29 of 33 canine *E. coli* from UTI produced type 1 fimbriae. Fimbriae which mediate mannose-resistant haemagglutination (MRHA) are implicated in the adherence of human uropathogenic *E. coli* to human uroepithelial cells and a number of researchers have examined canine uropathogenic strains for MRHA. The majority of canine strains were found to possess MRHA in studies by Garcia *et al.* (1988a, 1992) and Roos (1990). Wilson *et al.* (1988) reported that MRHA was not associated with canine isolates. The discrepancy may be explained by the observation by Garcia *et al.* (1988a) that canine isolates show MRHA with canine erythrocytes but not with human erythrocytes.

P fimbriae similar to those implicated in UTI in humans have been identified on canine *E. coli* UTI isolates (Westerlund *et al.*, 1987; Garcia *et al.*, 1988a,b, 1992). Although the fimbrial subunits were closely related to the F12 and F13 fimbriae of human uropathogenic strains, the adhesins were different. Differences were shown by the failure of the canine, but not the human isolates, to demonstrate MRHA with human erythrocytes and to agglutinate latex beads covered with the receptor for the P fimbriae. Garcia *et al.* (1988b) showed that canine isolates with F12- or F13-related fimbriae adhered to dog kidney epithelial cells but not to human bladder epithelial cells.

A high percentage of canine uropathogenic *E. coli* are haemolytic (Westerlund *et al.*, 1987; Wilson *et al.*, 1988; Zschock *et al.*, 1988; Schwarz, 1991). Percentages of isolates that were haemolytic ranged from 28% to 67%. Haemolysis is particularly associated with certain O groups and Wilson *et al.* (1988) noted that 70% of canine uropathogenic isolates of *E. coli* of O groups 2, 4 and 6 produced alpha-haemolysin. Alpha-haemolysin is a powerful cytotoxin and may be responsible for tissue damage.

Ability to scavenge iron in tissues through the action of the siderophore aerobactin is one characteristic of human uropathogenic *E. coli*. However, in one study of 33 *E. coli* strains from canine UTI, only a few strains were found to produce aerobactin (Westerlund *et al.*, 1987).

CNF-producing E. coli

In strains from diarrhoeic dogs, CNF1-production and chromosomally encoded alpha-haemolysin are closely associated (Prada *et al.*, 1991). Similar strains (serogroups O2, O4 and O6) were isolated from localized purulent processes (Pohl *et al.*, 1992). They produced aerobactin and were resistant to the bactericidal action of serum, but did not produce known adhesins or toxins other than CNF1.

Septicaemic E. coli

E. coli is a major cause of septicaemia in newborn puppies. Sager and Remmers (1990) carried out bacteriological cultures on 118 puppies which had died over an unstated period of time at an intensively operated dog breeding kennel. Bacterial septicaemia occurred in 74% of the cases and beta-haemolytic *E. coli* was one of the more commonly isolated organisms. They concluded that infections arose from contamination in the uterus, during passage through the birth canal or from mastitic milk of bitches.

Clinical signs

In newborn puppies EPEC were associated with watery diarrhoea and high mortality. Animals were dehydrated and emaciated. After experimental infection of neonatal puppies with an STa^{+} ETEC strain, Art (cited by

Broes, 1993) observed only a transitory diarrhoea. In puppies older than 3 months and in adult dogs, ETEC were associated with acute vomiting, diarrhoea and dehydration. Faeces were watery and contained blood. Relapses were common and diarrhoea often became chronic. *E. coli* infections were also associated with endometritis, pyometra and mastitis in sexually mature bitches and with infection of the male genital organs. Transmission of naturally occurring infection from males to females has been established.

Postmortem findings

Broes *et al.* (1988) reported watery and brownish black small intestinal contents in EPEC-infected animals. Numerous Gram-negative bacilli were found intimately attached to the epithelial lining in association with villous atrophy and varying degrees of crypt hyperplasia. Lesions were most severe in the ileum. The lamina propria was infiltrated with large numbers of histiocytes, plasmocytes and lymphocytes. ETEC infections were associated with gastroenteritis, whereas CNF^+ strains were isolated from purulent processes (pleuritis, pyometra, mastitis, prostatitis).

Diagnosis

Presently, there are no established methods in use in diagnostic laboratories for detection of EPEC or ETEC. Although not conclusive, isolation of alpha-haemolytic strains represents a first clue for pathogenic *E. coli* in dogs. A combination of serotyping and haemagglutination may be helpful as most pathogenic strains in dogs seem to belong to serogroups O2, O4, O6, O8 or O42 and show mannose-resistant haemagglutination. Differential diagnosis should exclude parvovirus infection, canine distemper and parasitic infections. Identification of uropathogenic *E. coli* is simple as quantitative culture of a properly collected sample of urine will yield large numbers of the organism.

Treatment

Nearly all *E. coli* strains involved with disease in dogs are resistant to one or more antimicrobial agent(s), which makes antibiotic sensitivity testing advisable.

E. coli Infections in Cats

E. coli form a normal part of the feline intestinal flora and is also often isolated from the preputium and the vagina of healthy cats. However,

E. coli is frequently involved with intestinal and extraintestinal infections. Unfortunately, few strains have been studied in detail, making definitive conclusions on their aetiological role difficult.

Characteristics associated with pathogenic E. coli *strains*

Lesions characteristic of attaching–effacing EPEC were reported in two diarrhoeic cats by Pospischil *et al.* (1987) and an SLT1-negative strain was isolated from these animals. During a Swedish study, 76% of 22 isolates of *E. coli* from diarrhoeic cats showed strong production of SLT1 compared with only 12% of 25 strains from healthy cats (Abaas *et al.*, 1989). This association suggests that VTEC may be causative agents of diarrhoea in cats. Most of the strains studied were haemolytic and belonged to serogroups O2, O4 and O6. Strains associated with septicaemic processes or with vaginal exudate produced aerobactin, were resistant to serum, fermented sorbose rapidly, and produced cytotoxic necrotizing factor 1 (CNF1). Some also produced colicin. They did not possess the genes for known adhesins or other toxins (Pohl *et al.*, 1992).

E. coli are an important cause of urogenital infections in cats (Wilson *et al.*, 1988; Apel *et al.*, 1989). Feline uropathogenic *E. coli* appear to share the characteristics of canine strains (Wilson *et al.*, 1988), which have been investigated more extensively. It is known that a high percentage of these *E. coli* are haemolytic. For example, Apel *et al.* (1989) found that among 188 bacterial isolates from the urine of diseased cats, 30.8% were non-haemolytic *E. coli* and 24.5% were haemolytic *E. coli*.

Clinical signs

No experimental infection studies with EPEC or VTEC have been reported. Most cats from which SLT1$^+$ strains were isolated, showed anorexia and had watery diarrhoea which persisted for several weeks. Illyutovich (cited by Sojka, 1965) infected cats with a septicaemic O111:H12 strain and observed fever, dyspepsia and anorexia which began 2–6 days postinfection and lasted for 5–15 days. Mortality was almost 50% and the inoculated strain was excreted in the faeces for 57–160 days postinfection. Septicaemia was present between 6 and 20 days postinfection.

Postmortem findings

EPEC and VTEC were isolated from cats showing catarrhal enteritis associated with petechiae, diffuse atrophy and focal villus fusion in the ileum. The mucosa was infiltrated with neutrophils and covered by an extensive layer of bacteria. Electron microscopy showed intimate attachment to both absorptive and goblet cells. CNF1$^+$ strains were isolated from cats with peritonitis, hepatic and renal degeneration, cystitis or vaginal exudation.

Treatment

Antibiotic treatment of *E. coli* diarrhoea reduced clinical signs, but was often followed by exacerbation in chronic cases when treatment was stopped.

E. coli Infections in Goats

Intestinal disorders

Infection by K99$^+$ ETEC is a significant cause of diarrhoea in newborn kids up to 2–3 weeks of age. However, cryptosporidiosis represents the main aetiological agent in this age group (Nagy *et al.*, 1983). Infected kids show profuse watery diarrhoea followed by dehydration and death. Diagnosis may be made by detection of K99 antigen in frozen sections by immunofluorescence or by slide agglutination with specific antisera.

EHEC strains have been isolated from 1- to 2-month-old diarrhoeic goats. They produced SLT1 and belonged to serotypes O157:K−:H− and O103:H2. They were not invasive, did not express known adhesins or produce other known toxins. Strain O103:H2 caused typical attaching and effacing lesions in large intestinal epithelial cells, did not attach to HEp-2 cells and was negative in the FAS test. The strain preferentially colonized the large intestine and caused severe chronic diarrhoea. Histology revealed multifocal villus atrophy and marked hyperplasia of crypt epithelium in the small intestine, whereas large numbers of coccobacilli adhered to the epithelial lining of caecum and colon (Duhamel *et al.*, 1992). As EHEC mainly affect 1- to 2-month-old goats, differential diagnosis should be made with coccidiosis which is the main intestinal pathogen of this age group.

Treatment of these intestinal disorders involves symptomatic measures in the first place: withdrawal of milk for the first 24 hours and administration of large volumes of water. If necessary, electrolytes are given. After 24 hours, milk is given again, but only half of the normal intake is made available. Oral or parenteral administration of antibiotics may be necessary, but treatment often comes too late.

Other diseases

Other strains of *E. coli* are associated with septicaemia or with chronic arthritis. Löliger (cited by Sojka, 1965) gave an account of experimental

E. coli orchitis produced with a strain isolated from the ejaculate of a goat. Suppurative inflammation of the epididymis may lead to seminal retention and sterility. Males with genital infection by haemolytic *E. coli* may transmit the infection to females, resulting in sterility. *E. coli* is, of course, an important agent of mastitis in goats.

E. coli Infections in Horses

Intestinal disorders

Diarrhoea is a common problem in foals, particularly during the first few weeks of life, but mortality is low. Rotavirus infection, salmonellosis and nutritional problems are the predominant causes of diarrhoea in foals. Enteric colibacillosis has not been documented until recently and probably does not constitute an important cause of diarrhoea. Good colostrum management, clean foaling areas and lack of overcrowding are the factors that contribute to a low incidence. However, there have been a few reports of *E. coli* associated with diarrhoea in foals. Holland *et al.* (1989) identified ETEC from a foal with diarrhoea. Ike *et al.* (1987) carried out a 5-year survey of bacteria in the faeces of 463 foals with diarrhoea and found that haemolytic *E. coli* were by far the most commonly suspected agent. They demonstrated that haemolytic *E. coli* were present in higher numbers in the faeces of foals with diarrhoea compared with the faeces of healthy foals. Isolates were commonly O101, and less frequently O8 or O147. These O groups are frequently implicated as ETEC in pigs, although in horses neither the fimbrial antigens nor the enterotoxins characteristic of these O groups in pigs were present. Thus, these strains are not ETEC and the nature of their role, if any, in diarrhoea requires further study.

In another study, no significant differences were found between *E. coli* serotypes in healthy and diseased foals. Tzipori *et al.* (1984) were not successful in inducing diarrhoea in newborn foals with isolates obtained from scouring foals. A $K99^+$ strain did not produce diarrhoea either. However, they presented evidence that horses possess receptors for the K88 pilus antigen of *E. coli* (not for K99) and reproduced profuse watery diarrhoea with a $K88^+$ LT^+ ETEC in a neonatal colostrum-deprived foal. As infection required a massive infectious dose and as degree of intestinal colonization was only limited, it was concluded that $K88^+$ ETEC are not likely to cause diarrhoea in foals reared under natural conditions. EPEC may be considered as potential pathogens in the horse as EPEC of human origin (O111:H−) caused characteristic ultrastructural damage to the epithelial brush border of equine small intestinal explants (Batt *et al.*, 1989).

Septicaemic disease

E. coli remains one of the most common organisms isolated in foals which die from septicaemia and generalized infection. Such strains differ from strains isolated from the faeces of clinically normal horses and possess virulence markers. Most septic strains were non-haemolytic and consistently showed resistance to killing by serum; some isolates produced aerobactin (Hirsh *et al.*, 1993). Moreover, a $CNF2^+$ strain was isolated from a case of metritis in a Belgian mare.

Concluding Remarks

It is clear that *E. coli* causes intestinal and extraintestinal infections in a wide variety of animal species. However, there has been very little effort to characterize the strains that are involved in disease in most species other than poultry, pigs, cattle and sheep. What is known indicates that there is remarkable host species specificity, that some defect in host defence is usually necessary for septicaemic disease, and that enteric disease is typically seen only in the neonatal and immediate postweaning periods.

References

Abaas, S., Franklin, A., Kühn, I., Ørskov, F. and Ørskov, I. (1989) Cytotoxin activity on Vero cells among *Escherichia coli* strains associated with diarrhea in cats. *American Journal of Veterinary Research* 50, 1294–1296.

Apel, J., Hamann, H.P. and Weiss, R. (1989) Occurrence and antibiotic resistance of bacterial pathogens in urine samples in cats. *Kleintierpraxis* 34, 467–468, 470–472.

Batt, R.M., Embaye, H., Hunt, J. and Hart, C.A. (1989) Ultrastructural damage to equine intestinal epithelium induced by enteropathogenic *Escherichia coli*. *Equine Veterinary Journal* 21, 373–375.

Broes, A. (1993) Les *Escherichia coli* pathogènes du chien et du chat. *Annales de Médecine Vétérinaire* 137, 377–384.

Broes, A., Drolet, R., Jacques, M., Fairbrother, J.M. and Johnson, W.M. (1988) Natural infection with an attaching and effacing *Escherichia coli* in a diarrheic puppy. *Canadian Journal of Veterinary Research* 52, 280–282.

Camguilhem, R. and Milon, A. (1989) Biotypes and O serogroups of *Escherichia coli* involved in intestinal infection of weaned rabbits: clues to diagnosis of pathogenic strains. *Journal of Clinical Microbiology* 27, 743–747.

Camguilhem, R. and Milon, A. (1990) Protection of weaned rabbits against experimental *Escherichia coli* O103 intestinal infection by oral formalin-killed vaccine. *Veterinary Microbiology* 21, 353–362.

Cantey, J.R. (1984) The rabbit model of *Escherichia coli* (strain RDEC-1) diarrhea.

In: Boedeker, E.C. (ed.) *Attachment of Organisms to the Gut Mucosa*, Vol. 1. CRC Press, Boca Raton, Florida, pp. 209–220.

Cantey, J.R. and Blake, R.K. (1977) Diarrhea due to *Escherichia coli* in the rabbit. A novel mechanism. *Journal of Infectious Diseases* 135, 454–462.

Duhamel, G.E., Moxley, R.A., Maddox, C.W. and Erickson, E.D. (1992) Enteric infection of a goat with enterohemorrhagic *Escherichia coli* (O103:H2). *Journal of Veterinary Diagnostic Investigation* 4, 197–200.

Garcia, E., Bergmans, H.E.N., Van der Bosch, J.F., Ørskov, I., Van der Zeijst, B.A.M. and Gaastra, W. (1988a) Isolation and characterisation of dog uropathogenic *Escherichia coli* strains and their fimbriae. *Antonie van Leeuwenhoek* 54, 149–163.

Garcia, E., Hamers, A.M., Bergmans, E.N., Van der Zeijst, B.A.M. and Gaastra, W. (1988b) Adhesion of canine and human uropathogenic *Escherichia coli* and *Proteus mirabilis* strains to canine and human epithelial cells. *Current Microbiology* 17, 333–337.

Garcia, E., Bergmans, H.E.N., Gaastra, W. and Van der Zeijst, B.A.M (1992) Nucleotide sequences of the major subunit of F9 and F12 fimbriae of uropathogenic *Escherichia coli*. *Microbial Pathogenesis* 13, 161–166.

Hirsh, D.C., Kirkham, C. and Wilson, W.D. (1993) Characteristics of *Escherichia coli* isolated from septic foals. *Veterinary Microbiology* 34, 123–130.

Holland, R.E., Sriranganathan, N. and DuPont, L. (1989) Isolation of enterotoxigenic *Escherichia coli* from a foal with diarrhea. *Journal of the American Veterinary Medical Association* 194, 389–391.

Ike, K., Kamada, M., Anzai, T., Imagawa, H., Kumanomido, T., Nakazawa, M., Kashiwazaki, M. and Kume, T. (1987) Some properties of *Escherichia coli* isolated from foals with diarrhea and mares with metritis. *Bulletin of Equine Research Institute* No. 24, 33–41.

Josse, M., Jacquemin, E. and Kaeckenbeeck, A. (1980) Présence chez le chien d'*Escherichia coli* productrices d'une entérotoxine thermostable (STa). *Annales de Médecine Vétérinaire* 124, 211–214.

Mainil, J., Jacquemin, E., Kaeckenbeeck, A., MacAldowie, C. and Taylor, D. (1991) Prevalence of enteropathogenic *Escherichia coli* in dog faeces. In: *Annual Conference of the Association of the Veterinary Teachers and Research Workers*. Abstract C23, Scarborough, UK.

McQueen, C.E., Boedeker, E.C., Le, M., Hamada, Y. and Brown, W.R. (1992) Mucosal immune response to RDEC-1 infection: study of lamina propria antibody-producing cells and biliary antibody. *Infection and Immunity* 60, 206–212.

Meier, C., Amtsberg, G. and Wittenbrink, M.M. (1983) Occurrence of bacterial pathogens in urine samples of dogs. *Effem Forschung fur Kleintierernahrung Report* No. 16, 7–13.

Milon, A. and Camguilhem, R. (1989) Essais de protection de lapereaux sevrés contre l'entérite à *Escherichia coli* O103: vaccinations des mères avec un vaccin inactivé. *Revue de Médecine Vétérinaire* 140, 389–395.

Milon, A., Esslinger, J. and Camguilhem, R. (1990a) Adhesion of *Escherichia coli*-strains isolated from diarrheic weaned rabbits to intestinal villi and HeLa cells. *Infection and Immunity* 58, 2690–2695.

Milon, A., Camguilhem, R. and Esslinger, J. (1990b) Vaccination du lapereau sevré contre la colibacillose O103: rôles du LPS et de l'adhésine. *Revue de Médecine Vétérinaire* 141, 969–975.

Morisse, J.P., Boilletot, E. and Maurice, R. (1985) Alimentation et modifications du milieu intestinal chez le lapin (AGV, NH3, pH, flore). *Recueuil de Médecine Vétérinaire* 161, 443–449.

Nagy, B., Nagy, G.Y., Pazlfi, V. and Bozso, M. (1983) Occurrence of cryptosporidia, rotavirus, coronavirus-like particles and $K99^+$ *Escherichia coli* in goat kids and lambs. In: *3rd International Symposium of the World Association of Veterinary Laboratory Diagnosticians*. Ames, Iowa, pp. 525–531.

O'Hanley, P.D. and Cantey, J.R. (1981) Immune response of the ileum to invasive *Escherichia coli* diarrheal disease in rabbits. *Infection and Immunity* 31, 316–322.

Okerman, L., Lintermans, P., Coussement, W. and Devriese, L.A. (1982) *Escherichia coli* ne produisent pas d'entérotoxine comme agent d'entérite chez le lapin avant le sevrage. *Recueuil de Médecine Vétérinaire* 158, 467–472.

Peeters, J.E. and Maertens, L. (1988) L'alimentation et les entérites post-sevrage. *Cuniculture* 15, 224–229.

Peeters, J.E., Charlier, G.J. and Halen, P.H. (1984a) Pathogenicity of attaching effacing enteropathogenic *Escherichia coli* isolated from diarrhoeic suckling and weanling rabbits for newborn rabbits. *Infection and Immunity* 46, 690–696.

Peeters, J.E., Geeroms, R. and Glorieux, B. (1984b) Experimental *Escherichia coli* enteropathy in weanling rabbits: clinical manifestations and pathological findings. *Journal of Comparative Pathology* 94, 521–528.

Peeters, J.E., Geeroms, R. Vroonen, C. and Pohl, P. (1988a) A selective citrate-sorbose medium for screening certain enteropathogenic attaching and effacing *Escherichia coli* in weaned rabbits. *Vlaams Diergeneeskundig Tijdschrift* 57, 264–270.

Peeters, J.E., Geeroms, R. and Ørskov, F. (1988b) Biotype, serotype and pathogenicity of attaching and effacing enteropathogenic *Escherichia coli* strains isolated from diarrheic commercial rabbits. *Infection and Immunity* 56, 1442–1448.

Peeters, J.E., Orsenigo, R., Maertens, L., Gallazzi, D. and Colin, M. (1993) Influence of two iso-energetic diets (starch vs fat) on experimental colibacillosis (EPEC) and iota-enterotoxaemia in early weaned rabbits. *World Rabbit Science* 1, 53–66.

Pohl, P., Mainil, J., Devriese, L.A., Haesebroek, F., Broes, A., Lintermans, P. and Oswald, E. (1992) *Escherichia coli* productrices de la toxine cytotoxique nécrosante de type 1 (CNF1) isolées à partir de processus pathologiques chez des chats et des chiens. *Annales de Médecine Vétérinaire* 137, 21–25.

Pohl, P.H., Peeters, J.E., Jacquemin, E.R., Lintermans, P.F. and Mainil, J.G. (1993) Identification of *eae*-sequences in rabbit enteropathogenic *Escherichia coli* (EPEC). *Infection and Immunity* 61, 2203–2206.

Pospischil, A., Mainil, J.G., Baljer, G. and Moon, H.W. (1987) Attaching and effacing bacteria in the intestines of calves and cats with diarrhea. *Veterinary Pathology* 24, 330–334.

Prada, J., Baljer, G., De Rycke, J., Steinrück, H., Zimmermann, S., Stephan, R. and Beutin, L. (1991) Characteristics of α-hemolytic strains of *Escherichia coli* isolated from dogs with gastroenteritis. *Veterinary Microbiology* 29, 59–73.

Prohaszka, L. (1980) Antibacterial effect of volatile fatty acids in enteric *E. coli* infections of rabbits. *Zentralblatt für Veterinärmedizin, Reihe B* 27, 631–639.

Reynaud, A. and Federighi, M. (1991) Study of virulence factors of *Escherichia coli* responsible for enteritis in rabbits. *Revue de Médecine Vétérinaire* 142, 817–821.

Roos, M. (1990) Comparison of potential virulence factors and sensitivity to antibiotics among *Escherichia coli* isolates from the urinary tract and rectum of dogs. Inaugural-Dissertation, Fachbereich Veterinarmedizin, Justus Liebig Universität, Giessen, Germany.

Sager, M. and Remmers, C. (1990) Contribution on perinatal mortality in the dog. Clinical, bacteriological and pathological investigations. *Tierarztliche Praxis* 18, 415–419.

Schwarz, J. (1991) Participation of *Escherichia coli* in diseases of the urogenital tract in dogs. 1. Information: Isolation of bacteria in cultures. *Kleintierpraxis* 36, 179–184.

Senior, D.F. (1985) Bacterial urinary tract infections: invasion, host defenses, and new approaches to prevention. *Compendium on Continuing Education for the Practicing Veterinarian* 7, 334–341, 344.

Sojka, W.J. (1965) Escherichia coli *in Domestic Animals and Poultry*. Commonwealth Agricultural Bureaux, Farnham Royal, UK, pp. 170–177.

Tzipori, S., Withers, M. and Hayes, J. (1984) Attachment of *E. coli*-bearing K88 antigen to equine brush-border membranes. *Veterinary Microbiology* 9, 561–570.

Van der Stock, J., de Schepper, J. and Devriese, L.A. (1981) Bacteriuria in the dog: a report of sixty cases. *Vlaams Diergeneeskundig Tijdschrift* 50, 109–117.

Wasteson Y., Olsvik, Ø., Skancke, E., Bopp, C.A. and Fossum, K. (1988) Heat-stable-enterotoxin-producing *Escherichia coli* strains isolated from dogs. *Journal of Clinical Microbiology* 26, 2564–2566.

Westerlund, B., Pere, A., Korhonen, T.K., Järvinen, A.K., Siitonen, A. and Williams, P.H. (1987) Characterization of *Escherichia coli* strains associated with canine urinary tract infections. *Research in Veterinary Science* 42, 404–406.

Wilson, R.A., Keefe, T.J., Davis, M.A., Browning, M.T. and Ondrusek, K. (1988) Strains of *Escherichia coli* associated with urogenital disease in dogs and cats. *American Journal of Veterinary Research* 49, 743–746.

Zschock, M., Hamann, H.P. and Weiss, R. (1988) Urinary tract diseases in the dog: bacteriological findings and antibiotic susceptibility *in vitro* of the most prevalent pathogens. *Kleintierpraxis* 33, 11–16.

Escherichia coli Diseases in Humans

13

J.P. NATARO AND M.M. LEVINE
Center for Vaccine Development, School of Medicine, University of Maryland at Baltimore, 10 South Pine Street, Baltimore, Maryland 21201, USA

Escherichia coli is the predominant facultative anaerobic constituent of normal colonic flora and usually successfully colonizes the newborn infant within hours of birth. Thereafter, for the remainder of a human's life, *E. coli* serves important intestinal physiological functions (Drasar and Hill, 1974). *E. coli* usually remains confined within the intestinal lumen as a harmless saprophyte, but, in the debilitated or immunosuppressed host or in the immunologically normal host with disruption of critical anatomical barriers, normal intestinal strains of *E. coli* are major causes of invasive opportunistic infections.

There also exists a subset of *E. coli* that possesses an array of specific virulence properties which allow them to overcome intact host defence mechanisms. Three distinct clinical entities result from infection with such inherently pathogenic strains of *E. coli*:

1. Urinary tract infections (UTI).
2. Diarrhoeal disease.
3. Neonatal sepsis/meningitis.

This chapter will focus on these three clinical entities and the bacteria which cause them.

E. coli in Urinary Tract Infection

Urinary tract infections (UTI) are important infections in all age groups. UTIs comprise a spectrum of clinical severity that includes asymptomatic and covert bacteriuria, cystitis and pyelonephritis (Kunin, 1970; Savage *et al.*, 1973). When infection is confined to the urinary bladder (cystitis), the patient is usually afebrile; lower abdominal discomfort, frequency and urgency of micturition, and dysuria are the principal symptoms (Stamm *et al.*, 1989). No defect in renal concentrating ability is present. Patients with acute pyelonephritis often have high fever, flank pain and tenderness, and constitutional symptoms. Patients with pyelonephritis typically exhibit a defect in renal concentrating ability.

Beyond the immediate discomfort and loss of productivity consequent to UTI, a major concern is that certain infected individuals can develop renal scarring, and rarely end stage renal failure, as a consequence of UTI. Children in the toddler and preschool age group (1–5 years of age) are probably at greatest risk of developing renal scarring since significant vesicoureteral reflux is not uncommonly seen in this age-group and such reflux appears to be a prerequisite for development of renal scars (Smellie and Normand, 1975; Berg and Johansson, 1983).

If urological anatomical abnormalities or stones are present, many Gram-negative bacteria in addition to *E. coli* commonly cause infection (Stamey, 1981). However, in the presence of an anatomically normal, unobstructed urinary tract, *E. coli* accounts for approximately 90% of UTIs (Winberg *et al.*, 1974; Gaymans *et al.*, 1976; Winterborn, 1977; Stamey, 1981).

Pathogenesis

Establishment of an *E. coli* urinary tract infection represents the culmination of a complex interaction between the bacterium and host defences (see reviews by Schoolnik, 1989; Stamm *et al.*, 1989; Johnson, 1991). All of the human urinary tract, except the distal urethra, is normally kept sterile by the unidirectional flushing action of urine. Any interference with this flow will increase the likelihood of UTI.

Only in the first 3 months of life are UTIs more common in males (Winberg *et al.*, 1974; Ginsburg and McCracken, 1982); thereafter, females are much more frequently affected. This notable sex ratio has been in part explained by the protective effect of the longer urethra in the male and the antibacterial properties of prostatic secretions. In the female, small amounts of urine can be extruded into the urethra with any increase in intra-abdominal pressure (e.g. coughing), thereby coming in contact with bacteria colonizing the urethra. Following return of intra-abdominal pressure to normal, the contaminated urine re-enters the bladder. Physical manipulation of the female urethra can likewise lead to entrance of bacteria from the urethra into the bladder. In female volunteers, 'milking' of the anterior urethra caused small numbers of bacteria to be demonstrable in bladder urine obtained by suprapubic puncture in nine of 24 women (Bran *et al.*, 1972). This observation helps explain the apparent increased incidence of cystitis in sexually active women in comparison with age-matched sexually abstinent females (Kunin and McCormack, 1968; Gaymans *et al.*, 1976; Fowler and Stamey, 1977).

The specific bacterial flora present in the vagina may play a role in the steps leading to UTI. Women with recurrent UTI are much more likely than other women to harbour *E. coli* in their periurethral areas (Stamey, 1981). Periurethral colonization with *E. coli* was found to precede and persist during UTI in women with recurrent UTI who were followed in longitudinal studies (Bailey *et al.*, 1973; Stamey, 1981). The same observation has been made for young girls with UTI (Bollgren and Winberg, 1976).

Using *E. coli* from UTI as a test organism, a quantitatively increased adherence has been observed when the bacteria are incubated with uroepithelial cells from patients with recurrent UTI as compared with uroepithelial cells from normal individuals (Svanborg-Edén *et al.*, 1976, 1978, 1982; Svanborg-Edén and Jodal, 1979; Schaeffer *et al.*, 1981, 1982; Reid and Sobel, 1987). Svanborg-Edén and co-workers have also shown that there are differences in the adhesive capacity of *E. coli* isolated from cases of pyelonephritis, cystitis, asymptomatic UTI and strains from stool cultures of healthy individuals (Svanborg-Edén *et al.*, 1976, 1978, 1982). *E. coli* strains manifesting the most adhesiveness for uroepithelial cells came from patients with pyelonephritis, followed in order by patients with cystitis, asymptomatic bacteriuria and normal colonic flora.

Evidence is now overwhelming that certain *E. coli* possess virulence factors that increase their ability to cause clinically significant UTI (Schoolnik, 1989; Johnson, 1991; Fig. 13.1). *E. coli* that cause UTI can be subdivided into pyelonephritis-associated and cystitis-associated strains. Approximately 70% of *E. coli* strains isolated from patients with pyelonephritis and 55% from persons with cystitis fall within O serogroups 1, 2, 4, 6, 7, 16, 18 and 75. Among K antigens, K1, K2, K3, K5, K12 and K13 are particularly common (Glynn *et al.*, 1971; Kaijser *et al.*, 1977).

Adherence factors

The ability of a bacterium to cause UTI is greatly enhanced by the presence of surface structures which promote adherence to urinary tract mucosa, facilitating resistance to the flushing action of the urinary stream (Hagberg *et al.*, 1983). Most clinically relevant *E. coli* adherence is thought to be mediated by fimbriae (also known as pili), hair-like protein organelles present on the surface of the bacterium (Hagberg *et al.*, 1981, 1983; Schoolnik, 1989). At least 60% of *E. coli* strains from the urine of patients with pyelonephritis possess a distinct class of fimbriae that enable the bacteria to haemagglutinate human P-antigen expressing erythrocytes in the presence of mannose (i.e. mannose-resistant haemagglutination, MRHA) (Svanborg-Edén and Hanson, 1978; Källenius *et al.*, 1981a, b, c;

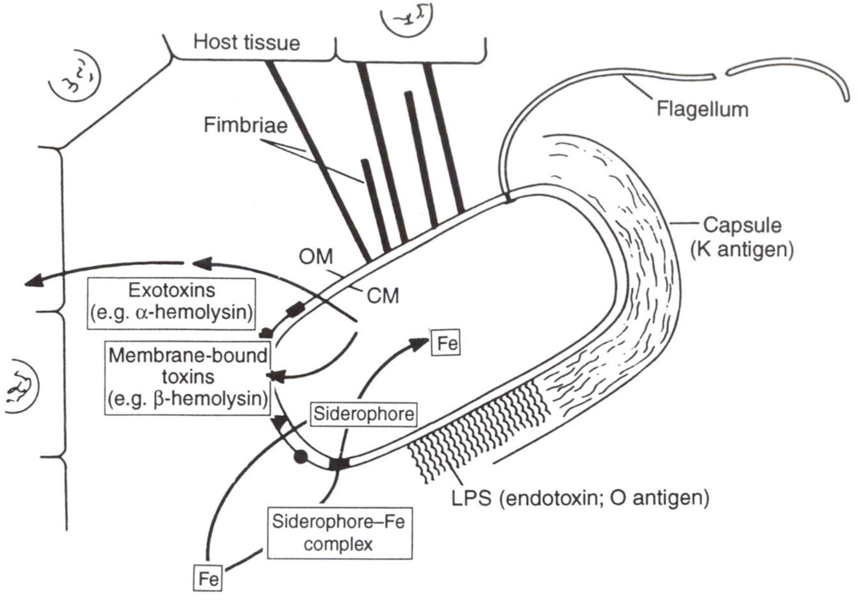

Fig. 13.1. Summary of putative virulence factors in uropathogenic *E. coli*. (Reproduced with permission from Johnson, 1991.)

Hagberg *et al.*, 1981; Korhonen *et al.*, 1982; Mäkelä and Korhonen, 1982; Svanborg-Edén *et al.*, 1982; Källenius *et al.*, 1983).

The erythrocyte antigen 'P', with which MRHA fimbriae interact, is a glycosphingolipid (or globoside) (Leffler and Svanborg-Edén, 1981; Källenius *et al.*, 1981a; Vaisanen *et al.*, 1981) which contains the specific disaccharide conformation α-D-Gal*p*-(1 → 4)-β-D-Gal*p* (Källenius *et al.*, 1981a). This globoside is contained in the structure of glycosphingolipids present on erythrocytes of all blood group P phenotypes except phenotype 'p'. Significantly, glycolipids containing the above disaccharide are also found on uroepithelial cells, the amount of glycolipid being related to the P blood group phenotype of the individual. Thus, the tendency of piliated pyelonephritogenic *E. coli* to adhere to uroepithelial cells is related to the individual's P blood group phenotype (Källenius *et al.*, 1981a, b). Adherence of P-fimbriated *E. coli* is significantly greater to uroepithelial cells of persons with P or P2 phenotype than to cells from p phenotype individuals. Moreover, the synthetic disaccharide α-D-Gal*p*-(1 → 4)-β-D-Gal*p* successfully blocks binding of pyelonephritogenic strains of *E. coli* to uroepithelial cells. The attachment of MRHA-fimbriated pyelonephritogenic *E. coli* to erythrocytes or uroepithelial cells can be increased by pretreating the cells with the purified carbohydrate portion of the glycosphingolipid receptor (Källenius *et al.*, 1981a, b).

Purified MRHA fimbriae prepared from pyelonephritogenic strains of *E. coli* adhere to uroepithelial cells and specific antiserum prepared against the pili can prevent attachment to uroepithelial cells of *E. coli* bearing the homologous pili (Korhonen *et al.*, 1981).

The physical structure and genetics of P fimbriae have been studied in great detail (Normark *et al.*, 1983; de Graaf and Mooi, 1986; Hacker, 1990) and are discussed in Chapter 16. Several lines of evidence suggest a role for P fimbriae in the pathogenesis of UTI (Lomberg *et al.*, 1983; Domingue *et al.*, 1985; Elo *et al.*, 1985; O'Hanley *et al.*, 1985a, b; Dowling *et al.*, 1987). The proportion of strains expressing P fimbriae declines progressively from as high as 70% among isolates from patients with pyelonephritis, to 36% among cystitis patients, 24% among asymptomatic bacteriuria patients and 19% among normal flora faecal strains (Johnson *et al.*, 1988; Johnson, 1991).

In addition to MRHA fimbriae, most UTI strains of *E. coli* also possess type 1 fimbriae, which mediate mannose-sensitive haemagglutination, (MSHA) (Eisenstein, 1988). Type 1 fimbriae are found in at least 70–80% of all *E. coli*, including normal stool isolates. It is believed that these fimbriae anchor *E. coli* to mucus in the large intestine (Ørskov *et al.*, 1980). These fimbriae also attach to urinary mucus and Tamm–Horsfall glycoprotein (Ørskov *et al.*, 1980). The ability of *E. coli* to attach to bladder mucus by means of type 1 somatic pili may be relevant to the pathogenesis of UTI and may in part account for localization of the infection (Hagberg *et al.*, 1983; Hultgren *et al.*, 1985). Indeed, adherence to urinary tract mucosa can be blocked with antitype 1 fimbrial monoclonal antibody, or with a mannose-containing receptor analogue; such interference inhibits the development of UTI (Abraham *et al.*, 1985; Aronson *et al.*, 1987).

Some *E. coli* isolated from UTI express MRHA but in the absence of P fimbriae; this phenomenon was originally referred to as X adherence (Hacker *et al.*, 1985). The majority of such strains express non-fimbrial, proteinaceous adhesins which bind to various portions of the Dr blood group antigen (Labigne-Roussel and Falkow, 1988; Nowicki *et al.*, 1988a, b, 1990). These factors may be difficult to visualize under electron microscopy but typically appear as coiled, fine fibrils lying close to the surface of the bacterium. The genes encoding these adhesins have been localized (Nowicki *et al.*, 1987; Hales *et al.*, 1988).

Dr family adhesins are most strongly epidemiologically associated with cystitis. Between 26% and 50% of cystitis isolates carry genes homologous with Dr family DNA probes, compared with 6–26% of pyelonephritis isolates, 6% of asymptomatic bacteriuria strains and 15–18% of faecal isolates (Israele *et al.*, 1987; Nowicki *et al.*, 1989; Johnson, 1991).

Some UTI isolates express other fimbrial adhesins, designated S, M and

G fimbriae. The role for any of these structures in the pathogenesis of UTI is as yet unclear. S fimbriae, known to be associated with neonatal sepsis and meningitis, have also been shown to confer adherence to renal cells (Korhonen *et al.*, 1986; Marre and Hacker, 1987).

Haemolysin

Most *E. coli* UTI isolates secrete a 110-kDa molecular weight protein toxin which lyses erythrocytes *in vitro* (Cavalieri *et al.*, 1984; Bhakdi *et al.*, 1988). The haemolysin molecule inserts itself into the lipid-containing membrane, forming a cytolethal pore (Bhakdi *et al.*, 1986; Menestrina *et al.*, 1987; Menestrina, 1988). In mouse and rat models of ascending and haematogenous UTI, haemolytic strains are more virulent, possibly by virtue of direct cytotoxicity as well as by the potential role of haemolysin in increasing availability of iron through haemolysis (Welch *et al.*, 1981; Waalwijk *et al.*, 1983; Smith and Huggins, 1985). Anti-haemolysin antibody titres are higher in patients with UTI than in asymptomatic control patients, and are highest in patients with severe infection (Seetharama *et al.*, 1988). Haemolysin production can be demonstrated in 49% of patients with pyelonephritis, 40% of those with cystitis, 20% of those with asymptomatic bacteriuria, and 12% of faecal isolates (Johnson, 1991).

Hacker *et al.* (1983) have shown that *E. coli* lacking the haemolysin are less virulent in rat models of UTI, while the virulence is restored when the cloned haemolysin gene is reintroduced, The precise role of the haemolysin in human infections, however, remains largely unknown.

Aerobactin

The level of free iron in host tissues is kept far below that needed by most bacteria for growth through the action of specific host iron binding proteins. Invasive bacterial pathogens, however, have evolved efficient mechanisms of scavenging free iron that is available and even competing with host proteins for bound iron. Bacterial molecules which effect this iron binding are called siderophores. Although *E. coli* produces several siderophores, the siderophore aerobactin is most closely associated with UTI (Bindereif and Neilands, 1985). Aerobactin is produced more frequently by pyelonephritis strains (73%) than faecal strains (41%) and environmental isolates (6%) (Johnson, 1991).

Other factors with potential relevance to UTI

Any pathogen which invades the urinary system encounters an array of host defences including the bactericidal action of serum and phagocytosis by polymorphonuclear cells. In mouse models, *E. coli* expressing the antiphagocytic K1 capsule are more virulent and more capable of causing UTI by the ascending route (Montgomerie, 1978). A greater proportion of human UTI isolates produce heavy capsules than do faecal *E. coli* isolates, and K1 isolates are disproportionately represented in pyelonephritis (Kaijser *et al.*, 1977).

Serum resistance in *E. coli* is mediated by a variety of factors (Bjorksten *et al.*, 1976), including capsular antigens (Cross *et al.*, 1984; Leying *et al.*, 1990), Col V (Aguero and Cabello, 1983) and TraT proteins (Aguero *et al.*, 1984). Serum-resistant strains are more virulent in animal models of UTI and are also more common among pyelonephritis strains and cystitis strains than among faecal isolates (Nicholson and Glynn, 1975; Bjorksten and Kaijser, 1978).

Epidemiology of UTI

UTIs occur throughout life, but occur with highest frequency in infancy, at the onset of sexual activity and again in old age. In the first 3 months of life UTI is more frequently found in males (Winberg *et al.*, 1974; Ginsburg and McCracken, 1982). After the neonatal period, UTIs are far more common in females (Roberts *et al.*, 1985). A peak of UTI occurs in females with the onset of sexual activity and in elderly males, in whom prostatic hypertrophy produces obstruction to urinary flow.

Asymptomatic bacteriuria is far more common than clinically apparent UTI. Screening studies in neonates suggest that as much as 1% of infants may have bacteriuria. Davies *et al.* (1974) studied the prevalence of bacteriuria in preschool children attending health clinics. Only one infection (asymptomatic) was recorded among 528 boys studied; the prevalence among girls was fourfold higher. The prevalence of asymptomatic or covert bacteriuria in school-age girls is 1–2% and is 0.03% in boys (Kunin, 1970; Savage *et al.*, 1973). It is estimated that 5–10% of girls develop covert bacteriuria during their school years. The annual incidence was computed by Kunin and McCormack (1968) to be 0.32 per 100 schoolgirls 5–12 years of age and by Savage *et al.* (1973) to be 0.9 per 100 girls 5–7 years of age.

The prevalence of significant bacteriuria in a population of healthy adult females over 14 years of age was 4.7% overall in a Dutch study (Gaymans *et al.*, 1976). The prevalence was lowest in 15–24 year olds and increased with age to peak in postmenopausal women. Many authorities believe that pregnancy is associated with an increased incidence of both asymptomatic and clinical UTI (Kunin, 1970).

UTI is found in a small proportion of infants and children who present with fever alone, although with a much higher frequency in girls than boys (Roberts *et al.*, 1985). Winberg *et al.* (1974) calculate that the risk of a child developing a clinical UTI prior to age 11 years is 2.8% for girls and

0.7% for boys. These workers also noted that the risk for recurrence of UTI was greater for girls than boys.

The critical question with respect to both symptomatic and asymptomatic UTI is whether irreversible damage occurs to the kidney, and if so, with what frequency (Smellie and Normand, 1975; Rapkin, 1977). Most studies now suggest that when renal damage occurs it is the result of renal scarring, which is almost exclusively associated with severe vesicoureteral reflux (Smellie and Normand, 1975; Rapkin, 1977; Winterborn, 1977). Renal scars seldom occur after the age of 5 years. Thus, it is infants and preschool children who are particularly at risk of reflux nephropathy. Reflux tends to disappear with increasing age, so only severe reflux in the preschool child carries a substantial risk (Berg and Johansson, 1983).

Vaccines Against UTI

Given the prevalence of UTI in all populations and the risk for renal damage, the development of vaccines against UTI (and specifically uropathogenic *E. coli*) is considered a priority (Kunin, 1986). Bacteria attacking the urinary tract encounter local secretory antibodies and, if they reach the renal parenchyma, systemic immune defences. In general, when infection is confined to the bladder, little or no antibody to *E. coli* O antigen is detected in serum and, when present, it is of the IgM class (Hanson *et al.*, 1977). With involvement of the upper urinary tract, serum IgG antibodies to the O antigen of the infecting *E. coli* are readily detectable (Hanson *et al.*, 1977). It has been suggested that the occurrence of serum IgG O antibody rises in pyelonephritis and is one measure of the greater tissue invasiveness of that form of UTI in contrast with cystitis (Hand and Smith, 1981). Local IgA and IgG antibodies to O antigen appear in the urine of patients with pyelonephritis (Hanson *et al.*, 1977).

The serum and local urinary antibody response to acidic polysaccharide K antigens is surprisingly meagre and frequently absent. Both serum and local urinary antibodies to MRHA pili appear following UTI (de Ree and van den Bosch, 1987). Studies by Rene and Silverblatt (1982) and Rene *et al.* (1982) showed that patients with pyelonephritis developed serum antibody to type 1 pili and that the levels of serum antibody to pili of the infecting strain were much lower in patients with cystitis; local antibodies in urine were not detectable.

Purified fimbrial vaccines

Fimbriae are potential immunogens because of their prominent surface localization and because antibodies directed against these adhesins may block interaction with urinary mucosa. However, attempts to use P fimbriae must take into account the considerable antigenic heterogeneity that exists among these structures (Clegg, 1982; Korhonen *et al.*, 1982).

O'Hanley (1990) and Roberts *et al.* (1984) assessed the ability of purified fimbriae injected parenterally to elicit protective responses in the urinary tract. Their data suggest that homologous protection could be demonstrated in the mouse model and that this protection correlated with the presence of urinary antifimbrial antibodies. Heterologous protection across P fimbrial types, however, has not been consistent. Lund *et al.* (1988) have proposed using the tip adhesin of P fimbriae as the vaccine antigen to minimize serological variation and maximize interference with epithelial colonization. Kaack *et al.* (1988) have investigated the possibility of immunizing mothers who may then transfer protective antibodies to their infants.

Patients with pyelonephritis appear to develop serum antibody responses to type 1 somatic pili (Rene and Silverblatt, 1982). This observation, coupled with the possible role of type 1 somatic pili in pathogenesis of UTI by attaching to urinary mucus, suggests that antibody to this antigen could be protective.

Capsular polysaccharide vaccines

Approximately 80–90% of the *E. coli* strains from cases of pyelonephritis fall within K types 1, 2, 3, 5, 12 and 13 (Kaijser *et al.*, 1977). Although antibodies to these polysaccharides are highly protective in experimental animal models (Kaijser and Ahlstedt, 1977; Kaijser *et al.*, 1978, 1983a, b), the antibody response to K antigens in the course of human UTI is often poor or absent (Hanson *et al.*, 1977; Hand and Smith, 1981). Similarly, inoculation of animals with purified K antigens often results in little or no antibody (Kaijser *et al.*, 1978; Schneerson *et al.*, 1982). Purified K13 polysaccharide, for example, failed to protect rats in the ascending pyelonephritis model (Kaijser *et al.*, 1978). However, multiple examples have now been reported wherein by coupling or associating a capsular polysaccharide with a protein carrier it is possible to elicit anticapsular antibodies. Scheerson *et al.* (1982) conjugated *E. coli.* K13 polysaccharide to bovine serum albumin. The conjugates stimulated serum IgG anti-K13 antibodies in rats and provided protection in the rat ascending pyelonephritis model.

E. coli in Enteric Disease

Characteristics of *E. coli* implicated in enteric diseases in humans are summarized in Table 13.1. Currently four distinct categories of diarrhoea-causing *E. coli* are clearly recognized as pathogens: enteropathogenic *E. coli* (EPEC), enterotoxigenic *E. coli* (ETEC), enteroinvasive *E. coli* (EIEC) and enterohaemorrhagic *E. coli* (EHEC) (Levine, 1987). In addition, two other categories (enteroaggregative and diffusely adherent *E. coli*) have been implicated in several epidemiological studies. Each category is distinct in its pathogenetic mechanisms, pathology, epidemiology and, generally, its characteristic O serogroups.

Enteropathogenic **E. coli**

Enteropathogenic *E. coli* (EPEC) cause a syndrome of watery diarrhoea, vomiting and fever in infants and young children. The spectrum of clinical illness ranges from self-limiting infant diarrhoea to a highly protracted syndrome of chronic enteritis accompanied by failure to thrive and wasting. EPEC occur within serogroups O55, O86, O111, O14, O119, O125, O126, O127, O128 and O142 (Levine, 1987; Donnenberg and Kaper, 1992). These *E. coli* adhere intimately to the intestinal epithelium and elicit a characteristic histopathological lesion in animal models (Polotsky *et al.*, 1977; Moon *et al.*, 1983) and in human patients (Ulshen and Rollo, 1980; Rothbaum *et al.*, 1982).

Pathogenesis of EPEC

In the 1940s and 1950s, investigators working in the UK, Europe and the USA incriminated *E. coli* of certain O:H serotypes as important causes of infant summer diarrhoea (Kauffman and du Pont, 1950). Neter (1959) coined the term enteropathogenic *E. coli* to refer to the serotypes of *E. coli* associated with infant diarrhoea between 1945 and 1953. Ewing and co-workers (1963) confirmed the findings of Neter and reported that strains within serogroups O26, O55, O86, O111, O125, O126, O127 and O128 were most commonly isolated from patients with diarrhoeal disease (O26 strains have subsequently been shown to belong to the enterohaemorrhagic category) (Levine, 1987).

In the late 1960s and early 1970s, however, two classes of *E. coli* capable of causing diarrhoea were described: ETEC and EIEC (DuPont *et al.*, 1971). In each instance a discrete virulence property was demonstrable, including epithelial cell invasiveness for EIEC and production of enterotoxins (LT or ST) for ETEC. Members of the EPEC serogroups were found to lack these properties (Sack *et al.*, 1975; Gross *et al.*, 1976; Gurwith *et al.*, 1977). Levine *et al.*. (1978) showed with volunteer studies that EPEC could cause diarrhoea by a mechanism distinct from those of ETEC and EIEC. The clinical syndrome included abdominal cramps, diarrhoea, nausea, vomiting and low-grade fever. One volunteer had copious diarrhoea, purged 5.6 litres of rice water stools, and required intravenous fluids to maintain hydration.

Table 13.1. Characteristics of *E. coli* implicated in enteric diseases in humans.

Category	Toxins	Invasion	Virulence plasmid	Adhesin	Clinical syndrome
Enterotoxigenic	LT, ST	–	Many	CFA/I, CFA/II, CFA/IV, others	Watery diarrhoea
Enteroinvasive	EIET[a]	+	140 MDa	Ipa's (?) dysentery	Watery diarrhoea
Enterohaemorrhagic	SLT-I, SLTT-II	– –	60 MDa	Intimin, fimbriae	Haemorrhagic colitis, HUS
Enteropathogenic	–	Limited	60 MDa	Bundle-forming pilus	Watery diarrhoea of infants
Enteroaggregative	EAST[a]	?	60 MDa[a]	AAF/I	Watery diarrhoea
Diffusely adherent	?	?	?	F1845[a]	Watery diarrhoea

[a] Role in pathogenesis unproven.

Early studies of pathogenesis demonstrated adherence of EPEC to the intestinal mucosa:

1. Polotsky *et al.* (1977) examined by light and electron microscopy the histopathological lesions evident when rabbit ligated intestinal loops were infected with classical EPEC strains.
2. Ulshen and Rollo (1980) described the histopathological lesion present in the intestinal biopsy from an infant with diarrhoea due to classic EPEC serotype O125ac:H21.
3. Rothbaum *et al.* (1982) described the histopathological lesions that existed in light and electron microscopic examination of infants infected with EPEC of serogroup O119 in the course of a protracted community outbreak.

Each of these three groups observed microcolonies of *E. coli* tightly adhering to villus tip cells. On electron microscopy a characteristic 'attaching and effacing' lesion was noted: EPEC were seen tightly adherent to epithelial cells with destruction of the brush border. Often the bacteria were found perched atop a pedestal formed from apical enterocyte membrane. Invasion of the mucosa is not a prominent feature of EPEC histopathological specimens, yet *in vitro* invasiveness has been shown (Donnenberg *et al.*, 1989).

Cravioto *et al.* (1979) reported that 80% of a large collection of EPEC strains adhered to HEp-2 cells in tissue culture in the presence of mannose (Fig. 13.2); normal flora *E. coli* and ETEC strains rarely showed adhesiveness for HEp-2 cells. Baldini and co-workers (1983) found that the HEp-2 adherence property of strain E2348/69, previously shown to be diarrhoeagenic in volunteers (Levine *et al.*, 1978), was encoded on a 60-MDa plasmid. Nataro *et al.* (1985b) showed that this was true of most EPEC and that HEp-2 adherence plasmids constituted a highly conserved family.

Colostrum-deprived piglets fed wild type EPEC developed pathognomonic EPEC histopathological lesions (Fig. 13.3), whereas piglets fed a plasmid-cured derivative did not. The role of the plasmid in the pathogenesis of EPEC was supported by volunteer studies in which 10^{10} E2348/69 or its plasmid-cured derivative were fed to a cohort of adult volunteers after gastric neutralization with bicarbonate (Levine *et al.*, 1985a). Ten individuals who received wild-type E2348/69 9 experienced clinical diarrhoea compared with only two of nine fed the plasmid-cured derivative ($P < 0.006$). The fact that two volunteers given the cured strain experienced diarrhoea demonstrated that chromosomal virulence factors were also present.

Baldini *et al.* (1983) and Nataro *et al.* (1987) localized the genes responsible for HEp-2 adherence in E2348/69 and identified a 1-kb DNA fragment which was shown to be a sensitive and specific gene probe for EPEC (Nataro *et al.*, 1985a). The factor responsible for HEp-2 adherence

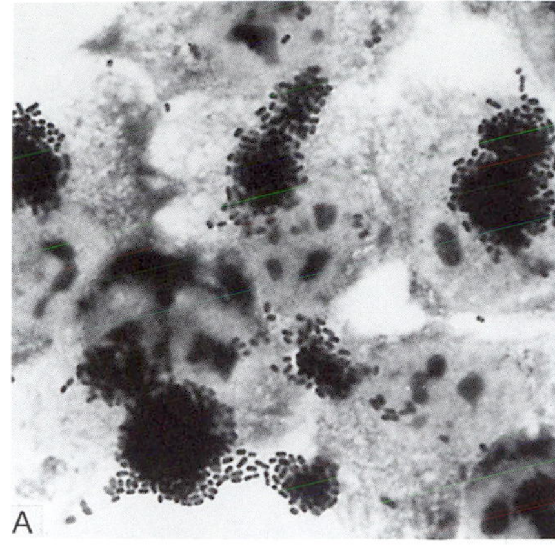

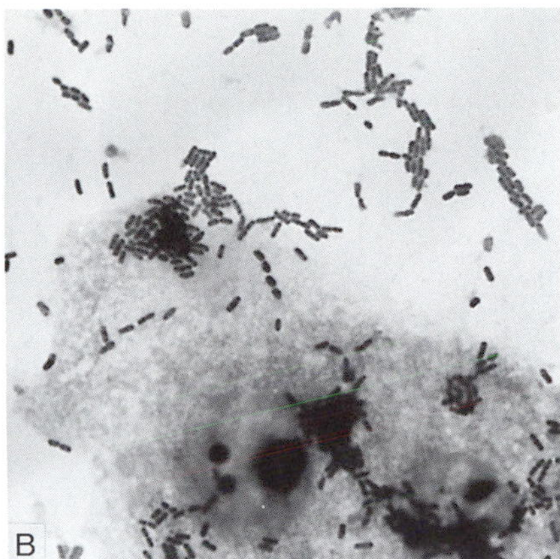

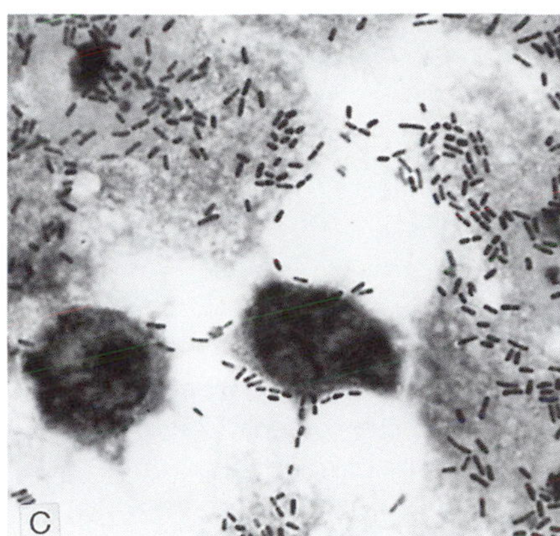

Fig. 13.2. HEp-2 adherence patterns. A fresh bacterial culture is incubated with a semiconfluent monolayer of HEp-2 cells for 3 hours, after which cells are fixed and stained. A, Localized adherence: bacteria form characteristic microcolonies on the surface of the HEp-2 cell. B, Aggregative adherence: bacteria adhere to each other away from cells as well as to the cell surface in a characteristic 'stacked brick' configuration. C, Diffuse adherence: bacteria are dispersed over the surface of the cell.

itself was later shown to be a bundle-forming pilus with homology to the family of type 4 fimbrial adhesins (Girón *et al.*, 1991a).

Jerse *et al.* (1990) conducted transposon Tn*phoA* mutagenesis of E2348/69 and identified a chromosomal locus required for the production of the attaching and effacing lesion. This gene, termed *eae* (and later *eaeA* when an adjacent gene was identified), was shown to encode a 94-kDa outer membrane protein, termed intimin (Jerse and Kaper, 1991). A deletion mutation in *eaeA* was constructed by Donnenberg and Kaper (1991) and fed to volunteers (Donnenberg *et al.*, 1992). In this study, ten out of ten volunteers fed the wild-type strain experienced diarrhoea compared to only four out of ten given the *eae* mutant strain.

More recently, several groups have elucidated other aspects of EPEC pathogenesis. Attachment and invasion of EPEC into eukaryotic cells is

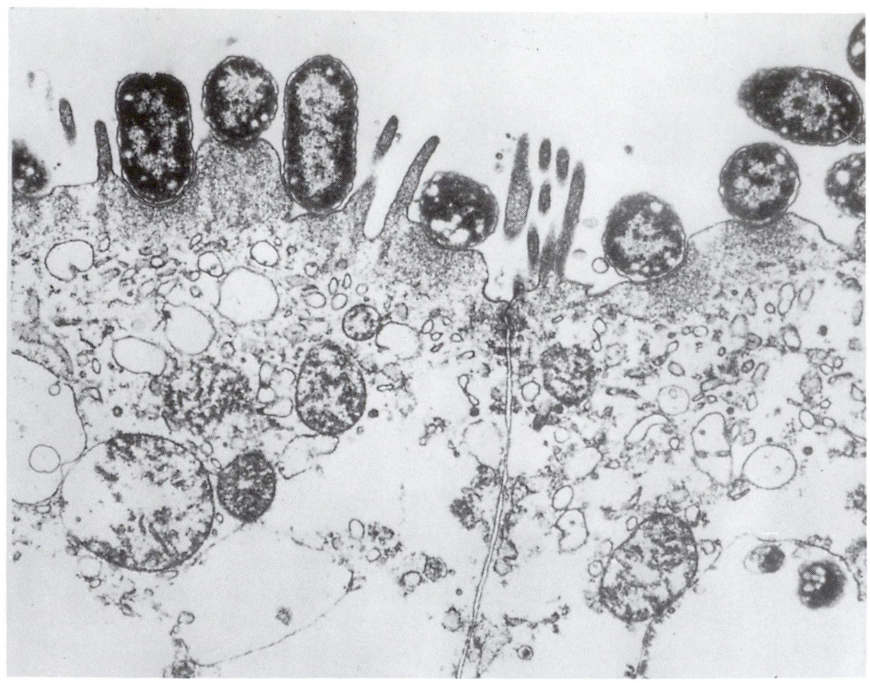

Fig. 13.3. Characteristic EPEC lesion obtained upon oral inoculation of gnotobiotic piglets. Note the intimate attachment of the bacteria to the enterocyte membrane with disruption of the apical cytoskeleton and other cytoplasmic contents. The appearance of a bacterium sitting on a 'pedestal' of cell membrane is quite characteristic. (Reproduced with permission from Baldini *et al.*, 1983.)

associated with rises in intracellular calcium concentrations (Baldwin *et al.*, 1991) and phosphorylation of cytoskeletal proteins (Finlay *et al.*, 1992), presumably leading to the destruction of the normal microvillar architecture. The precise mechanism by which these derangements lead to a net secretory state is still under investigation, yet it has been proposed by other investigators that alterations in enterocyte calcium levels can both decrease absorption and increase intestinal fluid secretion (Donowitz and Welsh, 1986).

Donnenberg and Kaper (1992) have proposed a three-step model of EPEC pathogenesis. The first step is initial mucosal encounter and colonization, mediated by the bundle-forming pilus. Following this initial colonization, the product of the *eaeA* locus, intimin, mediates an intimate attachment to the brush border; a second locus, *eaeB*, is also involved in forming the attaching and effacing lesion (Donnenberg *et al.*, 1993a). The third step involves disruption of the cytoskeleton and phosphorylation of cytoskeletal proteins (Chapter 20).

Epidemiology of EPEC

Three features characterize the epidemiology of EPEC infections (Levine and Edelman, 1984):

1. The occurrence of cases almost exclusively in the first 2 years of life.
2. The propensity to occur in epidemic form in infant nurseries in the developed world.
3. The high incidence of sporadic infant diarrhoea in the developing world.

Most of the early descriptions of EPEC were associated with outbreaks of neonatal diarrhoea in the UK and the USA. These outbreaks were often devastating, with high attack and fatality rates. The epidemiological features of these outbreaks are still not entirely clear, but the characteristics are highly suggestive of infant-to-infant transmission via the hands of nursing staff (Levine and Edelman, 1984). Since the 1950s, however, these outbreaks have become much less frequent, although they still occur (Robins-Browne *et al.*, 1980; Paulozzi *et al.*, 1986; Senerwa *et al.*, 1989).

It is not clear why natural EPEC infection is restricted to the first 2 years of life. Adult volunteer studies described above have shown severe diarrhoea with a very high attack rate. While it is true that these volunteers are naive with regard to EPEC and therefore are expected to be susceptible, the absence of EPEC as a cause of traveller's diarrhoea argues that the explanation involves more than just host experience.

At present, EPEC infection appears to be relatively uncommon in the USA. In contrast, in many developing countries, EPEC are among the most frequent causes of bacterial diarrhoea in infants (Levine and Edelman, 1984; Gomes *et al.*, 1989, 1991; Echeverria *et al.*, 1991a; Kain *et al.*, 1991). EPEC infections typically exhibit notable seasonality and are associated with warm season peaks (Levine and Edelman, 1984). This appears to be due to enhanced survival of EPEC as well as increased ability to proliferate to high inocula in contaminated weaning foods; transmission is most likely by contaminated food.

A number of reports stress the clinical severity of EPEC infections (Clausen and Christie, 1982; Rothbaum *et al.*, 1982). The studies of Gurwith and Williams (1977) and Gurwith *et al.* (1978) suggest that EPEC infections are clinically more severe than non-bacterial gastroenteritis or shigella infection. In addition, EPEC have sometimes been associated with persistent diarrhoeal cases (>14 days) in the developing world (Fagundes-Neto *et al.*, 1989).

Prior to the genetic studies of the 1980s, EPEC were defined strictly by serotype. The identification of the EAF plasmid and the use of the EAF DNA probe led to redefinition of the pathogen based on virulence determinants. Using the probe, Nataro *et al.* (1985a) showed that only EAF-positive members of recognized serogroups were associated with diarrhoea in Lima, Peru. Members of the classical serotypes may lack the EAF determinant; these appear to be epidemiologically less virulent (Echeverria *et al.*, 1991a). Members of serotypes not previously considered virulent may, however, possess EAF and cause diarrhoea with the classic attaching and effacing lesion (Pedroso *et al.*, 1993). Thus, a new definition emerges for the EPEC which considers the mechanisms of pathogenesis. Epidemiological and clinical detection of these organisms should thus be based on homology with EAF and EAE gene probes, with the characteristic pattern of localized adherence in the HEp-2 assay as a reasonable alternative.

Vaccines against EPEC

No vaccine against EPEC diarrhoea is currently available. It is not known whether clinical infections give rise to immunity or whether protection across serotypes exists. Serum and milk antibody to EPEC O antigens is common in nursing mothers.

In Germany (Linde and Koch, 1969) and Hungary (Kubinyi *et al.*, 1972, 1974; Rauss *et al.*, 1972), considerable work was carried out investigating oral vaccines to protect against EPEC. During the 1960s and 1970s, nosocomial infection was a serious problem for very young infants who were admitted to hospital. EPEC O111 and O55 were the predominant pathogens and the risk of nosocomial infection increased with the duration of hospital stay. To combat this problem, several oral vaccines were tested in infants for safety and immunogenicity, and two similar vaccines (Boivin extracts) were evaluated for efficacy in field trials (Kubinyi *et al.*, 1972, 1974; Rauss *et al.*, 1972; Mochmann *et al.*, 1974).

Two oral vaccines against EPEC that were shown to be safe in infants have undergone field trials:

1. A sodium deoxycholate Boivin extract vaccine prepared by Mochmann and co-workers (1974) from O111 and O55 EPEC strains.
2. A similar deoxycholate Boivin preparation produced from O111, O55 and O86 by Rauss and co-workers (1972).

Between 1969 and 1971 Rauss's Boivin extract vaccine was field-tested in Szeged, Hungary (Rauss *et al.*, 1972). The vaccine tablets each contained 0.5 mg of extract from O111, O55 and O86 *E. coli* (1.5 mg total); 0–12-month-old infants were randomized to receive three doses of vaccine or placebo orally over 6 days. For each subsequent week in the hospital the infants received a single weekly oral booster dose consisting of one tablet.

In total, 627 vaccinees and 1040 controls were compared for attack rates. Overall, 4.5% of vaccinees developed EPEC diarrhoea versus 7.6% in the control group, giving a vaccine efficacy of 41%. However, vaccine efficacy varied, depending on age, from 31% in neonates, to 55% in 1- to 2-month-old infants to 74% in infants 3 months or older. Unfortunately, the vaccine afforded the least protection in the age-group (neonates) in which nosocomial EPEC enteritis is most devastating.

The Boivin extract vaccine prepared by Mochmann and co-workers (1974) from O111 and O55 strains was field-tested in East Germany in 1970–1972. In this evaluation, infants were not randomly assigned to vaccine or control groups, so equivalency of risk and similarity of the groups cannot be assured. Nevertheless, EPEC O111 or O55 diarrhoeal infections occurred in only three of 6255 vaccinated children (0.48 cases/1000 infants) versus 15 cases in 12,870 unimmunized infants (1.14 cases/1000 infants). These vaccines are not in routine use at present anywhere in the world.

Now that specific adherence factors of EPEC have been characterized, future approaches to EPEC vaccine development include the presentation of BFP or intimin in a vaccine carrier strain or non-living carrier (such as a biodegradable microsphere).

Enterotoxigenic E. coli

ETEC are a major cause of diarrhoea in infants and young children in less-developed countries, in persons from industrialized countries who travel to less-developed areas, and in neonatal herd animals including piglets, lambs and calves (Levine, 1987). ETEC infection is characterized by watery diarrhoea, often accompanied by low-grade fever, abdominal cramps, malaise and vomiting. In its most severe clinical form ETEC infection can cause severe cholera-like purging of rice water stools leading to dehydration, even in adults.

Pathogenesis of ETEC

The basic pathogenetic paradigm for ETEC infection is thought to be colonization of the small bowel lumen with local production of secretogenic enterotoxins.

Toxins

ETEC are characterized by the ability to synthesize the heat-labile toxin (LT) and/or the heat-stable toxin (ST) (discussed in Chapter 14). Approximately 40% of ETEC strains isolated from cases of traveller's diarrhoea and from non-hospitalized infants in endemic areas are of the LT^+/ST^+ phenotype, another 40% have LT^-/ST^+ strains, and the remainder yield LT^+/ST^- organisms (Levine, 1987; Levine *et al.*, 1993). When village-based or outpatient studies are carried out in endemic areas, the most frequent isolates are LT^-/ST^+ (Black *et al.*, 1982a). In contrast, in hospitalized patients (presumably the most severe cases), LT^+/ST^+ strains predominate (Black *et al.*, 1981a, b).

LT is a high-molecular-weight protein that resembles cholera toxin (CT) in structure, function and mechanism of action. Both LT and CT are composed of one enzymatically active (ADP-ribosylating) A subunit joined to five receptor-binding B subunits. The receptors for LT B subunit found on enterocytes include GM_1 ganglioside and a second glycoprotein (Holmgren *et al.*, 1982). Following binding of LT to an enterocyte by its B subunits, the A subunit in some manner gains entrance to the cell. LT ADP-ribosylates the $G_{S\alpha}$ GTP-binding protein, leading to activation of adenylate cyclase in the enterocyte, and accumulation of cyclic AMP. The intracellular accumulation of cAMP elicits secretion by crypt cells and decreased absorption by villus tip cells.

LT from human ETEC (LT_h) is closely related to, but distinct from, LT found in porcine ETEC strains (LT_p) (Honda *et al.*, 1981; Geary *et al.*, 1982). Both LT_h and LT_p are immunologically related to CT (Clements and Finkelstein 1978).

The STs represent a group of enterotoxigenic molecules which are found in many enteric pathogens. Two distinct types are found in ETEC: STa and STb. The former has been strongly linked to diarrhoeal disease in humans and animals. The latter has been shown to be associated with diarrhoea in pigs.

STa is a small polypeptide whose mechanism is only partially understood. The toxin enters the cell after binding to a membrane receptor, suggested recently to be a glycoprotein (Hirayama *et al.*, 1992). STa activates the particulate intestinal guanylate cyclase activity leading to an intracellular accumulation of cyclic GMP and inducing a net secretory state in the enterocyte (Field *et al.*, 1978; Robins-Browne, 1980; Huott *et al.*, 1988; Visweswariah *et al.*, 1992).

Fimbriae

Uropathogenic *E. coli* benefit from the expression of adherence fimbriae in order to resist the flushing action of urine. Similarly, diarrhoeagenic *E. coli* also appear to have adapted adherence mechanisms to aid in colonization of the bowel (Klemm, 1985; de Graaf and Mooi, 1986). These structures are proteinaceous filaments but have been shown to exhibit several different morphologies (Fig. 13.4). One class appears rigid and tubular with a diameter of approximately 7 nm (e.g. CFA/I). A second distinct morphology is that of thinner, flexible, wiry structures, often called fibrillae or fimbrillae (e.g. CS3) (Levine *et al.*, 1984). More recently, structures which do not fall easily into either group have also been identified (Girón *et al.*, 1993). It is clear that all ETEC so far studied possess one, and usually more than one, of these surface structures.

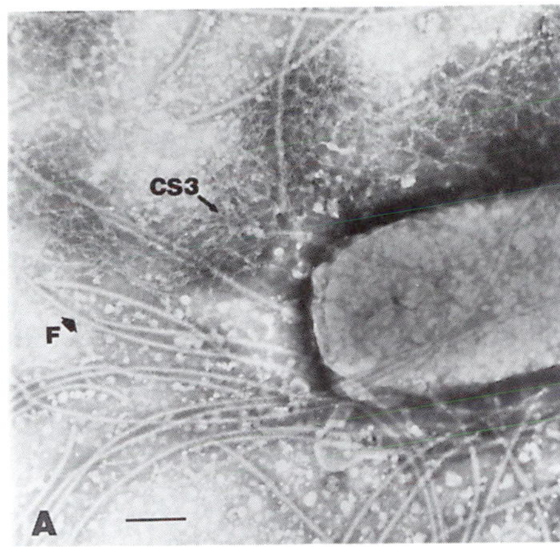

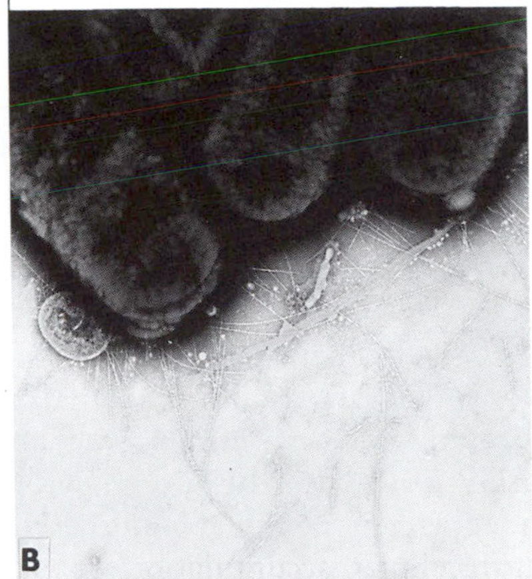

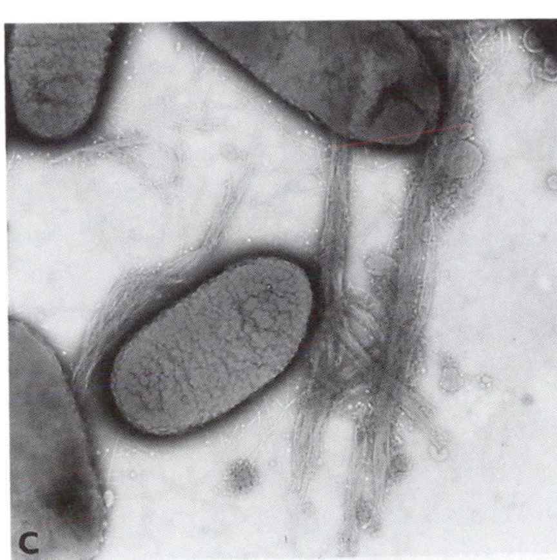

Fig. 13.4. Three morphologies of *E. coli* fimbriae seen by transmission electron microscopy. A, Flexible fibrillar morphology exemplified by the CS3 component of CFA/II. Note the typical narrow diameter, approximately 2–3 nm, and the mesh-like appearance. F = bacterial flagella. B, Rigid fimbrial morphology illustrated by ETEC fimbriae CFA/I. The diameter of individual fimbriae is approximately 7 nm. C, Bundle-forming morphology displayed by the EPEC bundle-forming fimbriae. Each bundle consists of many individual strands of about 2 nm. (Photomicrographs courtesy of Dr Jorge Girón.)

There exists a close correlation between presence of specific adhesion fimbriae and certain O serogroups. For example, CFA/I is found in O15, O25, O63, O78 and O128 strains, whereas CFA/II is seen in O6, O8, O80 and O85 strains, and CFA/IV (E8775) fimbriae are found in O25, O115 and O167 strains (Levine, 1987). CFA/I, CFA/II and CFA/IV fimbriae are virtually never encountered in non-enterotoxigenic normal flora strains. Fimbriae are discussed in detail in Chapter 16.

Epidemiology of ETEC

ETEC rarely cause infant or childhood diarrhoea in industrialized countries. The studies of Black *et al.* (1981b) in Bangladesh show that ETEC and rotavirus infection together are responsible for two-thirds of the cases of dehydrating infant diarrhoea in that country. This situation has been verified in many other developing countries (Donta *et al.*, 1977; Levine, 1987).

Prospective village-based studies of a cohort of children in Bangladesh (Black *et al.*, 1982a) showed that in the first 2 years of life each child suffers an average of six to seven separate episodes of diarrhoea per year. Approximately two episodes per child per year are due to ETEC. It was also shown that ETEC is the one enteropathogen that was significantly correlated with the development of clinical malnutrition.

ETEC infections in endemic areas are most common in warm seasons. Contaminated weaning foods are the primary mode of transmission (Black *et al.*, 1982b; Wood *et al.*, 1983). Bacteriological studies of traditional infant weaning foods have shown heavy contamination with faecal coliforms (Rowland *et al.*, 1978; Black *et al.*, 1982b); coliform counts increase with ambient temperature and with the hours of storage of the food.

In endemic areas incidence rates are highest in the first 2 years of life and diminish progressively thereafter until they are low in older children and adults (Levine *et al.*, 1979; Black *et al.*, 1981a; Levine, 1987). Serological and epidemiological evidence strongly supports the notion that acquired immunity is responsible for low incidence rates in adults. The prevalence of LT antitoxin and of anti-CFA antibodies is high in older children and adults, as are mean titres. In contrast, when adult travellers from industrialized countries visit ETEC-endemic less-developed areas, they are quite susceptible and attack rates for diarrhoea are high (NIH Consensus Conference Traveler's Diarrhea, 1985).

Traveller's diarrhoea may be defined as the acute diarrhoeal illness that occurs when persons from hygienic, industrialized countries travel to less-developed areas of the world. ETEC have been shown to cause 30–72% of the cases (NIH Consensus Conference Traveler's Diarrhea, 1985). Traveller's diarrhoea due to ETEC is typically transmitted via contaminated food and water vehicles. Person-to-person spread with ETEC is unusual (Levine *et al.*, 1980). Ingestion of antacids or hypochlorhydria predisposes to increased severity of disease.

Several additional sources of evidence argue that prior infection stimulates immunity. DuPont *et al.* (1976) noted that US students recently arrived to attend university in Mexico had high attack rates of ETEC diarrhoea, whereas US students resident in Mexico for at least 1 year and students from other Latin American countries had low attack rates. The most direct evidence, however, comes from volunteer studies of Levine *et al.* (1979, 1980). Volunteers who experienced clinical diarrhoea due to infection with ETEC strain H10407 (O78:H11, LT^+/ST^+) or B7A (O148:H28) were significantly protected when rechallenged 2 months later with the homologous organism.

Vaccines against ETEC

Enterotoxigenic *E. coli* comprise many different O:H serotypes, multiple antigenic types of fimbrial colonization factors and three different toxin phenotypes (LT only, ST only or both toxins). Any effective vaccine must therefore overcome the heterogeneity of ETEC surface structures. It is believed that broad-spectrum immunity in endemic areas derives from serial infections with strains bearing different antigens (Levine *et al.*, 1979). Protection appears to be mediated by secretory IgA (SIgA) antibody directed against fimbriae, other surface antigens and (LT). Heat-stable toxin (STa), a small peptide, does not elicit neutralizing antitoxin following natural infection. ETEC vaccine candidates include non-living antigen vaccines (toxoids, mixtures of inactivated whole bacteria and purified surface antigens) and several live oral vaccines.

Both serum and intestinal SIgA antibody responses to the homologous O antigen occur in approximately 90% of persons with clinical infections due to ETEC (Levine *et al.*, 1977, 1979, 1982; Evans *et al.*, 1978). The serum O antibody is predominantly in the IgM class and peaks 8–10 days after onset of infection.

Appearance of neutralizing or binding antitoxin to ST following ETEC infection in man has not been reported. In contrast, most persons who experience diarrhoea due to LT-producing strains of *E. coli* manifest significant rises in serum LT antitoxin (Evans *et al.*, 1978; Levine *et al.*, 1979, 1982). In experimental challenge studies in volunteers, rises in serum IgG antitoxin measured by enzyme-linked immunosorbent assay (ELISA) following ingestion of LT-producing *E. coli* were detected in 77% of ill persons (Levine *et al.*, 1985b). The serum antibody that appears following LT infection exhibits neutralizing activity. Rises in levels of SIgA antitoxin in intestinal fluid have also been described following experimental infection with LT-producing *E. coli* (Levine *et al.*, 1982, 1983).

Rises in serum IgG and intestinal SIgA antibody to CFA/I have been documented following infection with CFA/I-bearing strains (Evans *et al.*, 1978; Levine *et al.*, 1982). Levine *et al.* (1982) detected rises in serum IgG ELISA antibody to CFA/I in 67% of individuals infected with ETEC bearing CFA/I. In contrast, only one of 78 persons exhibited a rise in serum IgG ELISA antibody to type 1 somatic pili in the course of infection (Levine *et al.*, 1983).

TOXOIDS

The killed whole cell vibrio/CTB subunit combination oral cholera vaccine tested in Bangladesh conferred approximately 65% cross-protection against diarrhoea due to LT-producing *E. coli* in the 3 months following vaccination (Clemens *et al.*, 1988). This vaccine provided Finnish travellers with a comparable level of protection against traveller's diarrhoea due to

LT-producing *E. coli* (Peltola *et al.*, 1991). The protection is presumably due to the immunological cross-reactivity between LT and CT.

STa peptide can elicit binding and even neutralizing antitoxic antibody when conjugated to a carrier protein. Consequently, several groups have attempted to construct ST toxoids as either recombinant fusion proteins or as synthetic peptides. Klipstein *et al.* (1986) cross-linked synthetic ST to a synthetic immunodominant epitope of LT; when fed to a cohort of adult volunteers, this vaccine was well tolerated and elicited neutralizing intestinal SIgA anti-LT and anti-STa. Neither this nor any other ST toxoid has yet been tested for efficacy.

Purified colonization factor fimbriae as oral vaccines

Purified colonization factor fimbriae have been poorly immunogenic when fed orally because of the harmful effect of gastric juice on the fimbrial protein (Evans *et al.*, 1984). The possibility of delivering such antigens in biodegradable polymers has rekindled interest in this type of vaccine (Tacket *et al.*, 1993). These polymers may protect protein antigens, such as ETEC fimbriae, from gastric juice, thereby allowing successful oral immunization. Reid *et al.* (1993) have encapsulated CS1 and CS3 components of CFA/II into polylactide-polyglycolide microspheres. In volunteer studies, three doses of such a preparation conferred 30% protection against homologous challenge (Tacket *et al.*, 1993).

Inactivated fimbriated whole *E. coli* with or without toxoid

Inactivated ETEC bacteria, given alone or with toxoids, are also under investigation as oral vaccines (Evans *et al.*, 1988; Svennerholm *et al.*, 1989). Evans *et al.* (1988) protected volunteers from experimental challenge with a colicin-inactivated whole cell oral vaccine. Svennerholm *et al.* (1989) are currently testing an oral vaccine consisting of formalin-inactivated ETEC strains bearing different fimbrial colonization factor antigens, in combination with B subunit of CT. Another formalin-treated whole cell oral ETEC vaccine consisting of inactivated non-toxigenic *E. coli* bearing CFA/II fimbriae was only modestly immunogenic and did not protect volunteers from experimental challenge (Levine, 1990).

Passive protection

An orally administered preparation of milk immunoglobulin enriched for antibodies against ETEC has been shown to protect a cohort of adult volunteers (Tacket *et al.*, 1988). Pregnant cows were immunized by subcutaneous inoculation of LT, CT and inactivated ETEC whole cells. Milk was collected from the cows and concentrated, yielding a preparation containing 45% immunoglobulin. Ten volunteers received this preparation with buffer three times a day; control volunteers received a concentrate prepared without immunization. After 3 days, all volunteers were challenged with ETEC H10407 (CFA/I$^+$, ST$^+$, LT$^+$). Nine of ten control volunteers experienced diarrhoea compared with none of ten immunized volunteers ($P < 0.0001$).

Enteroinvasive E. coli

Enteroinvasive *E. coli* (EIEC) closely resemble *Shigella* in biochemical reactions, virulence properties, pathogenetic mechanisms and the clinical illness produced (DuPont *et al.*, 1971). Many EIEC are lactose negative and fall in O serogroups that crossreact with antisera directed against certain *Shigella* O antigens (Levine, 1987).

Pathogenesis of enteroinvasive E. coli

The ability to invade epithelial cells, including intestinal mucosa, is the pathognomonic feature of EIEC strains (DuPont *et al.*, 1971). This epithelial cell invasiveness can be assayed using the guinea-pig keratoconjunctivitis test: EIEC will cause purulent keratoconjunctivitis beginning 24 hours after inoculation into the conjunctival sac of a guinea-pig (DuPont *et al.*, 1971).

Shigella and EIEC harbour a 120- to 140-MDa plasmid that encodes genes required for epithelial cell invasiveness (Harris *et al.*, 1982; Sansonetti *et al.*, 1982; Hale *et al.*, 1983; Sansonetti, 1991). Loss of the plasmid results in loss of invasiveness and pathogenicity. Several regions of the *Shigella* plasmids have been characterized, including those encoding the invasion plasmid associated (Ipa) proteins. Ipa proteins are required for full invasiveness and are immunogenic (Hale, 1991). The roles of these and other plasmid-encoded genes are only partially understood.

Following invasion of epithelial cells of the distal ileum and colon, *Shigella* and EIEC lyse the phagosomal vacuole and multiply within the cytoplasm, causing cell destruction (Hale, 1991; Sansonetti, 1991). The bacteria move laterally via polymerization of cellular actin filaments (Bernardini *et al.*, 1989). The organisms then invade neighbouring enterocytes or pass into the lamina propria. All data thus far generated suggest that EIEC and *Shigella* use similar if not identical mechanisms.

Epidemiological and clinical observation of EIEC disease has suggested that a high proportion of EIEC infections result in watery diarrhoea, without the dysentery syndrome so characteristic of *Shigella* infection (Echeverria *et al.*, 1991b). For this reason, several investigators have searched for enterotoxins in EIEC. Fasano *et al.* (1990) have reported that when grown under iron-deprived conditions, EIEC secrete into the supernatant a 68–80 kDa moiety which elicits a secretory state in the Ussing chamber model.

Epidemiology of enteroinvasive E. coli

EIEC have been isolated from cases of diarrhoea in both industrialized and less-developed countries, although with low frequency. Most cases in industrialized countries relate to food-borne outbreaks (Marier *et al.*, 1973). This strongly suggests that contaminated food vehicles represent the major mode of transmission. Surveillance studies suggest that EIEC infections are more common in warm months (Levine *et al.*, 1993). Volunteer studies suggest that the typical inocula that occur in nature are probably 2 or 3 logs higher than those required for *Shigella* infection (DuPont *et al.*, 1971).

Enterohaemorrhagic E. coli

Enterohaemorrhagic *E. coli* (EHEC) have been associated with epidemic and endemic diarrhoea, haemorrhagic colitis and haemolytic uraemic syndrome (HUS). Recently, foodborne outbreaks in the USA have drawn attention to this organism as one of increasing importance.

Pathogenesis of EHEC

The pathogenesis of EHEC infection is poorly understood. Prototype EHEC strains, such as O157:H7 and O26:H11, elicit a characteristic intestinal lesion, most prominent in the large bowel. The lesion features haemorrhagic necrosis of the villus tips with little PMN infiltration.

Three potential virulence properties have been recognized in EHEC (Tzipori *et al.*, 1987; Yu and Kaper, 1992):

1. Shiga-like toxins 1 and 2 (SLTs), also known as verotoxins (VTs).
2. A 60-MDa plasmid involved in expression of unique fimbriae.
3. The *eae* gene product required for production of an attaching and effacing lesion (see EPEC).

A genetic construction with a specific deletion in the *eae* gene failed to elicit enteric disease in a gnotobiotic piglet model (Donnenberg *et al.*, 1993b). The role of the other two putative virulence factors is less clear.

Epidemiology of EHEC

The epidemiology of EHEC infection has undergone intense study in recent years. Several investigators have reported outbreaks in both paediatric and adult populations, often accompanied by lethal HUS (Carter *et al.*, 1987; Griffin and Tauxe, 1991). The frequency with which HUS accompanies EHEC colitis varies; in outbreak situations, the rate of HUS has been as high as 5–20% (Griffin and Tauxe, 1991). The factors which predispose the patient to developing this complication are not entirely known. Extremes of age, severity of initial presentation (fever, leucocytosis), previous gastrectomy and administration of antibiotics have been associated with the development of HUS (Lopez *et al.*, 1991).

EHEC have been reported to be endemic in parts of South America and Canada (Griffin and Tauxe, 1991). The increasing incidence of this infection in the USA was well demonstrated in Minnesota, where the incidence of HUS and EHEC rose dramatically during the 1980s (Martin *et al.*, 1990). The lethal nature of HUS as a complication of EHEC has brought wide public attention to outbreaks in the USA related to beef (Belongia *et al.*, 1991; Knight, 1993) and apple cider (Besser *et al.*, 1993). Knight (1993) estimates that *E. coli* O157:H7 is present in 1.0–2.5% of American meat and poultry samples, and less frequently in lamb and pork. Ground beef is considered to carry the highest risk. The occurrence of O157:H7 outbreaks has moved the US Food and Drug Administration to revise its recommendations for the cooking and handling of meat products.

Enteroaggregative E. coli

Cravioto's description of HEp-2 adherence was a major contribution to the understanding of *E. coli* infections (Cravioto *et al.*, 1979). Nataro *et al.* (1987) followed Cravioto's work by discerning three different phenotypes of *E. coli* adherence to HEp-2 cells (Fig. 13.2 above). Localized adherence (LA), in which the bacteria adhere to the HEp-2 cells in clusters, correlates with the EAF and is largely confined to classical EPEC O:H serotypes. In aggregative adherence (AA) bacteria adhere to the HEp-2 cells, to each other and to the glass coverslip. In diffuse adherence (DA), *E. coli* are dispersed over the surface of the HEp-2 cell.

The optimal method for performing the HEp-2 assay is a matter of some controversy. The method reported by Nataro *et al.* (1987), a single 3-hour incubation, differentiates LA, AA and DA. Others perform a 1-hour incubation, at which time the cells are washed and reincubated in fresh medium for 2 more hours, then washed again. This latter method, however, is unable to differentiate accurately LA, AA and DA (Vial *et al.*, 1990).

Organisms that exhibit AA, enteroaggregative *E. coli* (EAggEC), have been shown to cause diarrhoea in volunteer studies. Mathewson *et al.* (1986) fed *E. coli* JM221 to 16 volunteers: eight received a dose of 10^7 and eight received 10^{10} after neutralization with bicarbonate. Five of the volunteers fed the higher dose experienced enteric symptoms, including three with watery diarrhoea. At the time that JM221 was fed to volunteers, the strain was considered a diffusely adhering *E. coli*; Vial *et al.* (1988) later showed that this isolate was indeed enteroaggregative. Nataro *et al.* (1993) fed four different EAggEC isolates to groups of five volunteers each at doses of 10^{10}. Only one of the four strains, of serotype O44:H18, caused diarrhoea, eliciting liquid stools in four of five volunteers, two experiencing greater than one litre of diarrhoea each. These studies support the pathogenicity of EAggEC, but also suggest that not all strains are equally virulent.

Pathogenesis of EAggEC

The mechanisms by which EAggEC elicit enteric disease are not known. Studies in rabbit and rat ligated loops and in orally fed gnotobiotic piglets have revealed a similar pattern of histopathology in the small bowel (Fig. 13.5). Light microscopic examination of such sections reveals oedematous villi with infiltration of leucocytes and erythrocytes, often with necrosis of the villous tips and haemorrhage (Vial *et al.*, 1988; Tzipori, *et al.*, 1992). Eslava *et al.* (1993) have recently observed an outbreak of diarrhoea among infants in a Mexican village. The stools of all infants grew the same EAggEC strain, of serotype O147:H39. Ten infants died with severe diarrhoea; autopsy of these infants revealed a destructive lesion of

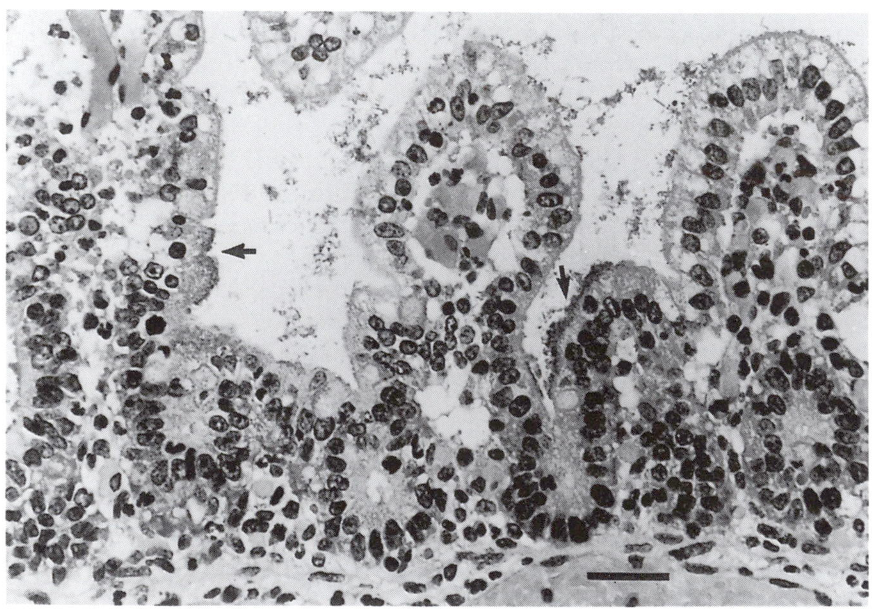

Fig. 13.5. EAggEC lesion shown by light microscopy of segment of ileum in gnotobiotic piglet fed enteroaggregative *E. coli* strain 17–2. Villi are oedematous and enterocytes themselves are swollen. The arrows point to aggregates of bacteria coating the villous surface. (Reproduced with permission from Tzipori *et al.*, 1992.)

the ileum strikingly similar to that observed in animal models. These data provide the first correlation between animal and human studies of EAggEC.

Nataro *et al.* (1992, 1993) have shown that the AA phenotype is plasmid associated, is genetically distinct from the bundle-forming pilus (BFP) of EPEC, and is apparently related to the presence of flexible, bundle-forming fimbriae termed Aggregative Adherence Fimbriae I (AAF/I).

Savarino *et al.* (1991) have identified an ST-like toxin in EAggEC isolates (called EAST1) whose gene is located on the large plasmid, closely linked to the gene cluster encoding AAF/I. The role of EAST1 in EAggEC diarrhoea is as yet undetermined. Baldwin *et al.* (1992) have reported a 120-kDa protein moiety in EAggEC supernatants with antigenic homology to the *E. coli* haemolysin. The protein elicited increases in intracellular calcium in cell cultures, an effect blocked when antibodies against the haemolysin were added to the system.

Vial *et al.* (1988) described plasmid-encoded lipopolysaccharide in at least one EAggEC strain and also identified surface fimbriae in several isolates. The surface lipopolysaccharide of some EAggEC strains is unusual in that the strains may be falsely found to be rough by standard tube agglutination. In fact, such isolates are resistant to rough-specific phages and yield a typical ladder configuration after lipopolysaccharide extraction.

Epidemiology of EAggEC

The epidemiology of EAggEC infections remains a subject of controversy. In several studies, EAggEC (defined by their characteristic HEp-2 adherence pattern) have been highly associated with persistent diarrhoea among infants and children in the developing world (Nataro *et al.*, 1987; Bhan *et al.*, 1989; Cravioto *et al.*, 1991; Wanke *et al.*, 1991). However, other studies have shown no such association (Girón *et al.*, 1991b). Some insight into a possible explanation for this phenomenon was provided by the volunteer studies of Nataro *et al.* (1993), which showed that not all EAggEC are equally virulent in volunteers; this pathogenetic heterogeneity may explain the lack of association of EAggEC in some areas. The molecular basis for the differences in virulence are not understood.

Diffuse-adherent **E. coli**

E. coli which exhibit the diffuse adherent (DA) pattern have been termed diffusely adherent *E. coli* (DAEC). The pathogenesis of DAEC is poorly understood. Bilge *et al.* (1989) have described a fimbrial structure (F1845) present in approximately 75% of DAEC strains; the role of this fimbria in pathogenesis is not yet proven.

Like EAggEC, association of DAEC with diarrhoea has been inconsistent. Recently, however, several studies have demonstrated that DAEC can be associated with diarrhoea in children outside of infancy (Girón *et al.*, 1991b; Levine *et al.*, 1993). Levine *et al.* (1993) followed a cohort of children 0–5 years in Santiago, Chile and showed that association of DAEC with diarrhoea increased with age. Children aged between 4 and 5 years had a relative risk of 2.1 for DAEC diarrhoea. This association with age may account for the lack of association in some previous studies, given that infants are the usual study population for diarrhoeal epidemiology.

E. coli in Sepsis and Meningitis

E. coli is a frequent cause of opportunistic sepsis in compromised hosts. Some strains, however, exhibit a high degree of virulence for systemic infection; such organisms are often isolated from cases of neonatal sepsis and meningitis. During the first month of life the incidence rate for meningitis is higher than at any other age. In a large perinatal study involving 54,535 live births, Overall (1970) reported that 24 cases of neonatal meningitis occurred, resulting in an incidence of 0.45 per 1000 live births.

Pathogenesis of neonatal meningitis

Less is known about the pathogenesis and specific virulence factors of systemic *E. coli* pathogens than about intestinal or urinary pathogens. Like most bacteria, it is thought that systemic *E. coli* follow a conserved strategy of infection:

1. Colonization of a mucosal site.
2. Evasion of host defences.
3. Multiplication.
4. Host damage.

The initial portal of entry in neonatal infections is most likely the gastrointestinal tract, where the bacteria invade or translocate through the intestinal epithelium. Upon entry into the circulation, systemic pathogens are much more likely than mucosal pathogens to encounter vigorous, highly effective host antibacterial responses and must, therefore, possess the ability to resist such host factors. In addition, some systemic *E. coli* may possess adherence factors (e.g. S fimbriae) which allow colonization and infection of the central nervous system. The full complement of virulence determinants is not yet characterized, but several putative factors have been described.

K1 capsule

From 40% to 80% of cases of neonatal meningitis are due to *E. coli* and approximately 80% of the strains possess K1 capsular antigen (McCracken *et al.*, 1974; Robbins *et al.*, 1974; Sarff *et al.*, 1975; Schiffer *et al.*, 1976; Glode *et al.*, 1977). The K1 antigen is an acidic polysaccharide, colominic acid (Silver and Vimr, 1990), which is a 2 → 8 α-linked homopolymer of *N*-acetylneuraminic (sialic) acid. *E. coli* K1 is identical in chemical structure to the group B acidic polysaccharide of *Neisseria meningitidis*, with which it shows complete immunological identity (Grados and Ewing, 1970). The virulence of K1-encapsulated *E. coli* is thought to be related to the ability of the K1 capsule to mask underlying structures of the bacterial cell surface; such 'masking' prevents development of specific antibody responses and the activation of the alternative complement system (Silver and Vimr, 1990). It has been proposed that the poor immunological recognition of K1-encapsulated bacteria may be due to the resemblance of this capsule to extracellular matrix proteins (Finne, 1982). Possession of K1 antigen alone is not sufficient to give a smooth *E. coli* the ability to become invasive and cause bacteraemia (Bjorksten *et al.*, 1976; Silver and Vimr, 1990).

At all ages, the colon of approximately 20–40% of individuals is colonized by *E. coli* strains bearing K1 polysaccharide as detected by rectal cultures (Sarff *et al.*, 1975; Schiffer *et al.*, 1976; Glode *et al.*, 1977). Full-term infants become colonized by transmission of *E. coli* K1 from their mothers (Sarff *et al.*, 1975). In approximately one in 2000–4000 neonates, the K1 *E. coli* invade the blood stream and are carried to the meninges. It is not entirely clear whether invasion occurs through nasopharyngeal (Sinai *et al.*, 1980) or intestinal mucosa, but the intestinal route appears more likely (Sarff *et al.*, 1975; Schiffer *et al.*, 1976; Glode *et al.*, 1977).

E. coli O1:K1 represents the most frequent O:K1 combination isolated from faecal cultures of healthy infants and pregnant women, accounting for 25–30% of the K1 strains present in the intestinal reservoir (Sarff *et al.*, 1975). In contrast, O1:K1 accounts for only 10% of *E. coli* K1 strains recovered from patients with neonatal meningitis. O18:K1 accounts for approximately 27% of strains isolated from neonatal meningitis but represents only 9–16% of isolates encountered in stool cultures. These observations demonstrate that additional virulence properties, including O antigen (or correlated with O antigen), work in tandem with the K1 polysaccharide to result in pathogenicity (Achtman *et al.*, 1982).

Silver and co-workers (1981) cloned the genes encoding production of K1 antigen. They transferred the genes to a non-pathogenic O75:K100 *E. coli* strain, the same O:K type that had been safely fed to a large number of volunteers. Thus an O75:K1 strain was created that lacked K100. When 10^7 organisms of this recombinant strain were fed to 5-day-old rats, bacteraemia did not occur (Silver and Vimr, 1990). In contrast an O18:K1 strain isolated from a neonate with meningitis and a naturally occurring O75:K1 pathogen isolated from a woman with pyelonephritis (*E. coli* strain LH) (Glode *et al.*, 1977) caused bacteraemia in 60% and 78%, respectively, of neonatal rats. All smooth *E. coli* strains colonized the intestine of rats equally well (Scannapieco *et al.*, 1982). These observations point out that K1 is indeed a critical antigen involved with ability to cause invasive disease, but other critical antigens and virulence properties must also exist. It is the net result of this array of virulence properties that results in invasiveness and the ability to cause bacteraemic infection.

Based on analogies with other polysaccharide-coated capsular bacteria such as *Haemophilus influenzae* type b (Sutton *et al.*, 1982), the K1 capsule may be critical in reducing the serum sensitivity of *E. coli*, particularly with respect to complement in the absence of antibody.

Fimbriae

Both intestinal and urinary isolates of *E. coli* express surface fimbriae which foster adherence to target sites of infection. Similarly, many systemic *E. coli* pathogens express structures termed S-fimbriae which have been shown to bind to sialyl galactoside units of cell surface glycoproteins (Ott *et al.*, 1986; Moch *et al.*, 1987). S-fimbriae are associated with increased adherence to vascular epithelium *in vitro* (Parkinnen *et al.*, 1989) and increased virulence in animal models (Hacker *et al.*, 1986). S-fimbriated *E. coli* isolates are found more frequently in cases of neonatal sepsis and meningitis in humans (Guerinia, 1983).

Other fimbriae may also be associated with systemic disease, although the roles for these other structures is less certain. Ngeleka *et al.* (1993) have suggested that F165[1] fimbriae may contribute to the ability of the bacterium to survive in the blood stream, although the mechanism by which this might occur is not known. Maslow *et al.* (1993) have shown that the majority of blood stream isolates of *E. coli* originating from the urinary tract, gastrointestinal tract or respiratory tract express either P, S or afimbrial adhesins.

Serum resistance

Bacterial resistance to the killing action of serum is measured by assessing bacterial regrowth after incubation in serum or growth capability in serial dilutions of serum. Technical differences can affect the results of serum resistance assays, and definitions in the literature vary. Nevertheless, it is clear that bacteria capable of systemic spread benefit from resistance to the non-specific killing action of human serum. Uropathogenic *E. coli* exhibit serum resistance more often than do normal flora *E. coli* (see above), but blood stream isolates exhibit even higher frequencies of serum resistance.

Among bacteraemic isolates, serum resistance is found most frequently among isolates causing the most severe infections leading to septic shock and death. This is particularly associated with K1 isolates (Guerinia *et al.*, 1983; Cross *et al.*, 1984, 1986).

Bacterial resistance to serum killing results from a combination of factors, including O and capsular polysaccharides and outer membrane proteins (Moll *et al.*, 1980). It appears that killing results from activation of the alternative complement pathway, leading to the formation of the membrane attack complex and access of lysozyme to the cell wall.

Epidemiology of sepsis and neonatal meningitis

Neonatal meningitis due to *E. coli* occurs in approximately one per 2000–3000 live births (Overall, 1970; Riley, 1972). Approximately 80% of the *E. coli* strains bear K1 antigen (Robbins *et al.*, 1974; Schiffer *et al.*, 1976; Glode *et al.*, 1977). Premature infants in a nursery with little contact with their mothers acquired *E. coli* K1 strains later than full-term infants, and acquisition appeared related to the nursery staff (Sarff *et al.*, 1975). *E. coli* K1 with identical O:H serotypes are typically found in maternal stool cultures and cerebrospinal fluid cultures of infants with *E. coli* meningitis.

The reason for the extreme susceptibility to *E. coli* meningitis in the neonatal period is not clear. Epidemiological clues suggest that this is due to host factors and not the consequences of age-related modes of transmission. Glode *et al.* (1977) measured IgG and IgM antibodies to K1 polysaccharide in sera of persons of various ages. IgG antibody was present in all age-groups, including newborns; the mean antibody level fell to its nadir at 6–12 months of age and rose progressively thereafter throughout childhood. IgM and anti-K1 antibodies were absent from the sera of newborns and young infants.

Vaccines against systemic E. coli *disease*

Because of the population at risk, the best approach to immunoprophylaxis of neonatal meningitis will entail vaccination of mothers during gestation in the hope of stimulating high levels of protective antibody that will readily cross the placenta and passively protect the neonate. With *H. influenzae* type B and group C meningococcus polysaccharides, IgG anticapsular antibody is highly protective; such antibody crosses the placenta and explains why these infections are rare in the first 2 months of life. It is not known whether IgG anti-K1 antibodies are also protective.

Since the group B meningococcal and K1 polysaccharides are chemically and immunologically identical, we can consider the acidic polysaccharide from either bacterial source as a potential immunizing agent against both pathogens. When purified group B meningococcal polysaccharide was given parenterally to adults, only one of 101 had a significant rise in anticapsular antibody (Wyle *et al.*, 1972). However, when a non-covalent complex of meningococcal group B polysaccharide and type 2 outer membrane protein was used as a combined immunizing agent, significant rises in bactericidal and anticapsular antibody were detected (Zollinger *et al.*, 1979). Two 120-μg doses of vaccine were administered subcutaneously 5 weeks apart to eight volunteers. All experienced mild local reactions, but no systemic untoward events were noted. Serum collected 2 weeks after the first dose of vaccine showed significant rises in anti-group B polysaccharide and anti-outer membrane protein antibodies in six of eight vaccinees. Unfortunately, the bactericidal activity of the postimmunization sera resided overwhelmingly in the IgM class; this would not be helpful if protection of infants depends on placental transfer of maternal antibody. Zollinger *et al.* (1982) extended these studies, comparing vaccines containing different ratios of polysaccharide to outer membrane protein. Combined vaccine containing a ratio of 1:1 or 1:3 (capsule:protein) was most effective in stimulating antibody.

Problems in developing anti-K1 vaccines are compounded by the fact that the polysialylated capsule shares immunological cross-reactivity with polysialylated proteins found in human tissues, including fetal brain (Finne *et al.*, 1983). Thus, poor immunogenicity may be a result of tolerance of the host to such polysialylated structures and stimulating an immune response may actually be harmful.

References

Abraham, S.N., Babu, J.P. Giampa, C.S., Hasty, D.L. Simpson, W.A. and Beachey, E.H. (1985) Protection against *E. coli*-induced urinary tract infections with hybridoma antibodies directed against type 1 fimbriae or complementary D mannose receptors. *Infection and Immunity* 48, 625–628.

Achtman, M., Mercer, A., Kusecek, B. and Pohl, A. (1982) Clonal patterns among K1 encapsulated *Escherichia coli*. In: Robbins, J., Hill, J.C. and Sadoff, J. (eds) *Bacterial Vaccines*. Thieme-Stratton, New York, pp. 233–241.

Aguero, M.E. and Cabello, F.C. (1983) Relative contribution of ColV and K1 antigen to the pathogenicity of *Escherichia coli. Infection and Immunity* 40, 359–368.

Aguero, M.E., Aron, L., DeLuca, A.G., Timmis, K.N. and Cabello, F.C. (1984) A plasmid-encoded outer membrane protein, TraT, enhances resistance of *E. coli* to phagocytosis. *Infection and Immunity* 46, 740–746.

Aronson, M., Medalia, O., Schori, L., Mirelman, D., Sharon, N. and Ofek, I. (1987) Prevention of colonization of the urinary tract of mice with *Escherichia coli* by blocking adherence with methyl-α-D-mannopyranoside. *Journal of Infectious Diseases* 139, 329–332.

Bailey, R.R., Gower, P.E., Roberts, A.P. and Stacey, G. (1973) Urinary tract infection in non-pregnant women. *Lancet* ii, 275–277.

Baldini, M.M., Kaper, J.B., Levine, M.M., Candy, D.C. and Moon, H.W. (1983) Plasmid-mediated adhesion in enteropathogenic *Escherichia coli. Journal of Pediatric Gastroenterology and Nutrition* 2, 8552–8558.

Baldwin, T.J., Ward, W., Aitken, A., Knutton, S. and Williams, P.H. (1991) Elevation of intracellular free calcium levels in HEp-2 cells infected with enteropathogenic *Escherichia coli. Infection and Immunity* 59, 1599–1604.

Baldwin, T.J., Knutton, S., Sellers, L., Manjarrez Hernandez, H.A., Aitken, A. and Williams, P.H. (1992) Enteroaggregative *Escherichia coli* strains secrete a heat-labile toxin antigenically related to *E. coli* hemolysin. *Infection and Immunity* 60, 2092–2095.

Belongia, E.A., MacDonald, K.L., Parham, G.L., White, K.E., Korlath, J.A., Lobato, M.N., Strand, S.M., Casale, K.A. and Osterholm, M.T. (1991) An outbreak of *Escherichia coli* O157:H7 colitis associated with consumption of precooked meat patties. *Journal of Infectious Diseases* 164, 338–343.

Berg, U.B. and Johansson, S.B. (1983) Age as a main determinant of renal functional damage in urinary tract infection. *Archives of Diseases in Childhood* 58, 963–969.

Bernardini, M.L., Mounier, J., d'Hauteville, H., Coquis-Rondon, M. and Sansonetti, P.J. (1989) Identification of *icsA*, a plasmid locus of *Shigella flexneri* that governs bacterial intra- and inter-cellular spread through interaction with F-actin. *Proceedings of the National Academy of Sciences of the United States of America* 86, 3867–3871.

Besser, R.E., Lett, S.M., Weber, J.T., Doyle, M.P., Barrett, T.J., Wells, J.G. and Griffin, P.M. (1993) An outbreak of diarrhoea and hemolytic uremic syndrome from *Escherichia coli* O157:H7 in fresh-pressed apple cider. *Journal of the American Medical Association* 269, 2217–2220.

Bhakdi, S., Mackman, N., Nicaud, J.M. and Holland, I.B. (1986) *Escherichia coli* hemolysin may damage target cell membranes by generating transmembrane pores. *Infection and Immunity* 52, 63–69.

Bhakdi, S., Mackman, N., Menestrina, G., Gray, L., Hugo, F., Seeger, W. and Holland, I.B. (1988) The hemolysin of *Escherichia coli. European Journal of Epidemiology* 4, 135–143.

Bhan, M.K., Raj, P., Levine, M.M., Kaper, J.B., Bhandari, N., Srivastava, R., Kumar, R. and Sazawal, S. (1989) Enteroaggregative *Escherichia coli* associated with persistent diarrhoea in a cohort of rural children in India. *Journal of Infectious Diseases* 159, 1061–1064.

Bilge, S.S., Clausen, C.R., Lau, W. and Moseley, S. (1989) Molecular characterization of a fimbrial adhesin, F1845, mediating diffuse adherence of diarrhoea-associated *Escherichia coli* to HEp-2 cells. *Journal of Bacteriology* 171, 4281–4289.

Bindereif, A. and Neilands, J.B. (1985) Aerobactin genes in clinical isolates of *Escherichia coli. Journal of Bacteriology* 161, 727–735.

Bjorksten, B. and Kaijser, B. (1978) Interaction of human serum and neutrophils with *Escherichia coli* strain: differences between strains isolated from urine of patients with pyelonephritis or asymptomatic bacteriuria. *Infection and Immunity* 22, 308–311.

Bjorksten, B., Bortolussi, R., Gothefors, L. and Quie P.G. (1976) Interaction of *E. coli* strains with human serum: lack of relationship to K1 antigen. *Journal of Pediatrics* 89, 892–897.

Black, R.E., Merson, M.H., Rowe, B., Taylor, P.R., Abdul Alim, A.R.M., Gross, R.J. and Sack, D.A. (1981a) Enterotoxigenic *Escherichia coli* diarrhoea: acquired immunity and transmission in an endemic area. *Bulletin of the World Health Organization* 59, 253–258.

Black, R.E., Merson, M.H., Huq, I., Abdul Alim, A.R.M. and Yunus, M. (1981b) Incidence and severity of rotavirus and *E. coli* diarrhoea in rural Bangladesh. Implications for vaccine development. *Lancet* i, 141–143.

Black, R.E., Brown, K.H., Becker, S., Abdul Alim, A.R.M.A. and Hug, I. (1982a) Longitudinal studies of infectious diseases and physical growth of children in rural Bangladesh. II. Incidence of diarrhoea and association with known pathogens. *American Journal of Epidemiology* 115, 315–324.

Black, R.E., Brown, K.H., Becker, S., Abdul Alim, A.R.M. and Merson, M.H. (1982b) Contamination of weaning foods and transmission of enterotoxigenic *Escherichia coli* diarrhoea in children in rural Bangladesh. *Transactions of the Royal Society of Tropical Medicine and Hygiene* 76, 259–264.

Bollgren, I. and Winberg, J. (1976) The periurethral aerobic flora in girls highly susceptible to urinary infection. *Acta Paediatrica Scandinavia* 65, 81–87.

Bran, J.L., Levison, M.E. and Kaye, D. (1972) Entrance of bacteria into the female urinary bladder. *New England Journal of Medicine* 286, 626–629.

Carter, A.O., Borczyk, A.A., Carlson, J.A.K., Harvey, B., Hockin, J.C., Karmali, M.A., Krishnan, C., Korn, D.A. and Lior, H. (1987) A severe outbreak of *Escherichia coli* O157 : H7-associated haemorrhagic colitis in a nursing home. *New England Journal of Medicine* 317, 1496–1500.

Cavalieri, S.J., Bohach, G.A. and Snyder, I.S. (1984) *Escherichia coli* α-hemolysin: characteristics and probable role in pathogenicity. *Microbiological Reviews* 48, 326–343.

Clausen, C.R. and Christie, D.L. (1982) Chronic diarrhoea in infants caused by adherent enteropathogenic *Escherichia coli. Journal of Pediatrics* 100, 358–361.

Clegg, S. (1982) Serologic heterogenicity among fimbrial antigens causing mannose resistant hemagglutination by uropathogenic *E. coli. Infection and Immunity* 35, 745–748.

Clemens, J.D., Harris, J., Sack, D., Chakraborty, J., Ahmed, F., Stanton, B., Khan, M.U., Kay, B.A., Huda, N., Khan, M.R., Yunus, M., Rao, M.R., Svennerholm, A.-M. and Holmgren, J. (1988) Field trial of oral cholera vaccines in Bangladesh: results of one year of follow-up. *Journal of Infectious Diseases* 158, 60–69.

Clements, J.D. and Finkelstein, R.A. (1978) Demonstration of shared and unique immunologic determinants in enterotoxins from *V. cholerae* and *E. coli. Infection and Immunity* 22, 709–713.

Cravioto, A., Gross, R.J., Scotland, S.M. and Rowe, B. (1979) An adhesive factor found in strains of *Escherichia coli* belonging to the traditional infantile enteropathogenic serotypes. *Current Microbiology* 3, 95–99.

Cravioto, A., Tello, A., Navarro, A., Ruiz, J., Villafan, H., Uribe, F. and Eslava,

C. (1991) Association of *Escherichia coli* HEp-2 adherence patterns with type and duration of diarrhoea. *Lancet* 337, 262–264.

Cross, A.S., Gemski, P., Sadoff, J.C., Ørskov, F. and Ørskov, I. (1984) The importance of the K1 capsule in invasive infections caused by *Escherichia coli*. *Journal of Infectious Diseases* 149, 184–193.

Cross, A.S., Kim, K.S., Wright, D.C., Sadoff, J.C. and Gemski, P. (1986) Role of lipopolysaccharide and capsule in the serum resistance of bacteremic strains of *Escherichia coli*. *Journal of Infectious Diseases* 154, 497–503.

Davies, J.M., Gibson, G.L., Littlewood, J.M. and Meadow, S.R. (1974) Prevalence of bacteriuria in infants and preschool children. *Lancet* ii, 7–10.

de Graaf, F.K. and Mooi, F.R. (1986) Fimbrial adhesins of *Escherichia coli*. *Advances in Microbial Physiology* 28, 66–143.

de Ree, J.M. and van den Bosch, J.F. (1987) Serological response to the P fimbriae of uropathogenic *Escherichia coli* in pyelonephritis. *Infection and Immunity* 55, 2204–2207.

Domingue, G.J., Roberts, J.A., Laucirica, R., Ratner, M.H., Bell, D.P., Suarez, G.M., Källenius, G. and Svenson, S. (1985) Pathogenic significance of P-fimbriated *Escherichia coli* in urinary tract infections. *Journal of Urology* 133, 983–989.

Donnenberg, M.S. and Kaper, J.B. (1991) Construction of an *eae* deletion mutant of enteropathogenic *Escherichia coli* by using a positive-selection suicide vector. *Infection and Immunity* 59, 4310–4317.

Donnenberg, M.S. and Kaper, J.B. (1992) Enteropathogenic *Escherichia coli*. *Infection and Immunity* 60, 3953–3961.

Donnenberg, M.S., Donohue-Rolfe, A. and Keusch, G.T. (1989) Epithelial cell invasion: an overlooked property of enteropathogenic *Escherichia coli* (EPEC) associated with the EPEC Adherence Factor. *Journal of Infectious Diseases* 160, 452–459.

Donnenberg, M.S., Tacket, C.O., Losonsky, G., Nataro, J.P., Kaper, J.B. and Levine, M.M. (1992) The role of the *eae* gene in experimental human enteropathogenic *Escherichia coli* (EPEC) infection. *Clinical Research* 40, 214A (abstract).

Donnenberg, M.S., Yu, J. and Kaper, J.B. (1993a) A second chromosomal gene necessary for intimate attachment of enteropathogenic *Escherichia coli* to epithelial cells. *Journal of Bacteriology* 175, 4670–4680.

Donnenberg, M.S., Tzipori, S., McKee, M.L., O'Brien, A.D., Alroy, J. and Kaper, J.B. (1993b) The role of the *eae* gene of enterohemorrhagic *Escherichia coli* in intimate attachment *in vitro* and in a porcine model. *Journal of Clinical Investigation* 92, 1412–1417.

Donowitz, M. and Welsh, M.J. (1986) Ca^{2+} and cyclic AMP in regulation of intestinal Na, K, and Cl transport. *Annual Review of Physiology* 48, 135–150.

Donta, S.T., Wallace, R.B. and Whipp, S.C. (1977) Enterotoxigenic *Escherichia coli* and diarrheal disease in Mexican children. *Journal of Infectious Diseases* 155, 482–485.

Dowling, K., Roberts, J.A. and Kaack, M.B. (1987) P-fimbriated *Escherichia coli* urinary tract infection: a clinical correlation. *Southern Medical Journal* 80, 1533–1536.

Drasar, B.S. and Hill, M.J. (1974) *Human Intestinal Flora*. Academic Press, London, pp. 36–43.

DuPont, H.L., Formal, S.B., Hornick, R.B., Snyder, M.J., Libonati, J.P., Sheahan, D.G., LaBrec, E.H. and Kalas, J.P. (1971) Pathogenesis of *Escherichia coli* diarrhoea. *New England Journal of Medicine* 285, 1–9.

DuPont, H.L., Olarte, J., Evans, D.G., Pickering, L.K., Galindo, E. and Evans, D.J. (1976) Comparative susceptibility of Latin American and US students to enteric pathogens. *New England Journal of Medicine* 295, 1520–1521.

Echeverria, P., Ørskov, F., Ørskov, I., Knutton, S., Scheutz, F., Brown, J.E. and Lexomboon, U. (1991a) Attaching and effacing enteropathogenic *Escherichia coli* as a cause of infantile diarrhoea in Bangkok. *Journal of Infectious Diseases* 164, 550–554.

Echeverria, P., Sethabutr, O. and Pitarangsi, C. (1991b) Microbiology and diagnosis of infections with *Shigella* and enteroinvasive *Escherichia coli. Reviews of Infectious Diseases* 13 (suppl. 4), S220–S225.

Eisenstein, B.I. (1988) Type 1 fimbriae of *Escherichia coli*: genetic regulation, morphogenesis, and role in pathogenesis. *Reviews of Infectious Diseases* 10, 341–344.

Elo, J., Tallgren, L.G., Vaisenen, V., Korhonen, T.K., Svenson, S.B. and Mäkelä, P.H. (1985) Association of P and other fimbriae with clinical pyelonephritis in children. *Scandinavian Journal of Urology and Nephrology* 19, 281–284.

Eslava, C., Villaseca, J., Morales, R., Navarro, A. and Cravioto, A. (1993) Identification of a protein with toxigenic activity produced by enteroaggregative *Escherichia coli. Abstracts of the 93rd General Meeting of the American Society for Microbiology*. American Society for Microbiology, Washington, DC, Abstr. B-105, p. 44.

Evans, D.G., Satterwhite, T.K., Evans, D.J., Jr and DuPont, H.L. (1978) Differences in serological responses and excretion patterns of volunteers challenged with enterotoxigenic *E. coli* with and without the colonization factor antigen. *Infection and Immunity* 19, 883–888.

Evans, D.G., Graham, D.Y., Evans, D.J., Jr and Opekun, A. (1984) Administration of purified colonization factor antigens (CFA/I, CFA/II) of enterotoxigenic *Escherichia coli* to volunteers. *Gastroenterology* 87, 934–940.

Evans, D.J., Jr, Evans, D.G., Opekun, A.R. and Graham, D.Y. (1988) Immunoprotective oral whole cell vaccine for enterotoxigenic *Escherichia coli* diarrhoea prepared by *in situ* destruction of chromosomal and plasmid DNA with colicin E2. *Federation of European Microbiological Societies Microbiology and Immunology* 47, 9–18.

Ewing, W.H., Davis, B.R. and Montague, T.S. (1963) *Studies on the occurrence of* Escherichia coli *Serotypes Associated with Diarrheal Disease*. US Department of Health, Education and Welfare, Washington, DC.

Fagundes-Neto, U., Ferreira, V., Patricio, F.R.S., Mostaco, V.L. and Trabulsi, L.R. (1989) Protracted diarrhea: the importance of enteropathogenic *Escherichia coli* (EPEC) strains and *Salmonella* in its genesis. *Journal of Pediatric Gastroenterology and Nutrition* 8, 207–211.

Fasano, A., Kay, B.A., Russell, R., Maneval, D.R. and Levine, M.M. (1990) Enterotoxin and cytotoxin production by enteroinvasive *Escherichia coli. Infection and Immunity* 58, 3717–3723.

Field, M., Graf, L.H., Laird, W.J. and Smith, P.L. (1978) Heat-stable enterotoxin of *Escherichia coli*: *in vitro* effects on guanylate cyclase activity, cyclic GMP concentration and ion transport in the small intestine. *Proceedings of the National Academy of Sciences of the United States of America* 75, 2800–2804.

Finlay, B.B., Rosenshine, I., Donnenberg, M.S. and Kaper, J.B. (1992) Cytoskeletal composition of attaching and effacing lesions associated with enteropathogenic *Escherichia coli* adherence to HeLa cells. *Infection and Immunity* 60, 2541–2543.

Finne, J. (1982) Occurrence of unique polysialyl carbohydrate units in glycoprotein of developing brain. *Journal of Biological Chemistry* 257, 11966–11970.

Finne, J., Leinonen, M. and Mäkelä, P.H. (1983) Antigenic similarities between brain components and bacteria causing meningitis. *Lancet* i, 355–357.

Fowler, J.E. and Stamey, T.A. (1977) Studies of introital colonization in women with recurrent urinary tract infections. VII. The role of bacterial adherence. *Journal of Urology* 117, 472–476.

Gaymans, R., Haverkorn, M.J., Valkenburg, H.A. and Goslings, W.R.O. (1976) A prospective study of urinary tract infections in a Dutch general practice. *Lancet* ii, 674–677.

Geary, S.J., Marchlewicz, B.A. and Finkelstein, R.A. (1982) Comparison of heat-labile enterotoxins from porcine and human strains of *E. coli*. *Infection and Immunity* 36, 215–220.

Ginsburg, C.M. and McCracken, G.H. (1982) Urinary tract infections in young infants. *Pediatrics* 69, 409–412.

Girón, J.A., Ho, A.S.Y. and Schoolnik, G.K. (1991a) An inducible bundle-forming pilus of enteropathogenic *Escherichia coli*. *Science* 254, 710–713.

Girón, J.A., Jones, T., Millan-Velasco, F., Castro-Munoz, E., Zarate, L., Fry, J., Frankel, G., Moseley, S.L., Baudry, B., Kaper, J.B., Schoolnik, G.K. and Riley, L.W. (1991b) Diffuse-adhering *Escherichia coli* (DAEC) as a putative cause of diarrhoea in Mayan children in Mexico. *Infection and Immunity* 163, 507–513.

Girón, J.A., Levine, M.M. and Kaper, J.B. (1993) Characterization of Longus, a novel pilus structure produced by enterotoxigenic *Escherichia coli*. *Abstracts of the 92nd Annual General Meeting of the American Society for Microbiology*. The American Society for Microbiology, Washington, DC, Abstr. B-260, p. 72.

Glode, M., Sutton, A., Moxon, E.R. and Robbins, J. (1977) Pathogenesis of neonatal *E. coli* meningitis: induction of bacteremia and meningitis in infant rats fed *E. coli* K1. *Infection and Immunity* 16, 75–80.

Glynn A., Brumfitt, W. and Howard, C.J. (1971) K antigens of *E. coli* and renal involvement in urinary tract infections. *Lancet* i, 514–516.

Gomes, T.A.T., Blake, P.A. and Trabulsi, L.R. (1989) Prevalence of *Escherichia coli* strains with localized, diffuse, and aggregative adherence to HeLa cells in infants with diarrhoea and matched controls. *Journal of Clinical Microbiology* 27, 266–269.

Gomes, T.A.T., Rassi, V., MacDonald, K.L., Ramos, S.R.T.S., Trabulsi, L.R., Vieira, M.A.M., Guth, B.E.C., Candeis, J.A.N., Ivey, C., Toledo, M.R.F. and Blake, P.A. (1991) Enteropathogens associated with acute diarrheal disease in urban infants in Sao Paulo, Brazil. *Journal of Infectious Diseases* 164, 331–337.

Grados, O. and Ewing, W.H. (1970) Antigenic relationship between *Escherichia coli* and *Neisseria meningitidis. Journal of Infectious Diseases* 122, 100–103.

Griffin, P.M. and Tauxe, R.V. (1991) The epidemiology of infections caused by *Escherichia coli* O157:H7, other enterohaemorrhagic *E. coli*, and the associated hemolytic uremic syndrome. *Epidemiological Reviews* 13, 60–98.

Gross, R.J., Scotland, S.M. and Rowe, B. (1976) Enterotoxin testing of *E. coli* causing epidemic infantile enteritis in the United Kingdom. *Lancet* i, 629.

Guerinia, N.G., Kessler, T.W., Guerinia, V.J., Neutra, M.R., Clegg, H.W., Langermann, S., Scannapieco, F.A. and Goldmann, D.A. (1983) The role of pili and capsule in the pathogenesis of neonatal infection with *Escherichia coli* K1. *Journal of Infectious Diseases* 148, 395–405.

Gurwith, M.J. and Williams, T.W. (1977) Gastroenteritis in children – a two-year review in Manitoba. I. Etiology. *Journal of Infectious Diseases* 136, 239–247.

Gurwith, M.J., Wiseman, D.A. and Chow, P. (1977) Clinical and laboratory assessment of the pathogenicity of serotyped EPEC. *Journal of Infectious Diseases* 135, 735–743.

Gurwith, M.J., Hinde, D., Gross, R. and Rowe, B. (1978) A prospective study of enteropathogenic *Escherichia coli* in endemic diarrheal disease. *Journal of Infectious Diseases* 137, 292–297.

Hacker, J. (1990) Genetic determinants coding for fimbriae and adhesins of extraintestinal *Escherichia coli. Current Topics in Microbiology and Immunology* 151, 1–27.

Hacker, J., Hughes, C., Hof, H. and Goebel, W. (1983) Cloned hemolysin genes from *Escherichia coli* that cause urinary tract infection determine different levels of toxicity in mice. *Infection and Immunity* 42, 57–63.

Hacker, J., Schmidt, G., Hughes, C., Knapp, S., Marget, M. and Goebel, W. (1985) Cloning and characterization of genes involved in production of mannose-resistant, neuraminidase-susceptible (X) fimbriae from a uropathogenic O6:K15:H31 *Escherichia coli* strain. *Infection and Immunity* 47, 434–440.

Hacker, J., Hof, H., Emody, L. and Goebal, W. (1986) Influence of cloned *Escherichia coli* hemolysin genes, S-fimbriae and serum resistance on pathogenicity in different animal models. *Microbial Pathogenicity* 1, 533–547.

Hagberg, L., Jodal, U., Korhonnen, T.K., Lidin-Janson, G., Lindberg, U. and Svanborg-Edén, C. (1981) Adhesion, hemagglutination and virulence of *E. coli* causing urinary tract infection. *Infection and Immunity* 31, 564–570.

Hagberg, L., Hull, R., Hull, S., Falkow, S., Freter, R. and Svanborg-Edén, C. (1983) Contribution of adhesins to bacterial persistence in the mouse urinary tract. *Infection and Immunity* 40, 265–272.

Hale, T.L. (1991) Genetic basis of virulence in *Shigella* species. *Microbiological Reviews* 55, 206–224.

Hale, T.L., Sansonetti, P.J., Schad, P.A., Austin, S. and Formal, S.B. (1983) Characterization of virulence plasmids and plasmid associated outer membrane proteins in *Shigella flexneri*, *Shigella sonnei*, and *Escherichia coli. Infection and Immunity* 40, 340–350.

Hales, B.A., Beverley-Clarke, H., High, N.J., Jann, K., Perry, R., Goldhar, J. and

Bounois, G.J. (1988) Molecular cloning and characterization of the genes for a non-fimbrial adhesin from *Escherichia coli. Microbial Pathogenesis* 5, 9–17.

Hand, W.L. and Smith, J.W. (1981) Immunology of enterobacterial infections. In: Nahmias A.J. and O'Reilly R.J. (eds) *Immunology of Human Infection, Part I.* Plenum Press, New York, pp. 221–248.

Hanson, L.Å., Ahlstedt, S., Fasth, A., Jodal, U., Kaijser, B., Larsson, P., Lindberg, U., Olling, S., Sohl-Åkerlund, A. and Svanborg-Eden, C. (1977) Antigens of *E. coli*, human immune response, and the pathogens of urinary tract infection. *Journal of Infectious Diseases* 136 (suppl.), S144–S149.

Harris, J.R., Wachsmuth, J.K., Davis, B.R. and Cohen, M.L. (1982) A high molecular weight plasmid correlates with *Escherichia coli* enteroinvasiveness. *Infection and Immunity* 37, 1295–1298.

Hirayama, T., Wada, A., Iwata, N., Takasaki, S., Shimonishi, Y. and Takeda, Y. (1992) Glycoprotein receptors for a heat-stable enterotoxin (STh) produced by enterotoxigenic *Escherichia coli. Infection and Immunity* 60, 4213–4220.

Holmgren, J., Fredman, P., Lindblad, M., Svennerholm, A.-M. and Svennerholm, L. (1982) Rabbit intestinal glycoprotein receptor for *Escherichia coli* heat-labile enterotoxin lacking affinity for cholera toxin. *Infection and Immunity* 38, 424–433.

Honda, T., Tsuji, T., Takeda, Y. and Miwatani, T. (1981) Immunologic non-identity of heat-labile enterotoxins from human and porcine enterotoxigenic *Escherichia coli. Infection and Immunity* 34, 337–340.

Hultgren, S.J., Porter, T.N., Schaeffer, A.J. and Duncan, J.L. (1985) Role of type 1 pili and effects of phase variation on lower urinary tract infections produced by *Escherichia coli. Infection and Immunity* 50, 370–377.

Huott, P.A., Liu, W., McRoberts, J.A., Giannella, R.A. and Dharmsathaphorn, K. (1988) Mechanism of action of *Escherichia coli* heat-stable enterotoxin in a human colonic cell line. *Journal of Clinical Investigation* 82, 514–523.

Israele, V., Darabi, A. and McCracken, G. (1987) The role of bacterial virulence factors and Tamm–Horsfall protein in the pathogenesis of *Escherichia coli* urinary tract infection in infants. *American Journal of Diseases of Children* 141, 1230–1234.

Jerse, A.E. and Kaper, J.B. (1991) The *eae* gene of enteropathogenic *Escherichia coli* encodes a 94 kDa membrane protein, the expression of which is influenced by the EAF plasmid. *Infection and Immunity* 59, 4302–4309.

Jerse, A.E., Yu, J., Tall, B.D. and Kaper, J.B. (1990) A genetic locus of enteropathogenic *Escherichia coli* necessary for the production of attaching and effacing lesions on tissue culture cells. *Proceedings of the National Academy of Sciences of the United States of America* 87, 739–743.

Johnson, J.R. (1991) Virulence factors in *Escherichia coli* urinary tract infection. *Clinical Microbiology Reviews* 4, 80–128.

Johnson, J.R., Moseley, S.M., Roberts, P.L. and Stamm, W.E. (1988) Aerobactin and other virulence genes among strains of *Escherichia coli* causing urosepsis: association with patient characteristics. *Infection and Immunity* 56, 405–412.

Kaack, M.B., Roberts, J.A., Baskin, G. and Patterson, G.M. (1988) Maternal immunization with P fimbriae for the prevention of neonatal pyelonephritis *Infection and Immunity* 56, 1–6.

Kaijser, B. and Ahlstedt, S. (1977) Protective capacity of antibodies against *E. coli* K antigens. *Infection and Immunity* 17, 286–389.

Kaijser, B., Hanson, L.Å., Jodal, U., Lidin-Janson, G. and Robbins, J.B. (1977) Frequency of *E. coli* K antigens in urinary tract infections in children. *Lancet* i, 663–664.

Kaijser, B., Larsson, P. and Olling, S. (1978) Protection against ascending *Escherichia coli* pyelonephritis in rats and significance of local immunity. *Infection and Immunity* 20, 78–81.

Kaijser, B., Larson, P., Nimmich, W. and Söderström, T. (1983a) Antibodies of *Escherichia coli* K and O antigens in protection against acute pyelonephritis. *Progress in Allergy* 33, 275–288.

Kaijser, B., Larsson, P., Olling, S. and Schneerson, R. (1983b) Protection against acute, ascending pyelonephritis caused by *Escherichia coli* in rats, using isolated capsular antigen conjugated to bovine serum albumin. *Infection and Immunity* 39, 142–146.

Kain, K.C., Barteluk, R.L., Kelly, M.T., Xin, H., Hua, G.D., Yuan, G., Proctor, E.M., Byrne, S. and Stiver, H.G. (1991) Etiology of childhood diarrhoea in Beijing, China. *Journal of Clinical Microbiology* 29, 90–95.

Källenius, G., Svenson, S.B., Möllby, R., Cedergren, B., Hultberg, H. and Winberg, J. (1981a) Structure of the carbohydrate part of the receptor on human epithelial cells for pyelonephritogenic *E. coli. Lancet* ii, 604–606.

Källenius, G., Möllby, R., Svenson, S. and Winberg, J. (1981b) Microbial adhesion and the urinary tract. *Lancet* ii, 866.

Källenius, G., Möllby, R., Svenson, S.B., Helin, I., Hultberg, H., Cedergren, B. and Winberg, J. (1981c) Occurrence of P-fimbriated *Escherichia coli* in urinary tract infection. *Lancet* ii, 1369–1372.

Källenius, G., Svenson, S.B., Hultberg, H., Möllby, R., Winberg, J. and Roberts, J.A. (1983) P-fimbriae of pyelonephritogenic *Escherichia coli*: significance for reflux and renal scarring – a hypothesis. *Infection* 1, 73–76.

Kauffman, F.D. and du Pont, A. (1950) *Escherichia coli* strains from infantile epidemic gastroenteritis. *Acta Pathologica Microbiologica Scandinavia* 27, 552–564.

Klemm, P. (1985) Fimbrial adhesins of *Escherichia coli. Reviews of Infectious Diseases* 7, 321–340.

Klipstein, F.A., Engert, R.F. and Houghten, R.A. (1986) Immunisation of volunteers with a synthetic peptide vaccine for enterotoxigenic *Escherichia coli. Lancet* i, 471–473.

Knight, P. (1993) Hemorrhagic *E. coli*: the danger increases. *ASM News* 59, 247–250.

Korhonen, T.K., Leffler, H. and Svanborg-Edén, C. (1981) Binding specificity of piliated strains of *Escherichia coli* and *Salmonella typhimurium* to epithelial cells, *Saccharomyces cerevesiae* cells and erythrocytes. *Infection and Immunity* 32, 796–804.

Korhonen, T.K., Väisänen, V., Saven, H., Hultberg, H. and Svenson, S.B. (1982) P-antigen recognizing fimbriae from human uropathogenic *Escherichia coli* strains. *Infection and Immunity* 37, 286–291.

Korhonen, T.K., Parkinnen, J., Hacker, J., Finne, J., Pere, A., Rhen, M. and

Holthofer, H. (1986) Binding of *Escherichia coli* S fimbriae to human kidney epithelium. *Infection and Immunity* 54, 322–327.

Kubinyi, L., Kiss, I. and Lendvai, K.G. (1972) Epidemiological evaluation of the efficiency of oral vaccination against enteropathogenic *Escherichia coli*. *Acta Microbiologica Academiae Scientarum Hungaricae* 19, 175–186.

Kubinyi, L., Kiss, I. and Lendvai, G. (1974) Epidemiological–statistical evaluation of oral vaccination against infantile *Escherichia coli* enteritis. *Acta Microbiologica Academiae Scientarum Hungaricae* 21, 187–191.

Kunin, C.M. (1970) A ten-year study of bacteriuria in schoolgirls. Final report of bacteriologic, urologic and epidemiologic findings. *Journal of Infectious Diseases* 122, 382–393.

Kunin, C.M. (1986) The prospects for a vaccine to prevent pyelonephritis. *New England Journal of Medicine* 314, 514.

Kunin, C.M. and McCormack, R.C. (1968) An epidemiological study of bacteriuria and blood pressure among nuns and working women. *New England Journal of Medicine* 278, 635–642.

Labigne-Roussel, A. and Falkow, S. (1988) Distribution and degree of heterogeneity of the afimbrial-adhesin-encoding operon (*afa*) among uropathogenic *Escherichia coli* isolates. *Infection and Immunity* 56, 640–648.

Leffler, H. and Svanborg-Edén, C. (1981) Glycolipid receptors for uropathogenic *Escherichia coli* on human erythrocytes and uroepithelial cells. *Infection and Immunity* 34, 920–929.

Levine, M.M. (1987) *Escherichia coli* that cause diarrhea: enterotoxigenic, enteropathogenic, enteroinvasive, enterohemorrhagic and enteroadherent. *Journal of Infectious Diseases* 155, 377–389.

Levine, M.M. (1990) Vaccines against enterotoxigenic *Escherichia coli* infections. In: Woodrow, G.C. and Levine, M.M. (eds) *New Generation Vaccines*. Marcel Dekker, New York, pp. 649–660.

Levine, M.M. and Edelman, R. (1984) Enteropathogenic *Escherichia coli* of classic serotypes associated with infant diarrhea: epidemiology and pathogenesis. *Epidemiological Reviews* 6, 31–51.

Levine, M.M., Caplan, E.S., Waterman, D., Cash, R., Hornick, R.B. and Snyder, M.J. (1977) Diarrhea caused by *Escherichia coli* that produce only heat-stable enterotoxin. *Infection and Immunity* 17, 78–82.

Levine, M.M., Bergquist, E.J, Nalin, D.R., Waterman, D.H., Hornick, R.B., Young, C.R. and Sotman, S. (1978) *E. coli* strains that cause diarrhea but do not produce heat-labile or heat-stable enterotoxins and are non-invasive. *Lancet* i, 1119–1122.

Levine, M.M., Nalin, D., Hoover, D.L., Bergquist, E.J., Hornick, R.B. and Young, C.R. (1979) Immunity to enterotoxigenic *Escherichia coli*. *Infection and Immunity* 23, 729–736.

Levine, M.M., Rennels, M.B., Cisneros, L., Hughes, T.P., Nalin, D.R. and Young, C.R. (1980) Lack of person-to-person transmission of enterotoxigenic *Escherichia coli* despite close contact. *American Journal of Epidemiology* 111, 347–355.

Levine, M.M., Black, R.E., Brinton, C.C., Clements, M.L., Fusco, P., Hughes, T.P., O'Donnell, S., Robins-Browne, R., Wood, S. and Young, C.R. (1982)

Reactogenicity, immunogenicity, and efficacy studies of *Escherichia coli* type 1 somatic pili parenteral vaccine in man. *Scandinavian Journal of Infectious Diseases Supplement* 33, 83–95.

Levine, M.M., Kaper, J.B., Black, R.E. and Clements, M.L. (1983) New knowledge on pathogenesis of bacterial enteric infections as applied to vaccine development. *Microbiological Reviews* 47, 510–550.

Levine, M.M., Ristaino, P., Marley, G., Smyth, C., Knutton, S., Boedeker, E., Black, R., Young, C., Clements, M.L., Cheney, C. and Patnaik, R. (1984) Coli surface antigens 1 and 3 of colonization factor antigen II-positive enterotoxigenic *Escherichia coli*: morphology, purification, and immune responses in humans. *Infection and Immunity* 44, 409–420.

Levine, M.M., Nataro, J.P., Karch, H., Baldini, M.M., Kaper, J.B., Black, R.E., Clements, M.L. and O'Brien, A.D. (1985a) The diarrheal response to some classic serotypes of enteropathogenic *Escherichia coli* is dependent on a plasmid encoding an enteroadherence factor. *Journal of Infectious Diseases* 152, 550–559.

Levine, M.M., Young, C.Y., Black, R.E., Takeda, Y. and Finkelstein, R.A. (1985b) Enzyme-linked immunosorbent assay to measure antibodies to purified heat-labile enterotoxins from human and porcine strains of *Escherichia coli* and to cholera toxin: application in serodiagnosis and seroepidemiology. *Journal of Clinical Microbiology* 21, 174–179.

Levine, M.M., Ferreccio, C., Prado, V., Cayazzo, M., Abrego, P., Martinez, J., Maggi, L., Baldini, M.M., Martin, W. Maneval, D., Kay, B., Guers, L., Lior, H., Wasserman, S.S. and Nataro, J.P. (1993) Epidemiologic studies of *Escherichia coli* diarrheal infections in a low socioeconomic level periurbal community in Santiago, Chile. *American Journal of Epidemiology* 138(10), 849–868.

Leying, H., Suerbaum, S., Kroll, H.P., Stahl, D. and Opferkuch, W. (1990) The capsular polysaccharide is a major determinant of serum resistance in K1-positive blood culture isolates of *Escherichia coli*. *Infection and Immunity* 58, 222–227.

Linde, K. and Koch, H. (1969) Oral immunization against coli enteritis with streptomycin-dependent *E. coli*. 3. Comparison of the effectivity of vaccines from killed and live streptomycin-dependent EC-O111 : B4 bacteria in active mice protection trial as well as by the inhibition of the settling of homologous streptomycin-resistant strains in the sterile intestine of mice. *Zentralblatt für Bakteriologie Parasitenkunde Infektionskrankheit und Hygiene* 211, 476–485.

Lomberg, H., Hanson, L.Å., Jacobson, B., Jodal, U., Leffler, H. and Svanborg-Edén, C. (1983) Correlation of P-blood group, vesicoureteral reflux, and bacterial attachment in patients with recurrent pyelonephritis. *New England Journal of Medicine* 308, 1189–1192.

Lopez, E.L., Devoto, S., Fayad, A., Canepa, C., Morrow, A.L. and Cleary, T.G. (1991) Association between severity of gastrointestinal prodrome and long-term prognosis in classic hemolytic–uremic syndrome. *Journal of Pediatrics* 120, 210–215.

Lund, B., Lindberg, F., Marklund, B.I. and Normark, S. (1988) Tip proteins of pili associated with pyelonephritis: new candidates for vaccine development. *Vaccine* 6, 110–112.

Mäkelä, H. and Korhonen, T. (1982) Bacterial adherence and urinary tract infection. *Lancet* i, 961.

Marier, R., Wells, J.G., Swanson, R.C., Dallhan, W. and Mehlman, I.J. (1973) An outbreak of enteropathogenic *Escherichia coli* foodborne disease traced to imported soft French cheese. *Lancet* ii, 1376–1378.

Marre, R. and Hacker, J. (1987) Role of S- and common type fimbriae of *Escherichia coli* in experimental upper and lower urinary tract infection. *Microbial Pathogenesis* 2, 223–226.

Martin, D.L., MacDonald, K.L., White, K.E., Soler, J.T. and Osterholm, M.T. (1990) The epidemiology and clinical aspects of the hemolytic uremic syndrome in Minnesota. *New England Journal of Medicine* 323, 1161–1167.

Maslow, J.N., Mulligan, M.E., Adams, K.S., Justis, J.C. and Arbeit, R.D. (1993) Bacterial adhesins and host factors: role in the development and outcome of *Escherichia coli* bacteremia. *Clinical Infectious Diseases* 17, 89–97.

Mathewson, J.J., Johnson, P.C., DuPont, H.L., Satterwhite, T.K. and Winsor, D.K. (1986) Pathogenicity of enteroadherent *Escherichia coli* in adult volunteers. *Journal of Infectious Diseases* 154, 524–527.

McCracken, G.H., Jr, Sarff, L.D., Globe, M.P., Mize, S.G., Schiffer, M.S., Robbins, J.B., Gotschlich, E.C., Ørskov, I. and Ørskov, F. (1974) Relationship between *E. coli* K1 capsular polysaccharide antigen and clinical outcome in neonatal meningitis. *Lancet* ii, 246–250.

Menestrina, G. (1988) *Escherichia coli* hemolysin permeabilizes small unilamellar vesicles loaded with calcium by a single-hit mechanism. *Federation of European Biological Societies Letters* 232, 217–220.

Menestrina, G., Mackman, N., Holland, I.B. and Bhakdi, S. (1987) *Escherichia coli* hemolysin forms voltage dependent ion channels in lipid membranes. *Biochimica et Biophysica Acta* 905, 109–117.

Moch, T., Hoschutzky, H., Hacker, J., Kroncke, K.D. and Jann, K. (1987) Isolation and characterization of the α-sialyl-β 2,3-galactosyl-specific adhesion from fimbriated *Escherichia coli. Proceedings of the National Academy of Sciences of the United States of America* 84, 3462–3466.

Mochmann, H., Ocklitz, H.W., Weh, L. and Heinrich, H. (1974) Oral immunization with an extract of *E. coli* enteritidis. *Acta Microbiologica Academiae Scientarum Hungaricae* 21, 193–196.

Moll, A., Manning, P.A. and Timmis, K.N. (1980) Plasmid-determined resistance to serum bactericidal activity: a major outer membrane protein, the TraT gene product, is responsible for plasmid-specified serum resistance in *Escherichia coli. Infection and Immunity* 28, 359–367.

Montgomerie, J.Z. (1978) Factors affecting virulence in *Escherichia coli* urinary tract infections. *Journal of Infectious Diseases* 137, 645–647.

Moon, H.W., Whipp, S.C., Argenzio, R.A., Levine, M.M. and Giannella, R.A. (1983) Attaching and effacing activities of rabbit and human enteropathogenic *Escherichia coli* in pig and rabbit intestines. *Infection and Immunity* 41, 1340–1351.

Nataro, J.P., Baldini, M.M., Kaper, J.B., Black, R.E., Bravo, N. and Levine, M.M. (1985a) Detection of an adherence factor of enteropathogenic *Escherichia coli* with a DNA probe. *Journal of Infectious Diseases* 152, 560–565.

Nataro, J.P., Scaletsky, I.C.A., Kaper, J.B., Levine, M.M. and Trabulsi, L.R.

(1985b) Plasmid-mediated factors conferring diffuse and localized adherence of enteropathogenic *Escherichia coli. Infection and Immunity* 48, 378–383.

Nataro, J.P., Kaper, J.B., Robins-Browne, R., Prado, V. and Levine, M.M. (1987) Patterns of adherence of diarrheagenic *Escherichia coli* rothbaum to HEp-2 cells. *Pediatric Infectious Disease Journal* 6, 829–831.

Nataro, J.P., Deng, Y., Maneval, D.R., German, A.L., Martin, W.C. and Levine, M.M. (1992) Aggregative adherence fimbriae I of enteroaggregative *E. coli* mediate adherence to HEp-2 cells and hemagglutination of human erythrocytes. *Infection and Immunity* 60, 2297–2304.

Nataro, J.P., Yikang, D., Girón, J., Savarino, S.J., Kothary, M.H. and Hall, R. (1993) Aggregative adherence fimbrial expression in enteroaggregative *Escherichia coli* requires two unlinked plasmid regions. *Infection and Immunity* 61, 1126–1131.

Neter, E. (1959) Enteritis due to enteropathogenic *Escherichia coli. Journal of Pediatrics* 55, 223–239.

Ngeleka, M., Jacques, M., Martineau-Doize, B., Harel, J. and Fairbrother, J.M. (1993) Pathogenicity of an *Escherichia coli* O115 : K'V165' mutant negative for $F165_1$ fimbriae in septicaemia of gnotobiotic pigs. *Infection and Immunity* 61, 836–843.

Nicholson, A.M. and Glynn, A.A. (1975) Investigation of the effect of K antigen in *Escherichia coli* urinary tract infections by use of a mouse model. *British Journal of Experimental Pathology* 56, 549–553.

NIH Consensus Conference Traveler's Diarrhea (1985) A balanced critical appraisal of the epidemiology, etiologies, presentation and treatment of traveler's diarrhea. *Journal of the American Medical Association* 253, 2700–2704.

Normark, S., Lark, D. and Hull, R. (1983) Genetics of digalactoside binding adhesin from a uropathogenic *Escherichia coli* strain. *Infection and Immunity* 41, 942–949.

Nowicki, B., Barrish, J.P., Korhonen, T., Hull, R.A. and Hull, S.I. (1987) Molecular cloning of the *Escherichia coli* O75X adhesin. *Infection and Immunity* 55, 3168–3173.

Nowicki, B., Moulds, J., Hull, R. and Hull, S. (1988a) A hemagglutinin of uropathogenic *Escherichia coli* recognizes the Dr blood group antigen. *Infection and Immunity* 56, 1057–1060.

Nowicki, B., Truong, L., Moulds, J. and Hull, R. (1988b) Presence of the Dr receptor in normal human tissues and its possible role in the pathogenesis of ascending urinary tract infection. *American Journal of Pathology* 133, 1–4.

Nowicki, B., Svanborg-Edén, C., Hull, R. and Hull, S. (1989) Molecular analysis and epidemiology of the Dr hemagglutinin of uropathogenic *Escherichia coli. Infection and Immunity* 57, 447–451.

Nowicki, B., Labigne, A., Moseley, S.L., Hull, R., Hull, S. and Moulds, J. (1990) The Dr hemagglutinin, afimbrial adhesins AFA-I and AFA-III, and F1845 fimbriae of uropathogenic and diarrhea-associated *Escherichia coli* belong to a family of hemagglutinins with Dr receptor recognition. *Infection and Immunity* 58, 279–281.

O'Hanley, P. (1990) Vaccines against *Escherichia coli* urinary tract infections. In: Woodrow, G.C. and Levine, M.M. (eds) *New Generation Vaccines*. Marcel Dekker, New York, pp. 631–647.

O'Hanley, P., Lark, D., Falkow, S. and Schoolnik, G. (1985a) Molecular basis of *Escherichia coli* colonization of the upper urinary tract in BALB/C mice. *Journal of Clinical Investigation* 75, 347–360.

O'Hanley, P., Low, D., Romero, I., Lark, D., Vosti, K., Falkow, S. and Schoolnik, G. (1985b) Gal-Gal binding and hemolysin phenotypes and genotypes associated with uropathogenic *Escherichia coli. New England Journal of Medicine* 313, 414–420.

Ørskov, I., Ørskov, F. and Birch-Anderson, A. (1980) Comparison of *Escherichia coli* fimbrial antigen F7 with type 1 fimbriae. *Infection and Immunity* 27, 657–666.

Ott, M., Hacker, J., Schmoll, T., Jarchau, T., Korhonen, T.K. and Goebel, W. (1986) Analysis of the genetic determinants coding for the S-fimbrial adhesion (sfa) in different *Escherichia coli* strains causing meningitis or urinary tract infections. *Infection and Immunity* 54, 646–653.

Overall, J.C., Jr (1970) Neonatal bacterial meningitis. *Journal of Pediatrics* 76, 499–511.

Parkinnen, J., Ristimaki, A. and Westerlund, B. (1989) Binding of *Escherichia coli* S fimbriae to cultured human epithelial cells. *Infection and Immunity* 57, 2256–2259.

Paulozzi, L.J., Johnson, K.E., Kamahele, L.M., Clausen, C.R., Riley, L.W. and Helgerson, S.D. (1986) Diarrhea associated with adherent enteropathogenic *Escherichia coli* in an infant and toddler center, Seattle, Washington. *Pediatrics* 77, 296–300.

Pedroso, M.Z., Freymuller, E., Trabulsi, L.R. and Gomes, T.A.T. (1993) Attaching–effacing lesion and intracellular penetration in HeLa cells and human duodenal mucosa by two *Escherichia coli* strains not belonging to the classical enteropathogenic *E. coli* serogroups. *Infection and Immunity* 61, 1152–1156.

Peltola, H., Sitonen, A., Kyronseppa, H., Mattila, L., Oksanen, P., Kataja, M.J. and Cadoz, M. (1991) Prevention of travelers' diarrhoea by oral B-subunit/whole-cell cholera vaccine. *Lancet* 338, 1285–1289.

Polotsky, Y.E., Dragunskaya, E.M., Seliverstova, V.G., Avdeeva, T.A., Chakhutinskaya, M.G., Ketyi, I., Vertenyi, A., Ralovich, B., Emody, L., Malovics, I., Safonova, N.V., Snigirevskaya, E.S. and Karyagina, E.I. (1977) Pathogenic effect of enterotoxigenic *Escherichia coli* and *Escherichia coli* causing infantile diarrhoea. *Acta Microbiologica Academiae Scientarum Hungaricae* 24, 221–236.

Rapkin, R.H. (1977) Urinary tract infection in childhood. *Pediatrics* 20, 508–511.

Rauss, K., Ketyi, I., Matusovits, E., Szendrei, L., Vertenyi A. and Varbiro B. (1972) Specific oral prevention of infantile enteritis. 3. Experiments with corpuscular vaccine. *Acta Microbiologica Academiae Scientarum Hungaricae* 19, 19–28.

Reid, G. and Sobel, J.D. (1987) Bacterial adherence in the pathogenesis of urinary tract infection: a review. *Reviews of Infectious Diseases* 9, 470–487.

Reid, R.H., Boedeker, E.C., McQueen, C.E., Davis, D., Tseng, L-Y., Kodak, J., Sau, K., Wilhemsen, C.L., Nellor, R., Dalal, P. and Bhagat, H.R. (1993) Preclinical evaluation of microencapsulated CFA/II oral vaccine against enterotoxigenic *E. coli. Vaccine* 11, 159–167.

Rene, P. and Sillverblatt, F.J. (1982) Serological response to *Escherichia coli* pili in pyelonephritis. *Infection and Immunity* 37, 749–754.

Rene, P., Dinolfo, M. and Silverblatt, F.J. (1982) Serum and urogenital antibody responses to *Escherichia coli* pili in cystitis. *Infection and Immunity* 38, 542–547.

Riley, H.D., Jr (1972) Editorial – Neonatal meningitis. *Journal of Infectious Diseases* 125, 420–425.

Robbins, J.B., McCracken, G.H., Jr, Gotschlich, E.C., Ørskov, F., Ørskov, I. and Hanson, L.Å. (1974) *Escherichia coli* K1 capsular polysaccharide associated with neonatal meningitis. *New England Journal of Medicine* 290, 1216–1220.

Roberts, J.A., Hardaway, K., Kaack, B., Fussell, E.N. and Baskin, G. (1984) Prevention of pyelonephritis by immunization with P-fimbriae. *Journal of Urology* 131, 602–607.

Roberts, K.B., Charney, E., Sweren, R.J., Ahonkhai, V.I., Bergman, D.A., Coulter, M.P., Fendrick, G.M., Lachman, B.S., Lawless, M.R., Pantell, R.H. and Stein, M.T. (1985) Urinary tract infection in infants with unexplained fever: a collaborative study. *Journal of Pediatrics* 103, 864–867.

Robins-Browne, R., Still, C.S., Miliotis, M.D., Richardson, M.D., Koornhof, H.J., Frieman, I., Schoub, B.D., Lecatsas, G. and Hartman, E. (1980) Summer diarrhea in African infants and children. *Archives of Diseases of Children* 55, 923–928.

Rothbaum, R., McAdams, A.J., Giannella, R. and Partin, J.C. (1982) A clinicopathologic study of enterocyte-adherent *Escherichia coli*: a cause of protracted diarrhea in infants. *Gastroenterology* 83, 441–454.

Rowland, M.G.M., Barrell, R.A.E. and Whitehead, R.G. (1978) Bacterial contamination in traditional Gambian weaning foods. *Lancet* i, 136–138.

Sack, R.B., Hirschhorn, N., Brownlee, I., Cash, R.A., Woodward, W.E. and Sack, D.A. (1975) Enterotoxigenic *Escherichia coli*-associated diarrheal disease in Apache children. *New England Journal of Medicine* 292, 1041–1045.

Sansonetti, P.J. (1991) Genetic and molecular basis of epithelial cell invasion by *Shigella* species. *Reviews of Infectious Diseases* 13 (suppl. 4), S285–S292.

Sansonetti, P.J., Kopecko, D.J. and Formal, S.B. (1982) Involvement of a plasmid in the invasive ability of *Shigella flexneri*. *Infection and Immunity* 35, 852–860.

Sarff, L.D., McCracken, G.H., Schiffer, M.S., Glode, M.P., Robbins, J.B., Ørskov, I. and Ørskov, F. (1975) Epidemiology of *Escherichia coli* K1 in healthy and diseased newborns. *Lancet* i, 1099–1104.

Savage, D.C.L., Wilson, M.I., McHardy, M., Dewar, D.A.E. and Fee, W.M. (1973) Covert bacteriuria of childhood: a clinical and epidemiological study. *Archives of Diseases in Childhood* 48, 8–20.

Savarino, S.J., Fasano, A., Robertson, D.C. and Levine, M.M. (1991) Enteroaggregative *Escherichia coli* elaborate a heat-stable enterotoxin demonstrable in an *in vitro* rabbit intestinal model. *Journal of Clinical Investigation* 87, 1450–1455.

Scannapieco, F.A., Guerina, N.G. and Goldmann, D.A. (1982) Comparison of virulence and colonizing capacity of *Escherichia coli* K1 and non-K1 strains in neonatal rats. *Infection and Immunity* 37, 830–832.

Schaeffer, A.J., Jones, J.M. and Dunn, J.K. (1981) Association of *in vitro Escherichia coli* adherence to vaginal and buccal epithelial cells with susceptibility of women to recurrent urinary tract infections. *New England Journal of Medicine* 304, 1062–1066.

Schaeffer, A.J., Jones, J.M., Falkowski, W.S., Duncan, J.L., Chmiel, J.S. and Plotkin, B.J. (1982) Variable adherence of uropathogenic *Escherichia coli* to epithelial cells from women with recurrent urinary tract infection. *Journal of Urology* 128, 1277–1230.

Schiffer, M.S., Oliveira, E., Glode, M.P., McCracken G.H., Sarff, L.M. and Robbins, J.B. (1976) A review: relation between invasiveness and the K1 capsular polysaccharide of *Escherichia coli. Pediatric Research* 10, 82–87.

Schneerson, R., Robbins, J.B., Egar, W., Zon, G., Sutton, A., Vann, W.F., Kaijser, B., Hanson, L.Å. and Ahlstedt, S. (1982) Bacterial capsular polysaccharide conjugates. In: Robbins, J., Hill, J.C. and Sadoff, J. (eds) *Bacterial Vaccines*. Thieme-Stratton, New York. pp. 311–321.

Schoolnik, G.K. (1989) How *E. coli* infect the urinary tract. *New England Journal of Medicine* 320, 804–805.

Seetharama, S., Cavalieri, S.J. and Snyder, I.S. (1988) Immune response to *Escherichia coli* alpha-hemolysin in patients. *Journal of Clinical Microbiology* 26, 850–856.

Senerwa, D., Olsvik, O., Mutanda, N., Lindqvist, K.J., Gathuma, J.M., Fossum, K. and Wachsmuth, K. (1989) Enteropathogenic *Escherichia coli* serotype O111:HNT isolated from pre-term neonates in Nairobi, Kenya. *Journal of Clinical Microbiology* 27, 1307–1311.

Silver, R.P. and Vimr, E.R. (1990) Polysialic acid capsule of *Escherichia coli* K1. In: Iglewski, B.H. and Clark, V.L. (eds) *Molecular Basis of Bacterial Pathogenesis*. San Diego: Academic Press, pp. 39–60.

Silver, R.P., Finn, C.W., Vann, W.F., Aaronson, W., Schneerson, R., Kretschmer, P.J. and Garon, C.F. (1981) Molecular cloning of the K1 capsular polysaccharide genes of *E. coli. Nature (London)* 289, 696–698.

Sinai, R.E., Marks, M.I., Powell, K.R. and Pai, C.H. (1980) Model of neonatal meningitis caused by *Escherichia coli* K1 in guinea pigs. *Journal of Infectious Diseases* 151, 193–197.

Smellie, J.M. and Normand, I.C.S. (1975) Bacteriuria, reflux and renal scarring. *Archives of Diseases in Childhood* 50, 581–585.

Smith, H.W. and Huggins, M.B. (1985) The toxic role of alpha-hemolysin in the pathogenesis of experimental *Escherichia coli* infection in mice. *Journal of Clinical Microbiology* 131, 395–403.

Stamey, T. (1981) Urinary tract infections in the female: a perspective. In: Remington, J.S. and Schwartz, M.N. (eds) *Current Clinical Topics in Infectious Diseases*. McGraw-Hill, New York, pp. 31–53.

Stamm, W.E., Hooton, T.M., Johnson, J.R., Johnson, C., Stapleton, A., Roberts, P.L. and Fihn, S.D. (1989) Urinary tract infections: from pathogenesis to treatment. *Journal of Infectious Diseases* 159, 400–408.

Sutton, A., Schneerson, R., Kendall-Morris, S. and Robbins, J.B. (1982) Differential complement resistance mediates virulence of *Haemophilus influenzae* type B. *Infection and Immunity* 35, 95–104.

Svanborg-Edén, C. and Hanson, L.Å. (1978) *Escherichia coli* pili as possible mediators of attachment to human urinary tract epithelial cells. *Infection and Immunity* 21, 229–237.

Svanborg-Edén, C. and Jodal, U. (1979) Attachment of *Escherichia coli* to urinary sediment epithelial cells from urinary tract infection-prone and healthy children. *Infection and Immunity* 26, 837–840.

Svanborg-Edén, C., Hanson, L.Å., Jodal, U., Lindberg, U. and Akerlund, A.S. (1976) Variable adherence to normal urinary tract epithelial cells of *E. coli* strains associated with various forms of urinary tract infections. *Lancet* ii, 490–492.

Svanborg-Edén, C., Eriksson, B., Hanson, L.Å., Jodal, U., Kaijser, B., Lidin-Janson, G., Lindberg, U. and Olling, S. (1978) *Escherichia coli* from children with various forms of urinary tract infection. *Journal of Pediatrics* 93, 398–403.

Svanborg-Edén, C., Hagberg, L., Hanson, L.Å., Lomberg, H., Ørskov, I. and Ørskov, F. (1982) Bacterial adherence and urinary tract infection. *Lancet* i, 961–962.

Svennerholm, A.-M., Holmgren, J. and Sack, D.A. (1989) Development of oral vaccines against enterotoxigenic *Escherichia coli* diarrhoea. *Vaccine* 7, 196–198.

Tacket, C.O., Losonsky, G., Link, H., Hoang, Y., Guesry, P., Hilpert, H. and Levine, M.M. (1988) Protection by milk immunoglobulin concentrate against oral challenge with enterotoxigenic *Escherichia coli. New England Journal of Medicine* 318, 1240–1243.

Tacket, C.O., Losonsky, G.A., Bhagat, H., Edelman, R.E., Reid, R., Boedeker, E.C. and Levine, M.M. (1993) Phase 1 study of an ETEC vaccine consisting of CFA/11 in biodegradable polymer microspheres. *Abstracts of the 93rd Annual General Meeting of the American Society for Microbiology*. The American Society for Microbiology, Washington, DC, Abstr. E60, p. 153.

Tzipori, S., Karch, H., Wachsmuth, K.I., Robins-Browne, R.M., O'Brien, A.D., Lior, H., Cohen, M.I., Smithers, J. and Levine, M.M. (1987) Role of 60-megadalton plasmid and Shiga-like toxins in the pathogenesis of infections caused by enterohemorrhagic *Escherichia coli* 0157:H7 in gnotobiotic pigs. *Infection and Immunity* 55, 3117–3125.

Tzipori, S., Montanaro, J., Robins-Browne, R.M., Vial, P., Gibson, R. and Levine, M.M. (1992) Studies with enteroaggregative *Escherichia coli* in the gnotobiotic piglet gastroenteritis model. *Infection and Immunity* 60, 5302–5306.

Ulshen, M.H. and Rollo, J.L. (1980) Pathogenesis of *Escherichia coli* gastroenteritis in man – another mechanism. *New England Journal of Medicine* 302, 99–101.

Väisänen, V., Elo, J., Hallgren, L.G., Siitoner, A., Mäkelä, P.H., Svanborg-Edén, C., Källenius, G., Svenson, S.B., Hultberg, H. and Korhonen, T. (1981) Mannose-resistant hemagglutination and P-antigen recognition are characteristic of *Escherichia coli* causing primary pyelonephritis. *Lancet* ii, 1366–1369.

Vial, P.A., Robins-Browne, R., Lior, H., Prado, V., Kaper, J.B., Nataro, J.P., Maneval, D., Elsayed, A. and Levine, M.M. (1988) Characterization of enteroadherent-aggregative *Escherichia coli*, a putative agent of diarrheal disease. *Journal of Infectious Diseases* 158, 70–79.

Vial, P.A., Mathewson, J.J., DuPont, H.L., Guers, L. and Levine, M.M. (1990)

Comparison of two assay methods for patterns of adherence to HEp-2 cells of *Escherichia coli* from patients with diarrhea. *Journal of Clinical Microbiology* 28, 882–885.

Visweswariah, S.S., Shanti, G. and Balganesh, T.S. (1992) Interaction of heat-stable enterotoxins with human colonic (T84) cells: modulation of the activation of guanylyl cyclase. *Microbial Pathogenesis* 12, 209–218.

Waalwijk, C., MacLaren, D.M. and de Graaf, J. (1983) *In vivo* function of hemolysin in the nephropathogenicity of *Escherichia coli. Infection and Immunity* 42, 245–249.

Wanke, C.A., Schorling, J.B., Barrett, L.J., Desouza, M.A. and Guerrant, R.L. (1991) Potential role of adherence traits of *Escherichia coli* in persistent diarrhea in an urban Brazilian slum. *Pediatric Infectious Disease Journal* 10, 746–751.

Welch, R.A., Dellinger, E.P., Minshew, B. and Falkow, S. (1981) Hemolysin contributes to virulence of extra-intestinal *Escherichia coli* infection. *Nature (London)* 294, 665–667.

Winberg, J., Andersen, H.J., Bergstrom, T., Jacobsson, B., Larson, H. and Lincoln, K. (1974) Epidemiology of symptomatic urinary tract infection in childhood. *Acta Paediatrica Scandinavia Supplement* 252, 1–20.

Winterborn, M.H. (1977) The management of urinary tract infections in children. *British Journal of Hospital Medicine* 17, 453–461.

Wood, L.V., Ferguson, L.E., Hogan P., Thurman, D., Morgan, D.R., DuPont, H.L. and Ericsson, C.D. (1983) Incidence of bacterial enteropathogens in foods from Mexico. *Applied and Environmental Microbiology* 46, 328–332.

Wyle, F.A., Artenstein, M.S., Brandt, B.L., Tramont, E.C., Kasper, D.L., Altieri, P., Berman, S.L. and Lowenthal, J.P. (1972) Immunologic response of man to group B meningococcal polysaccharide vaccines. *Journal of Infectious Diseases* 126, 514–522.

Yu, J. and Kaper, J.B. (1992) Cloning and characterization of the *eae* gene of enterohemmorrhagic *Escherichia coli* O157:H7. *Molecular Microbiology* 6, 411–417.

Zollinger, W.D., Mandrell, R.E., Grifiss, J.M., Altieri, P. and Berman, S. (1979) Complex of meningococcal group B polysaccharide and type 2 outer membrane protein immunogenic in man. *Journal of Clinical Investigation* 63, 836–848.

Zollinger, W.D., Mandrell, R.E. and Grifiss, J.M. (1982) Enhancement of immunologic activity by noncovalent complexing of meningococcal group B polysaccharide and outer membrane proteins. In: Robbins, J., Hill, J.C. and Sadoff, J. (eds) *Bacterial Vaccines*. Thieme-Stratton, New York, pp. 254–262.

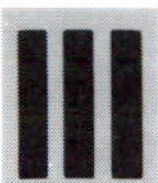

Virulence Factors of *Escherichia coli*

Escherichia coli Enterotoxins 14

C.L. Gyles
Department of Veterinary Microbiology and Immunology, University of Guelph, Guelph, Ontario, Canada N1G 2W1

Introduction

E. coli enterotoxins were discovered in the late 1960s as a result of use of the ligated intestine technique. This methodology was first reported in rabbits in studies with *Vibrio cholerae* by the French workers Violle and Crendiropoullo in 1915 and was rediscovered by Indian workers, De and Chatterje, in 1952. Not long thereafter, ligated segments of pig intestine were shown to respond with fluid secretion to strains of *E. coli* implicated in diarrhoeal disease in pigs (Moon *et al.*, 1966; Gyles and Barnum, 1967; Smith and Halls, 1967a). In 1967, Smith and Halls (1967b) presented good evidence that a heat-stable toxin induced the intestinal fluid response associated with porcine diarrhoeagenic strains of *E. coli*, and, in 1969, Gyles and Barnum reported their discovery of a heat-labile cholera-like enterotoxin from strains of *E. coli* isolated from diarrhoeic pigs. Subsequently, Smith and Gyles (1970) demonstrated differences between the two *E. coli* enterotoxins and called them LT (labile toxin) and ST (stable toxin).

When it became evident that there were two types of ST, they were called STa and STb (Burgess *et al.*, 1978); the former was methanol soluble and active in the intestine of infant mice and the latter was methanol insoluble and inactive in the infant mouse intestine but active in the intestine of weaned pigs. Later, So and McCarthy (1980) used the terms STI and STII as synonyms for STa and STb, respectively. In 1983 two types of STI were distinguished, and were called STIa and STIb (Moseley *et al.*, 1983). STIa consists of 18 amino acids, and STIb consists of 19 amino acids. Savarino and colleagues (1993) have recently reported another member of the STI family of enterotoxins. This toxin, called EAST1, is produced by enteroaggregative *E. coli* implicated in diarrhoea in children and will be discussed briefly in this chapter. Heat-stable enterotoxins related to STI of *E. coli* are also found in other species of bacteria including *Citrobacter freundii*, *Vibrio cholerae*, *V. mimicus* and *Yersinia enterocolitica*.

Strains of *E. coli* which produce one or more than one enterotoxin are called enterotoxigenic *E. coli* (ETEC). These *E. coli* are implicated in diarrhoeal disease in the young of a variety of animal species and in both young and adult humans. ETEC that are recovered from diarrhoeic calves and lambs typically produce STa (STI) as the only enterotoxin, but those implicated in diarrhoea in pigs produce various combinations of LT, STI and STII. It is not common for strains from animals to produce LT alone. ETEC isolated from the faeces of dogs with diarrhoea produce STI alone (Wasteson *et al.*, 1988) or STI and LT (Olson *et al.*, 1985) and ETEC recovered from chickens produce LT (Sekizaki *et al.*, 1985). Interestingly, the LT from chicken ETEC is identical to LT from human strains (Inoue *et al.*, 1993).

Since the recognition of *E. coli* enterotoxins in the 1960s, remarkable progress has been made and there is an abundant literature on association with disease, structure and physical features, receptor binding, biological activity, assays, immunology and genetics of *E. coli* enterotoxins.

Heat-labile Enterotoxins

Heat-labile enterotoxin I (LT-I)

Between 1969 and 1983 only one antigenic type of LT was recognized. However, in 1983, Green and colleagues reported a second antigenic type of LT, which was called LT-II to distinguish it from the original LT, which was referred to as LT-I. Most of this section on LT will be devoted to LT-I and the term LT will be used to refer to LT-I. Sometimes a distinction is made between LT from *E. coli* of porcine origin and LT from *E. coli* of human origin. Porcine LT is called LTp, P-LT or LTp-I and human LT is called LTh, H-LT or LTh-I (Holmes and Twiddy, 1983; Yamamoto and Yokota, 1983; Finkelstein *et al.*, 1987; Fukuta *et al.*, 1988).

Structure and physical features

LT was first purified by Clements and Finkelstein (1979) and characterized by Clements *et al.* (1980). These researchers demonstrated that LT bound firmly to gels containing agarose and could only be eluted with galactose and lactose. They established the structural similarity of LT to CT.

The LT subunits are synthesized separately and each contains an N-terminal hydrophobic leader sequence that is required for transport across the cytoplasmic membrane. The disulfide bond of the B subunit is required for generation of a structure that participates in assembly of holotoxin and A subunits promote pentamerization of the B subunits (Hardy *et al.*, 1988). The last four residues at the C-terminal of the A subunit are necessary for maintaining stability of the A1:B5 holotoxin complex and it has been suggested that these amino acids may serve as a stabilizing anchor (Sandkvist *et al.*, 1990; Streatfield *et al.*, 1992). The ten amino acids next to the last four at the C-terminal end play a role in promoting oligomerization of the B subunit.

LT in laboratory cultures is a periplasmic protein. Pre-LT A and pre-LT B are formed in the cytoplasm, transported through the cytoplasmic membrane, processed to form A and B subunits, then assembled into holotoxin molecules (Hofstra and Witholy, 1985). It is likely that, in the environment of the intestine, LT escapes through the outer membrane. Hunt and Hardy (1991) showed that LT and other periplasmic proteins of *E. coli* were released from growing bacteria by the addition to the culture medium of physiological concentrations of bile salts and that the amount released was increased if trypsin and iron starvation were superimposed on the exposure to bile salts.

The structure of LT has recently been reviewed (Spangler, 1992). It is an oligomeric protein of approximately 88 kDa, which consists of one A subunit of 30 kDa in association with five B subunits, each of 11.5 kDa (Hofstra and Witholy, 1985; Robertson, 1988; Sixma *et al.*, 1991). X-ray crystallography has shown that the toxin molecule consists of one A subunit above a central aqueous channel formed by the five B subunits (a doughnut-shaped arrangement). The B pentamer constitutes a highly stable arrangement with subunits held together by hydrogen bonding and salt bridges (Sixma *et al.*, 1993a). The A subunit is synthesized as a single polypeptide, but proteolysis shows that the molecule consists of a large enzymatically active peptide (A_1) and a small peptide (A_2) which connects the A subunit to the B pentamer. A_1 and A_2 are joined by a single disulfide bond which remains intact until the toxin enters a cell. A_2 traverses the central pore formed by the B pentamer and terminates in a hook-like structure. Two cysteine residues in the B subunit are located at the N- and C-terminals and form a S–S bond joining the two ends of the molecule. This disulfide bond is critical for maintenance of the native configuration of the B subunit.

Receptor binding

The LT B subunit pentamer binds the toxin to the lactose-containing oligosaccharide portion of ganglioside GM_1 in cell membranes (Griffiths *et al.*, 1986; Fukuta *et al.*, 1988; Schengrund and Ringler, 1989). Unlike CT which binds only GM_1 ganglioside, LT also binds a glycoprotein

(Holmgren *et al.*, 1982, 1985). LT also binds weakly to GM_2 and asialo-GM_1. The weakness of the binding to asialo-GM_1 indicates that optimal binding requires the free carboxyl group of sialic acid. Binding is multivalent, with each molecule capable of binding five GM_1 molecules. Studies involving both LT and CT have identified the binding site: by determining changes in fluorescence characteristics of tryptophan-88 (Trp-88) that are associated with binding of toxin to GM_1 (Moss *et al.*, 1977; De Wolf *et al.*, 1981); by analysis of site-specific mutants (Tsuji *et al.*, 1985); by magnetic resonance studies (Sillerud *et al.*, 1981); and, most recently, by X-ray crystallography (Sixma *et al.*, 1991, 1992, 1993a). These investigations indicate that Trp-88 of one B subunit and Gly-33 of an adjacent subunit are part of a cavity in which the binding site is located. One implication of these findings is that two subunits are required for binding.

Recently, X-ray crystallography has thrown light on the binding of LT to lactose (Sixma *et al.*, 1992). The data indicate extensive hydrogen bonding between galactose and B subunit residues Glu-51, Gln-61, Asn-90 and Lys-91 and van der Waals association between galactose and Trp-88 as well as His-57.

Toxin is internalized following binding of all five B subunits to the cell membrane, but several aspects of the process are not understood. It is not clear whether the A1 or A2 fragment is closer to the membrane or whether A alone or both A and B translocate across the membrane. However, X-ray crystallography has identified the location of the binding site of the terminal galactose of GM_1 and this is consistent with toxin binding to the enterocyte with the A1 fragment pointing away from the cell membrane (Sixma *et al.*, 1992). Reduction of the disulfide bond between A_1 and A_2 appears to be necessary for internalization. London (1992) has suggested that B subunit insertion into the membrane triggers marked conformational changes in the toxin molecule, and passage of the A subunit through the central pore of the B subunit pentamer described by Sixma *et al.* (1992). London (1992) proposed that the B subunit pentamer acts like an iris, so that a sliding action between B subunits results in opening of a large pore. Interestingly, there are many similarities in the B subunit arrangement of LT and verotoxins produced by *E. coli* (Sixma *et al.*, 1993b) although they differ with respect to size, amino acid sequence and binding targets. They are both pentamers with a doughnut-shaped arrangement, and with disulfide bridges that are critical to pentamer formation.

Biological activity

LT and CT possess the same enzymatic function, namely adenosine-diphospho-ribosyl transferase activity (Fishman, 1990). These toxins transfer adenosine diphosphate (ADP)-ribose from nucleotide adenine dinucleotide (NAD) to a major specific target and possibly other minor targets in the cell. The enzymatic activity resides in the A_1 fragment of the A subunit and neither the holotoxin nor the intact A subunit possesses substantial activity (Mekelanos *et al.*, 1979). Both proteolytic nicking and reduction must therefore take place before the toxin is functional. In studies on LT and Chinese hamster ovary (CHO) cells, Tsuji *et al.* (1984) showed that nicking of LT with trypsin resulted in a 50% reduction in the time for 50% elongation of the CHO cells and a reduction in the time during which bound toxin was susceptible to neutralization by antiserum.

LT possesses both NAD-glycohydrolase and ADP-ribosyl transferase activities. The A_1 subunit reacts with NAD to produce ADP-ribose and nicotinamide. Mutagenesis studies (Harford *et al.*, 1989) and comparisons with *Pseudomonas aeruginosa* exotoxin A, a well-characterized NAD-dependent ADP-ribosyl transferase (Sixma *et al.*, 1991, 1993a), have been used to identify active site residues in the A subunit of LT. These studies have shown that glutamine-112 is a component of the active site for binding NAD. There is evidence that LT, CT, pertussis toxin, exotoxin A of *P. aeruginosa* and diphtheria toxin, which are all NAD-dependent ADP-ribosyl transferases, have similar shapes in their NAD-binding sites (Domeninghini *et al.*, 1991).

LT transfers the ADP-ribose from NAD to an arginine residue in the 42-kDa stimulatory guanine nucleotide-binding regulatory protein subunit ($G_{s\alpha}$) of the adenylate cyclase system. ADP-ribosylation results in inability to turn off the system and persistent elevation of cyclic AMP (cAMP). The levels of cAMP in CHO cells exposed to toxin can increase several hundred-fold (Guerrant *et al.*, 1974). Activity requires the presence of guanine triphosphate (GTP) and is augmented *in vitro* by certain low-molecular-weight proteins called ADP-ribosylation factors (ARFs) (Moss and Vaughan, 1991). A_1 is first activated by associating with an ARF–GTP complex; then it transfers ADP-ribose from NAD to $G_{s\alpha}$. ADP-ribosylated $G_{s\alpha}$ binds GTP and complexes with the catalytic unit of adenylate cyclase to form an active complex, which converts ATP to cAMP. The complex remains activated because ADP-ribosylation inhibits the normal intrinsic GTPase activity of $G_{s\alpha}$. Furthermore, ADP-ribosylation of $G_{s\alpha}$ results in increased affinity of $G_{s\alpha}$ for GTP and decreased affinity for GDP, thereby promoting maintenance of the active state of the adenylate cyclase complex.

ADP-ribosylation of $G_{s\alpha}$ occurs in the brush border membrane of the intestinal epithelial cell. The ADP-ribosylated $G_{s\alpha}$ then travels across the cell to interact with the catalytic unit of adenylate cyclase, which is located in the basolateral border of the cell. There is some evidence to suggest that LT is processed through the Golgi prior to its activation of adenylate cyclase. Donta *et al.* (1993) found that Brefeldin A, an inhibitor of the trans-Golgi network, delayed the morphological effects of LT on Y1 mouse adrenal cells and caused both a delay and a reduction in the cAMP response to LT in these cells. Brefeldin A had no effect on the morphological activities of cAMP. Interestingly, ARFs have been localized to the Golgi.

The major clinical effect of LT is diarrhoea and the elevated levels of cAMP are proposed to be the basis for the diarrhoea. Normal intestinal ion-transport mechanisms are maintained by phosphorylation of proteins through activation of protein kinases and excessive stimulation of protein kinases is believed to be responsible for the electrolyte disturbances which characterize LT-mediated diarrhoea. LT is known to result in increased secretion of Cl^- from crypt cells and impaired absorption of Na^+ and Cl^- by cells at the tips of villi (Moriarty and Turnberg, 1986; Field *et al.*, 1989a, b). Water follows the electrolytes due to osmotic effects and a profuse watery diarrhoea results.

Although ADP-ribosylation of $G_{s\alpha}$ and the resulting increase in cAMP in enterocytes have long been proposed as the basis of the biological effects of CT and LT (Fig. 14.1A), several researchers have suggested that other mechanisms also operate to cause diarrhoea in response to these toxins (Fig. 14.1 B–D). Prostaglandin E_2 has been implicated (Fig. 14.1 pathways B and C). As early as 1972, Jacoby and Marshall (1972) and Finck and Katz (1972) reported that indomethacin and aspirin (drugs that block prostaglandin synthesis) inhibited CT-induced fluid secretion by intestinal tissue. Subsequently, indomethacin and ibuprofen were reported to inhibit CT-mediated synthesis of cAMP (Peterson *et al.*, 1988a, b). Later, Peterson and Ochoa (1989) showed that, following addition of CT to rabbit intestinal loops, PGE_2 was released into the lumen and correlated better with fluid accumulation than with cAMP.

It is clear that levels of cAMP and of prostaglandins are increased in response to CT and LT. Studies of kinetics of increases in levels of cAMP and prostaglandins in response to CT have not determined whether the initial increase in prostaglandin levels is due to increased cAMP (Peterson *et al.*, 1990). One explanation for the observations is that increased cAMP induces increased synthesis of prostaglandins, which stimulate adenylate cyclase resulting in further increases in cAMP. However, Peterson *et al.* (1990) note that phospholipase activity is increased in CT-treated cells and conclude that CT causes increased synthesis of prostaglandins because of stimulatory effects on arachidonic acid metabolism.

Other mechanisms may also contribute to diarrhoea due to LT or CT (Fig. 14.1). Enterochromaffin cells release their content of 5-hydroxytryptamine (5-HT) after exposure to CT (Nilsson *et al.*, 1983; Beubler and Horina, 1990). Beubler and Horina (1990) showed that a combination of ketanserin, which blocks 5-HT_2 receptors, and ICS 205–930, which blocks 5-HT_3 receptors, completely blocked CT-induced secretion in the rat intestine. The block in secretory response occurred despite

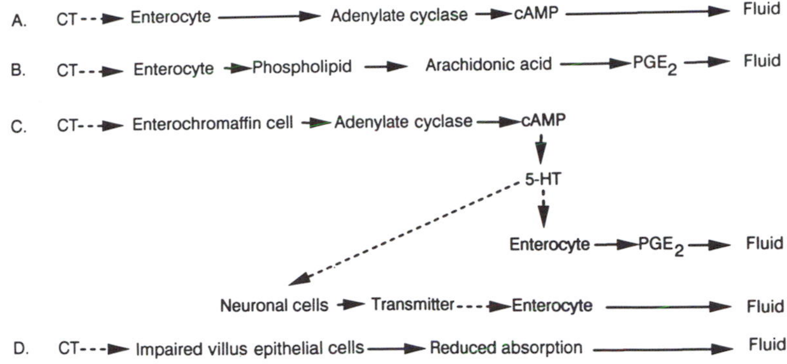

Fig. 14.1. Proposed pathways from cholera toxin (CT) to fluid accumulation in the intestine. The data are applicable to *E. coli* LT.

the failure of the drugs to reduce the elevated levels of cAMP in jejunal mucosa. They suggested that CT stimulation of adenylate cyclase in enterochromaffin cells induced release of 5-HT, which caused formation of prostaglandin E_2 via 5-HT_2 receptors and activation of neuronal structures via 5-HT_3 receptors. Thus, they proposed that a portion of the secretory effect was mediated by prostaglandin E_2 and the rest by an unknown transmitter released by enteric nerves. Peterson and Ochoa (1988) and Stephen and Osborne (1988) have provided evidence that LT and CT have effects on enterochromaffin cells, involving hormones such as serotonin and vasoactive intestinal peptide, which can increase secretion. Also, there is evidence for an increased rate of loss of villus cells exposed to CT, and loss of function and viability of absorptive cells has been suggested to contribute to diarrhoea.

Several biological assays are available for detection of LT. These include tests for fluid accumulation in ligated intestine of rabbits and pigs, intradermal tests for increased vascular permeability, and tests for cytotonic changes in cell cultures such as Chinese hamster ovary cells, Y1 mouse adrenal cells and Vero (African green monkey kidney) cells. Assays that involve the use of animals should not be used for routine testing and should be used only when no alternatives are available. If it is necessary to demonstrate the presence of biologically active toxin, the cell culture methods are very sensitive and effective. The recently described test for vacuole formation in HT29 cells is even more sensitive than the more traditional cell culture assays (Charanthia *et al.*, 1992). Bioassays based on measurement of increase in cAMP in cell lysate exposed to LT are available commercially and are very sensitive. There is no detectable gut damage in response to LT, since there is simply overstimulation of normal mechanisms. LT causes impaired cell function without any evidence of structural damage and is therefore said to be a cytotonic toxin, in contrast to cytotoxic toxins.

Both LT and CT possess mucosal adjuvant activity. It has been suggested that this effect may be due to the ability of the B subunit to bind intestinal epithelium, especially in Peyer's patches. However, the holotoxin is more effective than purified B subunit. Furthermore, mutations which result in loss of ADP-ribosyl transferase activity cause a loss in adjuvant property (Lycke *et al.*, 1992). However, since forskolin directly stimulates adenylate cyclase but has no immunostimulatory effects, stimulation of adenylate cyclase cannot be invoked to explain the stimulatory effects of the toxin on the immune response (Wilson *et al.*, 1993). Although adjuvant activity is not associated with the B subunit, its ability to bind to intestinal epithelial cells has generated interest in using it as a carrier for delivery of orally administered antigens to the intestinal epithelium (Aitken and Hirst, 1993; Nashar *et al.*, 1993).

There is a lag in the response of tissues to LT and CT, but the effect is prolonged since affected cells remain permanently affected. There was no observable fluid accumulation for 2 hours after inoculation of CT into mouse intestinal loops; a maximum was reached 8 hours after injection, and there was no significant decline in the subsequent 8-hour observation period (Hitotsubashi *et al.*, 1992a).

Immunology

The A and B subunits of LT are antigenically distinct (Gilligan *et al.*, 1983) and are also remarkably different in immunogenicity. There have been extensive studies on antigenic relationships among members of the CT–LT-I toxin family (Marchlewicz and Finkelstein, 1983; Takeda *et al.*, 1983a; Finkelstein *et al.*, 1987; Kazemi and Finkelstein, 1990). These toxins have common and unique antigenic determinants and enterotoxin-specific antibodies may sometimes account for a major portion of the neutralizing activity. Small differences in primary structure are sometimes associated with marked differences in neutralizing antibody specificities.

Immunization with intact toxin induces antibodies which react strongly with the B subunit and weakly or not at all with the A. Data from studies with CT indicate that monoclonal antibodies against the B subunit have potent neutralizing activity whereas antibodies against the A subunit have little or no neutralizing activity (Holmes and Twiddy, 1983; Lindholm *et al.*, 1983). The B subunit of LT is also thought to be immunodominant.

Toxoid vaccines based on the B subunit of LT have been tested by several laboratories and reported to be effective. Houghten and co-workers (1985) produced a completely synthetic toxoid vaccine by joining the 18-amino-acid sequence of STI to a 26-amino-acid sequence from the B subunit of LT. They found this toxoid to be immunogenic for both STI and LT. Following oral infection of piglets with an LT^+ ETEC on the first day of life, antibodies to LT were detectable in the intestine by day 7 (Olsson *et al.*, 1986).

Immunological tests that are specific and sensitive have been developed for detection of LT. These include latex particle agglutination (Finkelstein *et al.*, 1983; Yam *et al.*, 1992), immunodiffusion (Takeda *et al.*, 1983b) and GM_1-ELISA (Ristaino *et al.*, 1983) in which the receptor GM_1 is used to capture antigen. These tests are particularly suited to large-scale epidemiological studies.

Genetics

The structural genes for LT-I are on plasmids (Gyles *et al.*, 1974) but genes in the chromosome as well as DNA of the flanking regions may affect the level of expression of the plasmid-encoded genes (Neill *et al.*, 1983; Katayama *et al.*, 1990). In a study of extent of LT production by 76 LT^+ *E. coli* strains of human origin, Katayama *et al.* (1990) found that the level of toxin produced varied by a factor of 100. They determined that LT production was regulated at a transcriptional step and that DNA structure of the flanking regions may be involved in control of expression of the LT genes. Addition of zinc in concentrations of 10^{-6} M or 10^{-5} M resulted in significant increase in production of LT, without changes in bacterial growth (Sugarman and Epps, 1984). The presence of the antibiotics lincomycin and tetracycline in cultures of LT-positive *E. coli* results in an increase in cell-associated and extracellular LT (Yoh *et al.*, 1983).

The LT plasmids sometimes also encode resistance to antibacterial drugs (Gyles *et al.*, 1977). Nucleotide sequences of the genes for LT-I (Yamamoto *et al.*, 1983, 1984) have confirmed the close relationship of LTh-I and LTp-I by demonstrating more than 95% nucleotide sequence similarity. Homologies of 96%, 81% and 79% were reported for the B subunit genes of hLT and pLT, hLT and CT, and pLT and CT, respectively. Codon usage, G + C content, and divergence of the DNA sequences surrounding the toxin genes have suggested that the *E. coli* LT genes were derived from another organism, most likely *Vibrio cholerae*. Among porcine ETEC, LT-I genes are typically found in strains which also have genes for the K88 antigen. Among ETEC of human origin, LT-I genes are often associated with CFA-II (Echeverria *et al.*, 1986).

Several systems are now in common use for detection of LT genes. Hybridization methods involving non-radioactive DNA probes have been developed. In one recent study, a digoxigenin-labelled probe which detected genes for LT, STI and STII was reported to be sensitive, specific and reliable (Chapman and Daly, 1993). Polymerase chain reaction amplification procedures are also highly effective for detection of LT gene sequences (Woodward *et al.*, 1992). These methodologies are excellent for screening studies but do not indicate whether a functional gene is present.

Heat-labile enterotoxin II (LT-II)

LT-II differs from LT-I in that it is not neutralized by anti-CT or anti-LT-I. A variant of LT-II (LT-IIb) has been detected that is distinguishable in antigenicity and other characteristics from the prototype LT-IIa.

LT-II has a structure which is similar to that of LT-I (Guth *et al.*, 1986; Holmes *et al.*, 1986). The prototype LT-IIa consists of A and B polypeptides similar in size and in susceptibility to proteolytic cleavage compared with LT-I. LT-IIa and LT-IIb are similar in structure and are antigenically related but differ in some of their biological activities and in their pIs.

LT-II binds to a receptor which is different from GM1 ganglioside. Whereas LT-I binds best to GM1, LT-IIa binds best to GD1b, and LT-IIb binds best to GD1a (Fukuta *et al.*, 1988). Based on these observations as well as binding to other gangliosides, Fukuta and colleagues have suggested that LT-I binds to the terminal sugar sequence Galβ1–8GalNAcβ1–4(NeuAcα2–3)Gal, where GalNAc is *N*-acetylgalactosamine and NeuAc is *N*-acetylneuraminic acid; that LT-IIa binds to a sequence that is similar to that bound by LT-I except that it has a second NeuAc; and that LT-IIb binds a terminal NeuAcα2–3Galβ1–4GalNAc sequence. LT-IIa is not enterotoxic in rabbit, even in relatively large doses, and its role in disease has not been established.

LT-IIa is similar to LT-I in enzymatic activity and mode of activation of adenylate cyclase (Holmes *et al.*, 1986) but the specific activity of LT-IIa in Y1 mouse adrenal tumour cells is 25–50 times that of LT-I (Holmes *et al.*, 1986). *E. coli* cells which produce LT-IIa do so at a level less than 1% of the level of LT-I associated with LT-I-positive *E. coli*.

Genes coding for LT-II have been detected in *E. coli* from humans, cattle and buffalo (Seriwatana *et al.*, 1988). The structural genes for LT-II are chromosomal. The LT-IIa and LTh-I A subunit genes have 57% nucleotide sequence similarity but the B subunit genes lack significant sequence homology (Pickett *et al.*, 1989).

Heat-stable Enterotoxins

E. coli *heat-stable enterotoxin STI (STa)*

Structure and physical features

The two major types of ST appear to be completely unrelated and will therefore be discussed separately. What they have in common are heat stability, low molecular weight, secretion from the cell, and ability to interfere with water and electrolyte movement across the gut epithelium.

STI has a molecular weight of approximately 2000 (Lazure *et al.*, 1983). It is resistant to 100 °C for 15 min, is soluble in water and organic solvents, and resistant to proteolytic enzymes such as pronase, trypsin and chymotrypsin (Smith and Halls, 1967b; Alderete and Robertson, 1978). STI is acid resistant but susceptible to alkaline pH. It is completely inactivated by reducing and oxidizing agents which disrupt disulfide bonds (Robertson *et al.*, 1983). STIa and STIb share antigenic determinants and biologically active core sequences which reside in the C-terminal amino acid residues. The central sequence of 11 amino acids in both molecules is identical; they differ in the N-terminal end of the molecule. STIa molecules have an amino acid sequence consisting of Asn-Thr-Phe-**Tyr-Cys-Cys-Glu-Leu-Cys-Cys-Asn-Pro-Ala-Cys**-Ala-**Gly-Cys-Tyr**, whereas STIb molecules have a sequence of Asn-Ser-Ser-Asn-**Tyr-Cys-Cys-Glu-Leu-Cys-Cys-Asn-Pro-Ala-Cys**-Thr-**Gly-Cys-Tyr** (Moseley *et al.*, 1983; Sekizaki *et al.*, 1985; Thompson and Giannella, 1985; Stieglitz *et al.*, 1988). ST produced by chemical synthesis behaves exactly as ST produced by ETEC.

There is a characteristic central sequence of 13 amino acids with six cysteine residues which participate in disulfide bridge formation. The tertiary structure formed by the three disulfide bonds is critical and all three disulfide bonds are required for full biological activities (Okamoto *et al.*, 1987). Interestingly, conotoxins, which are small peptides recovered from sea snail venom, have amino acid sequence similarity with the active portion of STI.

Receptor binding

The sequence of events which ends in stimulation of intestinal secretion is initiated by binding of STI to specific receptors located on brush borders of intestinal epithelial cells. Several reports suggested that the STI receptor is separate from guanylyl cyclase and is associated with molecules of a variety of sizes. Cross-linking studies involving ^{125}I-STI and intestinal epithelial brush border membranes have identified labelled proteins of 49, 56, 68, 81, 133 and 153 kDa (De-Sauvage *et al.*, 1992) and molecules of 200 kDa (one type composed of 70 kDa and 70 kDa and a second type composed of 53 kDa and 77 kDa) (Hirayama *et al.*, 1992). None of these proteins showed guanylate cyclase activity. The receptors were glycoproteins but deglycosylation of the 70-kDa protein failed to affect receptor activity and the carbohydrate moieties were therefore not considered to be important for binding of STI. Purification of the receptor by ligand-affinity chromatography identified a major receptor protein subunit of 74 kDa (Hugues *et al.*, 1992). Cross-linking of the affinity-purified material to ^{125}I-STI showed binding predominantly to the 74 kDa protein, but some labelling of 164 and 45 kDa proteins. Thus, these studies indicate heterogeneity among intestinal epithelial brush border molecules that bind STI, with a 70–74 kDa protein appearing to be the main receptor protein.

Recently, the ST receptor cDNA was cloned from rat intestine (Schulz *et al.*, 1990) and from human intestine (De-Sauvage *et al.*, 1991). The deduced amino acid sequence and functional expression in mammalian cells showed that the receptor is a transmembrane guanylyl cyclase (GC-C) belonging to the atrial natriuretic peptide receptor family. The protein is estimated to be approximately 120 kDa. It consists of an extracellular receptor domain, a transmembrane domain and cytoplasmic domains which include a kinase homology domain and a guanylyl cyclase catalytic domain at the C-terminal region. Cross-linking of ^{125}I-STI to a recombinant cell line which expressed the cloned gene for the STI receptor resulted in the labelling of proteins with molecular masses of 153, 133, 81, 68, 56 and 49 kDa (De-Sauvage *et al.*, 1992). A polyclonal antibody against the extracellular domain of the receptor immunoprecipitated two proteins of approximately 140 and 160 kDa from the recombinant cell line as well as from T84 human colonic cells which endogenously express STI binding sites. The authors concluded that GC-C was the only receptor for STI on T84 cells.

Mann *et al.* (1993) demonstrated that a homologue of GC-C was also the STI receptor in the intestinal cell line Caco-2, but they showed that another intestinal cell line, IEC-6, had a receptor for STI that was not coupled to guanylyl cyclase. Although both cells bound STI, only the Caco-2 cells showed an increase in guanylyl cyclase following exposure to toxin.

Binding of toxin is maximal in villus preparations and decreases from villus to crypt. Nucleotides regulate binding of STI and receptor as well as guanylate cyclase activity in pig and rat intestinal brush border membranes. Adenine nucleotides decreased binding but stimulated guanylate cyclase (Gazzano *et al.*, 1991; Katwa *et al.*, 1992).

Biological activity

STI activates particulate guanylate cyclase in the brush border of intestinal epithelial cells in the jejunum and ileum, thereby leading to elevation of the levels of cGMP (Field *et al.*, 1978; Hughes *et al.*, 1978). STI does not bind to particulate guanylate cyclase from tissues other than intestinal tissue because other tissues lack the specific receptor.

Robertson (1988) reported that, although younger pigs are more sensitive to STI than are older pigs, there are no differences in guanylate cyclase activity in STI-stimulated intestinal epithelial brush border membranes from 7-day-old pigs compared with membranes from 7-week-old pigs. He concluded that sensitivity to STI was not the factor which determined age susceptibility to STI-positive ETEC in pigs. These findings were confirmed by Jaso-Friedmann and co-workers (1992), who reported no difference between enterocytes of 7-day-old and 7-week-old pigs with respect to the avidity of binding of ^{125}I-STI, number of receptors or increase in intracellular concentration of cGMP in response to STI. In contrast, Cohen *et al.* (1988) examined samples of small and large intestine of children of different ages and showed that the concentration of receptors for STI decreased rapidly with age, and that increased STI-mediated stimulation of guanylate cyclase was correlated with increased receptor density.

The rate of guanylate cyclase stimulation by STI is rapid, with maximal levels of cGMP observed within 5 minutes. Elevated cGMP causes increased fluid secretion by an unknown mechanism. The end result of STI action is inhibition of Na^+-coupled Cl^- absorption in villus tips, plus stimulation of electrogenic Cl^- secretion in crypt cells, which lead to excessive fluid in the lumen of the gut (Forte *et al.*, 1992).

Interestingly, the concentration of STI receptors is 3.5 times greater in the colon, compared with the ileum, and STI stimulates guanylyl cyclase in the colon of rats, resulting in a diminished capacity for absorption of fluid (Mezoff *et al.*, 1992). Thus, it is likely, that STI-induced diarrhoea represents the combined effects of fluid secretion in the small intestine and impaired absorption in the colon.

Nutritional status of the host may affect duration of action of STI. Cohen and colleagues (1992) showed that STI-induced intestinal secretion was prolonged in malnourished rats compared with normal, control rats. Jejunal brush border membranes from both sets of rats did not differ in STI receptor density, avidity of binding or guanylyl cyclase activation. Differences were found in rate of inactivation of STI.

Receptor activation by STI sets off a cascade that culminates in release of fluid and electrolytes into the intestinal lumen. Stimulation of particulate guanylyl cyclase results in an increase in intracellular cyclic GMP, most likely due to phosphorylation of STI receptor-guanylate cyclase or a closely related protein by protein kinase C (Crane *et al.*, 1992). Following the increase in intracellular cGMP, there is elevation of intracellular calcium and activation of the phosphatidylinositol pathway (de Jonge *et al.*, 1986).

Alternative mechanisms for fluid secretion have been proposed. Release of arachidonic acid, prostaglandins and leucotrienes has been suggested to be responsible for the derangements in fluid metabolism across the intestine. 5-Hydroxytryptamine (5-HT) has also been proposed as an important mediator in STI-induced fluid secretion; support for this concept comes from studies in the rat in which antagonists of 5-HT receptors inhibited STI-induced secretion without influencing STI-induced increase in cGMP (Beubler *et al.*, 1992).

STI is rapid acting, of short duration and highly potent. In mouse intestinal loops a fluid response is evident by 30 minutes postinoculation and is maximal at 2 hours. By 8 hours, the fluid has disappeared (Hitotsubashi *et al.*, 1992a). Only 6 ng of STI is required for a positive fluid response in the mouse intestine, compared with 200 ng of STII or CT.

STI also causes changes in the myoelectric activity of the small intestine. These changes could result in a loss of normal peristaltic activity (Giannella, 1983). Roussel *et al.* (1992) noted that the duration of the migrating myoelectric complex was longer in neonatal calves with STI-induced diarrhoea.

Bioassays for STI include ligated intestine tests in rabbits or pigs and an infant mouse assay in which toxin preparations are introduced into the stomach (Dean *et al.*, 1972). Increase in cGMP may also be measured as an indicator of STI activity.

Immunology

Antibodies are produced against STI only after association of the peptide with a carrier molecule. STI produced by ETEC strains of porcine, bovine and human origin are all neutralized by antiserum against a porcine ETEC (Robertson *et al.*, 1983). By investigating the reaction of monoclonal antibodies with chemically synthesized analogues of STI, Takeda *et al.* (1993) identified an antigenic site in the N-terminus, one in the core region, and a third in the C-terminus. They found that monoclonal antibodies that recognized the N-terminal residues (which are not essential for toxic activity) were most effective in neutralizing biological activity of STI and all neutralizing monoclonals appeared to neutralize by reacting with conformation-dependent epitopes.

Substitution of the amino acid at position 11 with either arginine or lysine results in a molecule that is non-toxic but retains its ability to stimulate neutralizing antibodies (Okamoto *et al.*, 1992). Sanchez *et al.* (1988) fused the B subunit of CT with a non-toxic decapeptide that was similar to STI and expressed the fused gene in an overexpression system. Neutralizing antibodies to STI were produced in response to vaccination with the purified decapeptide-CTB protein. Similarly, Clements (1990) fused the 3′ terminus of the STI gene to the gene for LT-B and produced a hybrid protein that stimulated antibodies which neutralized STI.

An ELISA for detection of STI has been reported by several researchers. Klipstein *et al.* (1984) produced a synthetic ST which was 15 times more antigenic than native STI and used this to produce hyperimmune serum in rabbits and goats. Using this antiserum, they developed a double sandwich ELISA that detected 140 pg ml^{-1} of STI. This concentration was 1/285 of the minimum concentration detected in the infant mouse assay. Lockwood and Robertson (1984) developed a competitive ELISA for STI which was similar in the concentration of STI that could be detected.

Genetics

Genes for STI are typically found on plasmids of a wide range of molecular sizes (Gyles *et al.*, 1974; Harnett and Gyles, 1985). Among porcine and bovine ETEC it is common to find genes for STI, colonizing fimbriae, drug resistance and production of colicin on a single plasmid (Harnett and Gyles 1985). Plasmids with genes for drug resistance and STI have been reported from ETEC of human and animal origins (Gyles *et al.*, 1977; Echeverria *et al.*, 1986). STI genes may be lost from an ETEC by loss of plasmid or by deletion of a DNA segment from the plasmid. Under the selective pressure applied by K99 antibodies in the intestine, genes for K99 and for STI may be lost during infection of pigs with ETEC (Mainil *et al.*, 1987).

Genetic studies demonstrated the existence of two types of STI. A plasmid gene for STI, called STIa, was cloned from a bovine isolate of *E. coli* and shown to be part of a transposon, Tn1681, which is flanked by inverted repeats of IS1 (So and McCarthy, 1980). Subsequently, STI genes from bovine, porcine and avian ETEC were also shown to be part of the same transposon (Sekizaki *et al.*, 1985).

A DNA probe from the porcine STIa gene failed to detect many ST-producing *E. coli* isolates of human origin (Moseley *et al.*, 1980), which were subsequently detected by a second DNA probe from a different ST gene (Moseley *et al.*, 1983) . The ST detected by this second probe was called STIb. Genes for both STIa and STIb may be carried by a single strain of ETEC of human origin (Moseley *et al.*, 1983).

Nucleotide sequence data and purification of the ST product showed that the gene for STIa encoded an 18-amino-acid product and the gene for STIb encoded a 19-amino-acid product (Aimoto *et al.*, 1982; Moseley *et al.*, 1983; Takao *et al.*, 1983; Sekizaki *et al.*, 1985; Stieglitz *et al.*, 1988; Okamoto and Takahara, 1990). STIa is sometimes referred to as STp (porcine STI) but is produced by animal and human isolates. STIb is sometimes called STh (human STI) and is produced by human isolates only.

DNA sequence and other data indicate that STIa is synthesized as a 72-amino-acid precursor molecule referred to as pre-pro-STI (Stieglitz *et al.*, 1988; Okamoto and Takahara, 1990). The 72-amino-acid structure consists of a 19-amino-acid signal peptide, followed by a 35-amino-acid pro sequence, then the 18-amino-acid STI. The function of the pro region is not known but it does not appear to be involved in transport of the peptide into the extracellular environment.

Synthesis of STI by *E. coli* is subject to catabolite repression and optimal yields are obtained in glucose-free media (Alderete and Robertson, 1977; Stieglitz *et al.*, 1988).

EAST1 – a relative of STI

Enteroaggregative *E. coli* (EAggEC) are implicated in diarrhoeal disease in children (Chapter 13) and it is not known whether similar types of *E. coli* cause disease in animals. Savarino *et al.* (1993) have shown that a low-molecular-weight heat-stable enterotoxin, called EAggEC heat-stable enterotoxin 1 (EAST1), is produced by these *E. coli*. These researchers have cloned and sequenced a DNA fragment from a plasmid in an EAggEC strain and have shown that it includes an open reading frame which encodes the EAST1 toxin. The sequence data indicate that EAST1 is a 38-amino-acid peptide with four cysteine residues. The EAST1 structural gene had high homology with the gene for STI and for guanylin, an analogue of STI found in mammalian tissue.

Heat-stable enterotoxin STII (STb)

STII is a 48-amino-acid peptide with disulfide bonds between Cys-10 and Cys-48 and between Cys-21 and Cys-36 (Fujii *et al.*, 1991). Anti-STII antibodies have been produced against STII conjugated with keyhole limpet haemocyanin. The antibodies neutralize STII but fail to neutralize STI or CT (Hitotsubashi *et al.*, 1992a).

STII does not alter intracellular levels of either cAMP or cGMP; nor does it alter Na^+ or Cl^- unidirectional fluxes (Weikel *et al.*, 1986). Its mechanism of action is not known. STII has been associated with mild histological damage to intestinal epithelium and it is conceivable that such damage could be responsible for impaired absorption of fluids (Whipp *et al.*, 1987). Several researchers have observed that STI causes a net, active secretion of HCO_3, which contributes to the secretory response (Argenzio *et al.*, 1984; Weikel and Guerrant, 1985; Weikel *et al.*, 1986). One recent report showed that the level of prostaglandin E_2 was increased in the fluid that accumulated in the mouse intestine in response to STII (Hitotsubashi *et al.*, 1992a) and that inhibitors of prostaglandin synthesis reduced the fluid response to STII. These findings have led to the suggestion that prostaglandin E_2 is a mediator of the fluid response. STII has also been shown to increase motility in mouse intestine by a direct action on ileal muscle cells (Hitotsubashi *et al.*, 1992b).

A more recent report (Dreyfus *et al.*, 1993) has suggested that STII acts by opening a G-protein-linked receptor-operated calcium channel in the plasma membrane. This conclusion was based on observations of a dose-dependent increase in intracellular Ca^{2+}, which was dependent on extracellular Ca^{2+} and which could be blocked by agents which impair GTP-binding regulatory function. Elevated intracellular Ca^{2+} can activate prostaglandin endoperoxidase synthetase and lead to formation of prostaglandins from arachidonic acid.

STII is rarely the only enterotoxin expressed by porcine ETEC. A recent study on the effects of an isogenic $STII^+$ and $STII^-$ pair of F41-positive *E. coli* showed that the presence of the genes for STII made no difference in the ability of the organism to induce diarrhoea in neonatal pigs (Casey *et al.*, 1993). The researchers concluded that STII did not contribute significantly to ETEC-induced diarrhoea in neonatal pigs.

STII is rapid acting and of moderate duration. In mouse intestinal loops, purified STII elicits an observable fluid response within 30 minutes after inoculation. Fluid accumulation is maximal at about 3 hours and gradually declines until the loop is negative at 16 hours (Hitotsubashi, 1992a).

For some considerable time STII appeared to be inactive in the intestine of animals other than pigs. However, recent reports have demonstrated that STII is susceptible to inactivation by trypsin in the gut, and that if it is protected from proteolysis it is active in the intestine of rats and mice (Whipp 1987, 1990; Hitotsubashi, 1992a). This discovery of susceptibility of laboratory rodents has facilitated studies on biological activity.

Production of STII appeared to be restricted to porcine ETEC, but genes for STII were reported in *E. coli* from two of 49 cytolethal distending toxin-producing strains of *E. coli*. When DNA probes are used to sample ETEC from pigs with diarrhoea, STII is the enterotoxin gene which is most frequently detected (Moon *et al.*, 1986). Handl *et al.* (1992) in Denmark also showed a very high frequency of occurrence of STII among porcine ETEC from weaned pigs. They found that 93% of ETEC from weaned pigs were positive for STII. There is one report of STII in *E. coli* strains from humans with diarrhoea (Lortie *et al.*, 1991).

The genes which encode STII are on plasmids, which are heterogeneous and may also determine other properties including LT, STI, colonization factors, drug resistance, colicin production and transfer functions (Gyles *et al.*, 1974; Harnett and Gyles, 1985). The nucleotide sequence of the gene for STII has been reported (Lee *et al.*, 1983; Picken *et al.*, 1983). The structural gene encodes a mature protein of 48 amino acids and a signal peptide of 23 amino acids (Dreyfus *et al.*, 1992). The STII gene is part of an approximately 9-kb transposon designated Tn4521 (Lee *et al.*, 1985; Hu *et al.*, 1987; Hu and Lee, 1988).

Concluding Comments

Since their discovery in the 1960s, much knowledge has accumulated about the enterotoxins of *E. coli*. The heat-labile enterotoxin, LT-I, has been most extensively investigated and its close relationship to CT has allowed extrapolation of information from the massive body of research on CT.

Recent X-ray crystallographic studies on LT-I have been exciting and have thrown light on molecular architecture as well as structure–function relationships. There is still a need to identify more clearly the mechanisms by which this toxin causes diarrhoea and to explore further the use of toxoids as vaccines. *E. coli* STI is a fascinating peptide, whose interaction with its receptor has been the subject of investigation in several laboratories. Identification of the receptor is likely to lead to a better understanding of its mechanism of action. *E. coli* STII is the least investigated of the enterotoxins, possibly because of the almost exclusive association with ETEC of porcine origin. However, one report of its association with ETEC of human origin and new observations on its mode of action are likely to stimulate more research on STII.

References

Aimoto, S., Takao, T., Shimonishi, Y., Hara, S., Takeda, T., Takeda, Y. and Miwatani, T. (1982) Amino acid sequence of heat-stable enterotoxin produced by human enterotoxigenic *Escherichia coli. European Journal of Biochemistry* 129, 257–263.

Aitken, R. and Hirst, T.R. (1993) Recombinant enterotoxins as vaccines against *Escherichia coli*-mediated diarrhoea. *Vaccine* 11, 235–240.

Alderete, J.F. and Robertson, D.C. (1977) Repression of heat-stable enterotoxin synthesis in enterotoxigenic *Escherichia coli. Infection and Immunity* 17, 629–633.

Alderete, J.F. and Robertson, D.C. (1978) Purification and chemical characterization of the heat-stable enterotoxin produced by porcine strains of enterotoxigenic *Escherichia coli. Infection and Immunity* 19, 1021–1030.

Argenzio, R.A., Liacos, J., Berschneider, H.M., Whipp., S.C. and Robertson, D.C. (1984) Effect of heat-stable enterotoxin of *Escherichia coli* and theophylline on ion transport in porcine small intestine. *Canadian Journal of Comparative Medicine* 48, 14–22.

Beubler, E. and Horina, G. (1990) 5-HT_2 and 5-HT_3 receptor subtypes mediate cholera toxin-induced intestinal fluid secretion in the rat. *Gastroenterology* 99, 83–89.

Beubler, E., Badhri, P. and Schirgi-Degen, A. (1992) 5-HT receptor antagonists and heat-stable *Escherichia coli* enterotoxin-induced effects in the rat. *European Journal of Pharmacology* 219, 445–450.

Burgess, M.N., Bywater, R.J., Cowley, C.M., Mullan, N.A. and Newsome, P. (1978) Biological evaluation of a methanol-soluble, heat-stable *Escherichia coli* enterotoxin in infant mice, pigs, rabbits, and calves. *Infection and Immunity* 21, 526–531.

Casey, T.A., Herring, C.J. and Schneider, R.A. (1993) Expression of STb enterotoxin by adherent *E. coli* is not sufficient to cause severe diarrhea in neonatal pigs. In: *Abstracts of the 93rd Annual General Meeting of the American*

Society for Microbiology. American Society for Microbiology, Washington, DC, Abstr. B-102, p. 44.

Chapman, P.A. and Daly, C.M. (1993) Evaluation of non-radioactive trivalent DNA probe (LT, ST1a, ST1b) for detecting enterotoxigenic *Escherichia coli*. *Journal of Clinical Pathology* 46, 309–312.

Charanthia, Z., Vanmaels, R. and Armstrong, G.D. (1992) A bioassay for cholera toxin involving HT29 cells. *Journal of Microbiological Methods* 14, 171–176.

Clements, J.D. (1990) Construction of a nontoxic fusion peptide for immunization against *Escherichia coli* strains that produce heat-labile and heat-stable enterotoxins. *Infection and Immunity* 58, 1159–1166.

Clements, J.D. and Finkelstein, R.A. (1979) Isolation and characterization of homogeneous heat-labile enterotoxins with high specific activity from *Escherichia coli* cultures. *Infection and Immunity* 24, 760–769.

Clements, J.D., Yancey, R.J. and Finkelstein, R.A. (1980) Properties of homogeneous heat-labile enterotoxin from *Escherichia coli*. *Infection and Immunity* 29, 91–97.

Cohen, M.B., Guarino, A., Shukla, R. and Giannella, R.A. (1988) Age-related differences in receptors for *Escherichia coli* heat-stable enterotoxin in the small and large intestine of children. *Gastroenterology* 94, 367–373.

Cohen, M.B., Nogueira, J., Laney, D.W., Jr and Conti, T.R. (1992) The jejunal secretory response to *Escherichia coli* heat-stable enterotoxin is prolonged in malnourished rats. *Pediatric Research* 31, 228–233.

Crane, J.K., Wehner, S., Bolen, E.J., Sando, J.J., Linden, J., Guerrant, R.L. and Sears, C.L. (1992) Regulation of intestinal guanylate cyclase by the heat-stable enterotoxin of *Escherichia coli* (STa) and protein kinase C. *Infection and Immunity* 60, 5004–5012.

De, S.N. and Chatterje, D.N. (1953) An experimental study of the mechanism of action of *Vibrio cholerae* on the intestinal mucous membrane. *Journal of Pathology and Bacteriology* 66, 559–562.

Dean, A.G., Ching, Y.-C., Williams, R.G. and Harden, L.B. (1972) Test for *Escherichia coli* enterotoxin using infant mice. Application in a study of diarrhea in children in Honolulu. *Journal of Infectious Diseases* 125, 407–411.

de Jonge, H.R., Bot, A.G.M. and Vaandrager, A.B. (1986) Mechanism of action of heat-stable enterotoxin. In: Falmagne, P., Alouf, J.E., Fehrenbach, F.J., Jelijaszewics, J. and Thelestram, M. (eds) *Bacterial Protein Toxins, Second European Workshop*. Gustav Fischer, Stuttgart, pp. 335–340.

De-Sauvage, F.J., Camerato, T.R. and Goeddel, D.V. (1991) Primary structure and functional expression of receptor for *Escherichia coli* heat-stable enterotoxin. *Journal of Biological Chemistry* 266, 17912–17918.

De-Sauvage, F.J., Horuk, R., Bennett, G., Quan, C., Burnier, J.P. and Goeddel, D.V. (1992) Characterization of the recombinant human receptor for *Escherichia coli* heat-stable enterotoxin. *Journal of Biological Chemistry* 267, 6479–6482.

De Wolf, M.S.J., Fridkin, M. and Kohn, L.D. (1981) Tryptophan residues of cholera toxin and its A protomers and B protomers. Intrinsic fluorescence and solute quenching upon interacting with the ganglioside GM_1, oligo-GM_1, or dansylated oligo-GM_1. *Journal of Biological Chemistry* 256, 5489–5496.

Domeninghini, M., Montecucco, C., Ripka, W.C. and Rappuoli, R. (1991)

Computer modelling of the NAD binding site of ADP-ribosylating toxins: active-site structure and mechanism of NAD binding. *Molecular Microbiology* 5, 23–31.

Donta, S.T., Beristan, S. and Tomicic, T.K. (1993) Inhibition of heat-labile cholera and *Escherichia coli* enterotoxins by brefeldin A. *Infection and Immunity* 61, 3282–3286.

Dreyfus, L.A., Urban, R.G., Whipp, S.C., Slaughter, C., Tachias, K. and Kupersztoch, Y.M. (1992) Purification of the STb enterotoxin of *Escherichia coli* and the role of selected amino acids in its secretion, stability and toxicity. *Molecular Microbiology* 6, 2397–2406.

Dreyfus, L.A., Harville, B., Howard, D.E., Shaban, R., Beatty, D.M. and Morris, S.J. (1993) Calcium influx mediated by the *Escherichia coli* heat-stable enterotoxin b (STb). *Proceedings of the National Academy of Sciences of the United States of America* 90, 3202–3206.

Echeverria, P., Seriwatana, J., Taylor., D.N., Changchawalit, S., Smyth, C.J., Twohig, J. and Rowe, B. (1986) Plasmids coding for colonization factor antigens I and II, heat-labile enterotoxin, and heat-stable enterotoxin A2 in *Escherichia coli. Infection and Immunity* 51, 626–630.

Field, M., Graf, L.H., Jr, Laird, W.J. and Smith, P.L. (1978) Heat-stable enterotoxin of *Escherichia coli*, *in vitro* effects on guanylate cyclase activity, cyclic GMP concentration, and ion transport in small intestine. *Proceedings of the National Academy of Sciences of the United States of America* 75, 2800–2804.

Field, M., Rao, M.C. and Chang, E.B. (1989a) Intestinal electrolyte transport and diarrheal disease. I. *New England Journal of Medicine* 321, 800–806.

Field, M., Rao, M.C. and Chang, E.B. (1989b) Intestinal electrolyte transport and diarrheal disease. II. *New England Journal of Medicine* 321, 879–883.

Finck, A.D. and Katz, R.L. (1972) Prevention of cholera-induced intestinal secretion in the cat by aspirin. *Nature* 238, 273–274.

Finkelstein, R.A., Yang, Z., Moseley, S.L. and Moon, H.W. (1983) Rapid latex particle agglutination test for *Escherichia coli* strains of porcine origin producing heat-labile enterotoxin. *Journal of Clinical Microbiology* 18, 1417–1418.

Finkelstein, R.A., Burks, M.F., Zupan, A., Dallas, W.S., Jacob, C.O. and Ludwig, D.S. (1987) Epitopes of the cholera family of enterotoxins. *Reviews of Infectious Diseases* 9, 544–561.

Fishman, P.H. (1990) Mechanism of action of cholera toxin. In: Moss, J. and Vaughan, M. (eds) *ADP-ribosylating Toxins and G Proteins*. American Society for Microbiology, Washington, DC, pp. 127–140.

Forte, L.R., Thorne, P.K., Eber, S.L., Krause, W.J., Freeman, R.H., Francis, S.H. and Corbin, J.D. (1992) Stimulation of intestinal Cl^- transport by heat-stable enterotoxin: activation of cAMP-dependent protein kinase by cGMP. *American Journal of Physiology* 263, C607–615.

Fujii, Y., Hayashi, M., Hitotsubashi, S., Fuke, Y., Yamanaka, H. and Okamoto, K. (1991) Purification and characterization of *Escherichia coli* heat-stable enterotoxin II. *Journal of Bacteriology* 173, 5516–5522.

Fukuta, S., Magnani, J.L., Twiddy, E.M., Holmes, R.K. and Ginsburg, V. (1988) Comparison of the carbohydrate-binding specificities of cholera toxin, and *Escherichia coli* heat-labile enterotoxins LTh-I, LT-IIa, and LT-IIb. *Infection and Immunity* 56, 1748–1753.

Gazzano, H.H., Wu, H.I. and Waldman, S.A. (1991) Activation of particulate guanylate cyclase by *Escherichia coli* heat-stable enterotoxin is regulated by adenine nucleotides. *Infection and Immunity* 59, 1552–1557.

Giannella, R.A. (1983) *Escherichia coli* heat-stable enterotoxin: biochemical and physiological effects on the intestine. *Progress in Food and Nutritional Science* 7, 157–165.

Gilligan, P.H., Brown, J.C. and Robertson, D.C. (1983) Immunological relationships between cholera toxin and *Escherichia coli* heat-labile enterotoxin. *Infection and Immunity* 42, 683–691.

Green, B.A., Neill, R.J., Ruyechan, W.T. and Holmes, R.K. (1983) Evidence that a new enterotoxin of *Escherichia coli* which activates adenylate cyclase in eucaryotic target cells is not plasmid mediated. *Infection and Immunity* 41, 383–390.

Griffiths, S.L., Finkelstein, R.A. and Critchley, D.R. (1986) Characterization of the receptor for cholera toxin and *Escherichia coli* heat-labile toxin in rabbit intestinal brush borders. *Biochemistry Journal* 238, 313–322.

Guerrant, R.L., Brunton, L.L., Schnaitman, T.C., Rebhun, L.L. and Gilman, A.G. (1974) Cyclic adenosine monophosphate and alteration of Chinese hamster ovary cell morphology: a rapid, sensitive *in vitro* assay of the enterotoxins of *Vibrio cholerae* and *Escherichia coli*. *Infection and Immunity* 10, 320–327.

Guth, B.E.C., Twiddy, E.M., Trabulsi, L.R. and Holmes, R.K. (1986) Variation in chemical properties and antigenic determinants among type II heat-labile enterotoxins of *Escherichia coli*. *Infection and Immunity* 54, 529–536.

Gyles, C.L. and Barnum, D.A. (1967) *Escherichia coli* in ligated segments of pig intestine. *Journal of Pathology and Bacteriology* 94, 189–194.

Gyles, C.L. and Barnum, D.A. (1969) A heat-labile enterotoxin from strains of *Escherichia coli* enteropathogenic for pigs. *Journal of Infectious Diseases* 120, 419–426.

Gyles, C.L., So, M. and Falkow, S. (1974) The enterotoxin plasmids of *Escherichia coli*. *Journal of Infectious Diseases* 130, 40–49.

Gyles, C.L., Palchaudhuri, S. and Maas, W. (1977) A conjugative plasmid carrying genes for enterotoxin production and drug resistance. *Science* 198, 198–199.

Handl, C.E., Olsson, E. and Flock, J.I. (1992) Evaluation of three different STb assays and comparison of enterotoxin pattern over a five-year period in Swedish porcine *Escherichia coli*. *Diagnostic Microbiology and Infectious Disease* 15, 505–510.

Hardy, S.J.S., Holmgren, J., Johansson, S., Sanchez, J. and Hirst, T.R. (1988) Coordinated assembly of multisubunit proteins: oligomerization of bacterial enterotoxins *in vivo* and *in vitro*. *Proceedings of the National Academy of Sciences of the United States of America* 85, 7109–7113.

Harford, S., Dykes, C.W., Hobden, A.N., Read, M.J. and Halliday, I.J. (1989) Inactivation of the *Escherichia coli* heat-labile enterotoxin by *in vitro* mutagenesis of the A-subunit gene. *European Journal of Biochemistry* 183, 311–316.

Harnett, N.M. and Gyles, C.L. (1985) Linkage of genes for heat-stable enterotoxin, drug resistance, K99 antigen, and colicin in bovine and porcine strains of enterotoxigenic *Escherichia coli. American Journal of Veterinary Research* 46, 428–433.

Hirayama, T., Wada, A., Iwata, N., Takasaki, S., Shimonishi, Y. and Takeda, Y. (1992) Glycoprotein receptors for a heat-stable enterotoxin (STh) produced by enterotoxigenic *Escherichia coli. Infection and Immunity* 60, 4213–4220.

Hitotsubashi, S., Fuji, Y., Yamanaka, H. and Okamoto, K. (1992a) Some properties of purified *E. coli* heat-stable enterotoxin II. *Infection and Immunity* 60, 4468–4474.

Hitotsubashi, S., Akagi, M., Saitou, A., Yamanaka, H., Fujii, Y. and Okamoto K. (1992b) Action of *Escherichia coli* heat-stable enterotoxin II on isolated sections of mouse ileum. *Federation of European Microbiological Societies Microbiology Letters* 90, 249–252.

Hofstra, H. and Witholy, B. (1985) Heat-labile enterotoxin in *Escherichia coli.* Kinetics of association of subunits into periplasmic holotoxin. *Journal of Biological Chemistry* 260, 16037–16044.

Holmes, R.K. and Twiddy, E.M. (1983) Characterization of monoclonal antibodies that react with unique and cross-reacting determinants of cholera enterotoxin and its subunits. *Infection and Immunity* 42, 914–923.

Holmes, R.K., Twiddy, E.M. and Pickett, C.L. (1986) Purification and characterization of type II heat-labile enterotoxin of *Escherichia coli. Infection and Immunity* 53, 464–473.

Holmgren, J., Fredman, P., Lindblad, M., Svennerholm, A.-M. and Svennerholm, L. (1982) Rabbit intestinal glycoprotein receptors for *Escherichia coli* heat-labile enterotoxin lacking affinity for cholera toxin. *Infection and Immunity* 38, 424–433.

Holmgren, J., Lindblad, M., Fredman, P., Svennerholm, L. and Myrvold, H. (1985) Comparison of receptors for cholera and *Escherichia coli* enterotoxins in human intestine. *Gastroenterology* 89, 27–35.

Houghten, R.A., Engert, R.F., Ostresh, J.M., Hoffman, S.R. and Klipstein, F.A. (1985) A completely synthetic toxoid vaccine containing *Escherichia coli* heat-stable toxin and antigenic determinants of the heat-labile toxin B subunit. *Infection and Immunity* 48, 735–740.

Hu, S.T. and Lee, C.H. (1988) Characterization of the transposon carrying the STII gene of enterotoxigenic *Escherichia coli. Molecular and General Genetics* 214, 490–495.

Hu, S.T., Yang., M.K., Spandau, D.F. and Lee, C.H. (1987) Characterization of the terminal sequences flanking the transposon that carries the *Escherichia coli* enterotoxin STII gene. *Gene* 55, 157–167.

Hunt, P.D. and Hardy, S.J.S. (1991) Heat-labile enterotoxin can be released from *Escherichia coli* cells by host intestinal factors. *Infection and Immunity* 59, 168–171.

Hughes, J.M., Murad, F., Chang, B. and Guerrant, R.L. (1978). Role of cyclic GMP in the activity of heat-stable enterotoxin of *E. coli. Nature* 271, 755–756.

Hugues, M., Crane, M.R., Thomas, B.R., Robertson, D., Gazzano, H., O'Hanley, P. and Waldman, S.A. (1992) Affinity purification of functional receptors for *Escherichia coli* heat-stable enterotoxin from rat intestine. *Biochemistry* 31, 12–26.

Inoue, T., Tsuji, T., Koto, M., Imamura, S. and Miyama, A. (1993) Amino acid sequence of heat-labile enterotoxin from chicken enterotoxigenic *Escherichia coli* is identical to that of human strain H1047. *Federation of European Microbiological Societies Microbiology Letters* 108, 157–161.

Jacoby, H.I. and Marshall, C.H. (1972) Antagonism of cholera enterotoxin by anti-inflammatory agents in the rat. *Nature* 235, 163–165.

Jaso-Friedmann, L., Dreyfus, L.A., Whipp, S.C. and Robertson, D.C. (1992) Effect of age on activation of porcine intestinal guanylate cyclase and binding of *Escherichia coli* heat-stable enterotoxin to porcine intestinal cells and brush border membranes. *American Journal of Veterinary Research* 53, 2251–2258.

Katayama, S., Ninomiya, M., Minami, J., Okabe, A. and Hayashi, H. (1990). Transcriptional control plays an important role for the production of heat-labile enterotoxin in enterotoxigenic *Escherichia coli* of human origin. *Microbiology and Immunology* 34, 11–24.

Katwa, L.C., Parker, C.D., Dybing, J.K. and White, A.A. (1992) Nucleotide regulation of heat-stable enterotoxin receptor binding and of guanylate cyclase activation. *Biochemistry Journal* 283, 727–735.

Kazemi, M. and Finkelstein, R.A. (1990) Study of epitopes of cholera enterotoxin-related enterotoxins by checkerboard immunoblotting. *Infection and Immunity* 58, 2352–2360.

Klipstein, F.A., Engert, R.F., Houghten, R.A. and Rowe, B. (1984) Enzyme-linked immunosorbent assay for *Escherichia coli* heat-stable enterotoxin. *Journal of Clinical Microbiology* 19, 798–803.

Lazure, C., Seidah, N.G., Chretien, M., Lallier, R. and St Pierre, S. (1983) Primary structure determination of *Escherichia coli* heat-stable enterotoxin of porcine origin. *Canadian Journal of Biochemistry and Cell Biology* 61, 287–292.

Lee, C.H., Moseley, S.L., Moon, H.W., Whipp, S.C., Gyles, C.L. and So, M. (1983) Characterization of the gene encoding heat-stable toxin II and preliminary molecular epidemiological studies of enterotoxigenic *Escherichia coli* heat-stable toxin II. *Infection and Immunity* 42, 264–268.

Lee, C.H., Hu, S.T., Swiatek, P.J., Moseley, S.L., Allen, S.D. and So, M. (1985) Isolation of a novel transposon which carries the *Escherichia coli* enterotoxin STII gene. *Journal of Bacteriology* 162, 615–620.

Lindholm, L., Holmgren, J., Wikstrom, M., Karlsson, U., Andersson, K. and Lycke, N. (1983) Monoclonal antibodies to cholera toxin with special reference to cross-reactions with *Escherichia coli* heat-labile enterotoxin. *Infection and Immunity* 40, 570–576.

Lockwood, D.E. and Robertson, D.C. (1984) Development of a competitive enzyme-linked immunosorbent assay (ELISA) for *Escherichia coli* heat-stable enterotoxin (STa). *Journal of Immunological Methods* 75, 295–307.

London, E. (1992) How bacterial protein toxins enter cells: the role of partial unfolding in membrane translocation. *Molecular Microbiology* 6, 3277–3282.

Lortie, L.A., Dubreuil, J.D. and Harel, J. (1991) Characterization of *Escherichia coli* strains producing heat-stable enterotoxin b (STb) isolated from humans with diarrhea. *Journal of Clinical Microbiology* 29, 656–659.

Lycke, N., Tsuji, T. and Holmgren, J. (1992) The adjuvant effect of *Vibrio cholerae* and *Escherichia coli* heat-labile enterotoxins is linked to their ADP-ribosylating activity. *European Journal of Immunology* 22, 2277–2281.

Mainil, J.G., Sadowski, P.L., Tarsio, M. and Moon, H.W. (1987) *In vivo* emergence of enterotoxigenic *Escherichia coli* variants lacking genes for K99 fimbriae and heat-stable enterotoxin. *Infection and Immunity* 55, 3111–3116.

Mann, E.A., Cohen, M.B. and Giannella, R.A. (1993) Comparison of receptors for *Escherichia coli* heat-stable enterotoxin: novel receptor present in IEC-6 cells. *American Journal of Physiology* 264, G172–G178.

Marchlewicz, B.A. and Finkelstein, R.A. (1983) Immunological differences among the cholera/coli family of enterotoxins. *Diagnostic Microbiology and Infectious Disease* 1, 129–138.

Mekelanos, J.J., Collier, R.J. and Romig, W.R. (1979) Enzymic activity of cholera toxin. II. Relationships to proteolytic processing, disulfide bond reduction, and subunit composition. *Journal of Biological Chemistry* 254, 5855–5861.

Mezoff, A.G., Giannella, R.A., Eade, M.N. and Cohen, M.B. (1992) *Escherichia coli* enterotoxin (STa) binds to receptors, stimulates guanyl cyclase, and impairs absorption in rat colon. *Gastroenterology* 102, 816–822.

Moon, H.W., Sorensen, D.K. and Sautter, J.H. (1966) *Escherichia coli* infection of the ligated intestinal loop of the newborn pig. *American Journal of Veterinary Research* 27, 1317–1325.

Moon, H.W., Schneider, R.A. and Moseley, S.L. (1986) Comparative prevalence of four enterotoxin genes among *Escherichia coli* isolated from swine. *American Journal of Veterinary Research* 47, 210–212.

Moriarty, K.J. and Turnberg, L.A. (1986) Bacterial toxins and diarrhoea. *Clinics in Gastroenterology* 15, 529–543.

Moseley, S.L., Huq, M.I., Alim, A.R.M.A., So, M., Samadpour-Motalebi, M. and Falkow, S. (1980) Detection of enterotoxigenic *Escherichia coli* by DNA colony hybridization. *Journal of Infectious Diseases* 142, 892–898.

Moseley, S.L., Samadpour-Motalebi, M. and Falkow, S. (1983) Plasmid association and nucleotide sequence relationships of two genes encoding heat-stable enterotoxin production in *Escherichia coli*. *Journal of Bacteriology* 156, 441–443.

Moss, J. and Vaughan, M. (1991) Activation of cholera toxin and *Escherichia coli* heat-labile enterotoxins by ADP-ribosylation factors, a family of 20 kDa nucleotide-binding proteins. *Molecular Microbiology* 5, 2621–2627.

Moss, J., Osborne, J.C., Fishman, P.H., Brewer, H.B. Vaughan, M. and Brady, R.O. (1977) Effect of gangliosides and substrate analogues on the hydrolysis of nicotinamide adenine dinucleotide by choleragen. *Proceedings of the National Academy of Sciences of the United States of America* 74, 74–78.

Nashar, T.O., Amin, T., Marcello, A. and Hirst, T.R. (1993) Current progress in the development of the B subunits of cholera toxin and *Escherichia coli* heat-labile enterotoxin as carriers for the delivery of heterologous antigens and epitopes. *Vaccine* 11, 235–240.

Neill, R.J., Twiddy, E.M. and Holmes, R.K. (1983) Synthesis of plasmid-coded heat-labile enterotoxin in wild-type and hypertoxinogenic strains of *Escherichia coli* and in other genera of Enterobacteriaceae. *Infection and Immunity* 41, 1056–1061.

Nilsson, O., Cassuto, J., Larsson, P.A., Jodal, M., Lidberg, P., Ahlman, H., Dahlstrom, A. and Lundgren, O. (1983) 5-Hydroxytryptamine and cholera secretion: a histochemical and physiological study in cats. *Gut* 24, 542–548.

Okamoto, K. and Takahara, M. (1990) Synthesis of *Escherichia coli* heat-stable enterotoxin STp as a pre-pro form and role of the pro sequence in secretion. *Journal of Bacteriology* 172, 5260–5265.

Okamoto, K., Okamoto, K., Yukitake, J., Kawamoto, Y. and Muyama, A. (1987) Substitutions of cysteine residues of *Escherichia coli* heat-stable enterotoxin by oligonucleotide-directed mutagenesis. *Infection and Immunity* 55, 2121–2125.

Okamoto, K., Yukitake, J., Okamoto, K. and Miyama, A. (1992) Enterotoxicity and immunological properties of two mutant forms of *Escherichia coli* STIp with lysine or arginine substituted for the asparagine residue at position 11. *Federation of European Microbiological Societies Microbiology Letters* 77, 191–196.

Olson, P., Hedhammao, A., Faris, A., Krovacek, K. and Wadstrom, T. (1985) Enterotoxigenic *Escherichia coli* (ETEC) and *Klebsiella pneumoniae* isolated from dogs with diarrhoea. *Veterinary Microbiology* 10, 577–589.

Olsson, E., Smyth, C.J., Soderlind, O., Svennerholm, A.M. and Mollby, R. (1986) Development of intestinal antibodies against *Escherichia coli* antigens in piglets with experimental neonatal diarrhoea. *Veterinary Microbiology* 12, 119–133.

Peterson, J.W. and Ochoa, L.G. (1989) Role of prostaglandins and cyclic AMP in the secretory effects of cholera toxin. *Science* 245, 857–859.

Peterson, J.W., Berg, W.D. and Ochoa, L.G. (1988a) Indomethacin inhibits cholera toxin-induced cyclic AMP accumulation in Chinese hamster ovary cells. *Federation of European Microbiological Societies Microbiology Letters* 49, 187–192.

Peterson, J.W., Ochoa, L.G. and Berg, W.D. (1988b) Inhibitory effect of ibuprofen on cholera toxin-induced cyclic AMP formation in Chinese hamster ovary cells. *Federation of European Microbiological Societies Microbiology Letters* 56, 139–144.

Peterson, J.W., Jackson, C.A. and Reitmeyer, J.C. (1990) Synthesis of prostaglandins in cholera toxin-treated Chinese hamster ovary cells. *Microbial Pathogenesis* 9, 345–353.

Picken, R.N., Mazaitus, A.J., Maas, W.K., Rey, M. and Heyneker, H. (1983) Nucleotide sequence of the gene for heat-stable enterotoxin II of *Escherichia coli*. *Infection and Immunity* 42, 269–275.

Pickett, C.L., Twiddy, E.M., Coker, C. and Holmes, R.K. (1989) Cloning, nucleotide sequence, and hybridization studies of the type IIb heat-labile enterotoxin gene of *Escherichia coli*. *Journal of Bacteriology* 171, 4945–4952.

Ristaino, P.A., Levine, M.M. and Young, C.R. (1983) Improved GM_1-enzyme-linked immunosorbent assay for detection of *Escherichia coli* heat-labile enterotoxin. *Journal of Clinical Microbiology* 18, 808–815.

Robertson, D.C. (1988) Pathogenesis and enterotoxins of diarrheagenic *Escherichia coli*. In: J.A. Roth (ed.) *Virulence Mechanisms of Bacterial Pathogens*. American Society for Microbiology, Washington, DC, pp. 241–263.

Robertson, D.C., Dreyfus, L.A. and Frantz, J.C. (1983) Chemical and immunological properties of *Escherichia coli* heat-stable enterotoxins. *Progress in Food and Nutritional Science* 7, 147–156.

Roussel, A.J., Woode, G.N., Waldron, R.C., Sriranganathan, N. and Jones, M.K.

(1992) Myoelectric activity of the small intestine in enterotoxin-induced diarrhea of calves. *American Journal of Veterinary Research* 53, 1145–1148.

Sanchez, J., Svennerholm, A.M. and Holmgren, J. (1988) Genetic fusion of a non-toxic heat-stable enterotoxin-related decapeptide antigen to cholera toxin B-subunit. *Federation of European Biological Societies Letters* 241, 110–114.

Sandkvist, M., Hirst, T.R. and Bagdasarian, M. (1990) Minimal deletion of amino acids from the carboxyl terminus of the B subunit of heat-labile enterotoxin causes defects in its assembly and release from the cytoplasmic membrane of *Escherichia coli. Journal of Biological Chemistry* 265, 15239–15244.

Savarino, S.J., Fasano, A., Watson, J., Martin, B.M., Levine, M.M., Guandalini, S. and Guerry, P. (1993) Enteroaggregative *Escherichia coli* heat-stable enterotoxin 1 represents another subfamily of *E. coli* heat-stable toxin. *Proceedings of the National Academy of Sciences of the United States of America* 90, 3093–3097.

Schengrund, C.L. and Ringler, N.J. (1989) Binding of *Vibrio cholera* toxin and the heat-labile enterotoxin of *Escherichia coli* to GM1, derivatives of GM1, and nonlipid oligosaccharide polyvalent ligands. *Journal of Biological Chemistry* 264, 13233–13237.

Schulz, S., Green, C.K., Yuen, P.S.T. and Garbers, D.L. (1990) Guanylyl cyclase is a heat-stable enterotoxin receptor. *Cell* 63, 941–948.

Sekizaki, T., Akashi, H. and Terakado, N. (1985) Nucleotide sequences of the genes for *Escherichia coli* heat-stable enterotoxin I of bovine, avian, and porcine origins. *American Journal of Veterinary Research* 46, 909–912.

Seriwatana, J., Echeverria, P., Taylor, D.N., Rasrinaul, L., Brown, J.E., Peiris, J.S. and Clayton, C.L. (1988) Type II heat-labile enterotoxin-producing *Escherichia coli* isolated from animals and humans. *Infection and Immunity* 56, 1158–1161.

Sillerud, L.O., Prestegard, J.H., Yu, R.K., Konigsmerg, W.H. and Shafer, D.E. (1981) Observation by ^{13}C NMR of interactions between cholera toxin and the oligosaccharide of ganglioside GM_1. *Journal of Biological Chemistry* 256, 1094–1097.

Sixma, T.K., Pronk, S.E., Kalk, K.H., Wartna, E.S., van Zanten, B.A.M., Witholt, B. and Hol, W.G.J. (1991) Crystal structure of a cholera toxin-related heat-labile enterotoxin from *E. coli. Nature (London)* 351, 371–377.

Sixma, T.K., Pronk, S.E., Kalk, K.H., van Zanten, B.A., Berghuis, A.M. and Hol, W.G. (1992) Lactose binding to heat-labile enterotoxin revealed by X-ray crystallography. *Nature (London)* 355, 561–564.

Sixma, T.K., Kalk, K.H., van Zanten, B.A., Dauter, Z., Kingma, J., Witholt, B. and Hol, W.G. (1993a) Refined structure of *Escherichia coli* heat-labile enterotoxin, a close relative of cholera toxin. *Journal of Molecular Biology* 230, 890–918.

Sixma, T.K., Stein, P.E., Hol, W.G. and Read, R.J. (1993b) Comparison of the B-pentamers of heat-labile enterotoxin and verotoxin-1: two structures with remarkable similarity and dissimilarity. *Biochemistry* 32, 191–198.

Smith, H.W. and Gyles, C.L. (1970) The relationship between two apparently different enterotoxins produced by enteropathogenic strains of *Escherichia coli* of porcine origin. *Journal of Medical Microbiology* 3, 387–401.

Smith, H.W. and Halls, S. (1967a) Observations by the ligated intestinal segment and oral inoculation methods on *Escherichia coli* infections in pigs, calves, lambs and rabbits. *Journal of Pathology and Bacteriology* 93, 499–529.

Smith, H.W. and Halls, S. (1967b) Studies on *Escherichia coli* enterotoxin. *Journal of Pathology and Bacteriology* 93, 531–543.

So, M. and McCarthy, B.J. (1980) Nucleotide sequence of the bacterial transposon Tn1681 encoding a heat-stable (ST) toxin and its identification in enterotoxigenic *Escherichia coli* strains. *Proceedings of the National Academy of Sciences of the United States of America* 77, 4011–4015.

Spangler, B.D. (1992) Structure and function of cholera toxin and the related *Escherichia coli* heat-labile enterotoxin. *Microbiological Reviews* 56, 622–647.

Stephen, J. and Osborne, M.P. (1988) Pathophysiological mechanisms in diarrhoeal disease. In: Donachie, W., Griffiths, E. and Stephen, J. (eds) *Bacterial Infections of Respiratory and Gastrointestinal Mucosae*. IRL Press, Oxford, pp. 149–170.

Stieglitz, H., Cervantes, L., Robledo, R., Covarrubias, L., Bolivar, F. and Kupersztoch, Y.M. (1988) Cloning, sequencing and expression in Ficoll generated minicells of an *Escherichia coli* heat-stable enterotoxin gene. *Plasmid* 20, 42–53.

Streatfield, S.J., Sandkvist, M., Sixma, T.K., Bagdasarian, M., Hol, W.G. and Hirst, T.R. (1992) Intermolecular interactions between the A and B subunits of heat-labile enterotoxin from *Escherichia coli* promote holotoxin assembly and stability *in vivo*. *Proceedings of the National Academy of Sciences of the United States of America* 89, 12140–12144.

Sugarman, B. and Epps, L.R. (1984) Zinc and the heat-labile enterotoxin of *Escherichia coli*. *Journal of Medical Microbiology* 18, 393–398.

Takao, T., Hitouji, T., Aimoto, S., Shimonishi, Y., Hara, S., Takeda, T., Takeda, Y. and Miwatani, T. (1983) Amino acid sequence of a heat-stable enterotoxin isolated from enterotoxigenic *Escherichia coli* strain 18D. *FEBS Letters* 152, 1–5.

Takeda, Y., Honda, T., Sima, H., Tsuji, T. and Miwatani, T. (1983a) Analysis of antigenic determinants in cholera enterotoxin and heat-labile enterotoxins from human and porcine enterotoxigenic *Escherichia coli*. *Infection and Immunity* 41, 50–53.

Takeda, Y., Honda, T. and Miwatani, T. (1983b) The use of the Biken test to detect enterotoxigenic '*Escherichia coli*' producing heat-labile enterotoxin. *Developments in Biological Standardization* 53, 113–121.

Takeda, T., Nair, G.B., Suzuki, K., Zhe, H.X., Yokoo, Y., De-Mol, P., Hemelhof, W., Butzler, J.P., Takeda, Y. and Shimonishi, Y. (1993) Epitope mapping and characterization of antigenic determinants of heat-stable enterotoxin (STh) of enterotoxigenic *Escherichia coli* by using monoclonal antibodies. *Infection and Immunity* 61, 289–294.

Thompson, M.R. and Giannella, R.A. (1985) Revised amino acid sequence for a heat-stable enterotoxin produced by an *Escherichia coli* strain (18D) that is pathogenic for humans. *Infection and Immunity* 47, 834–836.

Tsuji, T., Honda, T. and Miwatani, T. (1984) Comparison of effects of nicked and unnicked *Escherichia coli* heat-labile enterotoxin on Chinese hamster ovary cells. *Infection and Immunity* 46, 94–97.

Tsuji, T., Honda, T., Miwatani, T., Wakabayashi, S. and Matsubara, H. (1985)

Analysis of receptor-binding site in *Escherichia coli* enterotoxin. *Journal of Biological Chemistry* 260, 8552–8558.

Violle, H. and Crendiropoullo. (1915) Note on experimental cholera. *Comptes Rendus des Séances Societé de Biologie, Paris* 78, 331–332.

Wasteson, Y., Olsvik, O., Skancke, E., Bopp, C.A. and Fossum, K. (1988) Heat-stable-enterotoxin-producing *Escherichia coli* strains isolated from dogs. *Journal of Clinical Microbiology* 26, 2564–2566.

Weikel, C.S. and Guerrant, R.L. (1985) STb enterotoxin of *Escherichia coli* cyclic nucleotide-independent secretion. *Ciba Foundation Symposium* 112, 94–115.

Weikel, C.S., Nellans, H.N. and Guerrant, R.L. (1986) *In vivo* and *in vitro* effects of a novel enterotoxin, STb, produced by *Escherichia coli. Journal of Infectious Diseases* 153, 893–901.

Whipp, S.C. (1987) Protease degradation of *Escherichia coli* heat-stable, mouse-negative, pig-positive enterotoxin. *Infection and Immunity* 55, 2057–2060.

Whipp, S.C. (1990) Assay for enterotoxigenic *Escherichia coli* heat-stable toxin b in rats and mice. *Infection and Immunity* 58, 930–934.

Whipp, S.C., Kokue, E., Morgan, R.W. and Moon, H.W. (1987) Functional significance of histologic alterations induced by *Escherichia coli* heat-stable, mouse-negative, pig-positive enterotoxin (STb). *Veterinary Research Communications* 11, 41–55.

Wilson, A.D., Robinson, A., Irons, L. and Stokes, C.R. (1993) Adjuvant action of cholera toxin and pertussis toxin in the induction of IgA antibody response to orally administered antigen. *Vaccine* 11, 113–118.

Woodward, M.J., Carroll, P.J. and Wray, C. (1992) Detection of entero- and verocyto-toxin genes in *Escherichia coli* from diarrhoeal disease in animals using the polymerase chain reaction. *Veterinary Microbiology* 31, 251–261.

Yam, W.C., Lung, M.L. and Ng, M.H. (1992) Evaluation and optimization of a latex agglutination assay for detection of cholera toxin and *Escherichia coli* heat-labile enterotoxin. *Journal of Clinical Microbiology* 30, 2518–2520.

Yamamoto, T. and Yokota, T. (1983) Sequence of heat-labile enterotoxin of *Escherichia coli* pathogenic for humans. *Journal of Bacteriology* 155, 728–733.

Yamamoto, T., Tamura, T. and Yokota, T. (1984) Primary structure of heat-labile enterotoxin produced by *Escherichia coli* pathogenic for humans. *Journal of Biological Chemistry* 259, 5037–5044.

Yoh, M., Yamomoto, K., Honda, T., Takeda, Y. and Miwatani, T. (1983) Effects of lincomycin and tetracycline on production and properties of enterotoxins of enterotoxigenic *Escherichia coli. Infection and Immunity* 42, 778–782.

Escherichia coli Verotoxins and Other Cytotoxins

15

C.L. Gyles
Department of Veterinary Microbiology and Immunology, University of Guelph, Guelph, Ontario, Canada N1G 2W1

Verotoxins

Introduction

The name verotoxin (VT) was introduced into the literature in 1977 by Konowalchuk and colleagues who used the term to refer to an *E. coli* cytotoxin which was lethal for cultured Vero (African green monkey kidney) cells. In a study of 136 *E. coli* isolates, Konowalchuk *et al.* (1977) noted that ten were VT-positive and that seven of the ten were enteropathogenic *E. coli* (EPEC) associated with diarrhoeal disease in humans, one was an isolate from diarrhoea in pigs, and two were from food of animal origin. At about the same time, O'Brien and co-workers (in a preliminary report in 1977 and a full report in 1982) reported their discovery that certain EPEC strains produced a cytotoxin that was lethal for cultured HeLa cells. This *E. coli* cytotoxin shared a number of properties with Shiga toxin, namely the ability to inhibit protein synthesis in HeLa cells, enterotoxicity in rabbit intestine, and lethality for mice, and was therefore called Shiga-like toxin (SLT). Both groups of researchers suggested that VT (SLT) might play a role in diarrhoeal disease.

EPEC strain H30 was common to the investigations by both groups of researchers (Konowalchuk *et al.*, 1977; O'Brien *et al.*, 1982). One group had shown this strain to be VT positive and the other had demonstrated that it was SLT positive. Shortly afterwards, O'Brien and LaVeck (1983) purified SLT and demonstrated that Shiga toxin, produced by *Shigella dysenteriae*, and SLT produced by *E. coli* strain H30 were identical in physicochemical characteristics and biological properties.

Antigenic heterogeneity among verotoxins was recognized in the very first study by Konowalchuk and co-workers (1977). They showed that verotoxin produced by one porcine and one human *E. coli* isolate was not neutralized by antiserum which neutralized the VT of strain H30 and other strains of human origin. In the mid 1980s antigenic heterogeneity among VTs was rediscovered and examined more thoroughly. Several research groups characterized two antigenic types of VT (Scotland *et al.*, 1985; Karmali *et al.*, 1986; Strockbine *et al.*, 1986), called VT1 and VT2 (Scotland *et al.*, 1985), or SLTI and SLTII (Strockbine *et al.*, 1986). Subsequently, other antigenic types of SLT, all related to SLTII, were identified (Marques *et al.*, 1987; Gannon *et al.*, 1990; Ito *et al.*, 1990).

It is now evident that VTs consist of two groups, with VT1 (SLTI) constituting one group and VT2 (SLTII) and antigenically related toxins constituting a second group. Cytotoxicity of VT1 or SLTI is neutralized by antiserum to Shiga toxin or anti-VT1 toxin, but not by antiserum against VT2 (O'Brien *et al.*, 1982; Downes *et al.*, 1988; Head *et al.*, 1988). The limited immunological cross-reactivity between VT1 and VT2 is remarkable. Ito and co-workers (1988) found that neither anti-VT1 nor anti-VT2 hyperimmune serum detected the heterologous toxin in an enzyme-linked immunosorbent assay that detected as little as 20 pg of toxin per ml. However, monoclonal antibodies have been produced that react with the A subunits of VT1 and VT2 (Padhye *et al.*, 1989). Cytotoxicity of VT2 and antigenically related VTs is not neutralized by anti-Shiga toxin or anti-VT1 antiserum but there is cross-neutralization among members of this group of VTs. Members of group II include VT2 (SLTII), VT2c (SLTIIc) and SLTII variant (previously SLTIIv, now SLTIIe or VT2e), which is implicated in oedema disease of pigs (Smith *et al.*, 1983; Marques *et al.*, 1987; Gannon *et al.*, 1988; MacLeod *et al.*, 1991b). This toxin was called a variant because, unlike SLTII, it is inactive or weakly active on HeLa cells. SLTIIva (VT2d or SLTIId) is another variant, which is produced by an O128:B12 *E. coli* (strain H.I.8) recovered from diarrhoea in an infant (Konowalchuk *et al.*, 1977; Gannon *et al.*, 1990). The classification of these toxins into two groups, based on toxin neutralization, is supported by nucleotide sequence data. The SLT and VT systems of nomenclature for clearly characterized verotoxins and for the genes which encode them are shown in Table 15.1 and the two terms can now be used interchangeably.

Structure

Verotoxins have an A–B subunit structure, which has been determined by the identity of VT1 with Shiga toxin (Takao *et al.*, 1988), for which this structural organization has been clearly demonstrated (Donohue-Rolfe *et al.*, 1984), by nucleotide sequence data (De Grandis *et al.*, 1987; Gyles *et al.*, 1988; Weinstein *et al.*, 1988b; Gannon *et al.*, 1990) and by studies on purified toxins (O'Brien and LaVeck, 1983; Yutsudo *et al.*, 1987;

Table 15.1. Nomenclature[a] for verotoxins and Shiga-like toxins and the genes which encode them.

Gene product		Gene encoding cytotoxin	Reference strain(s)
SLT terminology	VT terminology		
SLT-I	VT1	*slt*-I	H19, H30
SLT-II	VT2	*slt*-II	933w, C600(pEB1)
SLT-IIv	VT2e	*slt*-IIv	412, S1191
SLT-IIc	VT2c	*slt*-IIc	E32511, B2F1, 7279
SLT-IId	VT2d	*slt*-IId	H.I.8

[a] The nomenclature for SLT-IId is proposed by the author.

Downes *et al.*, 1988; Ito *et al.*, 1988; Takao *et al.*, 1988; Oku *et al.*, 1989; MacLeod and Gyles, 1990; Head *et al.*, 1991). VTs all consist of an A subunit of approximately 33 kDa and several B subunits of approximately 7.5 kDa each. Cross-linking studies have shown that, in Shiga toxin, five B subunits are associated with each A subunit (Donohue-Rolfe *et al.*, 1984). X-ray crystallography has shown that a similar arrangement holds for VT1 (Stein *et al.*, 1992) and it is likely that an identical arrangement holds for the other VTs. Although VT1 and VT2 differ substantially in amino acid sequences, hybrid toxins formed by reassociation of VT1 B subunits with VT2 A subunits and of VT2 B subunits with VT1 A subunits are fully functional (Ito *et al.*, 1988; Head *et al.*, 1991).

The A subunit is the portion of the toxin molecule which possesses biological activity. Proteolysis and reduction of a disulfide bond convert the A subunit of Shiga toxin or VT into a large N-terminal A_1 fragment, which possesses enzymatic activity, and a small C-terminal A_2 fragment (Olsnes *et al.*, 1981; MacLeod *et al.*, 1991a). The A subunits of Shiga toxin and VT1 isolated from the bacteria may be in the nicked (O'Brien and LaVeck, 1983; MacLeod and Gyles, 1990) or unnicked form (Yutsudo *et al.*, 1987; Ito *et al.*, 1988).

The B subunit contains the binding site of the toxin molecule and is involved in binding VT to a glycolipid receptor in cell membranes. Stein *et al.* (1992) determined the crystal structure of the B subunit of VT1 and observed that the folding was very similar to that of the B oligomer of *E. coli* heat-labile enterotoxin (LT). Like LT, the B subunit pentamer is arranged to form a central pore, but, unlike LT, the pore is lined by neutral and non-polar amino acids. By analysing the amino acid sequences of VT1, VT2 and VT2e and locating the invariant residues on the VT1 B subunit pentamer, they identified a conserved cleft between adjacent B monomers and proposed that these may constitute five carbohydrate-binding sites on each pentamer. Their conclusions are supported by data from site-directed mutagenesis studies (Jackson *et al.*, 1990b).

Internalization of the toxin is believed to be effected by receptor-mediated endocytosis, followed by fusion with lysosomes, translocation to the Golgi apparatus and transfer to the cytosol (Sandvig *et al.*, 1992). Presumably, cleavage and reduction of the A subunit releases the enzymatically active A_1 fragment.

Physicochemical features

VTs are all heat-labile proteins, but there are differences among VTs in the degree of heat lability (Gannon and Gyles, 1990; MacLeod *et al.*, 1991a). VT2e is the most heat labile, and is completely inactivated after exposure to 65°C for 30 minutes; VT2d (SLTIIva) is the most heat resistant and shows no loss in activity after exposure to 75°C for 60 minutes. VT1 and VT2 are intermediate in their heat lability. VT2e loses cytotoxic activity after exposure to 2-mercaptoethanol or dithiothreitol, indicating that disulfide linkages in the intact molecule are critical for biological activity. VT2e is stable between pH 6 and 11 and its cytotoxicity is enhanced after exposure to trypsin (MacLeod *et al.*, 1991a).

The verotoxin molecules have a wide range of isoelectric points (pIs). Their respective pIs are: VT1, 7.0; VT2, 4.1 or 5.1; VT2e, 9.0 (O'Brien and LaVeck, 1983; Downes *et al.*, 1988; MacLeod *et al.*, 1991a). The high pI of VT2e raises the possibility that it may readily interact with surfaces on the basis of charge as well as receptor interactions.

Both the Shiga toxin of *S. dysenteriae* and the verotoxins of *E. coli* appear to occupy a periplasmic location in the bacterium (Donohue-Rolfe and Keusch, 1983; MacLeod and Gyles, 1989; MacLeod *et al.*, 1991a), but there are differences among the toxins with respect to their secretion. VT1 is highly cell associated, whereas VT2 is less highly cell associated (Strockbine *et al.*, 1986). There are conflicting reports on secretion of VT2e. Weinstein *et al.* (1989) have reported that VT2e is secreted to the exterior of the cell and that the B subunit is responsible for secretion. On the other hand, Macleod and Gyles (1989, 1990) have shown that VT2e is not secreted to any significant extent. It is possible that strain differences or differences in culture conditions may influence release of VTs from the periplasm. Subinhibitory concentrations of certain antibiotics have been shown to increase the secretion of VT1 *in vitro* (Walterspiel *et al.*, 1992).

Biological activities

Biological activities common to all VTs include cytotoxicity for Vero cells, lethality for mice and enterotoxicity in rabbit intestine. Following exposure to VTs, Vero cells take on a round, shrivelled appearance, which becomes evident at around 24 hours and is maximal at 3–4 days (Konowalchuk *et al.*, 1977). Vero cell cytotoxicity is the basis of the Vero cell assay that measures the cytotoxic effect (detachment of killed cells from monolayers) and is in widespread use for detection of VTs. In this test, one 50%-cytotoxic dose is given by approximately 1 pg of toxin. A similar CD_{50} value has been reported for VT1 and VT2 on HeLa cells (O'Brien and LaVeck, 1983; Downes *et al.*, 1988). A more rapid and sensitive assay is based on direct measurement of inhibition of protein synthesis by VTs. Inhibition of protein synthesis is detectable as early as 1 hour after exposure of Vero cells to toxin and permits detection of as little as 1 fg of toxin (MacLeod *et al.*, 1991a).

The receptor for VT1 and VT2 is globotriosyl ceramide (Gb3) (Lingwood *et al.*, 1987; Waddell *et al.*, 1988) whereas the preferred receptor for VT2e is globotetraosyl ceramide (Gb4) (De Grandis *et al.*, 1989; Samuel *et al.*, 1990). The minimum structure necessary for binding VT1 or VT2 is the terminal gal-$\alpha(1\rightarrow4)$-gal disaccharide; a terminal GalNAc residue $\beta(1\rightarrow3)$ linked to galactose is necessary for binding of VT2e. Susceptibility of a variety of cell lines to VTs has been shown to be related to presence or absence of the glycolipid receptor in the cell surface, indicating that these receptors are functionally significant. Waddell *et al.* (1990) used glycolipid incorporation experiments to demonstrate that Gb3 alone was a functional receptor for VT1. Distribution and concentration of the specific receptors in various tissues and in various animal species appear to be responsible for differences in target organs, and remarkable differences in susceptibility of various cell lines and tissues (Richardson *et al.*, 1992). For example, VT1, VT2 and VT2e are highly toxic for Vero cells, but VT2e is only weakly toxic for HeLa (cervical carcinoma) cells, whereas VT1 and VT2 are highly toxic for HeLa cells. These findings are explained by the observations that VT1 and VT2 bind to Gb3 whereas VT2e binds preferentially to Gb4 and that Vero cells contain similar levels of Gb3 and Gb4, whereas HeLa cells contain primarily Gb3 and little or no Gb4. Similarly, Madin–Darby bovine kidney (MDBK) cells that contain higher levels of Gb4 compared with Gb3 are significantly more susceptible to VTe than to VT1 and VT2 (DeGrandis *et al.*, 1989; Gannon and Gyles, 1990).

Binding affinity and binding to insusceptible cells may affect transport of verotoxin through the body and its availability for susceptible cells. For example, VT1 has greater binding affinity for Gb3 than does VT2 (Head *et al.*, 1991; Tesh *et al.*, 1993) and it has been suggested that the difference in binding affinity may enhance systemic spread of VT2, since it is less likely to bind to low levels of Gb3 present in intestinal epithelium. Also, binding of VT to P1 blood group antigen on mature red blood cells which do not undertake protein synthesis may reduce the amount of absorbed toxin that binds to susceptible vascular endothelial cells. Taylor *et al.*

(1990) have suggested that individuals who lack the P blood group antigen or express it poorly may be at greater risk for HUS than individuals who express this antigen well on red blood cells.

Vascular endothelial cells appear to be the host cells that are affected by VTs *in vivo* and the signs and symptoms of disease can be related to damage to these cells in target tissues (Kavi *et al.*, 1987; Karmali, 1989; MacLeod *et al.*, 1991a; Tesh *et al.*, 1991). Interestingly, there may be some species specificity in the action of VTs on vascular endothelium. VT2e is markedly more active on vascular endothelial cells of porcine origin than on similar cells of bovine origin (A. Valdivieso-Garcia and R.C. Clarke, Agriculture Canada, Guelph, 1993, personal communication). In experimental studies in rabbits, Richardson *et al.* (1992) used immunofluorescent staining to localize intravenously administered VT1 and showed that the highest levels of toxin were associated with binding to vascular endothelium in spinal cord, brain, caecum and colon, the tissues in which vascular lesions were observed. The underlying lesion in each organ was thrombotic microangiopathy. Some effects observed after exposure to VTs are likely to be secondary to the damage to endothelial cells. For example, VT-mediated decrease in synthesis of prostacyclin by endothelial cells (Karch *et al.*, 1988) may be responsible for inhibition of platelet aggregating activity, reported by Rose *et al.* (1985).

VTs are all lethal for mice, but appear to differ in the 50% lethal dose (LD_{50}). VT1 is less potent than VT2 in tests for mouse lethality. The LD_{50} dose for mice, by the intraperitoneal route, is 0.1–2 μg for VT1 (O'Brien and LaVeck, 1983; O'Brien and Holmes, 1987; Petric *et al.*, 1987; Tesh *et al.*, 1993) but 1.0 ng for VT2 (Tesh *et al.* 1993). In direct comparisons, the LD_{50} for VT2 has been reported to be 100–400 times less than that for VT1 (Gannon and Gyles, 1990; Tesh *et al.*, 1993). The mouse LD_{50} for VT2c is 2.7 ng (Oku *et al.*, 1989) and that for VT2e was approximately ten times less than for VT1 (Gannon and Gyles, 1990). Tesh *et al.* (1993) have shown that VT2 is more stable than VT1 and have suggested that greater potency may be due to greater resistance to intracellular processing or degradation.

Interestingly, in 1960 Gregory had demonstrated that extracts of *E. coli* from oedema disease of pigs were lethal for mice. This researcher, as well as Timoney (1960), had also noted the similarities between oedema disease toxin and Shiga toxin of *S. dysenteriae*.

Hind limb paralysis is often observed in mice and rabbits inoculated with VT and it is presumed that damage to the central nervous system is responsible for death. Although there is no direct evidence to support this supposition, appearance of extensive focal haemorrhagic capillary lesions and oedema in the brain in response to VTs in rabbits and pigs (Barrett *et al.*, 1989; MacLeod *et al.*, 1991b; Richardson *et al.*, 1992) is consistent with death due to central nervous system damage. Apparently, guinea pigs are refractory to VT2e (Schimmelpfennig and Weber, 1979).

VTs induce fluid accumulation in ligated segments of rabbit intestine and are therefore considered to be enterotoxic. Furthermore, the closely related Shiga toxin has been shown to be cytotoxic for human colonic and ileal epithelial cells in primary culture (Moyer *et al.*, 1987). Intragastric administration of VT to infant rabbits in controlled experiments has shown that diarrhoea and morphological changes, predominantly in the large intestine, are attributable to the toxin (Pai *et al.*, 1986). VT-mediated lesions in the large intestine have also been noted in response to toxin deposited in ligated segments of rabbit intestine (Keenan *et al.*, 1986) or administered intravenously (Barrett *et al.*, 1989). Interestingly, intestinal lesions are observed in the terminal ileum and colon of pigs following intravenous administration of VT2e to pigs but not after intraintestinal administration of toxin (MacLeod *et al.*, 1991a; Waddell and Gyles, 1993).

Several studies have been conducted to determine the mechanism by which VTs are enterotoxic. There is no alteration in levels of adenylyl cyclase or guanylyl cyclase in enterocytes in rabbits injected intraintestinally with VT. One suggested basis for fluid accumulation is impaired absorption caused by damage to and premature expulsion of mature columnar absorptive enterocytes at the tips of villi (Keenan *et al.*, 1986). It is likely that this contributes to enterotoxicity, but it is not clear whether there is a direct toxic effect of toxin on enterocytes, as suggested by Keenan and associates (1986). In support of a direct effect on intestinal epithelium, Kandel and colleagues (1989) have convincingly shown that Shiga toxin affects intestinal electrolyte transport in rabbit jejunal epithelium, causing an inhibition in absorption of NaCl, but no alteration in active anion secretion. They also demonstrated that villus cells, with more toxin binding sites, were more susceptible to inhibition of protein synthesis by Shiga toxin than were crypt cells. Other indirect mechanisms may also be involved since damage to villus epithelial cells is observed when VT2e is administered intravenously to pigs. The damage to epithelial cells appears to be the result of damage to the underlying vasculature (MacLeod *et al.*, 1991b). Furthermore, increased permeability of blood vessels could permit loss of fluids and cells into the lumen.

VT2e is poorly enterotoxic compared with the other VTs and pig intestine does not seem to respond to VTs with a fluid response as seen in rabbit intestine (Gannon and Gyles 1990; MacLeod *et al.*, 1991a). In the earliest tests of crude VT-positive preparations, VT from oedema disease strains of *E. coli* was found to have no enterotoxic effect in rabbit intestine (Konowalchuck *et al.*, 1977; Kashiwazaki *et al.*, 1980; Blanco *et al.*, 1983). However, failure was likely to be due to the use of insufficient quantities of toxin. MacLeod and Gyles (1990) used purified VT2e to induce fluid accumulation in rabbit intestine, but required a dose (75 μg) that was approximately 75 times the dose of VT1 or VT2. Diarrhoea is seen in some outbreaks of oedema disease in pigs but many strains of oedema disease *E. coli* are also enterotoxigenic; the diarrhoea could therefore be the result of enterotoxins produced by the *E. coli*. It is noteworthy that in experimental reproduction of oedema disease, Smith and Halls (1968) observed that diarrhoea preceded oedema disease when they used a strain that produced both VTe and enterotoxins.

Mechanism of action

Verotoxins inhibit protein synthesis in eukaryotic cells as a result of RNA *N*-glycosidase activity (Igarashi *et al.*, 1987; Endo *et al.*, 1988; Ogasawara *et al.*, 1988; Saxena *et al.*, 1989; Furutani *et al.*, 1990). The toxins cleave a specific *N*-glycosidic bond in 28S ribosomal RNA in 60S ribosomal subunits, thereby releasing a single adenine residue and preventing elongation-factor-1-dependent binding of aminoacyl-tRNA to ribosomes. The mechanism of action is the same as that of the plant toxin ricin (Igarashi *et al.*, 1987; Saxena *et al.*, 1989).

Identification of the active site of the VT molecule has been aided by comparison of the amino acid sequences of the A subunits of ricin and VTs. This comparison has shown that there are two regions of high homology (Hovde *et al.*, 1988; Jackson, 1990). X-ray crystallography of the ricin molecule demonstrated that these two regions lie within a cleft in the A chain which probably contains the active site of the molecule (Montfort *et al.*, 1987; Frankel *et al.*, 1989). Alterations in enzymatic activity resulting from changes in specific amino acids within these regions were investigated but did not provide conclusive data (Hovde *et al.*, 1988; Frankel *et al.*, 1989; Schlossman *et al.*, 1989; Jackson *et al.*, 1990a). Yamasaki *et al.* (1991) identified three regions that were conserved among A subunit molecules of VTs and ricin and noted that these regions were parts of the active site of the ricin molecule suggested by X-ray crystal diffraction. They carried out site-specific mutagenesis and determined that both glutamic acid 167 and arginine 170 of the A subunit of VT1 were important for enzymatic activity.

Jackson *et al.* (1990b) compared amino acid sequences of VT1, VT2 and VT2e and subjected certain conserved regions in the B subunit to site-specific mutagenesis. They demonstrated that a hydrophilic region near the N-terminus of the B subunit was involved in receptor binding and that a glutamine residue near the C-terminus was involved in extracellular localization. Perera *et al.* (1991) identified three amino acid residues in the B subunit of VT2 that were essential for toxin activity.

Binding of VT to its functional receptor is a critical aspect of its action on cells. In 1987, Lindberg *et al.* (1987) demonstrated that ^{125}I-Shiga toxin bound to glycolipids that contained Galα1-4Galβ (galabiose), located terminally or internally in oligosaccharides. In Keusch's laboratory, researchers examined the binding of ^{125}I-labelled Shiga toxin (equivalent to VT1) to separated glycolipids from microvillus membranes of enterocytes of rabbits of different ages and determined that toxin bound to Gb3, which was present in enterocytes from rabbits 20 days of age or older but not in younger rabbits (reviewed by Keusch *et al.*, 1991). The appearance of Gb3 in enterocyte membranes at around 20 days coincides with susceptibility of the rabbits to the enterotoxic action of Shiga toxin. Binding of Shiga toxin has also been demonstrated with purified glycolipids. Similar studies in Lingwood's laboratory demonstrated that VT2 bound specifically to Gb3 (Lingwood *et al.*, 1987; Waddell *et al.*, 1988).

Genetics

The genes for VT1 and VT2 are carried by temperate bacteriophages (Scotland *et al.*, 1983; Smith *et al.*, 1983, 1988). Isolation of bacteriophage particles and extraction of their DNA facilitated the cloning and nucleotide sequence determination for VT1 (Huang *et al.*, 1986; De Grandis *et al.*, 1987; Jackson *et al.*, 1987b). The VT1 operon includes two open reading frames which code for an A subunit and a smaller B subunit. Analyses of the nucleotide sequences for VTs indicate that A and B subunits are independently translated, since ribosomal binding sites precede the genes for both subunits. The deduced amino acid sequence of VT1 is not significantly different from that of Shiga toxin. Calderwood *et al.* (1987) and Strockbine *et al.* (1988) found that they differed by one amino acid in the B subunit. Takao *et al.* (1988) reported that the sequences were identical. Jackson *et al.* (1987a) determined the nucleotide sequence for VT2 from *E. coli* strain 933 and made comparisons with the sequences for VT1. The structural genes for the two toxins shared 57% nucleotide sequence homology in their A subunit genes and 60% in their B subunit genes.

The genes for VT2e appear not to be associated with bacteriophages (Smith *et al.*, 1983; Marques *et al.*, 1987). Smith *et al.* (1983) were able to transfer the genes for VT2e from an O141:K85,K88 strain of *E. coli* to *E. coli* K-12 by growing the two organisms together in broth. Subsequent investigation showed that the transferred genes were chromosomal and that transfer was associated with DNA rearrangements in the recipient strain (Chen, 1992). The genes for VT2e were cloned from total genomic DNA of two oedema disease strains of *E. coli* of serogroup O139 and their nucleotide sequence was determined (Gyles *et al.*, 1988; Weinstein *et al.*, 1988b). There was 91% overall nucleotide sequence similarity between the genes for VT2 and VT2e, with the A subunit genes having greater sequence similarity than the B subunit genes. Analysis of the nucleotide sequence of the cloned genes for VT2e showed that the DNA sequence of the B subunit was 98% homologous with that of the B subunit of VT2e but that the homology between the sequences of the A subunit genes was only 70.6% (Gannon *et al.*, 1990).

Initially, it appeared that strains of *E. coli* produced VT1 and/or VT2 (O'Brien and Holmes 1987) but it is now evident that some strains possess two operons of closely related VTs of the VT2 family. Ito and colleagues (1990) sequenced two separate DNA sequences from *E. coli* strain B2F1 (O91:H21) and compared these sequences with that of *slt*II. They found that the nucleotide sequences of the two VT operons of B2F1 had 99% homology with one another. The genes of the A and B subunits encoded by one operon, designated *vtx*2ha, had 98.6% and 95.5% nucleotide sequence homology, respectively, with the corresponding genes of the *slt*II operon. Also, Schmitt and co-workers (1991) demonstrated that five of 19 *E. coli* strains which produced VT2 had two copies of genes which hybridized with a DNA probe derived from *slt*II. Nucleotide sequencing of the genes for two toxins from one strain (E32511) showed that one operon was virtually identical with the *slt*II operon and the other encoded an A subunit that was identical to that of SLTII and a B subunit that was identical to that of *vtx*2ha from strain B2F1. This second operon was designated *slt*IIc. *E. coli* strain E32511, a reference strain, had previously been thought to encode a single type of verotoxin, called VT2 (Scotland *et al.*, 1985).

Recognition that some strains of the VT2 group contained the genes for more than one type of VT2 provided an explanation for some of the early confusion in the literature with regard to SLTII and VT2. Antiserum against 'SLTII' from strain 933 only partially neutralized 'VT2' from strain E32511, leading to the conclusion that the toxin called SLTII was different from the one called VT2. It is now clear that E32511 contains both SLTII and SLTIIc and that SLTIIc in crude toxin preparations from E32511 was not neutralized by anti-SLTII serum.

Little is known about regulation of synthesis of VTs. The genes for VT1 are iron regulated and the operon for VT1 is under the control of the *fur* regulatory system. Highest yields of VT1 are obtained when the bacteria are grown in media of low iron concentration (Calderwood and Mekalanos, 1987). In contrast, the genes for members of the VT2 group do not appear to be iron regulated (Weinstein *et al.*, 1988a; MacLeod and Gyles, 1989). Different levels of toxin production have been associated with verotoxigenic *E. coli* (VTEC) from different sources. Strains of *E. coli* that produce VT2e typically produce slightly lower levels of toxin (measured by Vero cell cytotoxicity) compared with strains that produce VT1, VT2, or both VT1 and VT2 (Gannon and Gyles, 1990). An *E. coli* strain of human origin (H.I.8) which produced a VT closely related to VT2e consistently produced even lower levels of VT (VT2d) than did oedema disease strains (Gannon *et al.*, 1990). When the genes were cloned and expressed in an *E. coli* K-12 background, the toxin titres increased 25-fold, probably because of the copy number of the plasmid vector (Gannon *et al.*, 1990). When a broth culture of strain H.I.8 was induced by exposure to mitomycin C, the levels of toxin that were produced increased approximately 3000-fold (Yee *et al.*, 1993). These observations are consistent with the existence of a repressor of toxin synthesis in the wild strain.

Physiological studies have shown that yield of VT2e in broth cultures is maximal at 37°C, with dramatic reductions at temperatures at 30°C and below as well as at 42°C. A marked increase in synthesis of VT2e also occurred at starting pH values of 8.5 and 8.0 compared with lower and higher pH values (MacLeod and Gyles, 1989).

Association with diseases

A simple hypothesis on the VTEC-mediated disease process that is consistent with data from natural and experimental disease (Chanter *et al.*, 1986; Richardson *et al.*, 1988, 1992; Schoonderwoerd *et al.*, 1988; Gannon *et al.*, 1989; Karmali, 1989; MacLeod *et al.*, 1991a; Zoja *et al.*, 1992) is that VTEC colonize the intestine and produce VT, which is absorbed into the circulation and damages tissues whose vascular endothelium is rich in specific receptors. Thus, in oedema disease in pigs, absorption of VT2e occurs in the ileum and the highest concentrations of receptors are found on small blood vessels in the brain, colonic mesentery, mucosa of the stomach and colon, and subcutaneous tissues of the forehead and eyelids. In calves, absorption of VT1 and/or VT2 occurs from the colon and damages blood vessels in the colonic mucosa. There is debate, however, about whether absorption into the local vasculature is necessary for diarrhoeal disease or whether there is a direct toxic effect on enterocytes.

VTEC are non-invasive but little is known about absorption of functionally active VT from the intestine and it appears that special conditions may be required for this to occur. For example, although rabbits and pigs are highly susceptible to intravenously administered VT, there is no evidence of verotoxaemia after oral or intraintestinal administration of VT (Waddell and Gyles, 1993), despite the presence of Gb3 in microvillous membranes of the enterocytes. However, VT2e administered orally to newborn preclosure pigs induces signs and symptoms of oedema disease and proves to be lethal (Waddell and Gyles, 1993). Alteration of the permeability of the ileum of weaned pigs by the addition of 5 mM sodium deoxycholate does cause absorption of active VT2e. Newborn conventional pigs to which O157:H7 VTEC were administered showed colonization of the colon and systemic effects of verotoxins (Gyles and Wilcock, 1987). Absorption may have occurred because of the permeability of the newborn intestine to proteins.

VTs are associated with both enteric and systemic disease. In humans, both enteric and systemic disease are usually seen; in cattle, only enteric disease is observed, and in pigs a predominantly systemic disease is recognized. Systemic disease requires absorption of active toxin into the circulation and may require that large amounts of toxin be present in the intestine and/or that unusual conditions of intestinal permeability exist.

Humans

Karmali (1989) presented a well-reasoned review of the evidence that implicates VTs in a number of disease syndromes in humans and animals. One VTEC-associated disease of humans which has no counterpart in animals is haemolytic uraemic syndrome (HUS), a combination of acute renal failure, thrombocytopenia and microangiopathic haemolytic anaemia, often preceded by diarrhoeal disease. A severe but strictly enteric form of disease is called haemorrhagic colitis, which results in a dysenteric syndrome. Mild diarrhoea and subclinical infection are other forms of human disease associated with VTEC.

The presence of VT-producing *E. coli* in the faeces or of faecal VT is strongly associated with disease in patients and there is remarkable similarity in clinicopathological and radiological features of HUS and haemorrhagic colitis (Karmali *et al.*, 1983, 1985; Grandsen *et al.*, 1986; Karmali, 1989). Karmali (1989) argues that these syndromes are different expressions of the same verotoxaemia. VT is produced in the intestine and a specific immune response to VT has been measured in patients. Interestingly, neutralizing antibodies to VT1, but not to VT2, appear to be widespread in the human population (Ashkenazi *et al.*, 1988). Similar observations have been made for sera from cattle in Ontario: approximately 80% of the samples had neutralizing antibodies to VT1 and about 5% had neutralizing antibodies to SLTII (R.C. Clarke, Agriculture Canada, Guelph, 1993, personal communication).

O157:H7 is the serotype of VTEC that is most frequently associated with disease in humans. It has been particularly associated with outbreaks of haemorrhagic colitis but is also involved in sporadic cases of haemorrhagic colitis and HUS in humans. This serotype and other serotypes of VTEC which cause haemorrhagic colitis are referred to as enterohaemorrhagic *E. coli* (EHEC). Tesh and O'Brien (1991) have reviewed evidence which suggests that VT2 may be the major cytotoxic factor of EHEC which contributes to colonic disease and acute renal failure. However, it is clear that strains which produce only VT1 have also been implicated in these diseases. In outbreaks of haemorrhagic colitis, HUS typically develops in 10–20% of individuals. Cattle appear to be a reservoir of organisms which cause disease in humans, and hamburger and milk have been implicated as vehicles of infection (Martin *et al.*, 1986; Borczyk *et al.*, 1987; Chapman *et al.*, 1989; Clarke *et al.*, 1989; Montenegro *et al.*, 1990; Read *et al.*, 1990). Emphasis on serotype O157:H7 sometimes obscures the fact that over 50 other serotypes of VTEC have been recovered from humans (reviewed by Karmali, 1989). Serotype O157:H7 and other serotypes of VTEC isolated from humans often exist in the intestine of normal cattle without inducing disease in them (Mohammad *et al.*, 1986; Clarke *et al.*, 1989; Read *et al.*, 1990; Wilson *et al.*, 1992). This is the case even though VTEC that are associated with disease in humans as well as those that are implicated in disease in calves produce VT1 and/or VT2 (Chanter *et al.*, 1986; Mainil *et al.*, 1987; Schoonderwoed *et al.*, 1988).

Cattle

In cattle, VTEC which produce VT1 and/or VT2 are implicated in both haemorrhagic colitis and diarrhoea. VTEC have been associated with calf diarrhoea on the basis of the higher frequency of their recovery from diarrhoe compared with normal calves (Mohammad *et al.*, 1985). They have also been recovered from calves in outbreaks of bloody diarrhoea (Chanter *et al.*, 1986; Mainil *et al.*, 1987; Schoonderwoerd *et al.*, 1988; Janke *et al.*, 1990). Bloody and non-bloody diarrhoea have been reproduced by inoculation of calves with isolates of the organisms recovered from diseased calves (Chanter *et al.*, 1984; Moxley and Francis, 1986). For further discussion, see Chapter 4.

Pigs

VTEC that cause oedema disease in pigs do not produce VT1 or VT2; they produce VT2e (Marques *et al.*, 1987; Gannon *et al.*, 1988). As early as 1949, Timoney demonstrated that oedema disease in pigs was the result of a toxaemia and reproduced the signs and lesions of the disease by intravenous injection of pigs with supernatants from centrifuged gut contents from pigs that had died of oedema disease. Shortly thereafter, it was shown that the toxic factor was a heat-labile toxin produced by certain strains of haemolytic *E. coli* (Erskine *et al.*, 1957). The toxin, termed edema disease principle (EDP), was partially purified by Clugston and Nielsen (1974) and used to reproduce the clinical and pathological features of oedema disease by intravenous injection of pigs.

In recent years, the EDP of *E. coli* has been shown to be a verotoxin (Dobrescu, 1983; Smith *et al.*, 1983; Linggood and Thompson, 1987; Marques *et al.*, 1987; Gannon *et al.*, 1988), characterized as SLTIIv (SLTIIe or VT2e) (Gannon and Gyles, 1990; MacLeod *et al.*, 1991b). The signs and symptoms of oedema disease have been reproduced by intravenous injection of pigs with purified VT2e (MacLeod *et al.*, 1991b). Prior to purification of VT2e, attempts to reproduce the disease by intravenous administration of toxin preparations were usually complicated by endotoxic shock which often resulted in death prior to development of signs of oedema disease (Clugston and Nielsen, 1974; Smith *et al.*, 1983).

Oedema disease, whether produced naturally or experimentally, has the same essential features of other diseases in which VTEC have been implicated (MacLeod *et al.*, 1991b). These features revolve around damage to small blood vessels in target organs. In oedema disease, the most common target tissues are the stomach, the eyelids, the cerebellum and the colon. On gross examination, oedema and haemorrhage are observed; on microscopic examination, lesions of oedema, haemorrhage and vasculitis are noted.

VT-producing *E. coli* isolated from pigs belong predominantly to three O serogroups: 138, 139 and 141 (Smith *et al.*, 1983; Gannon *et al.*, 1988). These *E. coli* are readily isolated from the faeces of normal or diseased weaned pigs and are typically haemolytic. Smith and co-workers (1983) found that all the O141:K85 and O141:K85,K88 isolates and about half the O138 and O139 isolates that they examined were VT^+. The role of VTEC in oedema disease is discussed in detail in Chapter 9.

Other species

There is little information on VTEC in other species. However, these organisms have been implicated in diarrhoea in cats (Abaas *et al.*, 1989) and dogs (Zschock *et al.*, 1989; J.D. Hammermueller, University of Guelph, Guelph, 1993, personal communication). Zschock *et al.* (1989) found that none of 45 strains of *E. coli* from diarrhoea in dogs in Germany produced VT, but Hammermueller (1993, personal communication) found VT-positive *E. coli* in association with diarrhoea in dogs in Ontario, Canada. Among *E. coli* from the faeces of 45 dogs with diarrhoea, four produced VT1 plus VT2 and six produced VT2 only; among 57 *E. coli* from the faeces of normal dogs, seven produced VT1 and none produced VT2. Interestingly, all four VT1-positive isolates from dogs with diarrhoea also produced VT2, STa or STb. VTEC have been implicated in diarrhoea in buffalo calves on the basis of their significantly greater frequency of isolation from diarrhoeic compared with healthy control calves (Mohammad *et al.*, 1985).

VTEC have been recovered from the faeces of healthy domestic animals of several species. Beutin *et al.* (1993) found VTEC in the faeces of 66% of sheep, 56% of goats, 21% of cattle, 14% of cats, 7.5% of pigs and 5% of dogs. No VTEC were found in the faeces of 144 chickens. The absence of VTEC from chicken faeces was also reported by Irwin *et al.* (1989) in Canada, who examined 500 samples.

Immunogenicity

VT1 and VT2 are highly immunogenic, but early studies suggested that VT2e was of low immunogenicity because crude preparations of VT2e elicited either no or low antibody titres in rabbits (Konowalchuk *et al.*, 1977; Schimmelpfenig and Weber, 1979; Smith *et al.*, 1983; Gannon and Gyles, 1990). However, it is likely that the apparent low immunogenicity was the result of low yields of toxin in the preparations. Dobrescu and van Wijnendaele (1979) obtained high levels of neutralizing antibody when they injected mice parenterally with a partially purified preparation of edema disease principle. When VT2e was purified, high levels of neutralizing antibody could readily be produced in pigs (MacLeod and Gyles, 1991; Waddell and Gyles, 1993). The apparently poor immunogenicity of SLTIIva (Gannon and Gyles, 1990) is due to low levels of production by the wild strain and high levels of neutralizing antibody can be obtained once the yield of toxin is increased by cloning the gene (Yee *et al.*, 1993).

VT1 and VT2 are cytotoxic for lymphocytes and lymphocytotoxicity has been reported in the spleen and intestinal-associated lymphoid tissue of mice inoculated intraperitoneally with VT (Padhye *et al.*, 1989). Furthermore, Cohen *et al.* (1990) showed that VT cytotoxicity is directed particularly against B lymphocytes committed to synthesis of IgA and IgG. They suggested that this may account for production of only IgM class anti-VT antibodies and failure of long-lasting anti-VT immunity against verotoxin-mediated diarrhoeal disease.

Other *E. coli* Cytotoxins

In addition to verotoxins, there are several other cytotoxins that are produced by *E. coli* and have a definite or probable role in diseases (Table 15.2). All, except for alpha-haemolysin, have been discovered in recent years.

Cytolethal distending toxin

A cytolethal distending toxin (CLDT), whose activity is lost following incubation at 70°C for 15 minutes, has been reported in culture filtrates of certain *E. coli* strains associated with diarrhoeal and other diseases in humans (Johnson and Lior, 1988) as well as in *Shigella dysenteriae* type 2 and *S. boydii* (Johnson and Lior, 1987). A similar activity was detected in *E. coli* O8 strains from diarrhoea in pigs, but culture filtrates had to be concentrated before the effect was observed (Johnson and Lior, 1987). CLDT caused progressive cell distension followed by cytotoxicity during incubation for 96–120 hours with low numbers of Vero, HeLa, HEp-2 and

Table 15.2. Cytotoxic protein toxins of *E. coli*.

Toxins	Biological effects	Types of disease
Verotoxins	Damage to vascular endothelium	HUS, HC, diarrhoea
CLDT	Cytotoxic for cell cultures	Diarrhoea
Vir cytotoxin	Cytotoxic for cell cultures	Bacteraemia
CNF	Cytotoxic for cell cultures	Diarrhoea, Bacteraemia
Alpha haemolysin	Cytotoxic for a variety of cell types	Bacteraemia, UTI
Enterohaemolysin	Lytic for eythrocytes	HUS, HC

UTI, urinary tract infection; HC, haemorrhagic colitis; CNF, cytotoxic necrotizing factor; HUS, haemolytic uraemic syndrome; CLDT, cytolethal distending toxin.

CHO cells. Cytotoxicity was more marked on HeLa, HEp-2 and CHO compared with Vero cells and was not evident for Y-1 adrenal cells. CHO cells were recommended for CLDT assays, since they did not respond to VT, which is produced by some CLDT-positive strains of *E. coli*. Similar toxin titres were found when culture supernatant and polymyxin B extracts were compared. CLDT caused erythema, but no necrosis in rabbit skin. The role of CLDT in disease is not known.

Vir cytotoxin and cytotoxic necrotizing factors

The Vir cytotoxin was discovered by Smith (1974), who reported that certain bovine and ovine septicaemic strains of *E. coli* of serotype O15:H21 and serogroup O78:K80 produced a toxin which was lethal for mice, rabbits and chickens. The Vir phenotype was uncommon among septicaemic strains of *E. coli* (Smith, 1974; Lopez-Alvarez and Gyles, 1980). The lethal effects of Vir cytotoxin suggested that it may play a role in bacteraemic disease in calves and lambs, but the low frequency of its occurrence indicated that the role was not a critical one. Later, De Rycke *et al.* (1987) isolated strains of Vir-positive *E. coli* with significant frequency from calves with diarrhoea.

Synthesis of this toxin was plasmid mediated and toxigenic strains produced a characteristic surface antigen. The plasmid responsible for production of toxin and the surface antigen was called Vir. Later, it was shown that the Vir plasmid behaved as an episome, that the surface antigen which it encoded was a pilus, and that some strains of *E. coli* produced toxin but no Vir pili (Lopez-Alvarez and Gyles, 1980; Lopez-Alvarez *et al.*, 1980). The Vir toxin was also called Vir cytotoxin because it caused a cytopathic effect in HeLa cells, characterized by multinucleation (Oswald *et al.*, 1989).

In the 1980s, a cytotoxic necrotizing factor (CNF) which induced formation of giant, polynucleated cells in HeLa and Vero cell cultures was detected in extracts of *E. coli* from diarrhoeal diseases in humans, pigs and calves (Caprioli *et al.*, 1984; Gonzalez and Blanco, 1985; De Rycke *et al.*, 1987, 1989), as well as in *E. coli* from septicaemia and urinary tract infections in humans (Alonso *et al.*, 1987; Caprioli *et al.*, 1987). Production of CNF was later associated with possession of P fimbriae and production of alpha haemolysin (Blanco *et al.*, 1990).

CNF is immunologically related to Vir cytotoxin (De Rycke *et al.*, 1987; Oswald *et al.*, 1989) and recent evidence indicates that these cytotoxins are sufficiently related as to be called CNF1 and CNF2, respectively (De Rycke *et al.*, 1990). Both toxins were lethal for mice and induced multinucleation in HeLa cells and necrosis in rabbit skin, but CNF2 was less potent in causing multinucleation and much more potent in causing skin necrosis than was CNF1. CNF2 induced a weak enterotoxic response in rabbit ileal loops. The toxicity of each type of CNF was partially neutralized by antibodies against the other type, but it was possible to distinguish between the two by an enzyme-linked immunosorbent assay (Tabouret and De Rycke, 1990). CNF1 is associated with a 115-kDa protein recognized by SDS–PAGE (De Rycke *et al.*, 1990) whereas CNF2 is associated with a 110-kDa protein (Oswald and De Rycke, 1990).

Pohl and colleagues (1992) found that 89% of a collection of 61 bovine strains of *E. coli* which produced CNF1 also produced aerobactin and were resistant to the bactericidal action of serum and that none of the strains had genes for enterotoxins or verotoxins, or for adhesins associated with *E. coli* strains implicated in diarrhoea. Most strains (60%) produced alpha-haemolysin. Of the 61 strains tested, 24 belonged to O serogroup 153, two to O78, two to O4, one to O15, one to O149 and one to O157; the remainder were either rough (two strains) or non-typeable (28).

Oswald *et al.* (1991) examined 43 bovine strains of CNF2-positive *E. coli* (36 from diarrhoeic calves and seven from extraintestinal infections) and found that the major O group to which strains belonged was O78; 79% of strains were serum resistant; 70% produced aerobactin; 9% produced haemolysin; and 53% adhered to calf villi. Nine per cent of strains hybridized with a gene probe for LT-IIa, and 53% hybridized with a probe for F17A fimbriae. Blanco and co-workers (1992) found that strains of *E. coli* that produced CNF2 were present in the faeces of healthy and diarrhoeic calves and that most of these strains belonged to O serogroups 1, 3, 15, 55, 88 and 123. Strains of serotype O55:H21 possessed the Vir pili whereas strains of O55:H4 produced P fimbriae.

De Rycke and Plassiart (1990) inoculated partially purified CNF2 into six lambs and examined the clinical signs and lesions that were produced. The signs that were observed consisted of neurological abnormalities and mucoid diarrhoea. Lesions of oedema and haemorrhage were noted in the central nervous system and foci of coagulation necrosis were detected in the myocardium. Available evidence suggests that CNF2 probably plays a role in extraintestinal infections in calves and lambs and may increase the severity of illness.

Alpha-haemolysin

Because of the frequent association of haemolytic *E. coli* with diarrhoea and oedema disease in pigs, Smith (1963) investigated haemolysins of *E. coli*. He found that one type of haemolysin was present in culture supernatants and a second was cell associated. He called these alpha-haemolysin and beta-haemolysin, respectively. Both haemolysins lysed erythrocytes from cattle, pig, horse, rabbit, guinea-pig and chicken. There has been considerable research on *E. coli* haemolysins over the past 10 years and readers are referred to reviews by Braun and Focareta (1991), Welch (1991) and Welch *et al.* (1992).

Smith (1963) observed that alpha-haemolysin was produced in the early logarithmic phase of growth and declined to an undetectable level by 48 hours' incubation. Alpha-haemolysin was highly heat labile: activity was completely lost after 10 minutes at 56°C, but pH had a marked influence on stability, which was much greater at acid pH values than at alkaline pH. A pH of 3 was found to be optimal for storage of alpha-haemolysin. Following intravenous administration to mice, alpha haemolysin induced haemoglobinuria and death, typically within 1–6 hours. Alpha-haemolysin was antigenic and neutralizing antibodies were readily detected in the serum of pigs and cattle, whose normal faecal flora typically contains alpha-haemolytic *E. coli*.

E. coli alpha-haemolysin is a pore-forming cytolysin (Bhakdi *et al.*, 1986). Passive influx of calcium and sucrose but not of the larger inulin and dextran into toxin-treated cells indicate generation of small pores in the plasma membrane by alpha-haemolysin. Calcium influx presumably changes intracellular metabolism substantially. Pores formed by the alpha-haemolysin allow dissipation of transmembrane ion gradients but the retention of cytoplasmic protein by the cells results in increased intracellular colloid-osmotic pressure. Water moves into the cell in response to the increased colloid-osmotic pressure which causes the cells to swell and lyse. Addition to the medium of osmoprotectants with large enough diameters protects the cells from the osmotic-induced changes. The toxin acts on a wide variety of cell types but little is known about binding to cell surfaces except that Ca^{2+} is required. Interestingly, chromosome-encoded alpha-haemolysin has higher activity than plasmid-encoded alpha-haemolysin and this has been attributed to a considerably longer mean lifetime of the pores caused by the chromosomally encoded toxin (Benz *et al.*, 1992).

E. coli alpha-haemolysin is now recognized as the prototype for a family of cytotoxins produced by several Gram-negative pathogens including *Actinobacillus pleuropneumoniae*, *A. actinomycetemcomitans*, *A. suis*, *Bordetella pertussis*, *Morganella morganii*, *Pasteurella haemolytica*, *Proteus mirabilis* and *P. vulgaris* (see reviews by Braun and Focareta, 1991; Welch, 1991). These cytotoxins belong to the RTX (repeats in toxin) gene family, characterized by amino acid sequences which include tandem repeats of a glycine rich, nine amino acid sequence. The repeated sequences are involved in binding of Ca^{2+} through the formation of a beta-turn-rich structure and are necessary for haemolytic activity.

Four genes (*hly*C, A, B and D) within a single operon (Noegel *et al.*, 1981; Felmlee *et al.*, 1985; Welch and Pellett, 1988) and a fifth unlinked gene (*tol*C) (Wandersman and Delepelaire, 1990) encode the products necessary for synthesis and secretion of the haemolysin. HlyA is a 110-kDa protein which is highly conserved at the genetic, protein and antigenic levels. HlyC is a 20-kDa protein. The haemolysin is encoded by *hly*A and is synthesized as an inactive prohaemolysin; the product of *hly*C is necessary for activation of the *hly*A gene product. Activation involves transfer of a fatty acid moiety from an acylated acyl carrier protein to pro-HlyA and the secreted haemolysin is believed to be a mixture, having a variety of acyl chains (Issartel *et al.*, 1991; Hughes *et al.*, 1992). The haemolysin requires special mechanisms for its transport because the molecule lacks an N-terminal signal peptide and does not follow the general Sec export pathway through the cytoplasmic membrane. The transporter proteins HlyB and HlyD and the outer membrane protein TolC are required for transport of the haemolysin into the extracellular environment. The C-terminal end of the HlyA molecule constitutes a recognition signal for the secretion system. HlyB, which is located in the cytoplasmic membrane, is probably responsible for transporting HlyA through the cytoplasmic membrane, using energy from ATP hydrolysis (Koronakis *et al.*, 1992; Braun *et al.*, 1993). It is likely that HlyD forms a bridge which spans the cytoplasmic and outer membranes and thereby effects the translocation of HlyA to the outer membrane. TolC is clearly required for export of HlyA but its role has not been identified. It has been suggested that it may be required for formation of a pore through which HlyA escapes or for formation of the apparatus for translocation from the cytoplasmic membrane to the outer membrane (Welch *et al.*, 1992).

The genes for alpha-haemolysin are sometimes located on plasmids in isolates of *E. coli* from pigs (Smith and Linggood, 1971), but are more often located in the chromosome (Welch, 1991). Codon usage and the low G + C content (39%) of the alpha-haemolysin operon suggest that these genes originated outside the genus (Felmlee *et al.*, 1985). In some strains of *E. coli*, transcription of the haemolysin genes is under iron regulation, mediated by the Fur protein.

Role in disease

Alpha-haemolysin plays an important role in the pathogenicity of extra-intestinal *E. coli* in humans. This conclusion is supported by epidemiological evidence and studies of transformed *E. coli* in animal models of disease. About 50% of *E. coli* that cause pyelonephritis and septicaemia in humans are haemolytic, whereas *E. coli* strains of the normal faecal flora are usually non-haemolytic. Hacker *et al.* (1983) showed that deletion of the *hly* determinant from a uropathogenic *E. coli* strain resulted in a marked reduction in toxicity for mice and that transfer of the cloned *hly* determinant from two uropathogenic *E. coli* strains into the Hly-negative strain restored its virulence. O'Hanley and co-workers (1991) used genetically defined *E. coli* strains that expressed digalactose binding and/or haemolysin in a rat model of pyelonephritis to show that haemolysin contributed to septicaemia and renal parenchymal injury. *E. coli* recovered from urinogenital tract infections in dogs and cats are also frequently haemolytic and it is likely that alpha-haemolysin plays a role in these diseases. Some experiments have suggested that haemolysin makes iron available for bacterial growth (Linggood and Ingram, 1982). However, there must be other mechanisms by which haemolysin contributes to disease. Smith and Huggins (1985) observed that there was no haemoglobinuria in mice that died shortly after intravenous inoculation of alpha-haemolysin, whereas haemoglobinuria was evident in mice that died later. Furthermore, haemolysis is not a feature of the extraintestinal infections in humans and animals in which haemolytic *E. coli* are causally implicated.

Alpha-haemolysin can cause marked changes in a variety of cell types. Cytocidal effects of alpha-haemolysin have been demonstrated for granulocytes, monocytes, endothelial cells, renal tubular epithelial cells and T lymphocytes (Bhakdi *et al.*, 1989; Jonas *et al.*, 1993), but damage to phagocytic cells probably plays a major role in promoting establishment of infection. Bhakdi *et al.* (1989) reported that alpha-haemolysin is the most potent leucocidin known to date, that the pores that are produced are not repaired by damaged polymorphonuclear leucocytes and allow efflux of small intracellular molecules including adenosine triphosphate (necessary for phagocyte function). Furthermore, the influx of Ca^{2+} into the cells causes exocytosis of granule contents by dying cells. In another study, partially purified haemolysin was cytotoxic for human peripheral leucocytes and activated neutrophil oxidative metabolism, causing an intense burst of chemiluminescence (Gadeberg and Orskov, 1984). Exposure of granulocytes to low doses of alpha-haemolysin induces leucotrienes from human polymorphonuclear granulocytes and chemotactic activity of the granulocytes (Scheffer *et al.*, 1985). Welch (1991) has reported that sublytic concentrations of alpha-haemolysin can impair the ability of macrophages to process and present antigens to T cells, and has suggested that more attention needs to be paid to the non-lytic, cytotoxic activities of alpha-haemolysin.

Alpha-haemolysin does not appear to play a role in enteric infections in pigs. Smith and Linggood (1971) cured porcine *E. coli* strains of their haemolysin plasmid and demonstrated that loss of ability to produce haemolysin had no observable effect on their ability to induce diarrhoea in newborn or weaned pigs or to induce oedema disease in weaned pigs. There was a marked increase in anti-haemolysin titres in the serum of pigs infected with haemolytic oedema disease strains of *E. coli* (Smith and Halls, 1968).

Enterohaemolysin

Enterohaemolysin is a poorly characterized haemolysin which is distinct from alpha- and beta-haemolysins and has been identified in association with verotoxigenic *E. coli* and certain EPEC (Beutin *et al.*, 1989). Activity is observed with washed, but not with unwashed sheep red blood cells. Almost 90% of verotoxigenic *E. coli* from various sources produced enterohaemolysin. The only group of VT^+ strains which were negative were porcine isolates, which produce alpha-haemolysin. Enterohaemolysin is a cell-associated, thermolabile haemolysin detected only in cells in the stationary phase of growth. There is some evidence that it may be a 60-kDa outer membrane protein (Beutin *et al.*, 1990). Production of enterohaemolysin is associated with a temperate bacteriophage in *E. coli* of O group 26. The mechanism of action appears to be that of a pore-forming cytolysin.

Concluding Comments

In recent years, there has been much new information about cytotoxic proteins produced by pathogenic *E. coli*, but several aspects of their interaction with animal and human hosts are still not understood. In the case of verotoxins, there is impressive evidence to implicate them in enteric and systemic disease, but the factors that influence production and release of toxin in the intestine, and the mechanisms by which active toxin is absorbed from the intestine are not known. Alpha-haemolysin is strongly associated with extraintestinal *E. coli* infections in humans, but the nature of its contribution to the disease process is still largely a matter of speculation. Nothing is known of the role, if any, of CLDT, CNF1, CNF2 and enterohaemolysin in diarrhoeal and systemic diseases.

References

Abaas, S., Franklin, A., Kuhn, I., Orskov, F. and Orskov, I. (1989) Cytotoxin activity on Vero cells among *Escherichia coli* strains associated with diarrhoea in cats. *American Journal of Veterinary Research* 50, 1294–1296.

Alonso, P., Blanco, J., Blanco, M. and Gonzalez, E.A. (1987) Frequent production of toxins by *Escherichia coli* strains isolated from human urinary tract infections. *Federation of European Microbiological Societies Microbiology Letters* 48, 391–396.

Ashkenazi, S., Cleary, T.G., Lopez, E. and Pickering, L.K. (1988) Anticytotoxin-neutralizing antibodies in immune globulin preparations: potential use in hemolytic-uremic syndrome. *Journal of Pediatrics* 113, 1008–1014.

Barrett, T.J., Potter, M.E. and Wachsmuth, I.K. (1989) Continuous peritoneal infusion of Shiga-like toxin II (SLT II) as a model for SLT II-induced diseases. *Journal of Infectious Diseases* 159, 774–777.

Benz, R., Dobereiner, A., Ludwig, A. and Goebel, W. (1992) Haemolysin of *Escherichia coli*: comparison of pore-forming properties between chromosome and plasmid-encoded haemolysins. *Federation of European Microbiological Societies Microbiology Immunology* 105, 55–62.

Beutin, L., Montenegro, M.A., Orskov, I., Orskov, F., Prada, J., Zimmermann, S. and Stephan, R. (1989) Close association of verotoxin (Shiga-like toxin) production with enterohemolysin production in strains of *Escherichia coli*. *Journal of Clinical Microbiology* 27, 2559–2564.

Beutin, L., Bode, L., Ozel, M. and Stephan, R. (1990) Enterohemolysin production is associated with a temperate bacteriophage in *Escherichia coli* O serogroup 26 strains. *Journal of Bacteriology* 172, 6469–6475.

Beutin, L., Geier, D., Steinruck, H., Zimmermann, S. and Scheutz, F. (1993) Prevalence and some properties of verotoxin (Shiga-like toxin)-producing *Escherichia coli* in seven different species of healthy domestic animals. *Journal of Clinical Microbiology* 31, 2483–2488.

Bhakdi, S., Mackman, N., Nicaud, J.-M. and Holland, I.B. (1986) *Escherichia coli* hemolysin may damage target cell membranes by generating transmembrane pores. *Infection and Immunity* 52, 63–69.

Bhakdi, S., Greulich, S., Muhly, M., Eberspacher, B., Becker, H., Thiele, A. and Hugo, F. (1989) Potent leukocidal action of *Escherichia coli* hemolysin mediated by permealization of target cell membranes. *Journal of Experimental Medicine* 169, 737–754.

Blanco, J., Gonzalez, E.A., Bernardez, I. and Regueiro, B. (1983) Differentiated biological activity of Vero toxin (VT) released by human and porcine *Escherichia coli* strains. *Federation of European Microbiological Societies Microbiology Letters* 20, 167–170.

Blanco, J., Alonso, M.P., Gonzalez, E.A., Blanco, M. and Garabal, J.I. (1990) Virulence factors of bacteraemic *Escherichia coli* with particular reference to production of cytotoxic necrotizing factor (CNF) by P-fimbriate strains. *Journal of Medical Microbiology* 31, 175–183.

Blanco, J., Blanco, M., Alonso, M.P., Garabal, J.I. and Gonzalez, E.A., (1992) Serogroups of *Escherichia coli* strains producing cytotoxic necrotizing factors

CNF1 and CNF2. *Federation of European Microbiological Societies Microbiology Letters* 75, 155–159.

Borczyk, A.A., Karmali, M.A., Lior H. and Duncan, L.M.C. (1987) Bovine reservoir for verotoxin-producing *Escherichia coli* O157:H7. *Lancet* i, 98.

Braun, V. and Focareta, T. (1991) Pore-forming bacterial protein hemolysins (cytolysins). *Critical Reviews in Microbiology* 18, 115–158.

Braun, V., Schonherr, R. and Hobbie, S. (1993) Enterobacterial hemolysins: activation, secretion and pore formation. *Trends in Microbiology* 1, 211–216.

Calderwood, S.B. and Mekalanos, J.J. (1987) Iron-regulation of Shiga-like toxin expression in *Escherichia coli* is mediated by the *fur* locus. *Journal of Bacteriology* 169, 4759–4764.

Calderwood, S.B., Auclair, F., Donohue-Rolfe, A., Keusch, G.T. and Mekalanos, J.J. (1987) Nucleotide sequence of the Shiga-like toxin genes of *Escherichia coli. Proceedings of the National Academy of Sciences of the United States of America* 84, 4364–4368.

Caprioli, A., Donneli, G. and Falbo, L. (1984) A cell division-active protein from *Escherichia coli. Biochemical and Biophysical Research Communications* 118, 587–593.

Caprioli, A., Falbo, V. and Ruggeri, F.M. (1987) Cytotoxic necrotizing factor production by haemolytic strains of *Escherichia coli* causing extra-intestinal infections. *Journal of Clinical Microbiology* 25, 146–149.

Chanter, A., Morgan, J.H., Bridger, J.C., Hall, G.A. and Reynolds, D.J. (1984) Dysentery in gnotobiotic calves caused by atypical *Escherichia coli. Veterinary Record* 114, 71.

Chanter, N., Hall, G.A., Bland, A.P., Hayle, A.J. and Parsons, K.R. (1986) Dysentery in calves caused by an atypical strain of *Escherichia coli* (S102-9). *Veterinary Microbiology* 12, 241–253.

Chapman, P.A., Wright, D.J. and Norman, P. (1989) Verotoxin-producing *Escherichia coli* infections in Sheffield: cattle as a possible source. *Epidemiology and Infection* 102, 439–445.

Chanter, N., Morgan, J.H., Bridger, J.C., Hall, G.A. and Reynolds, D.J. (1984) Dysentery in gnotobiotic calves caused by atypical *Escherichia coli. Veterinary Record* 114, 71.

Chen, J. (1992) Mapping of the chromosomal location of the genes for Shiga-like toxin II variant (SLT-IIv). MSc Thesis. University of Guelph, Guelph, Ontario, Canada.

Clarke, R.C., McEwen, S.A., Gannon, V.P., Lior, H. and Gyles, C.L. (1989) Isolation of verocytotoxin-producing *Escherichia coli* from milk filters in southwestern Ontario. *Epidemiology and Infection* 102, 253–260.

Clugston, R.C. and Nielsen, N.O. (1974) Experimental oedema disease of swine (*E. coli* enterotoxemia). I. Detection, and preparation of an active principle. *Canadian Journal of Comparative Medicine* 38, 22–28.

Cohen, A., Madrid-Marina, V., Estrov, Z., Freedman, M.H., Lingwood, C.A. and Dosch, H.-M. (1990) Expression of glycolipid receptors to Shiga-like toxin on human B lymphocytes: a mechanism for the failure of long-lived antibody response to dysenteric disease. *International Immunology* 2, 1–8.

De Grandis, S.A., Ginsburg, J., Toone, M., Climie, S., Friesen, J. and Brunton, J. (1987) Nucleotide sequence and promoter mapping of the *Escherichia coli* Shiga-like toxin operon of bacteriophage H-19B. *Journal of Bacteriology* 169, 4313–4319.

De Grandis, S., Law, H., Brunton, J. Gyles, C. and Lingwood, C.A. (1989) Globotetraosylceramide is recognized by the pig edema disease toxin. *Journal of Biological Chemistry* 264, 12520–12525.

De Rycke, J. and Plassiart, G. (1990) Toxic effects for lambs of cytotoxic necrotizing factor from *Escherichia coli. Research in Veterinary Science* 49, 349–354.

De Rycke, J., Guillot, J.F. and Boivin, R. (1987) Cytotoxins in nonenterotoxigenic strains of *Escherichia coli* isolated from feces of diarrheic calves. *Veterinary Microbiology* 15, 137–150.

De Rycke, J., Phan-thanh, L. and Bernard, S. (1989) Immunochemical identification and biological characterization of cytotoxic necrotizing factor of *Escherichia coli. Journal of Clinical Microbiology* 27, 983–988.

De Rycke, J., Gonzalez, E.A., Blanco, J., Oswald, E., Blanco, M. and Boivin, R. (1990) Evidence for two types of cytotoxic necrotizing factors in human and animal clinical isolates of *Escherichia coli. Journal of Clinical Microbiology* 28, 694–699.

Dobrescu, L. (1983) New biological effect of edema disease principle (*Escherichia coli* – neurotoxin), and its use as an *in vitro* assay for this toxin. *American Journal of Veterinary Research* 44, 31–34.

Dobrescu, L. and van Wijnendaele, F. (1979) Immunological studies in mice with swine edema disease principle (neurotoxin). *Zentralblatt für Veterinarmedizin* 26, 239–246.

Donohue-Rolfe, A. and Keusch, G.T. (1983) *Shigella dysenteriae* 1 cytotoxin, periplasmic protein releasable by polymyxin B and osmotic shock. *Infection and Immunity* 39, 270–274.

Donohue-Rolfe, A., Keusch, G.T., Edson, C., Thorley-Lawson, S. and Jacewicz, M. (1984) Pathogenesis of Shigella diarrhea IX. Simplified high yield purification of Shigella toxin and characterization of subunit composition and function by the use of subunit-specific monoclonal and polyclonal antibodies. *Journal of Experimental Medicine* 160, 1767–1781.

Downes, F.P., Barrett, T.J., Green, J.H., Aloisio, C.H., Spika, J.S., Strockbine, N.A. and Wachsmuth, I.K. (1988) Affinity purification and characterization of Shiga-like toxin II and production of toxin-specific monoclonal antibodies. *Infection and Immunity* 56, 1926–1933.

Endo, Y., Tsurugi, K., Yutsudo, T., Takeda, Y., Ogasawara, T. and Igarashi, K. (1988) Site of action of a Vero toxin (VT2) from *Escherichia coli* O157:H7 and of Shiga toxin on eukaryotic ribosomes. RNA N-glycosidase activity of the toxins. *European Journal of Biochemistry* 171, 45–50.

Erskine, R.G., Sojka, W.J. and Lloyd, M.K. (1957) The experimental reproduction of a syndrome indistinguishable from oedema disease. *Veterinary Record* 69, 301–303.

Felmlee, T., Pellett, S. and Welch, R.A. (1985) Nucleotide sequence of an *Escherichia coli* chromosomal haemolysin. *Journal of Bacteriology* 163, 94–105.

Frankel, A., Schlossman, D., Welsh, P., Hertler, A., Withers, D. and Johnston, S. (1989) Selection and characterization of ricin toxin A-chain mutations in *Saccharomyces cerevisiae. Molecular and Cellular Biology* 9, 415–420.

Furutani, M., Ito, K., Oku, Y., Takeda, Y. and Igarashi, K. (1990) Demonstration of RNA *N*-glycosidase activity of a Vero toxin (VT2 variant) produced by *Escherichia coli* O91 : H21 from a patient with the hemolytic uremic syndrome. *Microbiology and Immunology* 34, 387–392.

Gadeberg, O.V. and Orskov, I. (1984) *In vitro* cytotoxic effect of α-hemolytic *Escherichia coli* on human blood granulocytes. *Infection and Immunity* 45, 255–260.

Gannon, V.P.J. and Gyles, C.L. (1990) Characteristics of the Shiga-like toxin produced by *Escherichia coli* associated with porcine edema disease. *Veterinary Microbiology* 24, 89–100.

Gannon, V.P.J., Gyles, C.L. and Friendship, R.W. (1988) Characteristics of verotoxigenic *Escherichia coli* from pigs. *Canadian Journal of Veterinary Research* 52, 331–337.

Gannon, V.P.J., Gyles, C.L. and Wilcock, B.P. (1989) Effects of *Escherichia coli* Shiga-like toxins (verotoxins) in pigs. *Canadian Journal of Veterinary Research* 53, 306–312.

Gannon, V.P.J., Teerling, C., Masri, S.A. and Gyles, C.L. (1990) Molecular cloning and nucleotide sequencing of another variant of the *Escherichia coli* Shiga-like toxin II family. *Journal of General Microbiology* 136, 1125–1135.

Gonzalez, E.A. and Blanco, J. (1985) Production of cytotoxin VT in enteropathogenic and nonenteropathogenic *Escherichia coli* strains of porcine origin. *Federation of European Microbiological Societies Microbiology Letters* 26, 127–130.

Grandsen, W.R., Damm, M.A.S., Anderson, J.D., Carter, J.E. and Lior, H. (1986) Further evidence associating hemolytic uremic syndrome with infection by verotoxin producing *E. coli* O157 : H7. *Journal of Infectious Diseases* 154, 522–524.

Gregory, D.W. (1960) The (oedema disease) neuro-oedema toxin of haemolytic *Escherichia coli. Veterinary Record* 72, 1208–1209.

Gyles, C.L. and Wilcock, B. (1987) Response of conventional pigs to infection with verotoxigenic *Escherichia coli* O157 : H7. In: *Proceedings of the First International Symposium and Workshop on Verocytotoxin-producing* Escherichia coli *Infection*. Toronto, Canada.

Gyles, C.L., deGrandis, S.A., MacKenzie, C. and Brunton, J.L. (1988) Cloning and nucleotide sequence analysis of the genes determining verocytotoxin production in a porcine edema disease isolate of *Escherichia coli. Microbial Pathogenesis* 5, 419–426.

Hacker, J., Hughes, C., Hof, H. and Goebel, W. (1983) Cloned hemolysin genes from *Escherichia coli* that cause urinary tract infection determine different levels of toxicity in mice. *Infection and Immunity* 42, 57–63.

Head, S.C., Petric, M., Richardson, S., Roscoe, M. and Karmali, M.A. (1988) Purification and characterization of Verocytotoxin 2. *Federation of European Microbiological Societies Microbiology Letters* 51, 211–216.

Head, S.C., Karmali, M.A. and Lingwood, C.A. (1991) Preparation of VT1 and

VT2 hybrid toxins from their purified dissociated subunits. Evidence for B subunit modulation of A subunit function. *Journal of Biological Chemistry* 266, 3617–3621.

Hovde, C.J., Calderwood, S.B., Mekalanos, J.J. and Collier, R.J. (1988) Evidence that glutamic acid 167 is an active-site residue of Shiga-like toxin I. *Proceedings of the National Academy of Sciences of the United States of America* 85, 2568–2572.

Huang, A., deGrandis, S., Friesen, J., Karmali, M., Petric, M., Congi, R. and Brunton, J.L. (1986) Cloning and expression of the genes specifying Shiga-like toxin production in *Escherichia coli*. *Journal of Bacteriology* 166, 375–379.

Hughes, C., Issartel, J.P., Hardie, K., Stanley, P., Koronakis, E. and Koronakis, V. (1992) Activation of *Escherichia coli* prohemolysin to the membrane-targetted toxin by HlyC-directed ACP-dependent fatty acylation. *Federation of European Microbiological Societies Microbiology Immunology* 5, 37–43.

Igarashi, K., Ogasawara, T., Ito, K., Yutsudo, T. and Takeda, Y. (1987) Inhibition of elongation factor 1-dependent aminoacyl-tRNA binding to ribosomes by Shiga-like toxin I (VT1) from *Escherichia coli* O157 : H7 and by Shiga toxin. *Federation of European Microbiological Societies Microbiology Letters* 44, 91–94.

Irwin, R.J., McEwen, S.A., Clarke, R.C. and Meek, A.H. (1989) The prevalence of verocytotoxin-producing *Escherichia coli* and antimicrobial resistance patterns of non-verocytotoxin-producing *Escherichia coli* and *Salmonella* in Ontario broiler chickens. *Canadian Journal of Veterinary Research* 53, 411–418.

Issartel, J-P., Koronakis, V. and Hughes, C. (1991) Activation of *Escherichia coli* prohemolysin to the mature toxin by acyl carrier protein-dependent fatty acylation. *Nature (London)* 351, 759–761.

Ito, T., Yutsudo, T., Hirayama, T. and Takeda, Y. (1988) Isolation and some properties of A and B subunits of vero toxin 2 and *in vitro* formation of hybrid toxins between subunits of vero toxin 1 and vero toxin 2 from *Escherichia coli* O157 : H7. *Microbial Pathogenesis* 5, 189–195.

Ito, H., Terai, A., Kurazono, H., Takeda, Y. and Nishibuchi, M. (1990) Cloning and nucleotide sequencing of Vero toxin 2 variant genes from *Escherichia coli* O91 : H21 isolated from a patient with the hemolytic uremic syndrome. *Microbial Pathogenesis* 8, 47–60.

Jackson, M.P. (1990) Structure–function analyses of Shiga toxin and the Shiga-like toxins. *Microbial Pathogenesis* 8, 235–242.

Jackson, M.P., Neill, R.J., O'Brien, A.D., Holmes, R.K. and Newland, J.W. (1987a) Nucleotide sequence analysis and comparison of the structural genes for Shiga-like toxin I and Shiga-like toxin II encoded by bacteriophages from *Escherichia coli* 933. *Federation of European Microbiological Societies Microbiology Letters* 44, 109–114.

Jackson, M.P., Newland, J.W., Holmes, R.K. and O'Brien, A.D. (1987b) Nucleotide sequence analysis of the structural genes for Shiga-like toxin I encoded by bacteriophage 933J from *Escherichia coli*. *Microbial Pathogenesis* 2, 147–153.

Jackson, M.P., Deresiewicz, R.L. and Calderwood, S.B. (1990a) Mutational analysis of the Shiga toxin and Shiga-like toxin II enzymatic subunits. *Journal of Bacteriology* 172, 3346–3350.

Jackson, M.P., Wadolkowski, E.A., Weinstein, D.L., Holmes, R.K. and O'Brien, A.D. (1990b) Functional analysis of the Shiga toxin and Shiga-like toxin type II variant binding subunits by using site-directed mutagenesis. *Journal of Bacteriology* 172, 653–657.

Janke, B.H., Francis, D.H,. Collins, J.E., Libal, M.C., Zeman, D.H., Johnson, D.D. and Neiger, R.D. (1990) Attaching and effacing *Escherchia coli* as a cause of diarrhoea in young calves. *Journal of the American Veterinary Medical Association* 196, 897–901.

Johnson, W.M. and Lior, H. (1987) Production of Shiga toxin and a cytolethal distending toxin (CLDT) produced by serogroups of *Shigella* spp. *Federation of European Microbiological Societies Microbiology Letters* 48, 235–238.

Johnson, W.M. and Lior, H. (1988) A new heat-labile cytolethal distending toxin (CLDT) produced by *Escherichia coli* isolates from clinical material. *Microbial Pathogenesis* 4, 103–113.

Jonas, D., Schultheis, B., Klas, C., Krammer, P.H. and Bhakdi, S. (1993) Cytocidal effects of *Escherichia coli* hemolysin on human T lymphocytes. *Infection and Immunity* 61, 1715–1721.

Kandel, G., Donohue-Rolfe, A., Donowitz, M. and Keusch, G. (1989) Pathogenesis of Shigella diarrhoea. XVI. Selective targetting of Shiga toxin to villus cells of rabbit jejunum explains the effect of the toxin on intestinal electrolyte transport. *Journal of Clinical Investigation* 84, 1509–1517.

Karch, H., Bitzan, M., Pietsch, R., Stenger, K., Wulffen, H., Hessemann, J. and Dusing, R. (1988) Purified verotoxins of *Escherichia coli* O157:H7 decrease prostacyclin synthesis by endothelial cells. *Microbial Pathogenesis* 5, 215–221.

Karmali, M.A. (1989) Infection by verocytotoxin-producing *Escherichia coli. Clinical Microbiological Reviews* 2, 15–38.

Karmali, M.A., Steele, B.T., Petric, M. and Lim, C. (1983) Sporadic cases of haemolytic uraemic syndrome associated with faecal cytotoxin and cytotoxin-producing *Escherichia coli* in stools. *Lancet* i, 619–620.

Karmali, M.A., Petric, M., Corazon, L., Fleming, P.C., Arbus, G.S. and Lior, H. (1985) The association between idiopathic hemolytic uremic syndrome and infection by verotoxin producing *E. coli. Journal of Infectious Diseases* 151, 775–782.

Karmali, M.A., Petric, M., Louie, S. and Cheung, R. (1986) Antigenic heterogeneity of *Escherichia coli* verotoxins. *Lancet* i, 164–165.

Kashiwazaki, M., Ogawa, T., Isayama, Y., Akaike, Y., Tamura, K. and Sakazaki, R. (1980) Detection of vero cytotoxic strains of *Escherichia coli* isolated from diseased animals. *National Institute of Animal Health Quarterly (Japan)* 20, 116–117.

Kavi, J., Chant, I., Maris, M. and Rose, P.E. (1987) Cytopathic effect of verotoxin on endothelial cells. *Lancet* ii, 1035.

Keenan, K.P., Sharpnack, D.D., Collins, H., Formal, S.B. and O'Brien, A.D. (1986) Morphologic evaluation of the effects of Shiga toxin, and *E. coli* shiga-like toxin on the rabbit intestine. *American Journal of Pathology* 125, 69–80.

Keusch, G.T., Jacewicz, M., Mobassaleh, M. and Donohue-Rolfe, A. (1991) Shiga toxin: intestinal cell receptors and pathophysiology of enterotoxic effects. *Reviews of Infectious Diseases* 13 (Suppl. 4), S304–310.

Konowalchuk, J., Speirs, J.L. and Stavric, S. (1977) Vero response to a cytotoxin of *Escherichia coli. Infection and Immunity* 18, 775–779.

Koronakis, V., Stanley, P., Koronakis, E. and Hughes, C. (1992) The HlyB/HlyD-dependent secretion of toxins by Gram-negative bacteria. *Federation of European Microbiological Societies Microbiology Immunology* 105, 45–54.

Lindberg, A.A., Brown, J.E., Stromberg, N., Westling-Ryd, M., Schultz, J.E. and Karlsson, K.-A. (1987) Identification of the carbohydrate receptor for Shiga toxin produced by *Shigella dysenteriae* type 1. *Journal of Biological Chemistry* 262, 1779–1785.

Linggood, M. and Ingram, P. (1982) The role of alpha-haemolysin in the virulence of *Escherichia coli* for mice. *Journal of Medical Microbiology* 15, 23–36.

Linggood, M.A. and Thompson, J.M. (1987) Verotoxin production among porcine strains of *Escherichia coli* and its association with oedema disease. *Journal of Medical Microbiology* 25, 359–362.

Lingwood, C.A., Law, H., Richardson, S.E., Petric, M., Brunton, J.L., deGrandis, S. and Karmali, M. (1987) Glycolipid binding of natural and recombinant *Escherichia coli* produced Verotoxin *in-vitro*. *Journal of Biological Chemistry* 262, 8834–8839.

Lopez-Alvarez, J. and Gyles, C.L. (1980) Occurrence of the Vir plasmid among animal and human strains of invasive *Escherichia coli. American Journal of Veterinary Research* 40, 769–774.

Lopez-Alvarez, J., Gyles, C.L., Shipley, P. and Falkow, S. (1980) Genetic and molecular characteristics of Vir plasmids of bovine septicemic *E. coli. Journal of Bacteriology* 141, 758–769.

MacLeod, D.L. and Gyles, C.L. (1989) Effects of culture conditions on yield of Shiga-like toxin-IIv from *Escherichia coli. Canadian Journal of Microbiology* 35, 623–629.

MacLeod, D.L. and Gyles, C.L. (1990) Purification and characterization of an *Escherichia coli* Shiga-like toxin II variant. *Infection and Immunity* 58, 1232–1239.

MacLeod, D.L. and Gyles, C.L. (1991) Immunization of pigs with a purified Shiga-like toxin II variant toxoid. *Veterinary Microbiology* 29, 309–318.

MacLeod, D.L., Gyles, C.L. and Wilcock, B.P. (1991a) Reproduction of edema disease of swine with purified Shiga-like toxin II variant. *Veterinary Pathology* 28, 66–73.

MacLeod, D.L., Gyles, C.L., Valdivieso-Garcia, A. and Clarke, R.C. (1991b) Physiochemical and biological properties of purified *Escherichia coli* Shiga-like toxin II variant. *Infection and Immunity* 59, 1300–1306.

Mainil, J.F., Duchesnes, C.J., Whipp, S.C., Marques, L.R.M., O'Brien, A.D., Casey, T.A. and Moon, H.W. (1987) Shiga-like toxin production and attaching effacing activity of *Escherichia coli* associated with calf diarrhoea. *American Journal of Veterinary Research* 48, 743–748.

Marques, L.R.M., Peiris, J.S.M., Cryz, S.J. and O'Brien A.D. (1987) *Escherichia coli* strains isolated from pigs with edema disease produce a variant of Shiga-like toxin II. *Federation of European Microbiological Societies Microbiology Letters* 44, 33–38.

Martin, M.L., Shipman, L.D., Potter, M.E., Wachsmuth, I.K., Wells, J.G., Hedberg, K., Tauxe, R.V., Davis, J.P., Arnoldi, J. and Tilleli, J. (1986) Isolation of *Escherichia coli* 0157:H7 from dairy cattle associated with two cases of hemolytic uremic syndrome. *Lancet* ii, 1043.

Mohammad, A., Peiris, J.S.M., Wijewanta, E.A., Mahalingam, S. and Gunasekara, G. (1985) Role of verocytotoxigenic *Escherichia coli* in cattle and buffalo calf diarrhoea. *Federation of European Microbiological Societies Microbiology Letters* 26, 281–283.

Mohammad, A., Peiris, J.S.M. and Wijewanta, E.A. (1986) Serotypes of verocytotoxigenic *Escherichia coli* isolated from cattle and buffalo calf diarrhoea. *Federation of European Microbiological Societies Microbiology Letters* 35, 261–265.

Montenegro, M.A., Bulte, M., Trumpf, T., Aleksic, S., Reuter, G., Bulling, E. and Helmuth, R. (1990) Detection and characterization of faecal verotoxin-producing *Escherichia coli* from healthy cattle. *Journal of Clinical Microbiology* 28, 1417–1421.

Montford, W., Villafranca, J.E., Monzingo, A.F., Ernst, S.R., Katzin, B., Rutenber, B., Xuong, N.H., Hamlin, R. and Robertus, J.D. (1987) The three-dimensional structure of ricin at 2.8 Å. *Journal of Biological Chemistry* 262, 5398–5403.

Moxley, R.A. and Francis, D.H. (1986) Natural and experimental infection with an attaching and effacing strain of *Escherichia coli* in calves. *Infection and Immunity* 53, 339–346.

Moyer, M.P., Dixon, P.S., Rothman, S.W. and Brown, J.E. (1987) Cytotoxicity of Shiga toxin for primary cultures of human colonic and ileal epithelial cells. *Infection and Immunity* 55, 1533–1535.

Noegel, A., Rdest, U. and Goebel, W. (1981) Determination of the functions of hemolysin plasmid pHly152 of *Escherichia coli*. *Journal of Bacteriology* 145, 233–247.

O'Brien, A.D. and Holmes, R.H. (1987) Shiga and Shiga-like toxins. *Microbiological Reviews* 51, 206–220.

O'Brien, A.D. and LaVeck, G.D. (1983) Purification and characterization of a *Shigella dysenteriae* 1-like toxin produced by *Escherichia coli*. *Infection and Immunity* 40, 675–683.

O'Brien, A.D., Thompson, M.R., Cantey, J.R. and Formal, S.B. (1977) Production of a *Shigella dysenteriae*-like toxin by pathogenic *Escherichia coli*. In: *Abstracts of the Annual Meeting of the American Society for Microbiology*. ASM, Washington, DC, Abstr. B103.

O'Brien, A.D., LaVeck, G.D., Thompson, M.R. and Formal, S.B. (1982) Production of *Shigella dysenteriae* Type 1-like cytotoxin by *Escherichia coli*. *Journal of Infectious Diseases* 146, 763–769.

Ogasawara, T., Ito, K., Igarashi, K., Yutsudo, T., Nakabayashi, N. and Takeda, Y. (1988) Inhibition of protein synthesis by a vero toxin (VT2 or Shiga-like toxin II) produced by *Escherichia coli* O157:H7 at the level of elongation factor 1-dependent aminoacyl-tRNA binding to ribosomes. *Microbial Pathogenesis* 4, 127–135.

O'Hanley, P., Lalonde, G. and Ji, G. (1991) Alpha-hemolysin contributes to the pathogenicity of piliated digalactoside-binding *Escherichia coli* in the kidney:

efficacy of an alpha-hemolysin vaccine in preventing renal injury in the BALB/c mouse model of pyelonephritis. *Infection and Immunity* 59, 1153–1161.

Oku, Y., Yutsudo, T., Hirayama, T., O'Brien, A.D. and Takeda, Y. (1989) Purification and some properties of a Vero toxin from a human strain of *Escherichia coli* that is immunologically related to Shiga-like toxin II (VT2). *Microbial Pathogenesis* 6, 113–122.

Olsnes, S., Reisbig, R. and Eikled, K. (1981) Subunit structure of Shigella cytotoxin. *Journal of Biological Chemistry* 256, 8732–8738.

Oswald, E. and De Rycke, J. (1990) A single protein of 110 kDa is associated with the multinucleating and necrotizing activity coded by the Vir plasmid of *Escherichia coli. Federation of European Microbiological Societies Microbiology Letters* 66, 278–284.

Oswald, E., De Rycke, J., Guillot, J.F. and Boivin, R. (1989) Cytotoxic effect of multinucleation in HeLa cell cultures associated with the presence of Vir plasmid in *Escherichia coli* strains. *Federation of European Microbiological Societies Microbiology Letters* 58, 95–100.

Oswald, E., De Rycke, J., Lintermans, P., Van Muylem, K., Mainil, J., Doube, G. and Pohl, P. (1991) Virulence factors associated with cytotoxic necrotizing factor type two in bovine diarrhoeic and septicaemic strains of *Escherichia coli*. *Journal of Clinical Microbiology* 29, 2522–2527.

Padhye, V.V., Zhao, T. and Doyle, M.P. (1989) Production and characterization of monoclonal antibodies to Verotoxins 1 and 2 from *Escherichia coli* of serotype O157:H7. *Journal of Medical Microbiology* 30, 219–226.

Pai, C.H., Kelly, J.K. and Meyers, G. (1986) Experimental infection of infant rabbits with verotoxin-producing *Escherichia coli. Infection and Immunity* 51, 16–23.

Perera, L.P., Samuel, J.E., Holmes, R.K. and O'Brien, A.D. (1991) Identification of three amino acid residues in the B subunit of Shiga toxin and Shiga-like toxin type II that are essential for holotoxin activity. *Journal of Bacteriology* 173, 1151–1160.

Petric, M., Karmali, M.A., Richardson, S. and Cheung, R. (1987) Purification and biological properties of *Escherichia coli* Verocytotoxin. *Federation of European Microbiological Societies Microbiology Letters* 41, 63–68.

Pohl, P., Daube, G., Mainil, J., Lintermans, P., Kaeckenbeeck, A. and Oswald, E. (1992) Facteurs de virulence et phenotypes de soixante et une souches d'*Escherichia coli* d'origine bovine, productrices de la toxine cytotoxique necrosante de type 1 (CNF 1). *Annales de Recherche Veterinaire* 23, 83–91.

Read, S.C., Gyles, C.L., Clarke, R.C. and McEwen, S.A. (1990) Prevalence of verocytotoxigenic *Escherichia coli* in ground beef, pork, and chicken in southwestern Ontario. *Epidemiology and Infection* 105, 11–20.

Richardson, S.E., Karmali, M.A., Becker, L.E. and Smith, C.R. (1988) The histopathology of the hemolytic uremic syndrome associated with Verocytotoxin-producing *Escherichia coli* infections. *Human Pathology* 19, 1102–1108.

Richardson, S.E., Rotman, T.A., Jay, V., Smith, C.R., Becker, L.E., Petric, M., Olivieri, N.F. and Karmali, M.A. (1992) Experimental verocytotoxemia in rabbits. *Infection and Immunity* 60, 4154–4167.

Rose, P.E., Armour, J.A., Williams, B.B. and Hill, F.G.H. (1985) Verotoxin and neuraminidase induced platelet aggregating activity in plasma, their possible role in the pathogenesis of the hemolytic uremic syndrome. *Journal of Clinical Pathology* 38, 438–441.

Samuel, J.E., Perera, L.P., Ward, S., O'Brien, A.D., Ginsburg, V. and Krivan, H.C. (1990) Comparison of the glycolipid receptor specificities of Shiga-like toxin type II and Shiga-like toxin type II variants. *Infection and Immunity* 58, 611–618.

Sandvig, K., Garred, O., Prydz, K., Kozlov, J.V., Hansen, S.H. and van Deurs, B. (1992) Retrograde transport of endocytosed Shiga toxin to the endoplasmic reticulum. *Nature* 358, 510–512.

Saxena, S.K., O'Brien, A.D. and Ackerman, E.J. (1989) Shiga toxin, Shiga-like toxin II variant, and ricin are all single-site RNA N-glycosidases of 28S RNA when microinjected into *Xenopus* oocytes. *Journal of Biological Chemistry* 264, 596–601.

Scheffer, J., Konig, W., Hacker, J. and Goebel, W. (1985) Bacterial adherence and hemolysin production from *Escherichia coli* induces histamine and leukotriene release from various cells. *Infection and Immunity* 50, 271–278.

Schimmelpfennig, H. and Webver, R. (1979) Studies on the oedema disease producing toxin of *Escherichia coli* (*E. coli*-neurotoxin). *Fortschritte der Veterinarmedizin* 29, 25–32.

Schlossman, D., Withers, D., Welsh, P., Alexander, A., Robertus, J. and Frankel, A. (1989) Role of glutamic acid 177 of the ricin toxin A chain in enzymatic inactivation of ribosomes. *Molecular and Cellular Biology* 9, 5012–5021.

Schmitt, C.K., McKee, M.L. and O'Brien, A.D. (1991) Two copies of Shiga-like toxin II-related genes common in enterohemorrhagic *Escherichia coli* strains are responsible for the antigenic heterogeneity of the O157:H$^-$ strain E32511. *Infection and Immunity* 59, 1065–1073.

Schoonderwoerd, M., Clarke, R.C., van Dreumel, A.A. and Rawluk, S. (1988) Colitis in calves: natural and experimental infection with a verotoxin-producing strain of *Escherichia coli* O111:NM. *Canadian Journal of Veterinary Research* 562, 484–487.

Scotland, S.M., Smith, H.R., Willshaw, G.A. and Rowe, B. (1983) Vero cytotoxin production in strain of *Escherichia coli* is determined by genes carried on bacteriophage. *Lancet* ii, 216.

Scotland, S.M., Smith, H.R. and Rowe, B. (1985) Two distinct toxins active on Vero cells from *Escherichia coli* O157. *Lancet* ii, 885–886.

Smith H.R., Scotland, S.M., Willshaw, G.A., Wray, C., McLaren, I.M., Cheasty, T. and Rowe, B. (1988) Vero cytotoxin production and presence of VT genes in *Escherichia coli* strains of animal origin. *Journal of General Microbiology* 134, 829–834.

Smith, H.W. (1963) The haemolysins of *Escherichia coli*. *Journal of Pathology and Bacteriology* 85, 197–211.

Smith, H.W. (1974) A search for transmissible pathogenic characters in invasive strains of *Escherichia coli*: the discovery of a plasmid-mediated toxin and a plasmid-controlled lethal character closely associated with, or identical with, colicine V. *Journal of General Microbiology* 83, 95–111.

Smith, H.W. and Halls, S. (1968) The production of oedema disease amd diarrhoea in weaned pigs by the oral administration of *Escherichia coli*: factors that influence the course of the experimenatal disease. *Journal of Medical Microbiology* 1, 45–49.

Smith, H.W. and Huggins, M.B. (1985) The toxic role of alpha-haemolysin in the pathogenesis of experimental *Escherichia coli* infection in mice. *Journal of General Microbiology* 131, 395–403.

Smith, H.W. and Linggood, M.A. (1971) Observations on the pathogenic properties of the K88, Hly and Ent plasmids of *Escherichia coli* with particular reference to porcine diarrhoea. *Journal of Medical Microbiology* 4, 467–485.

Smith, H.W., Green, P. and Parsell, Z. (1983) Vero cell toxins in *Escherichia coli* and related bacteria: transfer by phage and conjugation and toxic action in laboratory animals, chickens and pigs. *Journal of General Microbiology* 129, 3121–3137.

Stein, P.E., Boodhoo, A., Tyrrell, G.J., Brunton, J.L. and Read, R.J. (1992) Crystal structure of the cell-binding B oligomer of verotoxin-1 from *E. coli. Nature (London)* 355, 748–750.

Strockbine, N.A., Marques, L.R.M., Newland, J.W., Smith, H.W., Holmes, R.K. and O'Brien, A.D. (1986) Two toxin-converting phages from *Escherichia coli* O157:H7 strain 933 encode antigenically distinct toxins with similar biologic activities. *Infection and Immunity* 53, 135–140.

Strockbine, N.A., Jackson, M.P., Sung, L.M., Holmes, R.K. and O'Brien, A.D. (1988) Cloning and sequencing of the genes for Shiga toxin from *Shigella dysenteriae* type 1. *Journal of Bacteriology* 170, 1116–1122.

Tabouret, M. and De Rycke, J. (1990) Detection of cytotoxic necrotising factor (CNF) in extracts of *Escherichia coli* strains by enzyme-linked immunosorbent assay. *Journal of Medical Microbiology* 32, 73–81.

Takao, T., Tanabe, T., Hong, Y., Shimonishi, Y., Kurazono, H., Yutsudo, T., Sasakawa, C., Yoshikawa, M. and Takeda, Y. (1988) Identity of molecular structure of Shiga-like toxin 1 (VT1) from *Escherichia coli* O157:H7 with that of Shiga toxin. *Microbial Pathogenesis* 5, 357–369.

Taylor, C.M., Milford, D.V., Rose, P.E., Roy, T.C. and Rowe, B. (1990) The expression of blood group P1 in post-enteropathic haemolytic ureamic syndrome. *Pediatric Nephrology* 4, 59–61.

Tesh, V.L. and O'Brien, A.D. (1991) Microreview. The pathogenic mechanisms of Shiga toxin and Shiga-like toxins. *Molecular Microbiology* 5, 1817–1822.

Tesh, V.L., Samuel, J.E., Perera, L.P., Sharefkin, J.B. and O'Brien, A.D. (1991) Evaluation of the role of Shiga toxin and Shiga-like toxins in mediating direct damage to human vascular endothelial cells. *Journal of Infectious Diseases* 164, 344–352.

Tesh, V.L., Burris, J.A., Owens, J.W., Gordon, V.M., Wadolkowski, E.A., O'Brien, A. and Samuel, J. (1993) Comparison of relative toxicities of Shiga-like toxins type I and type II for mice. *Infection and Immunity* 61, 3392–3402.

Timoney, J.F. (1949) Experimental production of oedema disease of swine. *Veterinary Record* 61, 710–712.

Timoney, J.F. (1960) An alternative method to repeated freezing and thawing for the preparation of an extract of haemolytic *Escherichia coli* which on intravenous injection in pigs mimics the syndrome of oedema disease. *Veterinary Record* 72, 1252.

Waddell, T. and Gyles, C.L. (1993) Sodium deoxycholate facilitates systemic absorption of Shiga-like toxin II variant from the intestine of the pig. In: *Abstracts of the 93rd Annual General Meeting of the American Society for Microbiology*. American Society for Microbiology, Washington, DC, Abstr. B-97, p. 43.

Waddell, T., Head, S., Petric, M., Cohen, A. and Lingwood, C. (1988) Globotriosyl ceramide is specifically recognized by the *Escherichia coli* verocytotoxin 2. *Biochemical and Biophysical Research Communications* 152, 674–679.

Waddell, T., Cohen, A. and Lingwood, C.A. (1990) Induction of verotoxin sensitivity in receptor-deficient cell lines using the receptor glycolipid globotriosylceramide. *Proceedings of the National Academy of Sciences of the United States of America* 87, 7898–7901.

Walterspiel, J.N., Ashkenazi, S., Morrow, A.L. and Cleary, T.G. (1992) Effect of subinhibitory concentrations of antibiotics on extracellular Shiga-like toxin I. *Infection* 20, 25–29.

Wandersman, C. and Delepelaire, P. (1990) TolC, an *Escherichia coli* outer membrane protein required for hemolysin secretion. *Proceedings of the National Academy of Sciences of the United States of America* 87, 4776–4780.

Weinstein, D.L., Holmes, R.K. and O'Brien, A.D. (1988a) Effects of iron and temperature on Shiga-like toxin I production by *Escherichia coli. Infection and Immunity* 56, 106–111.

Weinstein, D.L., Jackson, M.P., Samuel, J.E., Holmes, R.K. and O'Brien, A.D. (1988b) Cloning and sequencing of a Shiga-like toxin type II variant type from an *Escherichia coli* strain responsible for edema disease of swine. *Journal of Bacteriology* 170, 4223–4230.

Weinstein, D.L., Jackson, M.P., Perera, L.P., Holmes, R.K. and O'Brien, A.D. (1989) *In vivo* formation of hybrid toxins comprising Shiga toxin and the Shiga-like toxins and role of the B subunit in localization and cytotoxic activity. *Infection and Immunity* 57, 3743–3750.

Welch, R.A. (1991) Microreview. Pore-forming cytolysins of Gram-negative bacteria. *Molecular Microbiology* 5, 521–528.

Welch, R.A. and Pellett, S. (1988) The transcriptional organization of the *Escherichia coli* hemolysin. *Journal of Bacteriology* 170, 1622–1630.

Welch, R.A., Forestier, C., Lobo, A., Pellett, S., Thomas, W., Jr and Rowe, G. (1992) The synthesis and function of the *Escherichia coli* hemolysin and related RTX exotoxins. *Federation of European Microbiological Societies Microbiology Immunology* 105, 29–36.

Wilson, J.B., McEwen, S.A., Clarke, R.C., Leslie, K.E., Wilson, R.A., Waltner-Toews, D. and Gyles, C.L. (1992) Distribution and characteristics of verocytotoxigenic *Escherichia coli* isolated from Ontario dairy cattle. *Epidemiology and Infection* 108, 423–439.

Yamasaki, S., Furutani, M., Ito, K., Igarashi, K., Nischibuchi, M. and Takeda, Y. (1991) Importance of arginine at position 170 of the A subunit of vero toxin 1 produced by enterohemorrhagic *Escherichia coli* for toxin activity. *Microbial Pathogenesis* 11, 1–9.

Yee, A., deGrandis, S. and Gyles, C.L. (1993) Mitomycin C induced synthesis of a Shiga-like toxin from enteropathogenic *Escherichia coli* H.I.8. *Infection and Immunity* 61, 4510–4513.

Yutsudo, T., Nakabayashi, N., Hirayama, T. and Takeda, Y. (1987) Purification and some properties of a Verotoxin from *Escherichia coli* O157:H7 that is immunologically unrelated to Shiga toxin. *Microbial Pathogenesis* 3, 21–30.

Zoja, C., Corna, D., Farina, C., Sacchi, G., Lingwood, C., Doyle, M.P., Padhye, V.V., Abbate, M. and Remuzzi, G. (1992) Verotoxin glycolipid receptors determine the localization of microangiopathic process in rabbits given verotoxin-1. *Journal of Laboratory and Clinical Medicine* 120, 229–238.

Zschock, M., Herbst, W., Lange, H., Hamann, H.P. and Th. Schliesser (1989) Mikrobiologische untersuchengsergbnisse (bakteriologie und elektronmikroskopie) bei der diarrho des hundwelpen. *Tierarztliche Praxis* 17, 93–95.

Fimbriae of *Escherichia coli* 16

C.J. Smyth, M. Marron and S.G.J. Smith
Department of Microbiology, Moyne Institute, University of Dublin, Trinity College, Dublin 2, Ireland

Introduction

E. coli is the causative agent of both intestinal and extraintestinal infections. Extraintestinal infections caused by *E. coli* in man include urinary tract infections, newborn sepsis and meningitis, while in animals *E. coli* is a cause of mastitis in cattle, and septicaemia and enterotoxaemia in piglets. The adhesion of *E. coli* to host tissue at the site of infection is a prelude to these numerous infections. Attachment is mediated by rod-like or fibrillar surface appendages on the bacteria termed fimbriae or by adhesins that are difficult to demonstrate electron microscopically as morphological surface structures, often referred to as non-fimbrial or afimbrial adhesins. The fimbriae consist of a large number of copies of a structural subunit which confers antigenic specificity on the fimbriae and, in certain cases, a few copies of minor subunits, one being the adhesin with specific binding properties, the others being essential for presentation of the adhesin at the tip or on the surface of the fimbrial structure. While some non-fimbrial or afimbrial adhesins resemble capsular material surrounding bacterial cells as visualized by electron microscopy, other so-called non-fimbrial adhesins may be misnomers for structures which current staining procedures for electron microscopy do not reveal adequately.

In the initial stages of infection *E. coli* make contact with epithelial surfaces. The adhesins possessed by different pathogenic *E. coli* exhibit differential binding specificity to these epithelia. However, the binding properties of *E. coli* fimbriae are not restricted to epithelia. Basement membranes and extracellular matrix proteins are also targets for *E. coli* fimbriae. Indeed, host molecules, such as plasminogen and tissue-type plasminogen activator, have been shown to bind to *E. coli* fimbriae. Such binding does not appear to involve the adhesin sites of the fimbriae. This has led to the concept that fimbriae may also enhance *E. coli* virulence in a non-adhesive manner and should be thought of as multifunctional complexes.

While effective colonization of host tissues by pathogenic *E. coli* involves adhesin–receptor interaction to overcome host defence mechanisms such as urination, desquamation and peristaltic propulsion through the intestinal tract, other factors play a role in the establishment of infections at certain body sites. Motility may aid in penetration of mucus (Smyth, 1988). Lipopolysaccharides and capsules probably contribute to bile salt resistance and protection against host iron-binding proteins and non-specific serum factors such as complement (Mims, 1987; Woolcock, 1988). Acquisition of iron mediated by siderophores such as aerobactin and enterochelin may be important for survival (Griffiths *et al.*, 1988; Woolcock, 1988; Neilands, 1990). Moreover, although adherence mediated by fimbriae determines the site of infections, virulence factors such as haemolysin, heat-stable and heat-labile enterotoxins, Shiga-like toxins and cytotoxic necrotizing factor are responsible for the disease symptoms and the severity of the infection. Colonization of mucus is probably important to eventual adherence to and colonization of the underlying epithelium. Indeed, intestinal *E. coli* strains have been shown to utilize phosphatidylserine in mucus as a sole source of carbon and nitrogen, suggesting that the ability to grow in mucus may be essential to subsequent events (Krivan *et al.*, 1992).

Many reviews have been written on *E. coli* fimbriae associated with particular infections caused by this bacterium (Beachey, 1980; Savage and Fletcher, 1985; Sussman, 1985; Mirelman, 1986; Roth, 1988; Evans and Evans, 1990; Jann and Jann, 1990; Moon, 1990; Tennent *et al.*, 1990; Korhonen *et al.*, 1992a). This chapter will summarize information on *E. coli* fimbriae and focus on certain aspects of their biology, structure and genetics.

Fimbriae Found on Pathogenic *E. coli*

Nomenclature and distribution

The nomenclature of fimbriae is diverse and confusing. Although some attempts have been made to devise a system of F numbers to designate fimbrial antigens in the same way as O:K:H antigens of *E. coli*, most fimbriae are still referred to by their original names, albeit that some are well-recognized misnomers, e.g. K88 and K99 fimbriae, because of long-time usage in the literature and diagnostically. Terms such as CFA or PCF or CS fimbriae are descriptive terms coined to ascribe or infer function to surface-associated antigens in relation to infection.

Tables 16.1 and 16.2 catalogue the fimbriae and non-fimbrial or afimbrial adhesins described on pathogenic strains of *E. coli*. Type 1 fimbriae or common type fimbriae are produced by a wide range of *E. coli* strains. The other fimbrial and non-fimbrial adhesins are associated with infections in particular hosts and exhibit host-tissue specificity with respect to adhesive capacity. Electron microscopically most fimbriae are revealed as rigid rod-like structures of 5–7 nm in diameter (Fig. 16.1). Some fimbriae are thinner and flexible (2–4 nm), e.g. K88, K99 and CS3 fimbriae, and are sometimes referred to as fibrillae. Other adhesins are described as non-fimbrial or as afimbrial, e.g. the NFA-1 adhesin described as a capsule-like, fine fibrillar structure on the bacterial surface (Jann and Hoschützky, 1990). These fine meshes of fibrils are not unlike those of K88 fimbriae or CS3 fimbriae and might be more properly considered to be further types of fibrillar fimbriae. The term curli has been applied to 'novel' coiled, hair-like structures first described on strains of *E. coli* from bovine mastitis (Olsén *et al.*, 1989). Although the subunit protein curlin shares none of the common features of pilin molecules, it is debatable whether curli are distinct organelles or merely a new class of fimbriae.

It should also be noted that fimbrial and non-fimbrial adhesins can occur in combinations on *E. coli* strains (Table 16.3). This has been examined more thoroughly in enterotoxigenic *E. coli* than in strains of other infection origin.

Molecular architecture of fimbriae

Any model of fimbrial architecture must ultimately account for functional and biological properties of these structures. Models of fimbrial structure stem from electron microscopic, crystallographic and X-ray diffraction studies on type 1 fimbriae (Fig. 16.2) (Brinton, 1965, 1967). The supramolecular structure of this prototype rigid rod-like fimbria was described as a right-handed helical array of subunits of 17 kDa with 3.125 subunits per turn of the helix, a pitch of 2.3 nm, an outer diameter of 7 nm and an axial hole of 2.0–2.5 nm. Other rigid, rod-like fimbriae having the same overall morphological appearance to type 1 fimbriae were long assumed to comprise helical arrays of subunits, albeit that the numbers of subunits per turn and the pitch distances might vary because of differences in the molecular weights of the subunits (Smyth, 1986; Jann *et al.*, 1992).

The ultrastructure of the fibrillar types of fimbriae is less clear. Their different morphological appearance (Fig. 16.2) suggests a difference in subunit interaction on assembly into a supramolecular structure from that of the rigid, rod-like type of fimbria. Some electron micrographs suggest an open helical structure rather than a closed structure with an axial pore (Issacson, 1977; de Graaf *et al.*, 1980; de Graaf and Roorda, 1982; Jones and Isaacson, 1984; Isaacson, 1985). An open helical structure has been

Table 16.1. Characteristics of fimbrial and non-fimbrial adhesins of diarrhoeagenic and enterotoxaemic *E. coli*.

Class of *E. coli* fimbriae/adhesion antigens	Morphology[a]	Diameter (nm)	M_r subunit (kDa)	Genetic determinant	
				Locus	Location[b]
Enterotoxigenic[c]					
Human					
CFA/I (F2)	R	7	15.0	*cfa*	P
CFA/II (F3)					
CS1	R	7	16.8	*cso*	P
CS2	R	7	15.3		C
CS3	F	2–3	15.1	*cst*	P
CFA/III	R	7–8	18.0		P
CFA/IV					
CS4	R	6	17.0		P
CS5	R	5	21.0		P
CS6	NF		16.0	*css*	P
CS7	R	5	21.0		P
C17	R	6–7	17.0		P
PCFO9	F		27.0		P
PCFO148	F				P
PCFO159	R	7	19.0		P
PCFO166	R	7	15.5 or 17.0		P
2230	F		16.0		P
8786	NF		16.3		
Longus	R	7	22	*lng*	P
Animal					
K88 (F4)	F	2.1	27.6	*fae*	P
K99 (F5)	F	5	16.5	*fan*	P
987P (F6)	R	7	17.2	*fas*	P
F41	F	3.2	29.0		C
CS31A	F	2	26.8		P
CS1541	F	3–5	18.0, 19.0		
F17 (Fy)	R	3.4	20.0		C
F42			31.0		P
F141	R	5	17.0		
F165	R	4–6	17.5, 19.0		C
Enteropathogenic[d]					
BFP	R		19.5	*bfp*	C
FB171–14	F?	2–3	14.8		
FB171–15	R?	7	15.5		
FB171–16	R?	7	16.5		
AIDA-1	NF	2	100	*ada*	P
Enteroaggregative[e]					
GVVPQ	F	2–4	18		
AAF/1	F	2	14	*aaf*	P

Table 16.1. *continued*

Class of *E. coli* fimbriae/adhesion antigens	Morphology[a]	Diameter (nm)	M_r subunit (kDa)	Genetic determinant	
				Locus	Location[b]
Enteroinvasive[f]					
469–3	F	2	14		
Enterohaemorrhagic[g]					
O157:H7	R?		16		
Oedema disease[h]					
107	R	5	15.1	*fed*	C

[a] R = rigid, rod-shaped; F = fibrillar; NF = non-fimbrial.
[b] P = plasmid; C = chromosome.
[c] Data from de Graaf (1990), Smyth *et al.* (1991), Girón *et al.* (1994) and de Graaf and Gaastra (1994).
[d] Girón *et al.* (1991, 1993).
[e] Collinson *et al.* (1992); Nataro *et al.* (1992).
[f] Hinson *et al.* (1987).
[g] Karch *et al.* (1987).
[h] Imberechts *et al.* (1992).

proposed for *Bordetella pertussis* fimbriae with a 6.5 nm pitch distance and 2.5 repeating subunits per turn (Steven *et al.*, 1986). This serves as a useful model for the flexible, wiry fimbriae of *E. coli* (Fig. 16.2D and E).

The most significant contributions to current understanding of the macromolecular structure of fimbriae have come from analyses of the genetic determinants encoding biogenesis of fimbriae and from biochemical studies of dissociated fimbrial subunits (Mooi and de Graaf, 1985; Normark *et al.*, 1986; de Graaf, 1990; Hacker, 1990; Jann and Hoschützky, 1990; de Graaf and Gaastra, 1994). Specifically, genetic analyses of the determinants for P, S, type 1, CFA/I, K88 and K99 fimbriae have been particularly revealing. The general concept emerging from these studies is that the adhesive interaction of bacterial fimbriae can be mediated by major or minor fimbrial subunits, with the adhesin being located either at the tip of the fimbria or along the length of the macromolecular structure (Fig. 16.2).

In the case of P, S and type 1 fimbriae minor fimbrial subunits are the functional adhesins interacting with host tissue. P fimbriae have fibrils at the tips of the morphological rod structures composed of the major structural subunit PapA (Hultgren *et al.*, 1991; Hultgren and Normark, 1991; Kuehn *et al.*, 1992; Jones *et al.*, 1992; Jacob-Dubuisson *et al.*, 1993). This functional tip fibrillar complex presents the adhesin PapG to its receptor. While tip fibrils have not been revealed by electron microscopy on S fimbriae, minor subunits have been identified that are the adhesin and the

Table 16.2. Characteristics of fimbrial and non-fimbrial adhesins of extraintestinal *E. coli*.

Class of *E. coli* fimbriae/adhesion antigens	Morphology	Diameter (nm)	M_r subunit (kDa)	Genetic determinant	
				Locus	Location
Uropathogenic					
P group					
$F7_1$	R	7	20, 22	*fso*	C
$F7_2$	R	7	17, 20	*fst*	C
F8	R	7	19.5	*fei*	C
F9	R	7	21	*fni*	C
F11	R	7	18	*fel*	C
F12	R	7	16.8	*ftw*	C
F13	R	7	18.8, 19.5	*pap*	C
F14	R	7	20.5		C
Prs	R	7	19.5	*prs*	C
Prf	R	7	22	*prf*	C
Type 1	R	7	17	*fim, pil*	C
F1C	R	7	16.5, 17	*foc*	C
Dr	R	7	21	*dra*	C
S	R	7	16	*sfaI*	C
G	R	5–7	19.5		C
M	R	7	21	*bma*	C
Nfa-I	NF	–	21	*nfa*	C
Afa-I	NF	–	16	*afa*	C
Septicaemic/meningitis/colibacillosis					
S	R		16	*sfaII*	C
$F165_1$	R	5–8	19	*$F165_1$*	C
$F165_2$	R	5–8	17.5	*$F165_2$*	C
F11	R	7	18	*fel*	C

Data compiled from Hacker (1990), Fairbrother *et al.* (1988), Garcia *et al.* (1992), Harel *et al.* (1992), van den Bosch *et al.* (1993) and Hacker *et al.* (1993).

proteins involved in its functional presentation (Hacker, 1990; Hacker *et al.*, 1992). Type 1 fimbriae also possess a tip adhesin complex of minor subunits, although it has been proposed in this instance that these complexes are also present along the length of the fimbria composed of the structural subunits (Krogfelt and Klemm, 1988; Klemm and Krogfelt, 1991).

Other fimbriae, e.g. CFA/I, are composed of subunits of one type, viz. the structural subunit (Jann and Hoschützky, 1990, 1991; Jann *et al.*,

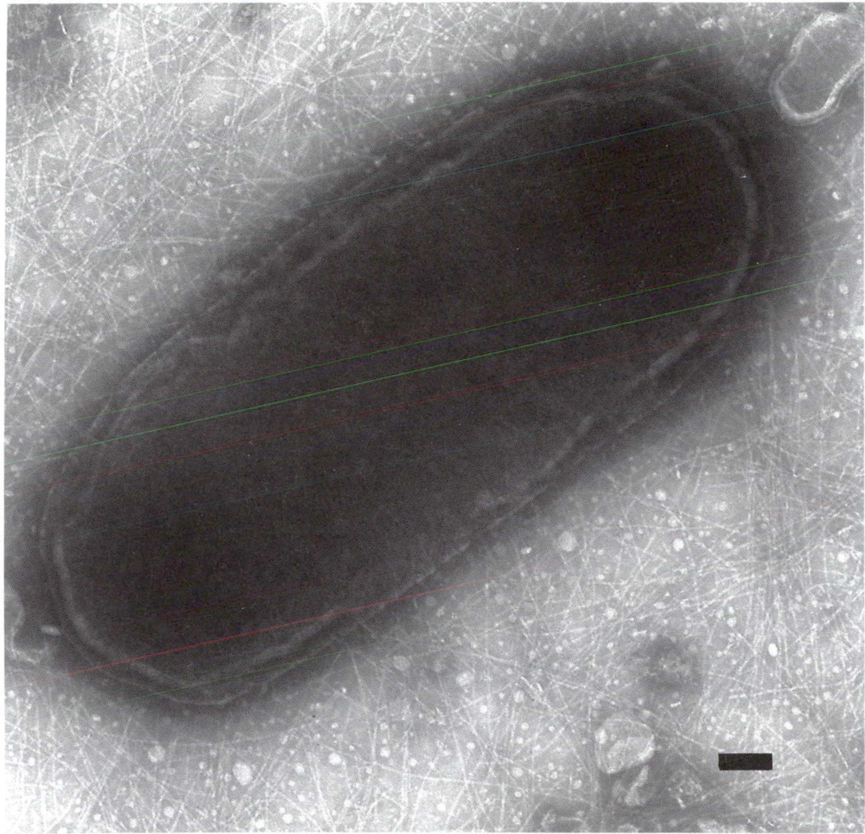

Fig. 16.1. Transmission electron micrograph of *E. coli* K-12 derivative (XL-1) expressing CS1 fimbriae from a recombinant plasmid encoding the CS1 fimbrial operon. Cells were negatively stained with 1% phosphotungstic acid. Scale bar = 100 nm.

1992; de Graaf and Gaastra, 1994). These subunits are either assembled in such a way that only the tip-located subunit has its receptor-binding domain exposed or such that all or many of the subunits of the fimbria possess exposed receptor-binding sites (Fig. 16.2B and C). In the case of K88 and K99 fimbriae which are fibrillar in nature, adhesive multivalency appears to allow for multiple interactions with host receptors, whereas in the case of CFA/I fimbriae, a tip-located structural subunit with an exposed receptor-binding site appears to be the adhesin.

Detailed genetic analysis of the *fae* and *fan* fimbrial operons has provided evidence for a role of minor subunits in their respective fimbrial structures. Three minor subunits, FanF, FanG and FanH, are required for initiation and elongation of K99 fimbriae. A model integrating them into

Table 16.3. Occurrence of combinations of adhesins/fimbriae on *E. coli*.[a]

Type of *E. coli*	Combination of adhesins/fimbriae[b]
Enterotoxigenic	K88 + 987P
	K88 + 987P + K99
	K88 + F41 + K99
	F41 + K99
	CS31A + K99
	K88 + CS31A + K99
	CS31A + K99 + F165
	F41 + 987P + K99 + F165
	F41 + 987P
	987P + F165
	CS1 + CS3
	CS2 + CS3
	CS4 + CS6
	CS5 + CS6
Uropathogenic	G + M
	$F7_1$ + $F7_2$ + F1A + F1C
	F12 + F13 + F14 + F1C
	F1A + F13
	S + Prf + NonF1A

[a] Type 1 fimbriae are not considered in this context.
[b] Data compiled from Hacker (1990); de Graaf and Gaastra (1994).

the K99 fimbria with the FanC structural/adhesin subunits has been proposed (Simons *et al.*, 1991). Likewise, in the case of K88 fimbriae, two minor subunits, FaeF and FaeH, have been shown to play an essential role in biogenesis (Bakker *et al.*, 1992). None of these minor subunits, respectively, possess adhesive capacity. Moreover, a minor tip-located subunit of K88 fimbriae designated FaeC does possess adhesive properties (de Graaf and Bakker, 1992; de Graaf and Gastra, 1994).

Wild-type strains with rigid rod-like P, S or type 1 fimbriae are often capsulated. Expression of the minor adhesin subunits at the tips of these fimbriae would ensure that the parts of these fimbriae involved in the adhesive process are exposed for receptor binding. In the case of the wiry fimbriae which surround the bacteria in a capsule-like manner, e.g. CS3 fimbriae or CS31A fimbriae, tip expression would not be crucial for adhesion (de Graaf and Gaastra, 1994).

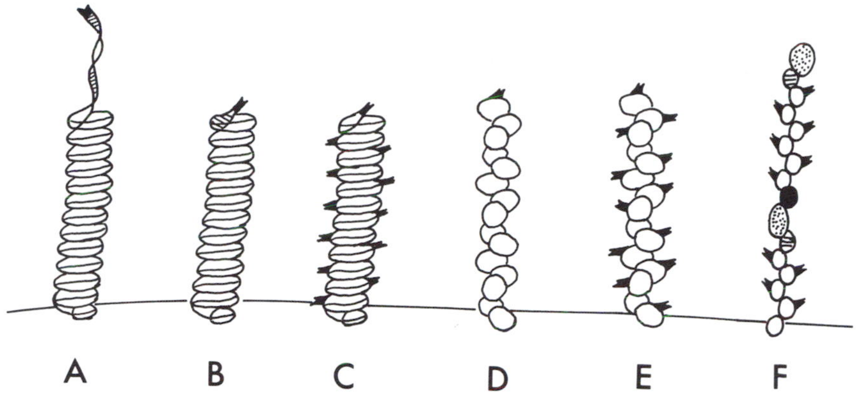

Fig. 16.2. Schematic representation of fimbrial structures in *E. coli*. The horizontal line represents the outer membrane surface of *E. coli*. The filled wedges represent the receptor binding sites of structural subunits or adhesin subunits. A, The P fimbria: PapA subunits are arranged in a helix to form a rigid rod-shaped structure with a terminal fibrillar structure consisting of the PapE minor subunit as its major component and PapF and PapK as minor components. The Galα1-4Gal adhesin PapG is at the terminus of the fibrillum. B, The S fimbria: SfaA subunits form the rigid rod-shaped structure with SfaS, the sialylgalactoside-binding adhesin, at its terminus possibly linked to a SfaA subunit by other minor subunits. The CFA/I fimbria: CfaB subunits form the rod-shaped fimbria, the terminal structural subunit being exposed to reveal its receptor-binding site. The type 1 fimbria: the rod-shaped fimbria consists of FimA subunits with minor subunits FimF and FimG linking the FimG mannose-specific adhesin to the FimA subunits. This may occur both terminally and by intercalation into the fimbria along its length. C, The SS142 fimbria: subunits form the rod-shaped fimbria, many of which have receptor-binding sites exposed along the length of the fimbria. D, Model of a fibrillar fimbria composed of structural subunits with the adhesin-binding site exposed on the terminal subunit. E, The K88 fimbria: a thin wiry fibrillar structure composed of FaeG subunits each with an exposed receptor-binding site forming a multivalent binding structure. F, The K99 fimbria: a thin wiry fimbria composed of FanC subunits (open) which act as adhesins. The FanF (dotted), FanG (hatched) and FanH (solid) minor subunits are involved in initiation of fimbrial biogenesis, elongation of the fimbria and positioning of FanC subunits to effect binding. The K88 fimbria may have a similar structure involving FaeC, FaeF and FaeH minor subunits. (Adapted from Krogfelt and Klemm, 1988; Jann and Hoschützky, 1991; Simons *et al.*, 1991; Bakker *et al.*, 1992; Jann *et al.*, 1992; Jones *et al.*, 1992).

Biogenesis of Fimbriae

Characterization of the genetic determinants encoding the biogenesis of *E. coli* fimbriae, sequencing of respective genes and comparison of the amino acid sequences of translated products have demonstrated common features. Fimbrial gene clusters encode:

1. Minor subunits.
2. Proteins involved in the transport of subunits across the periplasmic space, i.e. chaperones.
3. Proteins involved in directing assembly on the outer membrane, i.e. ushers.
4. Regulatory proteins (Mooi and de Graaf, 1985; Hultgren and Normark, 1991; Hultgren *et al.*, 1991; Jones *et al.*, 1992; Jacob-Dubuisson *et al.*, 1993).

Adhesins

Minor subunits which function as adhesins have so far only been described on *E. coli* associated with extraintestinal infections, viz. SfaS, PapG and FimH. Where fimbrial gene clusters have been fully characterized in enterotoxigenic *E. coli* (ETEC), there is no evidence to date for adhesive minor subunits in their fimbriae (de Graaf and Gaastra, 1994). Rather their component subunits appear to have dual adhesive and structural functions.

The reasons for this difference in functional organization are not known. It has been suggested that fimbriae with multiple adhesive sites might aid adherence to and colonization of intestinal mucus in initiation of ETEC infection by forming an 'adhesive capsule' around the ETEC bacteria. This 'adhesive capsule' could facilitate interaction with receptor molecules in the mucous gel which are probably more dispersed than the glycoconjugate receptors in the brush borders of enterocytes (de Graaf and Gaastra, 1994).

Chaperones

The role of a periplasmic chaperone in subunit translocation during fimbrial biogenesis was proposed initially in studies of K88 and K99 fimbrial biosynthesis (Mooi and de Graaf, 1985). The formation of chaperone–subunit complexes, comprising FanE and FanC, respectively, in the case of K99 fimbriae and FaeE and FaeG or the minor subunit FaeC, respectively, in the case of K88 fimbriae, was suggested to protect the subunits against proteolytic degradation by periplasmic proteases and to prevent premature assembly inside the bacterial cell.

The three-dimensional structure of the fimbrial chaperone PapD has been elucidated (Holmgren and Bränden, 1989; Jones *et al.*, 1992; Jacob-Dubuisson *et al.*, 1993). Shaped like a boomerang, it consists of two globular domains oriented towards one another. Each domain is a beta-barrel structure formed by two antiparallel beta-pleated sheets and has a topology similar to that of an immunoglobulin fold.

The amino acid sequences of several fimbrial chaperones are known and exhibit 30–40% identity and up to 60% similarity (Hultgren *et al.*, 1991; Jones *et al.*, 1992; Jacob-Dubuisson *et al.*, 1993; de Graaf and Gaastra, 1994; Kusters and Gaastra, 1994). A consensus sequence was derived from these analyses. When superimposed into the crystal structure of PapD, most of the invariant and conserved residues of the chaperone family were critical to maintenance of the structural integrity of the protein. Most of the invariant residues contributed to the hydrophobic core of the molecule. Site-directed mutagenesis has revealed that subunit recognition involves the conserved cleft of the molecule. Three invariant residues were found to form an internal salt bridge necessary to orient the two beta-barrel domains towards each other to form the binding cleft. Chaperones appear to form stable bimolecular complexes with fimbrial subunits, thereby maintaining the native conformation of subunits.

Whether all the fimbrial operons of human ETEC strains encode a chaperone is unclear (de Graaf and Gaastra, 1994). Operons encoding the fibrillar CS3 fimbriae and the non-fimbrial CS6 antigen possess genes encoding proteins with structural characteristics of PapD and FaeE, viz. CstC (the 27 kDa protein) and CssC, respectively. However, the gene cluster encoding CFA/I fimbriae does not appear to encode a chaperone.

Ushers

The terminal step in the biogenesis of fimbriae is assembly of subunits into a nascent fimbria in an ordered manner. A large outer membrane protein (80–95 kDa), which acts as a molecular usher, appears to be conserved in all fimbrial gene clusters of *E. coli* investigated thoroughly to date (Mooi and de Graaf, 1985; Jones *et al.*, 1992; de Graaf and Gaastra, 1994). Based on the P fimbrial system, the release of subunits from the chaperone–subunit complex appears to be ATP independent. The assembly of subunits into an ordered heterogeneous structure such as the P fimbria must be well choreographed. It has been proposed that the differing affinities of interaction of subunit-PapD complexes with PapC as well as the relative concentrations of each of the bimolecular complexes present in the periplasm ensures precise assembly. Comparison of the amino acid sequences of ushers derived from DNA sequences reveals a less pronounced genetic relationship than observed for the chaperones, with 25% identity and approximately 40% similarity (de Graaf and Gaastra, 1994; Kusters and Gaastra, 1994). Computer predictions of secondary structure indicate that ushers do not belong to the families of integral outer membrane proteins such as OmpA or the porins.

Host Receptors in Adherence

Principles

The concept that pathogenic bacteria bind to host tissues in a highly specific manner and that the selectivity and affinity of binding are determined by the presence of receptors on host cells that are recognized by ligand molecules (adhesins or lectins) on the bacterial surfaces forms the widely accepted basis for initiation of infection (Ofek and Beachey, 1980; Ofek and Sharon, 1990). The idea of 'tissue tropism' was advanced to emphasize the preference of a bacterium for certain tissues over others (Korhonen *et al.*, 1990, 1992b; Normark *et al.*, 1992). The restriction of infections caused by one particular type of pathogenic *E. coli* strain to one or a few animal species is further evidence of the specificity of such adherence. That susceptibility of a host to *E. coli* strains is genetically determined is well exemplified in the case of bacteria bearing K88 fimbriae and P fimbriae. Not all piglets are susceptible to infection with K88$^+$ ETEC (Rutter *et al.*, 1975; Sellwood *et al.*, 1975). Piglets which are resistant to infection lack the K88 receptor which is inherited in a simple Mendelian manner. A single locus with two alleles is involved, the allele specifying the receptor for K88 fimbriae being dominant over the non-receptor allele. K88 fimbriae exist as three serological variants designated K88ab, K88ac and K88ad. Up to five different pig phenotypes affect adherence of ETEC bearing K88 fimbrial variants (de Graaf and Gaastra, 1994).

The susceptibility of humans to infection with uropathogenic *E. coli* bearing P fimbriae correlates with the P blood group status of the individual (Leffler and Svanborg-Edén, 1986; Normark *et al.*, 1992). The quantity of this blood group glycolipid varies genetically from person to person. Relative susceptibility to colonization with P-fimbriate bacteria is related to the relative density of these receptors on host cells. Uroepithelial cells of individuals with the rare p$^-$ phenotype lack the receptor and fail to bind P-fimbriate bacteria.

The criteria that require to be fulfilled to establish that specific molecules on bacterial and host cells mediate adherence in a stereospecific adhesin–receptor interaction include demonstration that:

1. Adhesion to natural target host cells or *in vitro* model cell systems is inhibitable by:
(a) adhesin or receptor analogues;
(b) genetic manipulations of bacteria or host cells that alter expression of adhesin or receptor molecules, respectively;

(c) enzymes or chemicals that specifically modify or degrade adhesin or receptor structures;
(d) specific antibodies directed against the adhesin or receptor molecules;
(e) lectins of known specificity that bind to putative receptors.
2. The fimbriate bacteria bind to isolated receptor molecules or receptor analogues in a specific fashion (Ofek and Beachey, 1980).

Biochemical nature of receptors

The receptors for *E. coli* fimbriae appear with few exceptions to be glycoconjugates, both glycoproteins and glycolipids (Smyth, 1986; Karlsson *et al.*, 1992; de Graaf and Gaastra, 1994). The adhesin–receptor interaction occurs in a lectin-like fashion. The receptors are present in mucus, epithelial membranes and basement membranes. Table 16.4 summarizes current knowledge of receptor molecules or oligosaccharides

Table 16.4. Receptors for *E. coli* fimbriae.[a]

E. coli group	Adhesin	Receptor
Enterotoxigenic		
Type 1	FimH	Mannosides
K88	FaeG	Gal(β1-3)GalNAc Fuc(α1-2)Gal(β1-3/4)GlcNAc
K99	FanC	NeuGc-GM_3; NeuGc-SPG
F41		*N*-acetylgalactosamine; galactose
F17	F17-G	*N*-acetylglucosamine
CFA/I	CfaB	NeuAc-GM_2
CFA/II[CS1, CS2, CS3]		Asialo-GM_1
Uropathogenic		
P fimbriae	PapG(FsoG)	Gal(α1-4)Gal
Prs	PrsG	GalNAc(α1-3)Gal(α1-4)Gal
S fimbriae	SfaS	NeuAc(α2-3)Gal(β1-3)GalNAc (glycophorin A)
X fimbriae		NeuAc(α2-3)Gal; NeuAc
Dr	Dra	Type IV collagen
F1C		*N*-acetylgalactosamine, galactose
Others		
Curli	CsgA	Fibronectin
$F165_1$	$F165_1A$	Gal(α1-3)GalNAc (Forssman antigen)

[a] Data compiled from Smyth (1986), Mirelmann (1986), Olsén *et al.* (1989), Ofek and Sharon (1990), Olsén (1992), Harel *et al.* (1992), de Graaf and Gaastra (1994), Seignole *et al.* (1994).

involved in the adherence of *E. coli*. The receptor epitope of an oligosaccharide is often an internally located sugar sequence which is exposed such that the fimbrial lectin binds to it in a stereospecific manner. Glycolipids have perhaps received more attention than glycoproteins as receptors because the former only carry one oligosaccharide moiety per molecule in contrast to the latter which often carry several different saccharide chains linked to the same polypeptide sequence (Karlsson, 1989; Karlsson *et al.*, 1992). Moreover, glycolipids do not usually appear in body secretions. Glycolipids with a common minimally recognized sequence but with varying neighbouring groups are referred to as isoreceptors. However, as pointed out by Karlsson and co-workers (Karlsson *et al.*, 1991, 1992), binding of bacteria to isolated glycolipids on thin-layer plates or to microtitre wells coated with glycolipids may yield discrepant findings with respect to intact cells, such as erythrocytes or shedded epithelial cells, known to possess these glycolipids. The location of a binding epitope in the membrane may make it more selectively accessible than when placed in more random conformations on an *in vitro* assay surface.

Mammalian cell membranes contain diverse glycoconjugates expressing a plethora of oligosaccharide sequences. The nature and distribution of these oligosaccharides in the glycocalyx of cells over different species and tissues is probably the determining factor in 'tissue tropism' of pathogenic *E. coli* for host tissues and the haemagglutination patterns of strains against panels of erythrocyte species. However, the adhesin of a fimbria may evolve to fit the receptor architectures of isoreceptors on different mucosal surfaces.

For example, three distinct classes of G adhesin are found in P fimbriae (Normark *et al.*, 1992). These G adhesins are encoded by allelic variants of the same gene. Each class of G adhesin shows only 46–56% amino acid identity with the other two. $PapG_{J96}$ is only found on one strain J96. $PapG_{AD110}$ is frequent among strains from upper urinary tract infections (UTIs) in man. The third termed PrsG is common on strains causing human acute cystitis and is the only adhesin present on dog *E. coli* UTI isolates. These show differential binding to the globoseries of glycosphingolipid isoreceptors. PrsG mediates efficient binding to dog-derived MDCK cells, goat erythrocytes and sheep erythrocytes all of which contain GbO_5 (Forssman antigen) as the isoreceptor (GalNAcα1-3GalNAcβ1-3Galα1-4LacCer). Only the $PapG_{J96}$ adhesin agglutinated rabbit erythrocytes with GbO_3 as the dominant isoreceptor (Galα1-4LacCer), whereas $PapG_{AD110}$ promoted strong adherence to human bladder-derived T24 cells with GbO_4 as the dominant isoreceptor (GalNAcβ1-3Galα1-4LacCer). In human and canine uroepithelia GbO_4 and GbO_5, respectively, appear to be present in rather high amounts.

Receptor-binding sites of fimbrial adhesins

K88 fimbriae

The contribution of individual amino acid residues to the respective binding sites of the FaeG proteins of K88ab and K88ac fimbriae has been investigated. Hybrid *faeG* genes were constructed using unique restriction endonuclease sites in both *faeGab* and *faeGac* genes. In addition, site-directed mutagenesis was used to replace one or more K88ac-specific amino acid residues with their K88ab-specific counterparts at particular locations in the FaeGac subunit primary structure (de Graaf and Bakker, 1992; de Graaf and Gaastra, 1994).

These studies have identified hydrophobic phenylalanine or leucine residues in positions 134 and 147 and one or more amino acids with hydrophilic charged side chains at positions 136, 155 and 216 or in the hypervariable region of residues 163–174 as being essential to the receptor-binding site of the FaeG protein. Similar approaches have also permitted identification of residues involved in subunit–subunit interaction and serotype-specific epitopes.

K99, S and CFA/I fimbriae

FanC is the fimbrial subunit protein and adhesin of K99 fimbriae. Comparison of the primary structure of FanC with the amino acid sequences of other adhesins with sialic-acid-binding affinity, viz. the CfaB protein of CFA/I fimbriae and the SfaS protein of S-fimbriae, and of other proteins with identical specificity, e.g. the B subunit proteins of cholera and heat labile (LT) enterotoxins of *Vibrio cholerae* and *E. coli*, respectively, has revealed a consensus sequence which is probably involved in receptor binding (Table 16.5) (de Graaf and Gaastra, 1994). Site-directed mutagenesis has demonstrated that mutation of the lys-132 or arg-136 residue of the FanC protein and of lys-116 or arg-118 of the SfaS adhesin abolishes the binding properties of the respective fimbriae.

Binding to non-epithelial tissue and host proteins

Through analysing the binding of fimbriae to frozen tissue sections and immobilized mammalian glycoproteins, some fimbrial types have been shown to bind selectively to endothelium, basement membranes and matrix proteins (Korhonen *et al.* 1990, 1991, 1992b; Parkkinen, 1992). Type 1 and S-fimbriae bind by means of their lectin-like adhesins, FimH and SfaS, respectively. Type 1 fimbriae bind strongly to Tamm–Horsfall glycoprotein, which probably inhibits binding of type 1 fimbriate *E. coli* to epithelial cells *in vivo*, thereby precluding a role for these fimbriae in

Table 16.5. Putative consensus sequence for *N*-acetylneuramic acid-binding site of fimbrial adhesins and enterotoxins.[a]

Adhesin/enterotoxin subunit[b]	Amino acid sequence and numbered residues[c]
CfaB	^{56}K – K V I V K^{61}
CsoA	^{56}K – G V V V K^{61}
FanC	^{132}K – K D – D R^{136}
SfaS	^{116}K A R A V S K^{122}
CT-B	^{62}K – K A I E R^{67}
LT-B	^{62}K – K A I E R^{67}

[a] Data compiled from Lai (1977), Roosendaal *et al.* (1984), Leong *et al.* (1985), Hamers *et al.* (1989), Morschhäuser *et al.* (1990), Perez-Casal *et al.* (1990).
[b] CfaB, CFA/I fimbrial subunit; CsoA, CS1 fimbrial subunit; FanC, K99 major fimbrial subunit; SfaS, S fimbria adhesin subunit; CT-B, cholera enterotoxin B subunit; LT-B, *E. coli* LT enterotoxin B subunit.
[c] Residues of mature proteins are numbered.

ascending human urinary tract infection. However, type 1 fimbriate *E. coli* also bind to immobilized laminin, a major glycoprotein of basement membranes which forms a network of interactions with different cells and molecules. Recombinant *E. coli* strains expressing cloned type 1 fimbrial genes adhere in a mannose-inhibitable manner to immobilized laminin. Moreover, mutants lacking the *fimH* gene encoding the mannoside-specific fimbrial lectin do not bind.

S-fimbriae recognize sialylα2-3galactoside structures on human erythrocytes, the SfaS adhesin being the haemagglutinin. The target binding tissues *in vivo* were identified by incubating purified S-fimbriae on tissue sections followed by visualization of the bound fimbriae by indirect immunofluorescence, the specificity of binding being controlled by inhibition with sialyl lactose (NeuAcα2-3Galβ1-4Glc). Only brain and kidney revealed intense binding of S-fimbriae. The binding sites in the brain were the vascular endothelium and the epithelium of the choroid plexus and brain ventricles. In the kidney, binding occurred to the vascular endothelium and to the glomeruli.

Purified S-fimbriae can also bind plasminogen and tissue-type plasminogen activator (Hacker *et al.*, 1992; Korhonen *et al.*, 1992b; Parkkinen, 1992). Activation of plasminogen by tissue-type plasminogen activator is accelerated by immobilization of the plasminogen on the bacterial surface and also protects the bound plasmin from inhibition by α_2-antiplasmin

(Fig. 16.3). S-fimbriae immobilize plasminogen in a lysine-specific manner. A SfaS⁻ mutant displayed binding activity suggesting that this adhesin was not involved in plasminogen binding and activation. A minor subunit protein SfaG is involved in plasminogen binding and activation in a sialic-acid-independent manner. Enhancement of plasminogen activation was inhibited by ε-amino caproic acid indicating that the interactions were mediated by the lysine-binding sites of plasminogen and tissue-type plasminogen activator.

Dr fimbriae (X adhesin) are found on uropathogenic *E. coli* of O serovar 75 and haemagglutinate human erythrocytes bearing the Dr blood group antigen (Väisänen-Rhen *et al.*, 1984). The Dr antigen is part of the decay accelerating factor which regulates the complement cascade and protects erythrocytes from lysis by homologous complement. The DraA protein is the major subunit of Dr fimbriae and possesses adhesive and haemagglutinating capacity. Dr fimbriae adhere strongly to transitional epithelial cells of the ureter and to epithelial cells of the bladder and urethra. In the upper urinary tract Dr fimbriae bind to basement membranes and Bowman's capsule around the glomeruli. Analysis of the binding of Dr fimbriae to various basement membrane components revealed that type IV collagen was the target. The receptor region has been located to the amino terminal 7S fragment of the type IV collagen molecule. Chloramphenicol and *N*-acetyltyrosine are inhibitors of the binding properties of Dr fimbriae, indicating that binding does not depend on lectin-like protein–carbohydrate interaction (Korhonen *et al.*, 1992b).

In the case of P-fimbriae, binding has been demonstrated to immobilized fibronectin. This involves the amino- and carboxy-terminal fragments of fibronectin which are known to have common repeat sequences (Westerlund *et al.*, 1989; Korhonen *et al.*, 1992b). Fibronectin is an important glycoprotein constituent of extracellular fluids, connective tissues, basement membranes and on cell surfaces. P-fimbrial binding appears to involve protein–protein interaction and is independent of the RGDS-cell attachment domain of the fibronectin. Adherence assays with recombinant *E. coli* strains lacking one of the P-fimbrial components (PapA, PapE, PapF or PapG) revealed that deletion of the *papE* or *papF* gene decreased adherence to immobilized fibronectin. Thus, binding appears to be independent of the Galα1-4-specific lectin PapG. PapE (FsoE)- and PapF (FsoF)-dependent binding to fibronectin-containing regions of rat kidney tissue has been demonstrated (Westerlund *et al.*, 1991). The binding of P-fimbriae to fibronectin differs from the binding of Gram-positive bacteria to this glycoprotein in that P-fimbriae only bind to immobilized fibronectin and not to the soluble form, demonstrating that the binding is dependent on the conformation of the fibronectin molecules.

Curli present on *E. coli* isolated bovine mastitis also mediate binding to fibronectin. Electron microscopic analysis of *E. coli* expressing curli

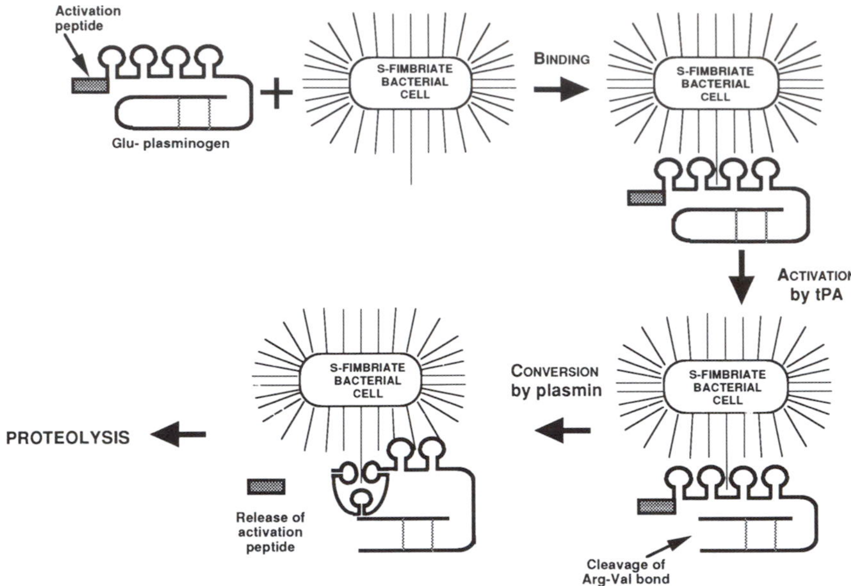

Fig. 16.3. Binding and activation of plasminogen on the surface of S-fimbriate *E. coli*. The native form of plasminogen is a single chain, glycoprotein serine protease of 91 kDa found in plasma and tissue fluids. Characteristic features of its structure are five loops called kringles in the amino-terminal portion of the molecule. These contain lysine-binding sites involved in interactions of plasminogen with fibrin and plasmin inhibitors. The carboxy-terminus contains the enzyme active site. Activation of plasminogen by tissue type plasminogen activator (tPA) occurs through hydrolysis of an Arg-Val peptide bond converting plasminogen to plasmin. The plasmin is able to modify itself by cleaving off a 8-kDa activation peptide at the amino terminus, thereby converting glutamic acid-plasmin to the lysine N-terminus form. Once bound to solid matrices by its lysine-binding sites (the kringle loops), plasmin is protected against physiological inhibitors. The 8-kDa aminoterminal activation peptide and the Arg-Lys bond are indicated by arrows. The narrow vertical lines indicate the disulfide bonds between the heavy and light chains of the plasmin. Conformational change in the kringle region of Lys-plasmin is emphasized. This leads to an increase in the affinity of binding and protection against inactivation. (Adapted from Kuusela *et al.*, 1992; Parkkinen, 1992.)

revealed binding of fibronectin along the entire curli. The binding was meta-periodate resistant indicating protein–protein interaction between the CsgA (*c*urlin *s*ubunit *g*ene) protein and fibronectin (Olsén *et al.*, 1989; Olsén, 1992).

Genetics of *E. coli* Adhesins

In general fimbrial operons exhibit a common theme in their organization, both in the arrangement of the genes involved in fimbrial biogenesis and in the regulation of the operon. However, variations occur with respect to the location of genes in the genome and the regulation of gene expression. Some of the unique features of these systems will be highlighted.

Enterotoxigenic E. coli

The structural organizations of the fimbrial operons of enterotoxigenic *E. coli* have been compared (Mooi and de Graaf, 1985; de Graaf, 1990; de Graaf and Gaastra, 1994). A feature of some of these gene clusters is the non-contiguous location of the structural genes and the genes involved in regulation. The production of CFA/I fimbriae requires expression from two regions on a high-molecular-weight plasmid which are separated by 40 kb of DNA (Smith *et al.*, 1982). Region 1 encodes the structural genes arranged as an operon which is regulated by a protein, CfaD, expressed from Region 2 of this plasmid (Savelkoul *et al.*, 1990). The major subunit, CfaB, and a putative usher, CfaC, as well as two additional proteins whose functions are unknown, constitute the structural operon (Jordi *et al.*, 1992b). Expression of CS1 and CS2 fimbriae of the CFA/II fimbrial complex is regulated by the Rns protein, which is related to CfaD (Caron *et al.*, 1989). The CS1 fimbrial operon is plasmid located, whereas the CS2 fimbrial operon is expressed from the bacterial chromosome. The Rns protein in the case of the CFA/II fimbrial complex is expressed from a distinct plasmid.

These arrangements of gene clusters contrast with the arrangements of the gene clusters of the K88 and K99 fimbriae expressed on animal ETECs (Simons *et al.*, 1991; Bakker *et al.*, 1992). In each instance both the structural and regulatory components are expressed from one contiguous operon. Furthermore, in both of these fimbrial systems a greater complexity is apparent in the numbers of genes involved in fimbrial biogenesis. Minor fimbrial subunits perform functions such as initiation and elongation of fimbriae (Simons *et al.*, 1991; Bakker *et al.*, 1992). In this respect, these operons more closely resemble the gene cluster arrangements for type 1, S and P fimbriae (Hacker, 1990; Hultgren *et al.*, 1991).

The CS3 fimbrial operon of the CFA/II fimbrial complex displays overlapping genes. Within the open reading frame for the putative usher protein, CstB, four other gene products are encoded. The expression of these four proteins is dependent on termination at an internal amber codon while expression of the usher protein requires suppression of this codon (Jalajakumari *et al.*, 1990). This complexity in translation has not been described for any other fimbrial operon.

Other diarrhoea-associated E. coli

The genetic organizations of the adhesins of EPECs have not been fully elucidated. The inducible bundle-forming pili (BFP) of EPECs are expressed from the *bfpA* locus on the 60 MDa EAF plasmid. These fimbriae mediate localized adherence of these bacteria to tissue culture cells and to microvilli in the early stages of EPEC infection. The EAF plasmid also encodes the *per* gene, the gene product of which regulates the expression of the chromosomally located *eae* gene (Donnenberg and Kaper, 1992). This *eae* gene encodes a 94-kDa outer membrane protein, intimin, responsible for the characteristic attaching and effacing lesion of EPEC infection. Intimin allows the bacterium to become closely attached to the enterocyte membrane. This triggers intracellular events leading to the accumulation of actin and other cytoskeletal proteins below the bacterium with the resultant formation of a pedestal on sloughing of the microvilli. The plasmid-mediated regulation of the chromosomally located *eae* gene resembles the genetic regulation of the CS2 fimbrial system. The AIDA-1 adhesin mediates the diffuse adherence phenotype of EPECs (Benz and Schmidt, 1992).

Recently, additional morphological types of fimbriae have been observed to be expressed on EPECs. The major subunits of these fimbriae share amino acid sequence homology with the major subunits of P fimbriae and type 1 fimbriae (Girón *et al.*, 1993). Based on this evidence it may be suggested that the operon organizations of these recently detected EPEC fimbriae may prove to be similar to those of the *pap* and *fim* operons.

The F1845 fimbriae of diarrhoea-associated *E. coli* are expressed from the *daa* operon which is arranged similarly to the operons of extraintestinal *E. coli*. Indeed, although not related to the *pap* operon, the *daa* operon exhibits similarities in regulation (Bilge *et al.*, 1993).

The genetics of the AAF/I fimbria of enteroaggregative *E. coli* are only beginning to be studied. Preliminary results show that two regions of a plasmid are required for its expression (Nataro *et al.*, 1992, 1993). This is reminiscent of the CFA/I fimbrial system. Indeed, sequencing of region 2 revealed that this region encodes a Rns (CfaD) homologue of 30 kDa.

Extraintestinal E. coli

The operons expressing the adhesins of extraintestinal *E. coli* are chromosomally located. The organizations of the *pap* and *sfa* operons have been studied in great detail (Hacker, 1990; Hultgren *et al.*, 1991). In contrast, the functions of all of the gene products expressed from the *dra*, *bma*, *afa* and *nfa* operons have not as yet been elucidated (Fig. 16.4). However, it seems valid to speculate from the arrangements of the different operons that gene products of similar molecular weight may perform similar functions in their respective operons. In particular, the high-molecular-weight protein in each operon may perform the role of the usher (Labigne-Roussel and Falkow, 1988; Ahrens *et al.*, 1993). On account of the notable similarity between the *afa* and *nfa* operons, which encode non-fimbrial adhesins and those expressing recognized fimbriae, electron microscope

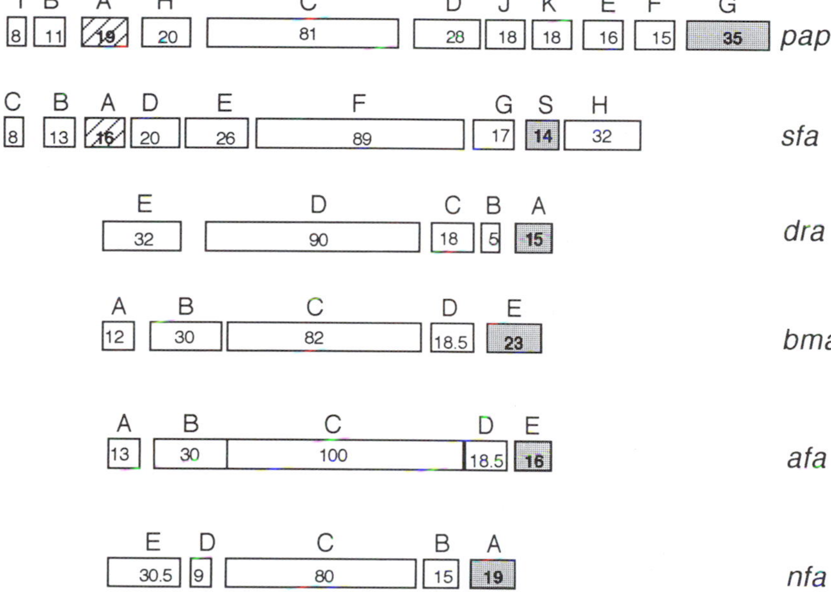

Fig. 16.4. Comparison of the gene products encoded on the operons for P fimbriae (*pap*), S fimbriae (*sfa*), Dr fimbriae (*dra*), M fimbriae (*bma*), Afimbrial adhesin I (*afa*) and Non-fimbrial adhesin-I (*nfa*). The boxes represent the gene products, the numbers indicate the molecular weights of the proteins in kilodaltons. The boxes with dots represent the adhesin gene products of each gene cluster. The hatched boxes represent the major structural subunits of the fimbrial systems. (Data is adapted from Hacker, 1990; Ahrens *et al.*, 1993.)

technology may not as yet be available to visualize all types of fimbrial structures present on bacterial surfaces.

Furthermore, only five proteins are expressed from each of the *dra*, *bma*, *afa* and *nfa* operons, in comparison with the *pap* operon, which encodes 11 proteins. The former operons probably encode the minimum number of gene products required for adhesin expression and in this respect resemble the CFA/I operon of human ETECs (Jordi *et al.*, 1992b; de Graaf and Gaastra, 1994).

Environmental Regulation of Expression of Fimbriae

The ability of *E. coli* to produce fimbriae confers on the bacterium a considerable advantage in terms of colonization. However, the production of fimbriae imposes a large stress on a bacterium when one considers that fimbrial subunits may account for approximately 5–10% of total cellular protein. The capacity to sense and to respond to environmental conditions that favour expression is essential. The expression of fimbriae may be subject to numerous regulatory systems, e.g. thermoregulation, osmoregulation, iron limitation and catabolite repression (Smyth and Smith, 1992). In general, fimbriae are best expressed *in vitro* at 37°C in low osmotic strength media at limiting concentrations of iron and glucose. These conditions approximate to those a bacterium encounters in the gut. The ability to transduce these signals such that fimbrial expression occurs is essential for pathogenesis and survival. A full exposition of all the regulatory schemes for fimbriae in *E. coli* is beyond the scope of this review. The reader is referred to Tables 16.6 and 16.7 and the references therein.

The evolution of studies on fimbriae in *E. coli* in the last 20 years can be divided into three phases, viz.:

1. The identification and purification of fimbriae.
2. The cloning and sequencing of fimbrial operons and the identification of dedicated regulators.
3. The demonstration that fimbrial operons are networked in regulons that are globally regulated (Dorman and Ní Bhriain, 1992).

P-fimbrial biogenesis exemplifies how local and global regulatory mechanisms modulate their expression. The P-fimbrial operon encodes two regulators, namely PapI and PapB. The *papI* gene is weakly transcribed and is essentially turned off below 26°C, since its promoter is temperature sensitive. The PapI protein activates expression of the *papB* gene and the PapB protein in concert with cAMP-CRP (cAMP receptor protein) in turn activates expression of its own promoter resulting in high level expression of the fimbrial subunit *papA* gene, since the *papA* and *papB* genes are read from the same promoter. This illustrates how a bacterium can sense

Table 16.6. Global regulation of fimbrial expression in *E. coli*.

Regulator	Fimbrial type	Mode of action	Reference
H-NS	P,S,CFA/I	Functions as transcriptional repressor; Mutants express fimbriae at restrictive temperatures	Göransson *et al.* (1990), Morschhäuser *et al.* (1993), Jordi *et al.* (1992a)
	Type 1	Higher inversion rates of *fimA* promoter	Kawula and Orndorff (1991)
Lrp	P	Modulation of phase variation	van der Woude *et al.* (1992); Nou *et al.* (1993)
	Type 1	Modulation of phase variation	Blomfield *et al.* (1993)
	S,F1485	Modulation of phase variation	van der Woude and Low (1994)
	K99	Positively regulated	Braaten *et al.* (1992)
	K88	Negative control in cooperation with FaeA	Huisman *et al.* (1994)
Crp	P	Functions as an antirepressor	Forsman *et al.* (1992)
	S	Positively regulated	Schmoll *et al.* (1990a)
Fur	CFA/I	Repression	Karjalainen *et al.* (1991)
RimJ	P	Thermoregulation	White Ziegler and Low (1992)
IHF	Type 1	Inversion of 314 bp sequence; positive regulation of *fimA*	Dorman and Higgins (1987)
RpoS	Curli	Antirepressor relieves repression mediated by H-NS	Olsén *et al.* (1993)

Table 16.7. Dedicated regulators of fimbrial expression.

Regulator	Fimbriae	Action	Reference
PapB	P	Positive, though at high concentrations is autoregulatory	Forsman *et al.* (1989)
PapI	P	Stimulates *papB* transcription	Båga *et al.* (1985)
SfaC/SfaB	S	Analogous to PapI and PapB	Schmoll *et al.* (1990b)
FimE	Type 1	Promotes inversion of phase switch DNA element upstream of *fimA* with preference for expression 'off'	McClain *et al.* (1991)
FimB	Type 1	Promotes inversion of phase switch fragment in either direction	McClain *et al.* (1991)
Crl	Curli	Transcriptional activator	Arnqvist *et al.* (1992)
FanA/FanB	K99	Antiterminators	Roosendaal *et al.* (1989)
FaeA/FaeB	K88	Related to PapI and PapB, respectively	de Graaf (1990); Huisman *et al.* (1994)
CfaD	CFA/I	Overcomes repression mediated by H-NS; a member of the AraC family of proteins	Jordi (1992); Jordi *et al.* (1992a); Savelkoul *et al.* (1990)
Rns	CS1/CS2	Positive regulator homologous to CfaD	Caron *et al.* (1989)
CsvR	CS5	Positive regulator homologous to CfaD	de Haan *et al.* (1991)
FapR	987P	Positive regulator homologous to CfaD	Klaasen and de Graaf (1990)

favourable environmental conditions and amplify these signals. Superimposed on this regulatory scheme is the action of H-NS and RimJ. Mutations in either of the genes encoding these proteins result in derepressed expression at non-permissive temperatures. Though the H-NS protein is produced at 37°C, it does not affect the expression of P-fimbriae. Recent data indicate that CRP acts as an antirepressor, relieving the transcriptional silencing caused by H-NS.

Another fimbrial operon which is subject to the repressive effects of H-NS is the CFA/I operon. The transcriptional silencing mediated by H-NS is overcome by CfaD. As indicated in Table 16.7, homologues of CfaD occur in other fimbrial systems and presumably their modes of action are analogous to that of CfaD. In addition catabolite repression and iron-regulated repression affect expression of the CFA/I fimbrial operon.

The emerging concept for fimbrial systems is the existence of one or two dedicated positive regulators and the transduction of environmental stimuli via pleiotropic regulators. Specific roles for alterations to DNA topology in the modulation of fimbrial expression have not yet been described (Dorman and Ní Bhriain, 1993). However, there are significant similarities to the regulation of other genes to suggest that the DNA topology of regions upstream of fimbrial operons dictates which regulatory proteins constellate at these sites. In turn, the composition of the resultant regulatory complexes determines the level of fimbrial expression.

Role of Fimbriae in *E. coli* Infection

The contribution of fimbriae in the binding of bacteria to the surface of epithelial cells of the host, involving stereospecific recognition between adhesin and receptor, is part of the accepted liturgy of bacterial pathogenesis. Potential contributions of fimbriae to virulence other than as attachment organelles have been evidenced in recent years.

The presence of bacterium-bound plasmin on S-fimbriate *E. coli* through the binding of plasminogen and tissue type plasminogen activator may contribute to the pathogenesis of sepsis and meningitis in newborn infants caused by these bacteria (Fig. 16.3 above) (Korhonen *et al.*, 1992b; Parkkinen, 1992). Plasmin can degrade non-collagenous glycoproteins of basement membranes. Pericellular activation of plasminogen is known to play a role in the penetration of extracellular matrices by invasive cancer cells. S-fimbriate bacteria have been shown to readily penetrate basement membrane preparations in the presence of plasminogen and tissue type plasminogen activator in the Matrigel invasion assay (Albini *et al.*, 1987; Parkkinen, 1992). S-fimbriae may also contribute to secondary organ colonization by blood-borne bacteria through binding to sialyl oligosaccharides of endothelial cells in the brain and kidney. Where the endothelium is fenestrated, the S-fimbriae may contact the subepithelial basement membrane. Adherence to laminin is also considered to be important in the invasion of tumour cells. The ability of S-fimbriate bacteria to adhere to the epithelium lining the choroid plexus and brain ventricles might provide a means of resisting mechanical clearance by cerebrospinal fluid flow (Parkkinen *et al.*, 1988).

The binding of P-fimbriae to fibronectin through protein–protein interactions indicates that these organelles bind by both lectin-dependent and lectin-independent specificities. Thus, these fimbriae may play a role not only in binding to uroepithelial cells but also in infection of the kidney (Westerlund *et al.*, 1989, 1991).

E. coli expressing curli interact with the 29-kDa amino-terminal part of fibronectin. Fibronectin interacts with many macromolecules including collagens, fibrinogen, fibrin, glycoaminoglycans and members of the integrin family. Fibronectin bound to curli may act as an adaptor molecule between *E. coli* and other matrix components. Indeed, fibronectin-coated *E. coli* expressing curli have been shown to bind to type I collagen in human skin sections (Fig. 16.5) (Olsén, 1992). Using PCR amplification with two *csgA*-specific primers, the *csgA* gene has been shown to be widespread in *E. coli* strains (Olsén, 1992). Fibronectin-binding was particularly prevalent in *E. coli* isolates from wound infections. Thus, curli may provide some colonization advantage for *E. coli* in lesions where serum-derived soluble fibronectin and exposed matrix proteins such as laminin and collagen are present.

The role of type 1 fimbriae in intestinal infections is controversial (Jayappa *et al.*, 1985; Orndorff and Bloch, 1990) as indeed is the role of phase variable expression of type 1 fimbriae. The binding of type 1 fimbriae to Tamm–Horsfall protein may facilitate bladder infection. However, such binding is proposed to preclude a role for these fimbriae in ascending urinary tract infection. The influence of type 1 fimbriae on the establishment of peritoneal *E. coli* infection was studied by May *et al.* (1993). The environment of the peritoneum presented to the bacteria differs from the gastrointestinal tract. In a rat peritonitis model type 1 fimbrial expression led to a diminution in the numbers of bacteria surviving within the peritoneum. As type 1 fimbriae are known to promote adhesion to phagocytic cells (Orndorff and Bloch, 1990), enhanced phagocytosis probably facilitated clearance. The data suggest that downregulation of type 1 fimbrial expression may be of benefit to *E. coli* in the peritoneum. Since *E. coli* is isolated in greater than 60% of intraperitoneal infections, it appears to be adept at making the transition from the environment of the gastrointestinal tract to that of the peritoneum.

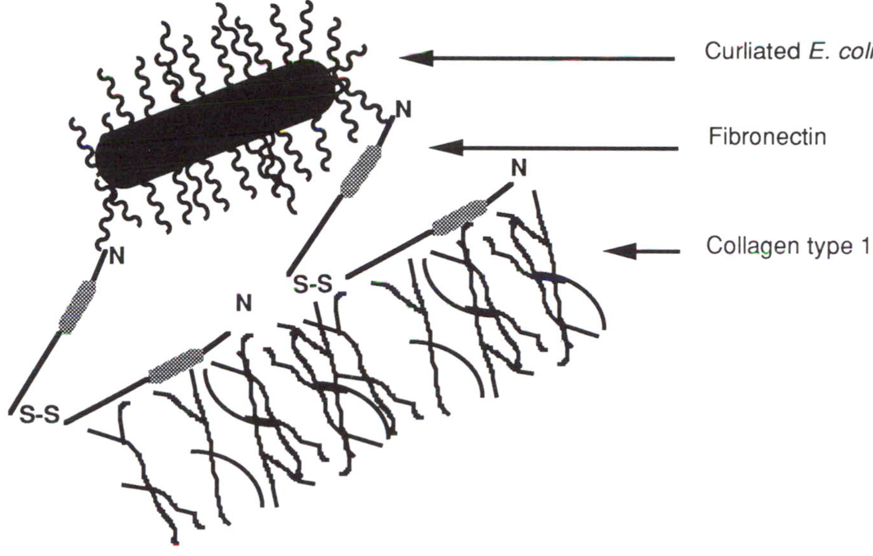

Fig. 16.5. Fibronectin acting as an adaptor molecule between *E. coli* expressing curli and type 1 collagen fibres. The fibronectin molecules are shown as dimers (222 kDa) held together by a disulfide bridge at the C-terminal portion of the molecule. N represents the proposed amino-terminal binding domains that interact with curli. The hatched boxes on the fibronectin molecules represents the collagen-binding domains comprising two 60 amino acid repeat regions distinct from the proposed 29-kDa amino-terminal bacterial binding domains. The fibronectin is a highly elongated protein. The two arms of the molecules are separated by an ~70° angle. The glycosylation of fibronectin comprises asparagine-linked oligosaccharide residues. (Adapted from Olsén, 1992.)

Concluding Comments

Molecular genetic analysis of pathogenic *E. coli* has enabled considerable strides to be made in our understanding of the functioning of fimbriae as adhesins. The next phase of analysis is to provide possible mechanisms for environmental control of fimbrial gene expression. Fimbriae may also prove to be useful carriers of peptide epitopes. Fimbriae are good immunogens. Insertion of totally foreign epitopes of viral surface proteins into type 1 fimbriae has already shown promise as a new antigen delivery system (Hedegaard and Klemm, 1989).

Acknowledgements

Work in the author's laboratory is supported by the Wellcome Trust and by the Health Research Board of Ireland. S.G.J.S. held a research assistantship from the Wellcome Trust. M.M. holds an HRB research studentship.

References

Ahrens, R., Ott, M., Ritter, A., Hoschützky, H., Bühler, T., Lottspeich, F., Boulnois, G.J., Jann, K. and Hacker, J. (1993) Genetic analysis of the gene cluster encoding nonfimbrial adhesin I from an *Escherichia coli* uropathogen. *Infection and Immunity* 61, 2505–2512.

Albini, A., Iwamoto, Y., Kleimen, H.K., Martin, G.R., Aaronson, S.A., Kozlowski, J.M. and McEwan, R.N. (1987) A rapid *in vitro* assay for quantitating the invasive potential of tumor cells. *Cancer Research* 47, 3239–3242.

Arnqvist, A., Olsén, A., Pfeifer, J., Russell, D.G. and Normark, S. (1992) The Crl protein activates cryptic genes for curli formation and fibronectin binding in *Escherichia coli* HB101. *Molecular Microbiology* 6, 2443–2452.

Båga, M. Göransson, M., Normark, S. and Uhlin, B.E. (1985) Transcriptional activation of a Pap pilus virulence operon from uropathogenic *Escherichia coli*. *European Molecular Biology Organization Journal* 4, 3887–3893.

Bakker, D., Willemsen, P.T.J., Willems, R.H., Huisman, T.T., Mooi, F.R., Oudega, B., Stegehuis, F. and de Graaf, F.K. (1992) Identification of minor fimbrial subunits involved in biosynthesis of K88 fimbriae. *Journal of Bacteriology* 174, 6350–6358.

Beachey, E.H. (ed.) (1980) *Bacterial Adherence, Receptors and Recognition Series B*, Vol. 6. Chapman & Hall, London.

Benz, I. and Schmidt, M.A. (1992) AIDA-1, the adhesin involved in diffuse adherence of the diarrhoeagenic *Escherichia coli* strain 2787 (O126:H27), is synthesized via a precursor molecule. *Molecular Microbiology* 6, 1539–1546.

Bilge, S.S., Apostol, J.M., Fullner, K.J., and Moseley, S.L. (1993) Transcriptional organization of the F1845 fimbrial adhesin determinant of *Escherichia coli*. *Molecular Microbiology* 7, 993–1006.

Blomfield, I.C., Calie, P.J., Eberhardt, K.J., McClain, M.S. and Eisenstein, B.I. (1993) Lrp stimulates phase variation of type 1 fimbriation in *Escherichia coli* K-12. *Journal of Bacteriology* 175, 27–36.

Braaten, B.A., Plakto, J.V., van der Woude, M.W., Simons, B.H., de Graaf, F.K., Calvo, J.M. and Low, D.A. (1992) Leucine-responsive regulatory protein controls the expression of both the *pap* and *fan* pili operons in *Escherichia coli*. *Proceedings of the National Academy of Sciences of the United States of America* 89, 4250–4254.

Brinton, C.C., Jr (1965) The structure, function, synthesis and genetic control of bacterial pili and a molecular model for DNA and RNA transport in Gram negative bacteria. *Transactions of the New York Academy of Sciences* 27, 1003–1054.

Brinton, C.C., Jr (1967) Contributions of pili to the specificity of the bacterial surface, and a unitary hypothesis of conjugal infectious heredity. In: Davis, B.D. and Warren, L. (eds) *The Specificity of Cell Surfaces*. Prentice-Hall, Englewood Cliffs, New Jersey, pp. 37–70.

Caron, J., Coffield, L.M. and Scott, J.R. (1989) A plasmid-encoded regulatory gene, *rns*, required for expression of the CS1 and CS2 adhesins of enterotoxigenic *Escherichia coli. Proceedings of the National Academy of Sciences of the United States of America* 86, 963–967.

Collinson, S.K., Emödy, L., Trust, T.J. and Kay, W.W. (1992) Thin aggregative fimbriae from diarrheagenic *Escherichia coli. Journal of Bacteriology* 174, 4490–4495.

de Graaf, F.K. (1990) Genetics of adhesive fimbriae of intestinal *Escherichia coli. Current Topics in Microbiology and Immunology* 151, 29–53.

de Graaf, F.K. and Bakker, D. (1992) Properties and synthesis of K88 fimbriae. In: Korhonen, T.K., Hovi, T. and Mäkelä, P.H. (eds) *Molecular Recognition in Host–Parasite Interactions, FEMS Symposium No. 61*. Plenum Press, New York, pp. 39–46.

de Graaf, F.K. and Gaastra, W. (1994) Fimbriae of enterotoxigenic *Escherichia coli*. In: Klemm, P. (ed.) *Fimbriae: Adhesion, Genetics, Biogenesis and Vaccines*. CRC Press, Boca Raton, pp. 57–88.

de Graaf, F.K. and Roorda, I. (1982) Production, purification and characterization of the fimbrial adhesive antigen F41 isolated from calf enteropathogenic *Escherichia coli* strain B41M. *Infection and Immunity* 36, 751–758.

de Graaf, F.K., Klemm, P. and Gaastra, W. (1980) Purification, characterization, and partial covalent structure of *Escherichia coli* adhesive antigen K99. *Infection and Immunity* 33, 877–883.

de Haan, L.A.M., Willshaw, G.A., van der Zeijst, B.A.M. and Gaastra, W. (1991) The nucleotide sequence of a regulatory gene present on a plasmid in an enterotoxigenic *Escherichia coli* strain of serotype O167:H5. *Federation of European Microbiological Societies Microbiology Letters* 83, 341–346.

Donnenberg, M.S. and Kaper, J.B. (1992) Enteropathogenic *Escherichia coli. Infection and Immunity* 60, 3953–3961.

Dorman, C.J. and Higgins, C.F. (1987) Fimbrial phase variation in *Escherichia coli*: dependence on integration host factor and homologies with other site-specific recombinases. *Journal of Bacteriology* 169, 3840–3843.

Dorman, C.J. and Ní Bhriain, N. (1992) Global regulation of gene expression during environmental adaptation: implications for bacterial pathogens. In: Hormaeche, C.E., Penn, C.W. and Smyth, C.J. (eds) *Molecular Biology of Bacterial Infection: Current Status and Future Perspectives, Society for General Microbiology Symposium No. 49*. Cambridge University Press, Cambridge, pp. 193–230.

Dorman, C.J. and Ní Bhriain, N. (1993) DNA topology and bacterial virulence gene regulation. *Trends in Microbiology* 1, 92–99.

Evans, D.J., Jr and Evans, D.G. (1990) Colonization factor antigens of human pathogens. *Current Topics in Microbiology and Immunology* 151, 129–145.

Fairbrother, J.M., Lallier, R., Leblanc, L., Jacques, M. and Larivière, S. (1988) Production and purification of *Escherichia coli* fimbrial antigen F165. *Federation of European Microbiological Societies Microbiology Letters* 56, 247–252.

Forsman, K., Göransson, M. and Uhlin, B.E. (1989) Autoregulation and multiple

DNA interactions by a transcriptional regulatory protein in *E. coli* pili biogenesis. *European Molecular Biology Organization Journal* 8, 1271–1277.

Forsman, K., Sondén, B., Göransson, M. and Uhlin, B.E. (1992). Antirepression function in *Escherichia coli* for the cAMP–cAMP receptor protein transcriptional activator. *Proceedings of the National Academy of Sciences of the United States of America* 89, 9880–9884.

Garcia, E., Bergmans, H.E.N., van der Zeijst, B.A.M. and Gaastra, W. (1992) Nucleotide sequences of the major subunits of F9 and F12 fimbriae of uropathogenic *Escherichia coli. Microbial Pathogenesis* 13, 161–166.

Girón, J.A., Ho, A.S.Y. and Schoolnik, G.K. (1991) An inducible bundle-forming pilus of enteropathogenic *Escherichia coli. Science* 254, 710–713.

Girón, J.A., Ho, A.S.Y. and Schoolnik, G.K. (1993) Characterization of fimbriae produced by enteropathogenic *Escherichia coli. Journal of Bacteriology* 175, 7391–7403.

Girón, J.A., Levine, M.M. and Kaper, J.B. (1994) Longus: a long pilus ultrastructure produced by human enterotoxigenic *Escherichia coli. Molecular Microbiology* 12, 71–82.

Göransson, M., Sondén, B., Nilsson, P., Dagberg, B., Forsman, K., Emanuelsson, K. and Uhlin, B.E. (1990) Transcriptional silencing and thermoregulation of gene expression in *Escherichia coli. Nature (London)* 344, 682–685.

Griffiths, E., Chart, H. and Stevenson, P. (1988) High-affinity iron uptake systems and bacterial virulence. In: Roth, J.A. (ed.) *Virulence Mechanisms of Bacterial Pathogens.* American Society for Microbiology, Washington, DC, pp. 121–137.

Hacker, J. (1990) Genetic determinants coding for fimbriae and adhesins of extraintestinal *Escherichia coli. Current Topics in Microbiology and Immunology* 151, 1–27.

Hacker, J., Morschhäuser, J., Ott, M. and Marre, R. (1992) Molecular investigation of *Escherichia coli* virulence in extraintestinal infections. In: Korhonen, T.K., Hovi, T. and Mäkelä, P.H. (eds) *Molecular Recognition in Host–Parasite Interactions, FEMS Symposium No. 61.* Plenum Press, New York, pp. 85–91.

Hacker, J., Kestler, H., Hoschützky, H., Jann, K., Lottspeich, F. and Korhonen, T.K. (1993) Cloning and characterization of the S fimbrial adhesin II complex of an *Escherichia coli* O18 : K1 meningitis isolate. *Infection and Immunity* 61, 544–550.

Hamers, A.M., Pel, H.J., Willshaw, G.A., Kusters, J.G., van der Zeijst, B.A.M. and Gaastra, W. (1989) The nucleotide sequence of the first two genes of the CFA/I fimbrial operon of human enterotoxigenic *Escherichia coli. Microbial Pathogenesis* 6, 297–309.

Harel, J., Forget, C., Saint-Amand, J., Daigle, F., Dubreuil, D., Jacques, M. and Fairbrother, J. (1992) Molecular cloning of a determinant coding for fimbrial antigen $F165_1$ a Prs-like fimbrial antigen from porcine septicaemic *Escherichia coli. Journal of General Microbiology* 138, 1495–1502.

Hedegaard, L. and Klemm, P. (1989) Type 1 fimbriae of *Escherichia coli* as carriers of heterologous antigenic sequences. *Gene* 85, 115–124.

Hinson, G., Knutton, S., Lam-Po-Tang, M.K.-L., McNeish, A.S. and Williams, P.H. (1987) Adherence to human colonocytes of an *Escherichia coli* strain isolated from severe infantile enteritis: molecular and ultrastructural studies for fibrillar adhesin. *Infection and Immunity* 55, 393–402.

Holmgren, A. and Bränden, C.-I. (1989) Crystal structure of chaperone protein PapD reveals an immunoglobulin fold. *Nature (London)* 342, 248–251.

Huisman, T.K., Bakker, D., Klaasen, P. and de Graaf, F.K. (1994) Leucine-responsive regulatory protein, IS*1* insertions, and the negative regulator FaeA control the expression of the *fae* (K88) operon in *Escherichia coli. Molecular Microbiology* 11, 525–536.

Hultgren, S.J. and Normark, S. (1991) Biogenesis of the bacterial pilus. *Current Opinion in Genes and Development* 1, 313–318.

Hultgren, S.J., Normark, S. and Abraham, S.N. (1991) Chaperone-assisted assembly and molecular architecture of adhesive pili. *Annual Review of Microbiology* 45, 383–415.

Imberechts, H., de Greve, H., Schlicker, C., Bouchet, H., Pohl, P., Charlier, G., Bertschinger, H., Wild, P., Vandekerckhove, J., van Damme, J., van Montagu, M. and Lintermans, P. (1992) Characterization of F107 fimbriae of *Escherichia coli* 107/86, which causes edema disease in pigs, and nucleotide sequence of the F107 major fimbrial subunit gene, *fedA*. *Infection and Immunity* 60, 1963–1971.

Isaacson, R.E. (1977) K99 surface antigen of *Escherichia coli*: purification and partial characterization. *Infection and Immunity* 15, 272–279.

Isaacson, R.E (1985) Pilus adhesins. In: Savage, D.C. and Fletcher, M. (eds) *Bacterial Adhesion*. Plenum Press, New York, pp. 307–336.

Jacob-Dubuisson, F., Kuehn, M. and Hultgren, S.J. (1993) A novel secretion apparatus for the assembly of adhesive bacterial pili. *Trends in Microbiology* 1, 50–55.

Jalajakumari, M.B., Thomas, C.J., Halter, R. and Manning, P.A. (1990) Genes for biosynthesis and assembly of CS3 pili of CFA/II enterotoxigenic *Escherichia coli*: novel regulation of pilus production by bypassing an amber codon. *Molecular Microbiology* 3, 1685–1695.

Jann, K. and Hoschützky, H. (1990) Nature and organization of adhesins. *Current Topics in Microbiology and Immunology* 151, 55–70.

Jann, K. and Hoschützky, H. (1991) Characterization and surface organization of *E. coli* adhesins. In: Ron, E.Z. and Rottem, S. (eds) *Microbial Surface Components and Toxins in Relation to Pathogenesis, FEMS Symposium No. 51*. Plenum Press, New York, pp. 3–10.

Jann, K. and Jann, B. (eds) (1990) Bacterial adhesins. In *Current Topics in Microbiology and.Immunology*, Vol. 151. Springer-Verlag, Berlin. pp. 1–209.

Jann, K., Ahrens, R., Bühler, T. and Hoschützky, H. (1992) Function and organization of *Escherichia coli* adhesins. In: Korhonen, T.K., Hovi, T. and Mäkelä, P.H. (eds) *Molecular Recognition in Host–Parasite Interactions, FEMS Symposium No. 61*. Plenum Press, New York, pp. 47–55.

Jayappa, H.G., Goodnow, R.A. and Geary, S.J. (1985) Role of *Escherichia coli* type 1 pilus in colonization of porcine ileum and its protective nature as a vaccine antigen in controlling colibacillosis. *Infection and Immunity* 48, 350–354.

Jones, C.H., Jacob-Dubuisson, F., Dodson, K., Kuehn, M., Slonim, L., Striker, R. and Hultgren, S.J. (1992) Adhesin presentation in bacteria requires molecular chaperones and ushers. *Infection and Immunity* 60, 4445–4451.

Jones, G.W. and Isaacson, R.E. (1984) Proteinaceous bacterial adhesins and their receptors. *CRC Critical Reviews in Microbiology* 10, 229–260.

Jordi, B.J.A.M. (1992) The mode of action of CfaD of *Escherichia coli* and VirF of *Shigella flexneri* and other members of the AraC family of positive regulators. *Molecular Microbiology* 6, 11.

Jordi, B.J.A.M., Dagberg, B., de Haan, L.A.M., Hamers, A.M., van der Zeijst, B.A.M., Gaastra, W. and Uhlin, B.E. (1992a) The positive regulator CfaD overcomes the repression mediated by histone-like protein H-NS (H1) in the CFA/I fimbrial operon of *Escherichia coli. European Molecular Biology Organization Journal* 11, 2627–2632.

Jordi, B.J.A.M., Willshaw, G., van der Zeijst, B.A.M. and Gaastra, W. (1992b) The complete nucleotide sequence of region 1 of the CFA/I fimbrial operon on human enterotoxigenic *Escherichia coli. DNA Sequence* 2, 257–263.

Karch, H., Heesemann, J., Laufs, R., O'Brien, A.D., Tacket, C.O. and Levine, M.M. (1987) A plasmid of enterohemorrhagic *Escherichia coli* O157:H7 is required for expression of a new fimbrial antigen and for adhesion to epithelial cells. *Infection and Immunity* 55, 455–461.

Karjalainen, T.K., Evans, D.G., Evans, D.J., Jr, Graham, D.Y. and Lee, C.-H. (1991) Iron represses the expression of CFA/1 fimbriae of enterotoxigenic *E. coli. Microbial Pathogenesis* 11, 317–323.

Karlsson, K.A. (1989) Current experience from the interaction of bacteria with glycosphingolipids. In: Switalski, L., Höök, M. and Beachey, E. (eds) *Molecular Mechanisms of Microbial Adhesion*. Springer-Verlag, New York, pp. 77–96.

Karlsson, K.-A., Ångström, J. and Teneberg, S. (1991) Characteristics of the recognition of host cell carbohydrates by viruses and bacteria. In: Wadström, T., Mäkelä, P.H., Svennerholm, A.-M. and Wolf-Watz, H. (eds) *Molecular Pathogenesis of Gastrointestinal Infections, FEMS Symposium No. 58.* Plenum Press, New York, pp. 9–21.

Karlsson, K.-A., Milh, M.A., Ångström, J., Bergström, J., Dezfoolian, H., Lanne, B., Leonardsson, I. and Teneberg, S. (1992) Membrane proximity and internal binding in the microbial recognition of host cell glycolipids: a conceptual discussion. In: Korhonen, T.K., Hovi, T. and Mäkelä, P.H. (eds) *Molecular Recognition in Host–Parasite Interactions, FEMS Symposium No. 61*. Plenum Press, New York, pp. 115–132.

Kawula, T.H. and Orndorff, P.E. (1991). Rapid site-specific DNA inversion in *Escherichia coli* mutants lacking the histone-like protein H-NS. *Journal of Bacteriology* 173, 4116–4123.

Klaasen, P. and de Graaf, F.K. (1990) Characterization of FapR, a positive regulator of expression of the 987P operon in enterotoxigenic *Escherichia coli. Molecular Microbiology* 4, 1779–1783.

Klemm, P. and Krogfelt, K.A. (1991) Molecular biology of *Escherichia coli* type 1 fimbriae. In: Wadström, T., Mäkelä, P.H., Svennerholm, A.-M. and Wolf-Watz, H. (eds) *Molecular Pathogenesis of Gastrointestinal Infections, FEMS Symposium No. 58*. Plenum Press, New York, pp. 87–92.

Korhonen, T.K., Virkola, R., Westurlund, B., Holthöfer, H. and Parkkinen, J. (1990) Tissue tropism of *Escherichia coli* adhesins in human extraintestinal infections. *Current Topics in Microbiology and Immunology* 151, 115–127.

Korhonen, T.K., Westerlund, B., Tarkkanen, A.-M., Sareneva, T., Virkola, R., Kuusela, P., Holthofer, H., van Die, I., Hoekstra, W., Allen, B.L. and Clegg, S. (1991) Binding of enterobacterial fimbria to proteins of basement membranes and connective tissue – a novel function for fimbriae. In: Ron, E.Z. and Rottem, S. (eds) *Microbial Surface Components and Toxins in Relation to Pathogenesis, FEMS Symposium No. 51*. Plenum Press, New York, pp. 11–21.

Korhonen, T.K., Hovi, T. and Mäkelä, P.H. (eds) (1992a) *Molecular Recognition in Host–Parasite Interactions, FEMS Symposium No. 61*. Plenum Press, New York.

Korhonen, T.K., Westerlund, B., Virkola, R., Tarkkanen, A.-M., Lähteenmäki, K., Kukkonen, M., Raunio, T., Adegoke, G., Miettnen, A. and Clegg, S. (1992b) Multifunctional nature of enterobacterial fimbriae. In: Korhonen, T.K., Hovi, T. and Mäkelä, P.H. (eds) *Molecular Recognition in Host–Parasite Interactions, FEMS Symposium No. 61*. Plenum Press, New York, pp. 93–100.

Krivan, H.C., Franklin, D.P., Wang, W., Laux, D.C. and Cohen, P.S. (1992) Phosphatidylserine found in intestinal mucus serves as a sole source of carbon and nitrogen for salmonellae and *Escherichia coli*. *Infection and Immunity* 60, 3943–3946.

Krogfelt, K.A. and Klemm, P. (1988) Investigation of minor components of *Escherichia coli* type 1 fimbriae: protein chemical and immunological aspects. *Microbial Pathogenesis* 4, 231–238.

Kuehn, M.J., Heuser, J., Normark, S. and Hultgren, S.J. (1992) P pili in uropathogenic *E. coli* are composite fibres with distinct fibrillar adhesive tips. *Nature (London)* 356, 252–255.

Kusters, J.G. and Gaastra, W. (1994) Fimbrial operons and evolution. In: Klemm, P. (ed.) *Fimbriae: Adhesion, Genetics, Biogenesis and Vaccines*. CRC Press, Boca Raton, pp. 189–207.

Kuusela, P., Ullberg, M., Kronvall, G. and Saksela, O. (1992) Binding and activation of plasminogen on the surface of *Staphylococcus aureus* and group A, C and G streptococci. In: Korhonen, T.K., Hori, T. and Mäkelä, P.H. (eds) *Molecular Recognition in Host–Parasite Interaction, FEMS Symposium No. 61*. Plenum Press, New York, pp. 153–162.

Labigne-Roussel, A. and Falkow, S. (1988) Distribution and degree of heterogeneity of the afimbrial-adhesin-encoding operon (*afa*) among uropathogenic *Escherichia coli* isolates. *Infection and Immunity* 56, 640–648.

Lai, C.-Y. (1977) Determination of the primary structure of cholera toxin B subunit. *Journal of Biological Chemistry* 252, 7249–7256.

Leffler, H. and Svanborg-Edén, C. (1986) Glycolipids as receptors for *Escherichia coli* lectins or adhesins. In: Mirelman, D. (ed.) *Microbial Lectins and Agglutinins: Properties and Biological Activity*. John Wiley & Sons, New York, pp. 83–111.

Leong, J., Vinal, A.C. and Dallas, W.S. (1985) Nucleotide sequence comparison between heat-labile toxin B-subunit cistrons from *Escherichia coli* of human and porcine origin. *Infection and Immunity* 48, 73–77.

May, A.K., Block, C.A., Sawyer, R.G., Spengler, M.D. and Pruett, T.L. (1993) Enhanced virulence of *Escherichia coli* bearing a site-targeted mutation in the major structural subunit of type 1 fimbriae. *Infection and Immunity* 61, 1667–1673.

McClain, M.S., Blomfield, I.C. and Eisenstein, B.I. (1991) Roles of *fimB* and *fimE* in site-specific DNA inversion associated with phase variation of type 1 fimbriae in *Escherichia coli. Journal of Bacteriology* 173, 5308–5314.

Mims, C.A. (1987) *The Pathogenesis of Infectious Disease*, 3rd edn. Academic Press, London.

Mirelman, D. (ed.) (1986) *Microbial Lectins and Agglutinins: Properties and Biological Activity*. John Wiley & Sons, New York.

Mooi, F.R. and de Graaf, F.K. (1985) Molecular biology of fimbriae of enterotoxigenic *Escherichia coli. Current Topics in Microbiology and Immunology* 118, 119–138.

Moon, H.W. (1990) Colonization factor antigens of enterotoxigenic *Escherichia coli* in animals. *Current Topics in Microbiology and Immunology* 151, 147–165.

Morschhäuser, J., Hoschützky, H., Jann, K. and Hacker, J. (1990) Functional analysis of the sialic acid-binding adhesin SfaS of pathogenic *Escherichia coli* by site-directed mutagenesis. *Infection and Immunity* 58, 2133–2138.

Morschhäuser, J., Uhlin, B.E. and Hacker, J. (1993) Transcriptional analysis and regulation of the *sfa* determinant coding for S-fimbriae of pathogenic *Escherichia coli* strains. *Molecular and General Genetics* 238, 97–105.

Nataro, J.P., Deng, Y., Maneval, D.R., German, A.L., Martin, W.C. and Levine, M.M. (1992) Aggregative adherence fimbriae I of enteroaggregative *Escherichia coli* mediate adherence to HEp-2 cells and hemagglutination of human erythrocytes. *Infection and Immunity* 60, 2297–2304.

Nataro, J.P., Yikang, D., Giron, J.A., Savarino, S.J., Kothary, M.H. and Hall, R. (1993) Aggregative adherence fimbria I expression in enteroaggregative *Escherichia coli* requires two unlinked plasmid regions. *Infection and Immunity* 61, 1126–1131.

Neilands, J.B. (1990) Molecular biology and regulation of iron acquisition by *Escherichia coli* K12. In: Iglewski, B.H. and Clark, V.L. (eds) *Molecular Basis of Bacterial Pathogenesis, The Bacteria*, Vol. 11. Academic Press, New York, pp. 205–248.

Normark, S., Båga, M., Göransson, M., Lindberg, F.P., Lund, B., Norgren, M. and Uhlin, B.-E. (1986) Genetics and biogenesis of *Escherichia coli* adhesins. In: Mirelman, D. (ed.) *Microbial Lectins: Properties and Biological Activity*. John Wiley & Sons, New York, pp. 113–143.

Normark, S., Marklund, B.-I., Nyholm, P.-G., Pascher, I. and Strömberg, N. (1992) Bacterial adherence and host tropism in *Escherichia coli*. In: Korhonen, T.K., Hovi, T. and Mäkelä, P.H. (eds) *Molecular Recognition in Host–Parasite Interactions, FEMS Symposium No. 61*. Plenum Press, New York, pp. 133–138.

Nou, X., Skinner, B., Braaten, B., Blyn, L., Hirsch, D. and Low, D. (1993) Regulation of pyelonephritis-associated pili phase-variation in *Escherichia coli*: binding of the PapI and the Lrp regulatory proteins is controlled by DNA methylation. *Molecular Microbiology* 7, 545–553.

Ofek, I. and Beachey, E.H. (1980) General concepts and principles of bacterial adherence in animals and man. In: Beachey, E.H. (ed.) *Bacterial Adherence,*

Receptors and Recognition Series B, Vol. 6. Chapman & Hall, London, pp. 1–29.

Ofek, I. and Sharon, N. (1990) Adhesins as lectins: specificity and role in infection. *Current Topics in Microbiology and Immunology* 151, 91–113.

Olsén, A. (1992) Regulatory and Functional Studies of Curli, a Novel Surface Organelle of *Escherichia coli* that Mediates Binding to Soluble Matrix Proteins. *Umeå University Medical Dissertation, New Series No. 356, PhD Thesis*. University of Umeå, Sweden.

Olsén, A., Jonsson, A. and Normark, S. (1989) Fibronectin binding mediated by a novel class of surface organelles on *Escherichia coli. Nature (London)* 338, 652–655.

Olsén, A. Arnqvist, A., Hammar, M., Sukupolvi, S. and Normark, S. (1993) The RpoS sigma factor relieves H-NS-mediated transcriptional repression of *csgA*, the subunit gene of the fibronectin-binding curli in *Escherichia coli. Molecular Microbiology* 7, 523–536.

Orndorff, P.E. and Bloch, C.A. (1990). The role of type 1 pili in the pathogenesis of *Escherichia coli* infections: a short review and some new ideas. *Microbial Pathogenesis* 9, 75–79.

Parkkinen, J. (1992) *Escherichia coli* fimbriae: oligosaccharide-specific binding to host tissues and enhancement of plasminogen activation. In: Korhonen, T.K., Hovi, T. and Mäkelä, P.H. (eds) *Molecular Recognition in Host–Parasite Interactions, FEMS Symposium No. 61*. Plenum Press, New York, pp. 163–171.

Parkkinen, J., Korhonen, T.K., Pere, A., Hacker, J. and Soinila, S. (1988) Binding sites in the rat brain for *Escherichia coli* S fimbriae associated with neonatal meningitis. *Journal of Clinical Investigation* 81, 860–865.

Perez-Casal, J., Swartley, J.S. and Scott, J.R. (1990) Gene encoding the major subunit of CS1 pili of enterotoxigenic *Escherichia coli. Infection and Immunity* 58, 3594–3600.

Roosendaal, E., Gaastra, W. and de Graaf, F.K. (1984) The nucleotide sequence of the gene encoding the K99 subunit of enterotoxigenic *Escherichia coli. Federation of European Microbiological Societies Microbiology Letters* 22, 253–258.

Roosendaal, B., Damoiseaux, J., Jordi, W. and de Graaf, F.K. (1989) Transcriptional organization of the DNA region controlling expression of the K99 gene cluster. *Molecular and General Genetics* 215, 250–256.

Roth, J.A. (ed.) (1988) *Virulence Mechanisms of Bacterial Pathogens*. American Society for Microbiology, Washington, DC.

Rutter, J.M., Burrows, M.R., Sellwood, R. and Gibbons, R.A. (1975) A genetic basis for resistance to enteric disease caused by *E. coli. Nature (London)* 257, 135–136.

Savage, D.C. and Fletcher, M. (eds) (1985) *Bacterial Adhesion*. Plenum Press, New York.

Savelkoul, P.H.M., Willshaw, G.A., McConnell, M.M., Smith, H.R., Hamers, A.M., van der Zeijst, B.A.M. and Gaastra, W. (1990) Expression of CFA/I fimbriae is positively regulated. *Microbial Pathogenesis* 8, 91–99.

Schmoll, T., Morschhäuser, J., Ott, M., Ludwig, B., van Die, I. and Hacker, J. (1990a) Complete genetic organization and functional aspects of the *Escherichia coli* S fimbrial adhesin determinant: nucleotide sequence of the genes *sfa B, C, D, E, F. Microbial Pathogenesis* 9, 331–343.

Schmoll, T., Ott, M., Oudega, B. and Hacker, J. (1990b) Use of a wild-type gene fusion to determine the influence of environmental conditions on the expression of the S fimbrial adhesin in an *Escherichia coli* pathogen. *Journal of Bacteriology* 172, 5103–5111.

Seignole, D., Grange, P., Duval-Iflah, Y. and Mauricout, M. (1994) Characterization of O-glycan moieties of the 210 and 240 kDa pig intestinal receptors for *E. coli* K88ac fimbriae. *Journal of General Microbiology* 140 (in press).

Sellwood, R., Gibbons, R.A., Jones, G.W. and Rutter, J.M. (1975) Adhesion of enteropathogenic *Escherichia coli* to pig intestinal brush borders: the existence of two pig phenotypes. *Journal of Medical Microbiology* 8, 405–411.

Simons, L.H., Willemsen, P.T.J., Bakker, D., de Graaf, F.K. and Oudega, B. (1991) Localization and function of FanH and FanG, minor components of K99 fimbriae of enterotoxigenic *Escherichia coli. Microbial Pathogenesis* 11, 325–336.

Smith, H.R., Willshaw, G.A. and Rowe, B. (1982) Mapping of a plasmid, coding for colonization factor antigen I and heat-stable enterotoxin production, isolated from an enterotoxigenic strain of *Escherichia coli. Journal of Bacteriology* 149, 264–275.

Smyth, C.J. (1986) Fimbrial variation in *Escherichia coli*. In: Birkbeck, T.H. and Penn, C.W. (eds) *Antigenic Variation in Infectious Diseases, Special Publications of the Society for General Microbiology*, Vol. 19. IRL Press, Oxford, pp. 95–125.

Smyth, C.J. (1988) Flagella: their role in virulence. In: Owen, P. and Foster, T.J. (eds) *Immunochemical and Molecular Genetic Analysis of Bacterial Pathogens*. Elsevier, Amsterdam, pp. 3–11.

Smyth, C.J. and Smith, S.G.J. (1992) Bacterial fimbriae: variation and regulatory mechanisms. In: Hormaeche, C.E., Penn, C.W. and Smyth, C.J. (eds) *Molecular Biology of Bacterial Infection: Current Status and Future Perspectives, Society for General Microbiology Symposium No. 49*. Cambridge University Press, Cambridge, pp. 267–297.

Smyth, C.J., Boylan, M., Matthews, H.M. and Coleman, D.C. (1991) Fimbriae of human enterotoxigenic *Escherichia coli* and control of their expression. In: Ron, E.Z. and Rottem, S. (eds) *Microbial Surface Components and Toxins in Relation to Pathogenesis*. Plenum Press, New York, pp. 37–53.

Steven, A.C., Bisher, M.E., Trus, B.L., Thomas, D., Zhang, J.M. and Cowell, J.L. (1986) Helical structure of *Bordetella pertussis* fimbriae. *Journal of Bacteriology* 167, 968–974.

Sussman, M. (ed.) (1985) *The Virulence of* Escherichia coli, *Special Publications of the Society for General Microbiology, No. 13*. Academic Press, London.

Tennent, J.M., Hultgren, S., Marklund, B.-I., Forsman, K., Göransson, M., Uhlin, B.E. and Normark, S. (1990) Genetics of adhesin expression in *Escherichia coli*. In: Iglewski, B.H. and Clark, V.L. (eds) *Molecular Basis of Bacterial Pathogenesis, The Bacteria*, Vol. 11. Academic Press, New York, pp. 79–110.

Väisänen-Rhen, V. (1984) Fimbria-like haemagglutinin of *Escherichia coli* O75 strains. *Infection and Immunity* 46, 401–407.

van den Bosch, J.F., Hendricks, J.H.I.M., Gladigau, I., Willems, H.M.C., Storm,

P.K. and de Graaf, F.K. (1993) Identification of F11 fimbriae on chicken *Escherichia coli* strains. *Infection and Immunity* 61, 800–806.

van der Woude, M.W. and Low, D.A. (1994) Leucine-responsive regulatory protein and deoxyadenosine methylase control the phase variation and expression of the *sfa* and *daa* pili operons in *Escherichia coli. Molecular Microbiology* 11, 605–618.

van der Woude, M.W., Braaten, B.A. and Low, D.A. (1992) Evidence for global regulatory control of pilus expression in *Escherichia coli* by Lrp and DNA methylation: model building based on the analysis of *pap. Molecular Microbiology* 6, 2429–2435.

Westerlund, B., Kuusela, P., Vartio, T., van Die, I and Korhonen, T.K. (1989) A novel lectin-independent interaction of P fimbriae of *Escherichia coli* with immobilized fibronectin. *Federation of European Biochemical Societies Letters* 243, 199–204.

Westerlund, B., van Die, I., Kramer, C., Kuusela, P., Holthöfer, H., Tarkkanen, A.-M., Virkola, R., Riegman, N., Bergmans, H., Hoekstra, W. and Korhonen, T.K. (1991) Multifunctional nature of P fimbriae of uropathogenic *Escherichia coli*: mutations in *fsoE* and *fsoF* influence fimbrial binding to renal tubuli and immobilized fibronectin. *Molecular Microbiology* 5, 2965–2975.

White-Ziegler, C.A. and Low, D.A. (1992) Thermoregulation of the *pap* operon: evidence for the involvement of RimJ, the N-terminal acetylase of the ribosomal protein S5. *Journal of Bacteriology* 174, 7003–7012.

Woolcock, J.B. (1988) Bacterial resistance to humoral defense mechanisms: an overview. In: Roth, J.A. (ed.) *Virulence Mechanisms of Bacterial Pathogens*. American Society for Microbiology, Washington, DC, pp. 73–93.

17

Structure, Function and Synthesis of Surface Polysaccharides in *Escherichia coli*

C. Whitfield, W.J. Keenleyside and B.R. Clarke
Department of Microbiology, University of Guelph, Guelph, Ontario, Canada N1G 2W1

Introduction

The surface of *E. coli* is composed primarily of polysaccharides which are involved in critical interactions with the environment. In many cases, surface polymers are essential for survival within the host and constitute key determinants of virulence. The objective of this chapter is to provide an overview of cell surface polysaccharides in *E. coli*. Where possible, we will relate their structure and surface organization to various functions and biological effects in the host. In addition, we will discuss the mechanisms involved in the synthesis and regulation of these components but space limitations and the broad scope of this review preclude a detailed analysis of these areas.

Structure and Attachment of Cell Surface Polysaccharides in *E. coli*

Overview of the surface architecture of E. coli

The architecture of the cell wall of *E. coli* is typical of Gram-negative bacteria. The characteristic outer membrane of *E. coli* (Chapter 18) has received detailed attention and studies using genetically characterized derivatives of the laboratory strain, *E. coli* K-12, have contributed models for outer membrane structure and function in other bacteria. However, the cell surface of *E. coli* K-12 is significantly different from that of recent clinical isolates of *E. coli*, particularly with respect to the polysaccharide components. The outer membrane contains the unique and complex

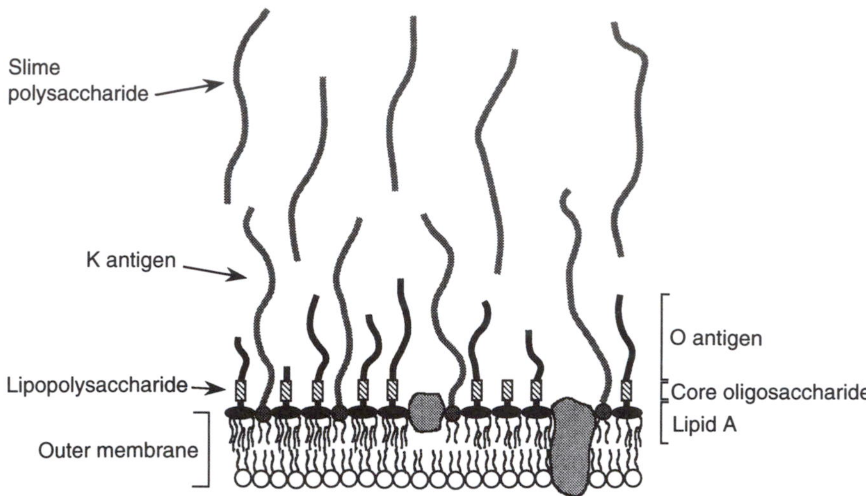

Fig. 17.1. Schematic representation of the outer membrane of *E. coli*.

glycolipid, lipopolysaccharide (LPS), which is composed of three structurally distinct domains (Fig. 17.1). Lipid A is the hydrophobic portion of LPS and replaces phospholipids in the outer leaflet of the outer membrane, to form an atypical lipid bilayer. A variable length hydrophilic polysaccharide known as the O-polysaccharide (or O-antigen) can be attached to lipid A via the core oligosaccharide. Most clinical isolates of *E. coli* produce 'smooth' LPS (S-LPS) containing O-antigen. In contrast, the LPS molecule in *E. coli* K-12 terminates with the core oligosaccharide and is termed 'rough' (R-LPS). The smooth and rough terminology historically describes the morphology of bacterial colonies expressing the respective type of LPS.

Many *E. coli* strains produce an additional polysaccharide layer termed the K-antigen, which can mask the underlying O-antigen in serological (agglutination test) analyses. This layer forms a capsule, which can be visualized under the electron microscope. K-antigens are therefore also known as capsular polysaccharides (CPSs). Due to their anionic nature, capsules can be stained with electropositive stains such as ruthenium red or labelled with cationized ferritin. Capsules are highly hydrophilic and tend to collapse under the dehydrating conditions used in preparation of samples for electron microscopy. However the structure can be stabilized by pretreatment with capsule-specific antiserum (Fig. 17.2), or by using the recently developed freeze-substitution method for sample preparation (Beveridge and Graham, 1991).

The O and K antigens are structurally diverse. There are 173 O and 80 K antigens in the international scheme (Ørskov and Ørskov, 1992). The

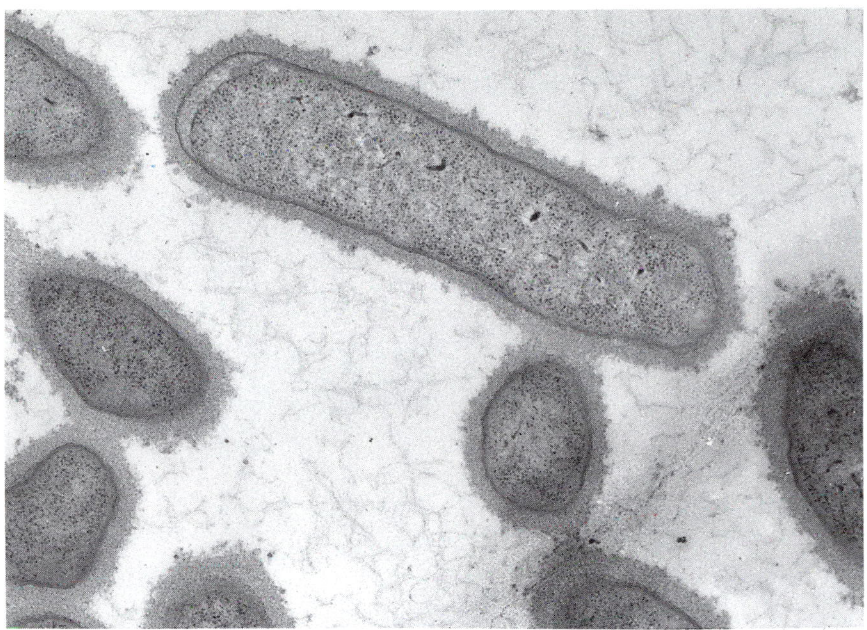

Fig. 17.2. Electron micrograph of *E. coli* O9:K30:H12. The K30 capsular layer has been stabilized using a K30-specific monoclonal antibody.

structures of the repeating units of many of these polysaccharides have been reported (Dutton and Parolis, 1989). The O and K antigens occur naturally in selected combinations. While these polysaccharides confer serotype specificity within the species, identical polymers may occur in the O antigens and capsular polysaccharides of other bacterial species. *E. coli* also produces two cell surface polysaccharides that are not serotype specific (Table 17.1). The enterobacterial common antigen (ECA) is produced by all Enterobacteriaceae, except *Erwinia chrysanthemi* (Kuhn *et al.*, 1988). The slime polysaccharide, colanic acid (M, or mucoid antigen), is produced by several *E. coli* strains and by strains of *Salmonella* and *Aerobacter cloacae* (Markovitz, 1977).

Chemistry of E. coli *lipopolysaccharides*

The lipid A portion of LPS is essential for outer membrane integrity. Lipid A consists of a β-glucosaminyl-1,6-glucosamine backbone in which the glucosamine residues are phosphorylated by a phosphomonoester group at position 4′ and a phosphoryl group at position 1 (Fig. 17.3). Six fatty acid residues are found in lipid A. Four β-hydroxymyristoyl chains are attached

Table 17.1. *E. coli* cell surface polysaccharides[a] which do not confer serotype specificity.

Polysaccharide	Structure
Colanic acid	*O* Ac ↓ 2/3 →4)-α-L-Fuc*p*-(1→3)-β-D-Glc*p*-(1→3)-β-L-Fuc*p*-(1→ 4 ↑ 1 β-D-Gal*p*-(1→4)-β-D-Glc*p*A-(1→3)-β-D-Gal*p* ‖ Pyr
Enterobacterial Common Antigen (ECA)	→4)-β-D-ManNAcA-(1→4)-α-D-GlcNAc-(1→3)-α-D-Fuc4NAc-(1→

[a] Structures reviewed in Kenne and Lindberg (1983).

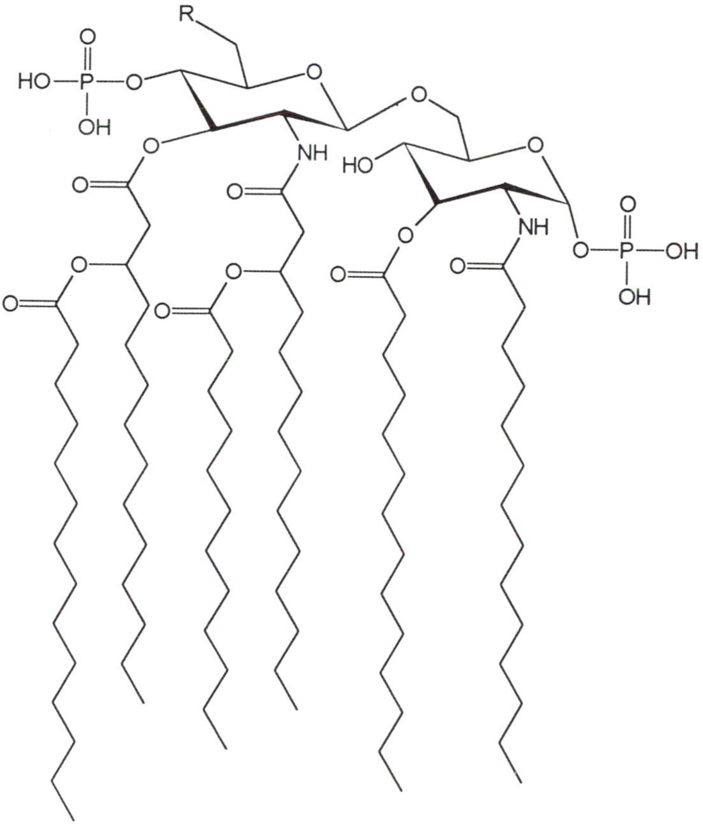

Fig. 17.3. Structure of lipid A from *E. coli* K-12.

directly to the diglucosamine backbone at positions 2, 3, 2′ and 3′ and the remaining two are esterified to the non-reducing end of the hydroxymyristoyl residues (Qureshi and Takayama, 1990; Raetz, 1990).

The core oligosaccharide contains a conserved inner region nearest lipid A and a more variable outer region, culminating in an attachment point for O antigen. Any truncation of the LPS core results in an inability to attach O antigen. The inner core contains 3-keto-deoxy-D-*manno*-octulosonic acid (KDO) and L-*glycero*-D-*manno*-heptose (Table 17.2). KDO was originally thought to be unique to LPS but is now known to occur in certain *E. coli* K antigens (see below). The outer core contains a number of hexose residues and variation in this region gives rise to five recognized core types in *E. coli* (Table 17.3). However, this may not represent all *E. coli* core types found in nature. Studies on adherent and non-adherent

Table 17.2. *E. coli* inner core regions from chemotypes R3[a] (Haishima *et al.*, 1992) and K-12 (Holst *et al.*, 1991) LPS.

Chemotype	Structure
R3	(GlcN) ↓ 7 Hep 1 ↓ 7 OUTER CORE→3)-Hep-(1→3)-Hep-(1→5)-KDO-(2→LIPID A 4 ↑ 2 KDO 4 ↑ 2 (KDO)
K-12	L-α-D-Hep*p* 1 ↓ 7 OUTER CORE→3)-L-α-D-Hep*p*-(1→3)-L-α-D-Hep*p*-(1→5)-KDO-2→LIPID A

[a] In the R3 inner core, a partially *N*-acetylated glucosamine residue and a side-chain terminal KDO are present in non-stoichiometric amounts.

Table 17.3. Structure of the hexose-containing outer regions of *E. coli* LPS core oligosaccharides.[a]

```
Core type       Structure

E. coli R1      α-D-Galp-(1→2)-α-D-Glcp-(1→3)-α-D-Glcp-(1→
                    2              3
                    ↑              ↑
                    1              1
                α-D-Galp       β-D-Glcp

E. coli R2      α-D-Glcp-(1→2)-α-D-Glcp-(1→3)-α-D-Glcp-(1→
                    2                              6
                    ↑                              ↑
                    1                              1
                α-D-GlcpNAc                    α-D-Galp

E. coli R3      α-D-Glcp-(1→2)-α-D-Galp-(1→3)-α-D-Glcp-(1→
                    2              3
                    ↑              ↑
                    1              1
                α-D-Glcp       α-D-GlcpNAc

E. coli R4      α-D-Galp-(1→2)-α-D-Glcp-(1→3)-α-D-Glcp-(1→
                    2                              4
                    ↑                              ↑
                    1                              1
                α-D-Galp                       β-D-Galp

E. coli K-12    α-D-Glcp-(1→2)-α-D-Glcp-(1→3)-α-D-Glcp-(1→
                    6                              6
                    ↑                              ↑
                    1                              1
        GlcpNAc or L-α-D-Hepp                  α-D-Galp
```

[a] The structures are from Jansson *et al.* (1981). The R3 structure was described in more detail in Haishima *et al.* (1992). The modified version of the *E. coli* K-12 core was described by Holst *et al.* (1991); either GlcNAc or Hep residues can substitute the terminal hexose.

strains of *E. coli* O119 have shown that the same O antigens can be attached to two core types. Compositional analysis of one core type indicated a novel structure with variation in the 'conserved' inner heptose region (Bradley *et al.*, 1991). The possible attachment of the same O antigen to structurally different core types has been recognized for some time (Schmidt *et al.*, 1969). In a recent study, the R1 chemotype was detected in 123 of 180 *E. coli* clinical isolates, making it the most prevalent core (Gibb *et al.*, 1992). There also appears to be a relationship between the core chemotype and the O and K antigen. For example, R1 core is found in strains which express the O1, O4, O6, O8 and O18 O antigens and the K1 and K5 K antigens. The reasons for this association are unclear but chemical compatibility between the core and O antigen has been suggested as one explanation (Gibb *et al.*, 1992). Although O polysaccharides can be attached to heterologous LPS cores in strains carrying cloned *rfb* (O antigen biosynthesis) genes (see below), efficiency of the attachment of a specific O antigen may be determined by core type. This may, in turn, offer a selective advantage to strains with the appropriate combination.

The O polysaccharides of *E. coli* include homo- and heteropolysaccharides and contain a variety of hexoses, methyl pentoses and amino sugars (Table 17.4). Some polysaccharides (e.g. O111) contain dideoxyhexoses, which are common constituents of *Salmonella* O polysaccharides. Antigenic changes can occur due to alteration in the sugar sequence (e.g. O1A and O1B) or the linkage sequence (e.g. O1B and O1C or O8, O9 and O9a) (Table 17.4). Some *E. coli* O antigens are identical to structures produced by other bacteria. Thus, the O8 and O9 polysaccharides are identical to the *Klebsiella* O5 and O3 antigens, respectively (Kenne and Lindberg, 1983; Dutton and Parolis, 1989).

Work with *Salmonella enterica* serovar Typhimurium and *E. coli* O111 first illustrated that the length of O polysaccharide attached to lipid A core is highly variable (Goldman and Leive, 1980; Munford *et al.*, 1980; Palva and Mäkelä, 1980; Hitchcock and Brown, 1983). This phenomenon is now known to be widespread in bacterial genera. Hetereogeneity in LPS is readily observed in silver-stained sodium dodecyl sulfate–polyacrylamide gels (SDS–PAGE), in which characteristic ladder patterns result from lipid A core molecules substituted with increasing lengths of O polysaccharide (Fig. 17.4). Each 'rung' in the ladder reflects addition of a repeating unit and the interband spacing reflects the size of the repeating unit. The amount of capping of lipid A core with O polysaccharide is variable and therefore most strains with S-LPS also contain some R-LPS, which is evident as a fast migrating fraction on SDS–PAGE (Fig. 17.4).

Chemistry of E. coli *K antigens*

Chemical and genetic criteria have been used to subdivide *E. coli* K antigens (Table 17.5) (Jann and Jann, 1992). All K antigens are acidic polymers. Group I K antigens contain a variety of hexoses and methyl pentoses. Hexuronic acids provide the principal negatively charged components, although pyruvate residues are also common (Table 17.6). Group IA K antigens resemble polysaccharides produced by *Klebsiella*. For example, the capsular polysaccharides in *E. coli* K30 and *Klebsiella* K20 are identical (Choy and Dutton, 1973; Chakraborty *et al.*, 1980). Several *E. coli* group I K antigens also show serological cross-reactions with pneumococcal polysaccharides (Heidelberger *et al.*, 1968). The slime

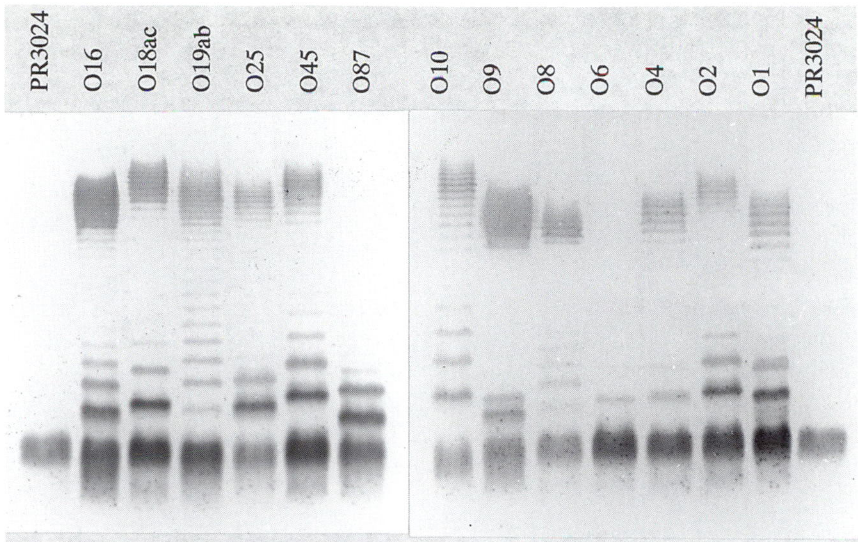

Fig. 17.4. SDS–polyacrylamide gel showing LPS profiles from different *E. coli* O-serotypes. The serotype is indicated above each lane. Strain PR3024 is an O-deficient derivative with a complete core oligosaccharide and is included to indicate the mobility of R-LPS. Note the strain-dependent banding patterns in the O-substituted LPS molecules and the differences in interband spacing which reflect the chemical structure of the O-polysaccharide repeating unit.

polysaccharide colanic acid (Table 17.1), which is widely distributed in *E. coli* strains, resembles group IA K antigens in its chemical structure. Colanic acid is not expressed in *E. coli* strains with other group IA K antigens, but it can be produced simultaneously with group IB K antigens (Jayaratne *et al.*, 1993). K antigens in group IB are distinguished from those of group IA by the presence of amino sugars. Some are not true polysaccharides because they contain amino acid substituents (e.g. K40, K49; Table 17.6). Group IB K antigens have no obvious counterparts in other bacteria. The group IA and IB K antigens are expressed with a limited range of O antigens, predominantly O8 and O9 (Jann and Jann, 1992; Table 17.5).

E. coli group II K antigens are expressed with a wide range of O antigens. Group II K antigens contain a variety of negatively charged components, including KDO, sialic acid (Neu5*p*NAc) and hexuronic acids (Table 17.7). Some group II K antigens are polymers which contain ribitol-phosphate (e.g. K18) or glycerol-phosphate (e.g. K2a) and resemble the teichoic acids of Gram-positive bacteria. Several group II K antigens are similar to capsular polysaccharides in *Neisseria meningitidis* and

Table 17.4. Structures of representative *E. coli* O-polysaccharides.[a]

Serotype	Structure
O1A/O1A1	→3)-α-L-Rha*p*-(1→3)-β-L-Rha*p*-(1→4)-β-D-Glc*p*NAc-(1→3)-α-L-Rha*p*-(1→ 2 ↑ 1 β-D-Man*p*NAc
O1B	→2)-α-L-Rha*p*-(1→2)-α-D-Gal*p*-(1→3)-β-D-Glc*p*NAc-(1→3)-α-L-Rha*p*-(1→ 2 ↑ 1 β-D-Man*p*NAc
O1C	→2)-α-L-Rha*p*-(1→3)-α-D-Gal*p*-(1→3)-β-D-Glc*p*NAc-(1→3)-α-L-Rha*p*-(1→ 2 ↑ 1 β-D-Man*p*NAc
O7	→3)-α-D-Glc*p*NAc-(1→3)-β-D-Qui*p*4NAc-(1→2)-α-D-Man*p*-(1→4)-β-D-Gal*p*-(1→ 3 ↑ 1 α-L-Rha*p* Qui*p*4NAc = 4-acetamido-4,6-dideoxy-D-glucopyranose

O8	→3)-β-D-Man*p*-(1→2)-α-D-Man*p*-(1→2)-α-D-Man*p*-(1→
O9	→3)-α-D-Man*p*-(1→3)-α-D-Man*p*-(1→2)-α-D-Man*p*-(1→2)-α-D-Man*p*-(1→2)-α-D-Man*p*-(1→
O9a	→3)-α-D-Man*p*-(1→3)-α-D-Man*p*-(1→2)-α-D-Man*p*-(1→2)-α-D-Man*p*-(1→
O18ac	→2)-α-L-Rha*p*-(1→4)-α-Gal*p*-(1→6)-α-Glc*p*-(1→3)-α-GlcpNAc-(1→ 3 ↑ 1 β-Glc*p*NAc
O111	α-Col*p* 1 ↓ 3 →3)-β-D-Glc*p*NAc-(1→4)-α-D-Glc*p*-(1→4)-α-D-Gal*p*-(1→ 6 ↑ 1 α-Col*p* Col=3,6-dideoxy-L-*xylo*-hexose

[a] With the exception of the O1A/O1A1 (Jann *et al.*, 1992a) and the O1B and O1C (Gupta *et al.*, 1992) polysaccharides, the structures shown are reviewed by Dutton and Parolis (1989).

Table 17.5. Grouping of *E. coli* K-antigens.[a]

Characteristic	Group IA	Group IB	Group II
Acidic component	GlcA, GalA Pyr	GlcA, NeuNAc	GlcA, NeuNAc KDO, ManNAcA, phosphate
Expressed below 20°C	Yes	Yes	No
Coexpression with O-groups	O8, O9, O20	O8, O9, O20	Many
Coexpression with colanic acid	No	Yes	Yes
Terminal lipid residue	Lipid A-core	Lipid A-core	L-Glycerophosphate
Removal of lipid at pH 5–6/100°C	No	No	Yes
Biosynthesis genetic loci	near *his* and *rfb*, with a possible additional locus near *trp*	near *his* and *rfb*?	*kps* near *serA*
Elevated levels of CMP-KDO synthetase	No	No?	Yes
Structural resemblance to CPS from	*Klebsiella* spp.	None known	*Neisseria meningitidis* and *Haemophilus influenzae*

[a] Modified from Jann and Jann (1992).

Haemophilus influenzae. For example, the K1 polysaccharide is identical to the capsular polysaccharide of *N. meningitidis* type b (McGuire and Binkley, 1964), but the same structure is also found in *Pasteurella haemolytica* A2 (Adlam *et al.*, 1987) and *Moraxella nonliquefaciens* (Devi *et al.*, 1991). Group II K antigens can also be co-expressed with colanic acid (Goebel, 1963; Keenleyside *et al.*, 1993).

As with O antigens, serotype specificity in K antigens can be altered by changes in linkage (Table 17.7). For example, the K1 and K92 antigens are both homopolymers of sialic acid and are distinguished only by the alternating $\alpha 2 \rightarrow 9$ linkage found in K92. Addition of side groups also has a profound effect. The K23, K18 and K20 polysaccharides contain the same carbohydrate backbone; the antigenicity is altered by the presence or position of O-acetyl residues.

It is important to note that the K-12 designation for the well-characterized *E. coli* laboratory strain is unrelated to capsule type. *E. coli* K-12 can produce colanic acid under appropriate conditions (see below) but lacks genes for group II K antigens. However, there are other *E. coli* strains which do produce a serotype K-12 (group II) capsular polysaccharide.

Surface attachment of E. coli *polysaccharides*

Two modes of cell attachment have been proposed for the surface polysaccharides of *E. coli* (Table 17.8). Several *E. coli* group II K antigens have a diacylglycerol residue attached via a phosphodiester linkage to their reducing terminus. This terminal lipid moiety was first detected in *E. coli* K92 and *N. meningitidis* groups A, B and C capsular polysaccharides (Gotschlich *et al.*, 1981). The same lipid is probably present in *H. influenzae* capsules (Egan *et al.*, 1982; Kuo *et al.*, 1985). Thus a series of polysaccharides with similar repeating unit structures terminate in a similar phospholipid. In *E. coli* K12 and K82 K antigens, the L-glycerophosphatidyl residue is linked to the polysaccharide via a KDO residue, which forms the reducing terminus of the polysaccharide but is not part of the repeating unit structure (Schmidt and Jann, 1982). The distribution of the KDO-containing form of linkage unit has not been established. Interestingly, one form of ECA containing the longest polysaccharide chains, also has a terminal L-glycerophosphatidyl residue. This form of ECA is termed ECA_{PG}, to reflect its linkage to phosphatidyl glycerol (Kuhn *et al.*, 1988). The terminal phospholipid has been implicated in surface active phenomena, including micelle formation and, presumably, attachment (Gotschlich *et al.*, 1981; Kuhn *et al.*, 1988). However, only 20–50% of *E. coli* group II K antigen chains are lipid substituted (Jann and Jann, 1990). This may be a consequence of the acid labile linkage between the polymer and the lipid. It is not clear whether the lipid-free polymers are

Table 17.6. Structures of representative *E. coli* group I K-antigens.[a]

Serotype	Structure
Group IA	
K27	→4)-α-D-Glc*p*-(1→4)-β-D-Glc*p*A-(1→3)-α-L-Fuc*p*-(1→ 3 ↑ 1 α-D-Gal*p*
K28	→3)-α-D-Glc*p*-(1→4)-β-D-Glc*p*A-(1→4)-α-L-Fuc*p*-(1→ 4 2/3 ↑ ↑ 1 OAc (70%) β-D-Gal*p*
K29	→2)-α-D-Man*p*-(1→3)-β-D-Glc*p*-(1→3)-β-D-Glc*p*A-(1→3)-α-D-Galp-(1→ 4 ↑ 1 β-D-Glc*p*-(1→2)-α-D-Man*p* ‖ Pyr
K30	→2)-α-D-Man*p*-(1→3)-β-D-Gal*p*-(1→ 3 ↑ 1 β-D-Glc*p*A-(1→3)-α-D-Gal*p*

Group IB	
K9	→3)-β-D-Gal*p*-(1→3)-β-D-Glc*p*NAc-(1→4)-α-D-Gal*p*-(1→4)-α-Neu*p*5Ac-(1→ ↑ *O*Ac
K40	→4)-β-D-Glc*p*A-(1→4)-α-D-Glc*p*NAc-(1→6)-α-D-Glc*p*NAc-(1→ 6 ↑ L-serine (amide)
K44	→4)-β-D-Glc*p*A-(1→3)-α-L-Rha*p*-(1→4)-α-D-Glc*p*NAc-(1→6)-β-D-Gal*p*NAc-(1→
K49	→4)-β-D-Glc*p*A-(1→6)-β-D-Gal*p*-(1→6)-β-D-Glc*p*-(1→3)-β-D-Glc*p*NAc-(1→ 6 ↑ L-threonine (75%), L-serine (25%) (amide)

[a] For a review of these and other structures, the reader is referred to Dutton and Parolis (1989).

Table 17.7. Structures of representative *E. coli* group II K-antigens.[a]

Serotype	Structure
K1	→8)-α-Neu*p*5Ac-(2→
K2a	O O ‖ ‖ [-O-P-O→4)-α-D-Gal*p*-(1→2)-Glycerol-(1→]$_{2n}$---[O-P-O→5)-α-D-Gal*f*-(1→2)-Glycerol-(1→]$_n$ | | OH OH
K4	→4)-β-D-Glc*p*A-(1→3)-β-D-Glc*p*NAc-(1→ 3 ↑ 1 β-D-Fru*f*
K5	→4)-β-D-Glc*p*A-(1→4)-α-D-Glc*p*NAc-(1→
K7	→3)-β-D-Man*p*NAcA-(1→4)-β-D-Glc*p*-(1→ 6 ↑ *O*Ac

K13	→3)-α-D-Rib*f*-(1→7)-β-KDO*p*-(2→ 4 ↑ *O*Ac
K18	O ‖ →2)-β-D-Rib*f*-(1→2)-D-Ribitol-(5-O-P-O- 3 | ↑ OH *O*Ac
K20	→3)-β-D-Rib*f*-(1→7)-β-KDO*p*-(2→ 5 ↑ *O*Ac
K23	→3)-β-D-Rib*f*-(1→7)-β-KDO*p*-(2→
K92	→8)-α-Neu*p*5Ac-(2→9)-α-Neu*p*5Ac-(2→

[a] For a review of these and other K-antigen structures the reader is referred to Dutton and Parolis (1989).

Table 17.8. Mode of surface association of *E. coli* cell surface polysaccharides.

Polysaccharide	Terminal residue
O-antigen	Lipid A-core
Low-molecular-weight ECA (ECA_{LPS})	Lipid A-core
High-molecular-weight ECA (ECA_{PG})	L-Glycerophosphate
Group II K-antigen	L-Glycerophosphate
Low-molecular-weight group I K-antigen (K_{LPS})	Lipid A-core
High-molecular-weight group I K-antigen	None?
Colanic acid	None?

retained at the cell surface by ionic interactions or if most are released to the surroundings.

Lipid A core acts as the anchor for the O antigenic surface polysaccharides of Gram-negative bacteria and, in *E. coli*, it also serves as an attachment point for several different polysaccharides. For example, a second form of ECA (ECA_{LPS}) is found linked to lipid A core. Unlike ECA_{PG}, ECA_{LPS} contains short polysaccharide chains and is found only in strains with R1, R4 and K-12 core chemotypes. ECA_{PG} can only be attached to lipid A core in strains deficient in O antigen, perhaps indicating competition of different polysaccharides for the same anchor (Kuhn *et al.*, 1988).

Lipid A core has also been implicated in the surface expression of *E. coli* group I K antigens. At least some of the K40 (group IB) polysaccharide is linked to lipid A (Jann *et al.*, 1992b) and short oligosaccharides of K30 (group IA) antigen are also linked in this fashion (Homonylo *et al.*, 1988; Whitfield *et al.*, 1989; MacLachlan *et al.*, 1993). To indicate the serological classification as a K antigen, rather than O antigen, and in keeping with ECA designations, we have termed this form of K antigen K_{LPS}. In strains lacking the authentic O antigen, the acidic K_{LPS} would be considered as an LPS molecule from a serological standpoint. Interestingly, there are a number of polysaccharide structures which are considered as group I K antigens when co-expressed with an O antigen but are O antigens when expressed alone. Examples include the IB K antigens K87 (=O32), K85 (=O141) and K9 (=O104) (Jann and Jann, 1990). The O and K antigens are therefore often operationally defined and there is clearly no chemical feature of a polysaccharide which could unequivocally place it as either a K or an O antigen.

Only a portion of the group I K antigen on the cell surface terminates in lipid A core (Jann *et al.*, 1992b). A survey of strains containing group I K antigens in this laboratory has indicated that, in general, group IB K_{LPS} contains longer polysaccharide chains. K_{LPS} in group IA strains is limited to one or two repeating units of K antigen and some serotypes produce no detectable K_{LPS}, despite the presence of a well-developed capsular structure (MacLachlan *et al.*, 1993). By constructing mutants in *E. coli* K30 with truncated lipid A cores, we have shown that high molecular weight group I K antigen is assembled on the cell surface by a pathway which is LPS independent (MacLachlan *et al.*, 1993). The loss of K_{LPS} resulting from the core defect has no effect on the ability of the cell to form a capsule structure which is indistinguishable from the wild type, when examined by electron microscopy. It is not clear whether an alternative anchor links the high-molecular-weight capsular group I K antigen to the cell surface. A phospholipid is an obvious possibility, and this would provide a common theme between ECA and K antigens. The situation in group I K antigens therefore resembles the so-called 'O-antigen capsule' first described in *E. coli* O111 (Goldman *et al.*, 1982, 1984). In some isolates, O111 polysaccharide is attached to lipid A core as a conventional O antigen but additional O111 polysaccharide is also exported in an LPS-free capsular form. This same phenomenon was confirmed by subsequent studies and extended to serotypes O55 and O127 (Peterson and McGroarty, 1985); this may be a frequent feature in *E. coli* strains.

Colanic acid is widely distributed in *E. coli* and bears structural resemblance to the group IA K antigens. We have found no evidence of an LPS-associated colanic acid fraction in *E. coli*. Unlike *E. coli* K antigens, the high-molecular-weight form of colanic acid shows only loose association with the cell surface. Thus, although colanic acid is sometimes called a capsular polysaccharide, it is more properly referred to as slime polysaccharide. There is no requirement for a terminal molecule involved in surface attachment of colanic acid.

Functions of *E. coli* Cell Surface Polysaccharides

The roles played by the LPS O antigen and the capsular K antigen polysaccharides in the pathogenesis of *E. coli* infections are now well documented. Interestingly, there are no reports of a role for ECA or colanic acid in virulence. Since *E. coli* has a dual lifestyle (inside and outside the host), it is conceivable that these polymers assume more importance when the bacterium is outside the host.

Resistance to serum killing

Complement-mediated serum killing is an important host defence mechanism. Depending on the nature of the cell surface, bacteria can activate complement by either the classical or the alternative pathway (Joiner, 1985; Frank *et al.*, 1987). Although the initial steps differ, the final product of both pathways is the membrane attack complex (MAC), an amphiphilic protein complex capable of inserting into the outer membrane of *E. coli* (Joiner *et al.*, 1985) and other Gram-negative bacteria, to cause bacterial lysis. While the classical pathway is initiated by the formation of an antigen–antibody complex, the alternative pathway is of primary importance during the preimmune phase of an infection when specific antibodies are absent. The alternative pathway is initiated by the non-specific binding of the serum protein C3b, to a target structure on the bacterial cell surface (Horstmann, 1992). Once bound, C3b may be activated by interacting with factor B to form the C3 convertase C3bBb; this initiates assembly of the MAC. Alternatively, bound C3b can be inactivated to iC3b by factor I, with factor H serving as a cofactor. Manipulation of these steps is crucial in the ability of a bacterium to withstand non-specific serum killing. As is true for many Gram-negative pathogens, O- and K-antigenic polysaccharides of *E. coli* play important roles in circumventing the bactericidal effects of the complement system (Taylor, 1983; Joiner, 1985; Frank *et al.*, 1987; Cross *et al.*, 1988; Cross, 1990). However, it should be emphasized that serum resistance is multifactorial.

Resistance to serum killing is an important virulence factor of *E. coli* isolated from septicaemia (McCabe *et al.*, 1978). Although the molecular aspects underlying this phenomenon have not been well characterized, some survival strategies have been elucidated which are common to *E. coli* and other Gram-negative bacteria (Joiner *et al.*, 1983; Frank *et al.*, 1987; Taylor and Robinson, 1980).

The chemical structure, length and distribution of the O-polysaccharide are important determinants of serum resistance, particularly in unencapsulated bacteria. In general, C3b and C5b-9 are preferentially bound by long *E. coli* O-polysaccharide chains at a distance from the membrane target for the MAC (Joiner *et al.*, 1984; Porat *et al.*, 1987; Tomás *et al.*, 1988; Porat *et al.*, 1992). Consequently, the O antigen is believed to prevent the MAC from inserting into the cell membrane, possibly through steric hindrance, or by affecting the configuration of the MAC formation. However, Stawski *et al.* (1990) investigated 194 *E. coli* reference strains for serum sensitivity and showed that possession of S-LPS was not sufficient for serum resistance in all O serotypes.

E. coli O111 is a well studied EPEC serogroup which is not associated with a K antigen, but produces an O-antigen capsule (see above). These strains normally require the presence of specific antibody for effective serum killing (Joiner *et al.*, 1983). By serial passage in serum, Goldman *et al.* (1984) isolated *E. coli* O111 variants which still bound antibody and activated complement, but were either partially or completely serum resistant. Completely resistant strains lost the O-antigen capsule, contained 50% more LPS than the parent, and covered approximately 30% more lipid A core with O antigen. In contrast, the partially resistant strains retained the O-antigen capsule, exhibited the same degree of coverage of lipid A core, but contained 40% more LPS than the parent. Previous studies by these workers suggested that O111-specific antibody promoted serum-killing by binding C3b, and focusing MAC formation at critical membrane sites. It was therefore suggested that increasing the amount and coverage of lipid A core prevented access of the MAC to these sites and induced deposition of complement at sites which are at a distance from the target site. *E. coli* O6, O18ac (Porat *et al.*, 1987) and O83 (Stawski *et al.*, 1990) strains also acquire a serum-resistant phenotype by altering the length and coverage of lipid A core. This may therefore represent a common strategy. There are several examples where the same O antigen gives serum resistance in one strain and not in another. This has been well documented for *E. coli* O6 (Cross *et al.*, 1986; Stawski *et al.*, 1990), O8 (Taylor and Robinson, 1980; Stawski *et al.*, 1990) and O9 (McCallum *et al.*, 1989; Stawski *et al.*, 1990). These results may also relate to variation in the coverage of lipid A core.

As is generally the case with invasive *E. coli*, most K1 isolates are associated with a limited number of O antigens (Ørskov and Ørskov, 1992). The prevalence of certain O and K serotypes in invasive *E. coli* infections is thought to reflect the selection of bacterial clones which exhibit a functional relationship between the O and K antigens (Achtman and Pluschke, 1986; Cross, 1990). Pluschke and co-workers studied the serum resistance of different O1:K1, O7:K1 and O18:K1 *E. coli* isolates from neonatal meningitis, septicaemia and urinary tract infections and showed that the O7 and O18 O polysaccharides, but not the O1 polysaccharide, contribute to the serum resistance of *E. coli* K1 (Pluschke *et al.*, 1983; Pluschke and Achtman, 1984). The purified O7 and O18 LPS had a reduced ability to bind C3b compared to the O1 LPS. These properties were correlated with chemical differences between the O1, O7 and O18 polysaccharides, rather than differences in length or distribution.

The expression of some K antigens is also correlated with serum resistance and, in many instances, the capsular layer acts in concert with the O polysaccharide in conferring protection. The K1, K92 (Table 17.6) and K9 (Table 17.7) polysaccharides of *E. coli* all contain sialic acid and all contribute to serum resistance (Stevens *et al.*, 1978, 1983; Van Dijk *et al.*, 1979; Stawski *et al.*, 1990). K1 strains account for approximately 80% of *E. coli* isolates from neonatal meningitis (Robbins *et al.*, 1974) and bacteraemia (Cross *et al.*, 1984) in humans. While the importance of the

E. coli K1 antigen as a virulence determinant has been recognized for some time, its role in conferring serum resistance has been controversial. One explanation for the apparently contradictory data has come from studies involving quantitation of K1 CPS (Vermeulen *et al.*, 1988; Leying *et al.*, 1990). These studies revealed that, depending on the strain, a threshold level of K1 polysaccharide may be required to confer serum resistance. Furthermore, in *E. coli* O18:K1 Bort, the O18 LPS phenotype appeared to play a role in conferring protection below the critical K1 level (Vermeulen *et al.*, 1988). Interestingly, some K1 strains produce R-LPS or SR-LPS (Cross *et al.*, 1984; Kusecek *et al.*, 1984). The inhibitory effect of sialic acid polymers on the activation of the alternative pathway has been well documented (Michalek *et al.*, 1988) and the process in *E. coli* K1 is best characterized (Silver and Vimr, 1990). The inhibitory effect of sialic acid-containing polymers is generally believed to result from their ability to preferentially bind factor H, rather than factor B (Michalek *et al.*, 1988). In addition, it appears that the K1 CPS binds C3b poorly (Van Dijk *et al.*, 1979), suggesting more than one mechanism for inhibiting the alternative pathway.

A small number of *E. coli* group II K antigens lack sialic acid but still confer some protection against serum killing. However in most cases, full protection requires the co-expression of selected O antigens. Although relatively few quantitative studies have been reported, it is reasonable to assume that, as with the K1 antigen, the degree of protection afforded by a particular capsule type may also be a function of the size and distribution of the capsular layer. Glynn and Howard (1970) studied four O6:K13 strains and reported a quantitative relationship between serum resistance and the amount of K13 CPS (a group II K antigen). In contrast, Stawski *et al.* (1990) failed to demonstrate such a relationship in a quantitative analysis of six O6:K13 strains and not all O^+:K13 serotypes examined were found to be serum resistant. These results further illustrate the variation within a single K serotype of *E. coli*.

In general, the group I K antigens of *E. coli* appear to function primarily in conferring resistance to phagocytosis (see below). This certainly appears to be the case for several group IA K antigens (e.g. K27, K30), which play no measurable role in resistance to complement-mediated serum killing (Taylor and Robinson, 1980; Opal *et al.*, 1982; McCallum *et al.*, 1989). In contrast, Stawski *et al.* (1990) observed that loss of K87 expression in a spontaneously occurring capsule-deficient mutant of *E. coli* O8:K87 resulted in a serum-sensitive phenotype, while loss of K9 expression in an O9:K9 strain led to a partial reduction in the level of resistance. These results suggest that, at least in these two serotypes, the K9 and K87 capsules may play a minor role in conferring serum resistance. In K9 this effect may be due to the sialic acid in its chemical structure. Interestingly, the K9 and K87 polysaccharides are both group IB K antigens (Jayaratne *et al.*, 1993). In view of the evidence for linkage to lipid A core in the group IB K antigens (Jann *et al.*, 1992b; MacLachlan *et al.*, 1993), it would be interesting to determine if the loss of K9 and K87 expression in these mutants resulted in altered O-antigen expression or coverage, by altering availability of lipid A core.

Recent studies with *E. coli* O115:K"V165":F165, suggest that this strain produces a capsule which does not resemble a typical *E. coli* K antigen, but behaves more like an O-antigen capsule. However, there is no structural similarity between this capsule and the O115 polysaccharide (Ngeleka *et al.*, 1992). Analysis of 'acapsular' variants indicates that this polysaccharide layer confers serum resistance. There may therefore be further mechanisms for serum resistance in *E. coli*.

Protection against phagocytosis

Ingestion by a phagocytic cell generally requires opsonization. This process involves binding of complement and/or antibody to the bacterial surface; the bound components can then interact with specific receptors on phagocytic cells (Horwitz and Silverstein, 1980). The majority of invasive *E. coli* isolates are encapsulated and most of these strains are poorly phagocytized (Van Dijk *et al.*, 1979). The capsule is the most important antiphagocytic factor produced by *E. coli*, although the basis for this property is not well characterized. Encapsulated *E. coli* K29 (group IA) are not ingested even if attached to the surface of phagocytic cells by lectins; unencapsulated derivatives are efficiently ingested under these conditions (Horwitz and Silverstein, 1980). Negative charge and hydrophilicity are physical properties of K antigens which are believed to play a role in the inhibition of contact with the negatively charged phagocytic cells. Those capsules which are more highly charged, or are more hydrophilic, are generally more resistant (Horwitz, 1982; Moxon and Kroll, 1990).

In addition to their physicochemical properties, certain structural features of K antigens contribute to the antiphagocytic phenotype. Phagocytic cells possess receptors for C3b- as well as the C3b-degradation products iC3b, and C3d,g; B lymphocytes possess receptors for the C3d degradation product of C3b (Hostetter, 1986). Consequently, capsules which fail to activate complement confer resistance to both opsonophagocytosis and serum killing (see above). Studies with *Streptococcus pneumoniae* have demonstrated that structural differences among capsular serotypes correlate with differences in binding and degradative processing of C3b (Hostetter, 1986). Based on these observations, one can speculate that differences in C3b processing, combined with different binding affinities for the bound C3b ligands, may affect interactions with phagocytes and lymphocytes. The degree of protection conferred by the capsular layer varies depending upon the serotype. The group II K1 capsule is the most potent inhibitor of phagocytosis among *E. coli* capsules (Bortolussi *et al.*, 1979, 1983; Cross *et al.*, 1984). This can be directly attributed to the failure of K1 capsule to activate complement and to bind C3b efficiently (see above). Surpisingly, the K5 capsule of *E. coli* does not appear to confer protection against phagocytosis (Cross *et al.*, 1986), despite the fact that *E. coli* K5 strains are highly pathogenic, and are frequently isolated from cases of neonatal meningitis, bacteraemia and urinary tract infections. The K5 serotypes associated with these infections are limited however (O75:K5:H5, O6:K5:H1, O18ac:K5:H$^-$), and the invasive nature of these strains may be a function of other surface properties, including the O antigen.

One would expect that in some situations, LPSs which do not activate complement might also confer some protection against phagocytosis. This has been demonstrated for some unencapsulated mutants of *S. enterica* serovar Typhimurium (Stendahl and Edebo, 1972). In studies with different *E. coli* K1 isolates (Cross *et al.*, 1984), smooth strains were found to be more resistant to opsonophagocytosis than rough K1 strains. In general however, *E. coli* O antigens do not appear to play a significant role in protection against phagocytosis.

The group IA *E. coli* K29 capsule (Table 17.6) does not activate complement and inhibits or masks the interaction of phagocytic cells with underlying structures which do fix complement (Horwitz and Silverstein, 1980). This steric effect of *E. coli* capsules is not well understood. In some cases, the capsule may prevent the interaction of phagocytes with antibody bound to the underlying O antigen. This is not always the case; antibodies to the O18 antigen opsonized encapsulated *E. coli* O18:K1 and were protective against challenge in an animal model (Pluschke and Achtman, 1985; Kaufman *et al.*, 1986; Kim *et al.*, 1986; Cryz *et al.*, 1990, 1991). Similarly, monoclonal anti-O4 antibodies effectively opsonized *E. coli* O4:K12:H$^-$ *in vitro* (Abe *et al.*, 1988). Curiously, an antibody shown to be protective against *E. coli* O18:K1 (Kaufman *et al.*, 1986) did not protect against lethal challenge with *E. coli* O18:K5 (Cross *et al.*, 1988). These contradictory results may reflect the importance of capsule coverage or the length of the O antigen relative to capsule and the ability of O antigen to extend beyond the capsule periphery.

The protective effect of the capsular layer is generally lost with the development of an immune response. However, the structures of K1 and K5 polysaccharides prevent an effective immune response from being raised in neonates and young children. This is due to a phenomenon which has been termed bacterial camouflage (Jann and Jann, 1985) or mimicry (Horwitz and Silverstein, 1980). These structures are not recognized as foreign antigens, due to their similarity to host structures. The K1 antigen is subject to form variation in which the polymer is *O*-acetylated. The non-acetylated K1 polymer is non-immunogenic but addition of *O*-acetyl groups renders it weakly immunogenic (Ørskov *et al.*, 1979). However, the (non-acetylated) polysialic-acid-containing K92 polymer (Table 17.7) is immunogenic (Egan *et al.*, 1982). Non-immunogenicity is therefore confined to the non-acetylated α-2,8-linked polysialic acid. This is thought to be due to structural identity between the K1 repeating unit structure and carbohydrates found on the embryonic neural adhesion molecule N-CAM (Jann and Jann, 1992). Passive immunization with monoclonal antibodies which react with K1 polysaccharide does provide protection against challenge with *E. coli* O18ac:K1 in an animal model (Kim *et al.*, 1985). The K4 and K5 capsules may also mimic host components (Jann and Jann, 1990, 1992) (Table 17.6). The K5 polysaccharide resembles the first polymeric intermediate in heparin synthesis. Removal of the fructosyl side-group from the K4 polysaccharide, which can occur under physiological conditions, eliminates the immunodominant K4 epitope and results in formation of a polymer similar to chondroitin. Such structural mimicry may not be confined to K antigens. For example, the *E. coli* O2 O polysaccharide is serologically cross-reactive with kidney tissue (Holmgren *et al.*, 1971) and other uncharacterized cross-reactions have been reported between *E. coli* and blood group antigens (Drach *et al.*, 1971).

Once ingested by a phagocytic cell, the bacterium is subjected to the action of antimicrobial molecules. The bactericidal permeability-increasing protein (BPI) is a cationic protein which interacts with regions of lipid A core and mediates intragranulocyte killing of Gram-negative bacteria. The O-polysaccharide offers some protection against BPI in *E. coli* and *S. enterica* serovar typhimurium (Weiss *et al.*, 1980). Protection is dependent on O-antigen chain length in a fashion similar to resistance to complement-mediated serum killing. Environmentally induced increases in O-chain length in *E. coli* O9 and O111 result in increased resistance to BPI *in vitro* (Weiss *et al.*, 1986).

Sepsis and the biological effects of LPS

Septic shock resulting from bacteraemia is a leading cause of morbidity and mortality among hospitalized individuals. Most of the symptoms observed during Gram-negative sepsis are attributed to LPS (endotoxin). Furthermore, many of the effects characteristic of septic shock, such as hypotension, fever, metabolic acidosis and disseminated intravascular coagulation, can be induced by introducing LPS into experimental animals (Gilbert, 1960; Crutchley *et al.*, 1967; Morrison and Ulevitch, 1978). The lipid A portion of LPS is primarily responsible for these biological responses and it is clear that the precise chemistry of lipid A from a given bacterium is important in the generation of these effects (Qureshi and Takayama, 1990; Raetz, 1990).

The cascade of events leading to septic shock is complex. LPS stimulates expression of numerous cellular mediators that either directly or indirectly cause the symptoms of sepsis. Tumour necrosis factor-α (TNFα), interleukin 1 (IL-1), IL-6, IL-8 and platelet activating factor (PAF) are produced by cells such as macrophages and endothelial cells. Some of these mediators may stimulate their own expression to amplify the inflammatory response. In response to TNFα, IL-1 and PAF, arachidonic acid metabolism results in synthesis of leucotrienes, thromboxane A2 and prostaglandins. In addition, T cells are stimulated to secrete interferon-γ, IL-2, IL-4 and granulocyte-monocyte colony-stimulating factor (Bone, 1993). All of these mediators may promote septic shock by affecting the vascular endothelium leading to increased vascular permeability. Furthermore, modulation of the coagulation pathway may lead to fibrin deposition and clot formation (Nawroth and Stern, 1986). Neutrophil activation and adherence to the endothelium is promoted by many of the mediators described above and by complement components C3a and C5a (Sherry and Cerami, 1988; Bone, 1991, 1993). Aggregation of these neutrophils and their subsequent degranulation may cause damage to the vascular endothelium. The initial effects caused by mediator release may aid in defence against invading pathogens and in repair of tissues. Down-modulation of the sepsis cascade can occur (Bone, 1991, 1993) and LPS can be processed by hepatic Kupffer cells to a less toxic molecule which may be cleared through hepatocyte uptake (Treon *et al.*, 1993). However, if the affecting stimuli persist causing continuous localized inflammation, overstimulation may occur or down-regulation may be compromised and septic shock may ensue.

The primary event initiating the sepsis cascade may be interaction of LPS with host macrophages (Glode *et al.*, 1976; Mathison and Ulevitch, 1979). Once stimulated by LPS, macrophages secrete TNFα (cachectin) (Beutler *et al.*, 1985a; Mahoney *et al.*, 1985). A role for TNFα as the central mediator of septic shock is supported by studies in which anti-TNFα antibodies were shown to protect mice and rabbits from the lethal effects of LPS (Beutler *et al.*, 1985b; Tracey *et al.*, 1987a; Mathison *et al.*, 1988). In addition, exposure of mice, rats, guinea-pigs, and dogs to recombinant TNFα mimics many of the effects of LPS exposure (Tracey *et al.*, 1986, 1987b; Remick *et al.*, 1987; Stephens *et al.*, 1988). However, mediators such as IL-1 and PAF may also produce symptoms similar to those observed during sepsis (Bessin *et al.*, 1983; Lefer *et al.*, 1984; Oppenheimer *et al.*, 1986). Therefore, other mediators may act in combination with TNFα early in sepsis.

One important aspect of LPS-induced shock is the physical interaction of LPS with immune cells. An LPS binding protein (LBP) has been identified in the plasma of humans and rabbits (Tobias *et al.*, 1985, 1986). This protein is synthesized in hepatocytes (Ramadori *et al.*, 1990) and is present in normal serum at a concentration of $<0.5\ \mu g\ ml^{-1}$ (Schumann *et al.*, 1990). However, in response to LPS exposure, serum levels of LBP may reach 50 μg ml^{-1} (Schumann *et al.*, 1990). LBP acts as a carrier protein, binding specifically to the lipid A region of LPS (Tobias *et al.*, 1989). This binding enhances interaction of LPS and whole bacterial cells (through opsonization) to macrophages (Wright *et al.*, 1989; Martin *et al.*, 1992). Immunodepletion of LBP from rabbit blood decreased the response of blood cells to LPS *ex vivo* (Schumann *et al.*, 1990). However, this response was not completely inactivated, suggesting the existence of a low sensitivity LBP-independent response to LPS.

The LPS/LBP complex binds to macrophages via the surface glycoprotein CD14 (Wright *et al.*, 1990). Blocking CD14 with CD14-specific monoclonal antibodies prevents secretion of TNFα from the macrophages (Wright *et al.*, 1990). Soluble CD14 can neutralize monocyte activation by LPS (Schutt *et al.*, 1992) and shedding of CD14 by human monocytes has been suggested as a mechanism of modulating CD14-dependent activation (Bazil and Strominger, 1991). In addition, murine monocytes that have been transfected with the genes for human and rabbit CD14 are hypersensitive to LPS/LBP (Lee *et al.*, 1992) and transgenic mice overexpressing human CD14 are hypersensitive to LPS-induced shock (Ferrero *et al.*, 1993). However, LPS-dependent monocyte activation is not completely dependent on CD14 (Wright *et al.*, 1990; Lee *et al.*, 1992) and other LPS receptors have been suggested (Lei and Morrison, 1988a, b; Hampton *et al.*, 1988; Chen *et al.*, 1990; Golenbock *et al.*, 1990; Kirkland *et al.*, 1990). Coupling of LPS/LBP interaction with CD14 to mediator expression may require a signalling mechanism involving protein kinases (Lauener *et al.*, 1990). However, the precise mechanism(s) involved in LPS-induced immune cell activation is not understood.

Preadministration of sublethal amounts of LPS can result in endotoxin tolerance in mice (Freudenberg and Galanos, 1988). LPS from *Rhodobacter sphaeroides* is non-toxic and does not stimulate TNFα production in cell lines or in mice (Takayama *et al.*, 1989; Qureshi *et al.*, 1991b). Also, this non-toxic LPS is antagonistic against the activity of toxic LPS from *E. coli* (Qureshi *et al.*, 1991a). Similarly, synthetic LPS derivatives such as lipid X and lipid IV_A (see below) also protect against endotoxaemia (Proctor *et al.*, 1986; Tobias *et al.*, 1989; Qureshi and Takayama, 1990; Raetz, 1990; Lam *et al.*, 1991). These results may reflect competition for available LPS receptors, although other factors such as corticosteroid induction are also involved (Zuckerman and Qureshi, 1992).

LPS molecules from diverse Gram-negative bacteria contain cross-reactive epitopes, due to conserved structures in the lipid A and inner core region. This led to the use of LPS from rough mutants of *S. enterica* serovar Minnesota (strain R595) and *E. coli* O111:B4 (strain J5) as immunogens for production of broadly cross-reactive monoclonal antibodies (Mutharia *et al.*, 1984; Bogard *et al.*, 1987). It has been proposed that similar human monoclonal antibodies could be used for passive protection, and combined with antibiotic therapy, this would afford an effective treatment for sepsis in a broad range of nosocomial infections (Ziegler *et al.*, 1982). Several reports have supported the efficacy of passive protection against bacterial cells and LPS, although the precise mechanism underlying the protection is not clear (Teng *et al.*, 1985; Ziegler *et al.*, 1991). However, other researchers have reported conflicting results in a mouse lethal challenge model, using both polyclonal and monoclonal antibodies against *E. coli* J5 LPS (Greisman and Johnston, 1987; Baumgartner *et al.*, 1990). Although promising, the long-term success of this therapeutic approach has yet to be established (Bone, 1993).

Synthesis and Genetics of Cell Surface Polysaccharides

A large number of genes is devoted to the assembly and regulation of cell surface polysaccharides in *E. coli*. These are distributed among several chromosomal loci (Fig. 17.5). Biochemical and molecular genetic

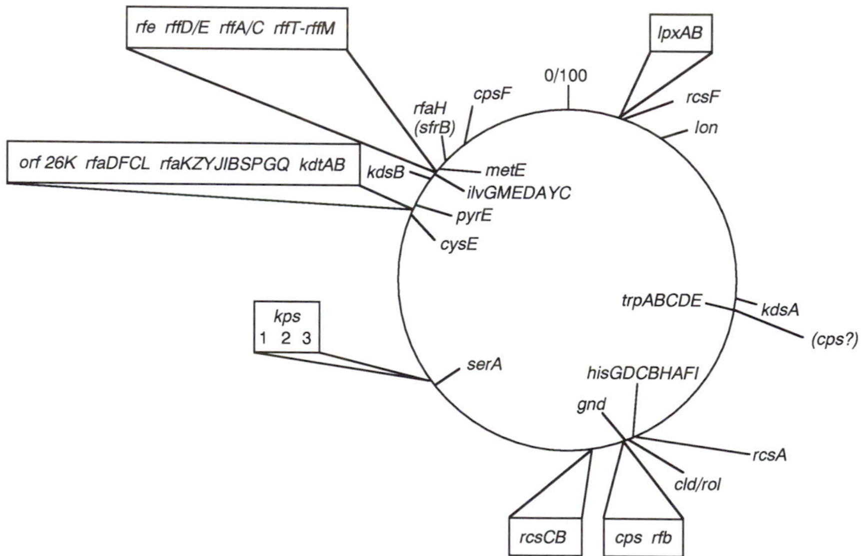

Fig. 17.5. Location of genes necessary for the synthesis and expression of cell surface polysaccharides in *E. coli*. The 100-minute chromosomal map is shown. Genes which are involved only in polysaccharide synthesis are identified on the outside of the circular map; relevant adjacent markers are indicated inside the circle. Note that individual strains of *E. coli* do not necessarily contain all of the genes shown.

approaches have resulted in significant progress in our understanding of the biogenesis of cell surface components and the functions of many of the gene products involved are now known. The biosynthesis of cell surface polysaccharides can also involve products of genes which are not confined to a role in polysaccharide assembly. For example, the galactosyl precursor (UDP-Gal) required for synthesis of LPS core and many polysaccharides is produced by GalE, an enzyme required for metabolism of galactose via the Leloir pathway (Mäkelä and Stocker, 1984; Whitfield and Valvano, 1993). As might be expected, given the similarities in polysaccharide structure, there are common themes in the biosynthesis of cell surface polysaccharides (Whitfield and Valvano, 1993). All are synthesized using precursors available in the cytoplasm and the initial steps are either cytoplasmic or occur at the cytoplasmic face of the cell membrane. Polysaccharides are exported (translocated) to the cell surface at a limited number of sites; these sites are often located above membrane adhesions (Bayer Junctions), at which the cytoplasmic and outer membranes come into contact. The arguments for (and against) a role for membrane adhesions in cell surface assembly have been reviewed in detail elsewhere (Whitfield and Valvano, 1993). An overview of our current knowledge of *E. coli* systems follows.

Lipopolysaccharide biosynthesis

The three parts of the LPS molecule have distinct structures and properties and this is reflected in the biosynthetic pathway. The hydrophilic O polysaccharide is synthesized separately from lipid A core and the two parts are joined at a later stage. Many of the events leading to formation of the LPS molecule have been described but the terminal steps involving translocation of the completed molecule across the periplasm and outer membrane, and proper insertion on the cell surface, have not been resolved. Aspects of these processes have been reviewed in more detail elsewhere (Jann and Jann, 1984; Mäkelä and Stocker, 1984; Schnaitman and Klena, 1993; Whitfield and Valvano, 1993). The genes for the enzymes involved in LPS synthesis are found at several chromosomal loci (Fig. 17.5).

Lipid A synthesis

The pathway for lipid A synthesis was resolved following the identification of monosaccharide precursors which accumulate in some phosphatidylglycerol-deficient mutants of *E. coli* (reviewed by Raetz, 1990). The initial precursor is the activated sugar UDP-GlcNAc (uridine diphospho-*N*-acetyl glucosamine). The pathway begins with fatty acid acylation of UDP-GlcNAc at positions 2 and 3 to produce UDP-2,3-diacylglucosamine. The UMP (uridine monophosphate) residue is then removed to form the precursor, lipid X. These reactions are catalysed by a series of cytoplasmic enzymes, including the products of *lpx*A (UDP-GlcNAc acyltransferase) and *lpx*B (lipid A disaccharide synthase) (Raetz, 1990). The diglucosamine backbone of lipid A is assembled by joining a lipid X molecule to a second molecule of UDP-2,3-diacylglucosamine. The UDP residue is then removed resulting in lipid IV_A (tetraacyl diglucosamine-1-phosphate). The addition of KDO residues to lipid IVA precedes the final acylation reactions.

Synthesis of the core oligosaccharide

CMP-KDO (cytidine monophospho-KDO) provides the precursor for the KDO residues in the inner core. Two cytoplasmic enzymes, KdsA and KdsB, catalyse the conversion of arabinose-5-phosphate via KDO-8-phosphate to CMP-KDO (Raetz, 1990). Addition of KDO residues to lipid IV_A is mediated by a cytoplasmic enzyme KdtA (Clementz, 1992). Interestingly, KdtA is a bifunctional transferase and adds two KDO residues. The resulting KDO_2-lipid IV_A is then fully acylated and a final KDO residue, phosphoryl residues and heptose moieties are subsequently added (Raetz, 1990). The inner KDO region of LPS core is essential for survival so mutants lacking the KDO residues are not viable (Raetz, 1990). Attempts have been made to exploit the conserved and essential KDO residues as novel targets for antibacterial agents. Inhibitory KDO analogues have been designed which block LPS synthesis (Goldman *et al.*, 1987; Hammond *et al.*, 1987), resulting in accumulation of lipid IV_A and other metabolites (Goldman *et al.*, 1988) and impaired virulence of *E. coli* (Hammond, 1992).

The *rfa* gene cluster contains structural genes for synthesis of the remainder of the LPS core. The *rfa* locus contains as many as 17 open reading frames and the genes are arranged in three different transcriptional units (Roncero and Casadaban, 1992; Schnaitman and Klena, 1993). *rfa* gene products include sugar transferase enzymes and enzymes required for the formation of LPS core-specific precursors, such as ADP-heptose. The activities of some of the enzymes have been resolved directly, some have activities inferred from better characterized counterparts in *S. enterica* serovar Typhimurium, while the functions of others are still unknown (Table 17.9). The lipid A-KDO_2 acts as an acceptor for sequential transfer of the remaining core sugars, and the order of transfer is predicted by the structure of the core oligosaccharide (Tables 17.2 and 17.3). Although mutants which lack LPS regions distal to the heptosyl residues are viable in the laboratory, these bacteria have altered expression of outer membrane proteins, flagella and pili, and are classically sensitive to hydrophobic compounds (Parker *et al.*, 1992). Any *rfa* mutation results in a defective core oligosaccharide and prevents the addition of O polysaccharide, giving R-LPS as the completed product.

Table 17.9. Genes required for the biosynthesis of the core oligosaccharide of *E. coli* K-12 LPS.

Gene	Enzymatic activity of gene product	Reference
kds A	3-deoxy-D-*manno*-octulosonic acid-8-phosphate synthetase	Woisetchläger and Högenauer, 1987
kds B	CTP:CMP-KDO cytidyltransferase (CMP-KDO synthetase)	Goldman and Kohlbrenner, 1985
kdt A	KDO transferase	Clementz and Raetz, 1991
rfa B	UDP-galactose:(glucosyl) LPS α1,6-galactosyltransferase	Pradel *et al.*, 1992
rfa C	ADP-heptose:(3-deoxy-D-*manno*-octulosonyl) LPS α1,5-heptosyltransferase	Chen and Coleman, 1993
rfa D	ADP-L-glycero-D-*manno*-heptose-6-epimerase	Pegues *et al.*, 1990
rfa E	unknown	
rfa F	ADP-heptose:(heptosyl) LPS α1,3-heptosyltransferase	Raetz, 1990
rfa G	UDP-glucose:(heptosyl) LPS α1,3-glucosyltransferase	Creeger and Rothfield, 1979 Parker *et al.*, 1992
rfa I	UDP-glucose:(glucosyl) LPS α1,3-glucosyltransferase	Pradel *et al.*, 1992
rfa J	UDP-glucose:(glucosyl) LPS α1,2-glucosyltransferase	Pradel *et al.*, 1992
rfa K	UDP-*N*-acetylglucosamine:(glucosyl) LPS β1,6-*N*-acetylglucosaminyl transferase	Klena *et al.*, 1992b
rfa L	O-antigen ligase	Klena *et al.*, 1992b
rfa Q	unknown	Pradel *et al.*, 1992
rfa S	unknown	Pradel *et al.*, 1992
rfa Y	unknown	Klena *et al.*, 1992b
rfa Z	unknown	Klena et al., 1992b

O-polysaccharide synthesis

The O polysaccharide is synthesized separately using membrane-bound enzymes and a lipid carrier termed undecaprenol phosphate. Most of the bacterial glycosyl transferase enzymes which participate in the polymerization process are peripheral membrane proteins, presumably located at the cytoplasmic face of the cell membrane, since the precursors are available within the cytoplasm (Whitfield and Valvano, 1993). Assembly of O polysaccharides is therefore a transmembrane pathway with the final polymerized molecule being attached to completed lipid A core at the periplasmic face of the cytoplasmic membrane (McGrath and Osborn, 1991). The *rfa*L gene product is involved in the ligation of O antigen to lipid A core. Although ligase activity has not been directly demonstrated, *rfa*L-defective strains are unable to transfer polymerized undecaprenol-linked O polysaccharide to lipid A core; such strains have R-LPS (Mäkelä and Stocker, 1984; Klena *et al.*, 1992a; Schnaitman and Klena, 1993).

Two polymerization pathways have been established for O polysaccharides. The best characterized pathway is in *S. enterica* serovar Typhimurium, where growth of the O-polysaccharide chain occurs at the reducing terminus. In this pathway, repeating units of O polysaccharide are synthesized first as undecaprenyl pyrophosphate-linked intermediates. During chain elongation, the polysaccharide grows by increments of one repeating unit. Partially polymerized polymers are transferred as a block from one lipid carrier to a single repeating unit attached to a second carrier. The nascent chains therefore remain attached to undecaprenyl-pyrophosphate until fully polymerized (reviewed in Jann and Jann, 1984; Schnaitman and Klena, 1993; Whitfield and Valvano, 1993). Mutations in the *rfc* gene result in an SR-LPS which comprises a single repeating unit of O antigen attached to lipid A core (Naide *et al.*, 1965), indicating that the Rfc protein is required for the polymerization process. To date, no examples of this type of mechanism have been directly described in *E. coli*. However, there are several heteropolysaccharide O antigens in *E. coli* (e.g. O111) which contain structures similar to the O antigens of *S. enterica* serovar Typhimurium and these represent candidates for this type of assembly mechanism. More importantly, functional homologues of Rfc have recently been identified in both *E. coli* O7 and K-12 (M.A. Valvano, University of Western Ontario, London, Ontario, December 1993, personal communication).

The second polymerization method involves growth of the polysaccharide at the non-reducing terminus and occurs by a fundamentally different process. This mechanism is best known in the *E. coli* O8 and O9 polysaccharides. These are homopolymers of mannose (Table 17.4) and the mannose-containing repeating units are thought to be assembled and polymerized by a sequential series of sugar transfers using mannosyl transferase enzymes. There is no requirement for a polymerase enzyme in this scheme (Jann and Jann, 1984). During elongation, α-glucosyl-pyrophosphoryl-undecaprenol appears to serve as an acceptor for mannosyl residues (Jann *et al.*, 1982; Weisgerber and Jann, 1982). Following polymerization, the α-glucosyl residue is transferred with the O antigen and ligated to a lipid A-precore acceptor; the precore lacks its terminal glucosyl residue and is therefore completed by this reaction (Weisgerber *et al.*, 1984). Expression of the O8 and O9 O polysaccharides is dependent on a function provided by the *rfe* gene (Schmidt *et al.*, 1976; Jann *et al.*, 1979; Meier-Dieter *et al.*, 1990); *rfe* mutants are unable to form α-glucosyl-pyrophosphorylundecaprenol (Jann *et al.*, 1982). As will be described below, Rfe appears to be a GlcNAc transferase which is involved in the biosynthesis of ECA, although this is difficult to reconcile with its role in O-polysaccharide assembly.

The *rfb* gene cluster of *E. coli* contains genes for the biosynthesis of O polysaccharide. These include structural genes for enzymes involved in the synthesis of O-specific sugar precursors, repeating unit assembly and polymerization. To date, the *rfb* genes of *E. coli* serotypes O1 (Ding *et al.*, 1991), O2 (Neal *et al.*, 1991), O4 (Haraguchi *et al.*, 1991), O7 (reviewed in Valvano, 1992), O9 (Kido *et al.*, 1989), O75 (Batchelor *et al.*, 1991), O101 (Heuzenroeder *et al.*, 1989) and O111 (Bastin *et al.*, 1991) have been cloned and the O polysaccharides expressed in *E. coli* K-12 recipients (reviewed in Valvano, 1992; Whitfield and Valvano, 1993). Some of the biosynthetic functions are suggested by the phenotypes of mutations in the cloned *rfb* gene clusters and detailed analysis of the genes and their products is now possible. Although *E. coli* K-12 strains have R-LPS, a functional *rfb* gene cluster was recently assembled from two different lines of K-12 strains. Serological analysis indicates that *E. coli* K-12 is a descendant of a strain which types as O16, with cross-reaction with O17 (Liu and Reeves, 1994).

ECA Synthesis

The biosynthesis of the repeating unit of ECA has been examined in detail and the process resembles that of O polysaccharides. The genetic determinants for ECA are located at the *rfe* and *rff* loci (Meier and Mayer, 1985) (Fig. 17.5). The ECA gene cluster contains the structural genes for three glycosyl transferases and for enzymes involved in synthesis of ECA-specific precursors; at least seven genes are involved, based on complementation analyses (Meier-Dieter *et al.*, 1992). Mutations in many of the genes have been identified and the function of the gene products characterized (Barr and Rick, 1987; Meier-Dieter *et al.*, 1992) (Table 17.10). The trisaccharide repeating unit of ECA (Table 17.1) is assembled on undecaprenol monophosphate by sequential addition of glycosyl residues. Each of the

Table 17.10. Enzymes involved in ECA biosynthesis in *E. coli*. The data is taken from Meier-Dieter *et al.* (1990, 1992) and references therein.

Gene	Enzyme	Function
rff E	UDP-GlcNAc-2-epimerase	UDP-ManNAcA precursor synthesis
rff D	UDP-ManNAc dehydrogenase	UDP-ManNAcA precursor synthesis
rff A	TDP-4-keto-6-deoxy-D-Glc transaminase	TDP-D-Fuc4NAc precursor synthesis
rfe	GlcNAc transferase	Undecaprenol-pyrophosphoryl-GlcNAc (Lipid I) formation
rff M	ManNAcA transferase	Undecaprenol-pyrophosphoryl-GlcNAc-ManNAcA (Lipid II) formation
rff T	Fuc4NAc transferase	Undecaprenol-pyrophosphoryl-GlcNAc-ManNAcA-Fuc4NAc (Lipid III) formation
rff C	Unknown	ECA elongation?

specific transferases has been identified and the undecaprenol-linked intermediates, lipids I–III, have been characterized (Barr and Rick, 1987; Barr *et al.*, 1989; Meier-Dieter *et al.*, 1990, 1992) (Table 17.10). The nucleotide sequence of the *rfe* gene has been determined (Ohta *et al.*, 1991; Meier-Dieter *et al.*, 1992) and biochemical data suggest that Rfe is most likely a UDP-GlcNAc : undecaprenyl-phosphate GlcNAc-1-phosphate transferase which forms the first undecaprenol-linked intermediate, lipid I (Meier-Dieter *et al.*, 1992). The precise mechanism involved in ECA polymerization has not been determined and the stage at which ECA_{PG} and ECA_{LPS} are added to their respective lipid termini is unknown. However, it has been shown that *rfaL* is required for formation of ECA_{LPS} (Kuhn *et al.*, 1988), indicating that O antigen and ECA_{LPS} share pathways for attachment to lipid A core and, presumably, for subsequent translocation and surface expression.

K-antigen Synthesis

Several criteria which are used to subdivide the K antigens of *E. coli* are based on genetics and are reflected in the biosynthesis pathways. Serologically distinct group II K antigens are synthesized by enzymes encoded by allelic gene clusters at the *kps* locus. *kps* was formerly termed *kps*A (Ørskov and Nyman, 1974), and maps near *ser*A (Vimr, 1991) (Fig. 17.5). The 17 kbp *kps* gene cluster from serotype K1 represents the first capsule genes to be cloned and expressed in *E. coli* K-12 (Silver *et al.*, 1981); several *kps* clusters from other serotypes have now been cloned and examined (reviewed in Boulnois and Roberts, 1990). It has been known for some time that the group I and group II K antigens' genes are not allelic (Ørskov and Ørskov, 1962; Ørskov *et al.*, 1976), indicating significant differences between the group I and II K antigens. In general, the synthesis of the group I K antigens has received relatively little attention, whereas assembly of group II K antigens has been analysed in some detail.

Group I K antigens

The (*cps*) genes for the biosynthesis of the group IA K27 (Schmidt *et al.*, 1977) and K30 (Laakso *et al.*, 1988; Whitfield *et al.*, 1989) CPS are located near *his* and are adjacent to the *rfb* locus. Transfer of the *his*-linked *cps* genes from *E. coli* K27 and K30 to *E. coli* K-12 confers expression of the K antigen. However, in serotype K27, an additional uncharacterized *trp*-linked locus may also be involved (Schmidt *et al.*, 1977). Although it is assumed that the group IB K-antigen biosynthesis genes map near *his* by analogy to group IA, direct data to support this hypothesis is not available. The essential *cps* genes involved in the biosynthesis of colanic acid in *E. coli* K-12 appear to be allelic with those for the group IA K antigens in *E. coli* (Keenleyside *et al.*, 1992). The *cps* genes comprise five complementation groups (Trisler and Gottesman, 1984), but detailed analysis is not available. Recent studies in the authors' laboratory have shown that the RfbK and RfbM enzymes encoded by the *rfb* gene locus in *E. coli* O9:K30 provide the mannosyl precursor (GDP-Man) used in biosynthesis of both O9 and K30 polysaccharides (Jayaratne *et al.*, 1994). Thus there is cooperation between biosynthetic pathways for different cell surface polysaccharides.

Although the precise pathway for biosynthesis of the group I K-antigens is not known, structural similarity to *Klebsiella* CPS has led to speculation that similar biosynthetic pathways may be used. The CPS in *Klebsiella aerogenes* is polymerized using undecaprenol-linked intermediates and it is thought that a block-wise assembly is used, reminiscent of *S. enterica* serovar Typhimurium O polysaccharides (Sutherland and Norval, 1970; Troy *et al.*, 1971). Preliminary studies on colanic acid biosynthesis in *E. coli* K-12 are consistent with an identical mechanism to that established for *Klebsiella* (Johnson and Wilson, 1977).

Group II K-antigens

The genetics and biosynthesis of the group II K antigens have been extensively researched and many details of the processes have been resolved. In most *E. coli* strains with group II K antigens, the *kps* genes form a cluster with a conserved organization. The cluster can be divided into three regions, based on the general functions of the respective gene products (Silver *et al.*, 1984; Boulnois *et al.*, 1987). Similar modular organization of CPS gene clusters occurs in *N. meningitidis* and *H. influenzae*, which produce polysaccharides structurally related to *E. coli* group II antigens (Table 17.4) (reviewed in Whitfield and Valvano, 1993).

The central region (region 2) of *kps* contains genes which encode functions involved in assembly and polymerization; these processes are best understood in *E. coli* K1 and K5. Region 2 varies in size and composition, depending on the chemistry of the K-antigen repeating unit (Roberts *et al.*, 1988; Boulnois and Roberts, 1990; Boulnois *et al.*, 1992). The K1 (Kundig *et al.*, 1971; Rohr and Troy, 1980) and K5 (Finke *et al.*, 1991) group II K antigens are polymerized at the non-reducing terminus. *In vitro* synthesis of the K1 polysaccharide using membrane preparations was first described in the 1960s and the substantial progress in this area has been reviewed elsewhere (Troy, 1992; Whitfield and Valvano, 1993). The sialyltransferase enzyme (NeuS; polyST) elongates naturally occurring polysialyl polymers within the membrane, as well as exogenous acceptors consisting of polysialic acid (Kundig *et al.*, 1971; Troy and McCloskey, 1979). A single enzyme catalyses both reactions (Steenbergen *et al.*, 1992) and the enzyme acts in a processive fashion (Steenbergen and Vimr, 1990; Steenbergen *et al.*, 1992). The polyST enzymes from *E. coli* K1 and K92 are very similar. However, the K92 polyST is a further example of a bifunctional enzyme which confers dual linkage specificity (Table 17.7) within the final product (Vimr *et al.*, 1992).

The polyST enzyme is not by itself sufficient for initiation of K1 polysaccharide synthesis (Steenbergen *et al.*, 1992) and the initiating reaction is unknown. The initial sialic acid residue appears to be transferred to an acceptor molecule which does not contain sialic acid (Rohr and Troy, 1980). Undecaprenol monophosphoryl sialic acid residues have been identified (Troy *et al.*, 1975), but it is not clear whether these molecules act only as intermediate donors of sialic acid (Troy and McCloskey, 1979) or serve as acceptors for growing polymers. Polypeptides have also been reported at the terminus of some polysialic acid chains (Troy and McCloskey, 1979; Rodŕiguez-Aparicio *et al.*, 1988; Weisgerber and Troy, 1990) and these residues may play a role either in polymerization or export processes. No undecaprenol-linked intermediates have been identified in the biosynthesis of the *E. coli* K5 polymer (Finke *et al.*, 1991). The presence of KDO in the linkage between the polymer and terminal phospholipid may require a different biosynthetic mechanism. Alternatively, growth of the polymer on an undecaprenol-linked KDO residue may create a labile linkage preventing extraction of intact intermediates. If biosynthesis proceeds by a rapid sequential process, high-molecular-weight undecaprenol-linked polymers could quickly form and these molecules would also be difficult to isolate by conventional procedures.

Regions 1 and 3 of the biosynthetic cluster flank the central region and encode functions conserved among different *kps* clusters. Functions encoded by regions 1 and 3 are therefore not specific to a particular polysaccharide structure (Roberts *et al.*, 1986, 1988). Region 1 gene products are involved in translocation of polysaccharide from the periplasm to the cell surface (Boulnois *et al.*, 1987; Silver *et al.*, 1987; Bronner *et al.*, 1993; Pazzani *et al.*, 1993) and at least one protein (KpsD) involved in this process is located in the periplasm (Silver *et al.*, 1987). Export of group II K antigens to the cell surface occurs at discrete areas (Krönke *et al.*, 1990b) which coincide with zones of adhesion, where the cytoplasmic and outer membrane come into contact. Some mutants in region 1 accumulate fully modified polymer in the periplasm (Krönke *et al.*, 1990a). Other region 1 functions include modification of the polysaccharide with the terminal lipid and KDO residues (Boulnois and Roberts, 1990). The presence in region 1 of a structural gene for an additional copy of CMP-KDO synthetase (KpsU; Pazzani *et al.*, 1993) explains the characteristic elevated activity of this enzyme in strains with group II K antigens (Table 17.4) (Finke *et al.*, 1989a, b).

Polysaccharide accumulates in the cytoplasm of cells with de-energized membranes (Krönke *et al.*, 1990b) or in cells harbouring mutations in region 3 *kps* genes from *E. coli* K5 (Krönke *et al.*, 1990a). Intracellular polysaccharide lacks the phospholipid anchor (Krönke *et al.*, 1990a; Troy, 1992; Bronner *et al.*, 1993). *kps* region 3 contains two genes, *kps*M and *kps*T. Homology between KpsM and KpsT and ATP-binding cassette transporters has led to the proposal that region 3 gene products are required to translocate newly synthesized polysaccharide to the periplasm from their site of synthesis at the cytoplasmic face of the cell membrane (Smith *et al.*, 1990; Pavelka *et al.*, 1991).

Recent examination of *E. coli* K10 and K54 *ser*A-linked *kps* clusters indicated that some *kps* clusters lack conserved regions 1 and 3 (Boulnois *et al.*, 1992). The origin and function of these clusters are particularly intriguing questions.

Regulation of Expression of Cell Surface Polysaccharides in *E. coli*

Many of the biological functions of cell surface polysaccharides are influenced by both their presence and amount. Consequently, factors regulating these components have significant effects on the virulence of *E. coli*. Recently, some of the regulatory systems have begun to be identified.

Regulation of LPS

Although the SDS–PAGE profile of LPS is characteristic for a given strain of *E. coli*, environmental conditions do affect LPS expression. Altered growth rates or culture under stress conditions have a profound influence on the SDS–PAGE profile, particularly in the amount of LPS core capped with O antigen (Weiss *et al.*, 1986; Nelson *et al.*, 1991). Selection for serum-resistance in *E. coli* O111 (Goldman *et al.*, 1984) and O6 and O18ac (Porat *et al.*, 1987) results in strains which cap more lipid A core with O polysaccharide and show an increase in O-polysaccharide chain length. Given the role of LPS in serum resistance, any increase in the amount of S-LPS or increase in O-polysaccharide chain length would significantly enhance the pathogenicity of *E. coli*. In one report, structural changes in the *E. coli* O157 O antigen also resulted from altered growth rates (Dodds *et al.*, 1987). The extent of this phenomenon within *E. coli* LPS and its potential effect on virulence is unknown.

In many *E. coli* LPS, the distribution of O-polysaccharide chain lengths is multimodal (Kusecek *et al.*, 1984). It has been suggested that the varying chain lengths of O antigen attached to lipid A core reflect properties of the O-antigen polymerase and/or ligase (Goldman and Hunt, 1990). However, other factors are also now known to be involved. Recently, a gene termed *rol* (*r*egulator of *O*-chain *l*ength), or *cld* (O-*c*hain *l*ength *d*etermination) has been identified in *E. coli* O75 (Batchelor *et al.*, 1991, 1992), *E. coli* O111 (Bastin *et al.*, 1993) and *S. enterica* serovar Typhimurium (Batchelor *et al.*, 1992; Bastin *et al.*, 1993). *rol*/*cld* mutants have unregulated O-antigen chain lengths. Rol/Cld is distinct from the O-antigen polymerase although it is conceivable that Rol/Cld and the polymerase interact to modulate the LPS phenotype (Batchelor *et al.*, 1992; Bastin *et al.*, 1993). The factors affecting the activity of Rol/Cld are presently unknown, but are central to the pathogenesis of *E. coli*.

The *rfa*H (also termed *sfr*B) gene regulates the expression of LPS core by acting at the level of transcription of the *rfa* core biosynthesis genes in *E. coli* and *S. enterica* serovar Typhimurium (Creeger *et al.*, 1984; Brazas *et al.*, 1991; Pradel and Schnaitman, 1991). RfaH was originally proposed to act as a transcription antiterminator, but recent studies support a role as a positive regulator of core synthesis in both *E. coli* (Pradel and Schnaitman, 1991) and *S. enterica* serovar Typhimurium (Brazas *et al.*, 1991). RfaH also regulates the F factor *tra* operon (Beutin *et al.*, 1981). In *S. enterica* serovar Typhimurium, an *rfa*H defect results in R-LPS with heterogeneous core structure (Lindberg and Hellerqvist, 1980). Any modulation of core synthesis by RfaH will also affect the availability of attachment points for O polysaccharide. This, in turn, has profound effects on pathogenicity.

Regulation of K-antigen expression

Expression of CPS is influenced by growth conditions. One of the characteristic features of *E. coli* group II K antigens is the temperature sensitivity of their expression (Ørskov *et al.*, 1984) (Table 17.5). It is known that the level of CMP-KDO synthetase in strains with group II K antigens is reduced at CPS-restrictive temperatures (Finke *et al.*, 1989b). While this may not be sufficient by itself to prevent K-antigen synthesis, the effect may reflect complex regulation of the *kps* cluster. Details of the regulation system have yet to be determined. Synthesis of K antigen, a key virulence determinant, only at temperatures experienced in the host is an intriguing phenomenon.

The expression of many group I K antigens is regulated by the *rcs* (*r*egulator of *c*apsule *s*ynthesis) gene system. This system has been best described in studies by S. Gottesman's laboratory, which have focused on colanic acid regulation in *E. coli* K-12 (Gottesman and Stout, 1991). The *rcs* system comprises several regulatory proteins, including an environmentally responsive two-component regulatory system. Two-component regulatory systems are found in many bacteria where they control a variety of physiological functions, including several virulence determinants. Response to environmental cues is mediated by a series of phosphorylation reactions, often originating with autophosphorylation of a sensor (or kinase) protein and culminating in the modification of the activity of a transcriptional activator protein (effector) by phosphotransfer. The sensor in group I capsule regulation is thought to be RcsC, a protein which spans the cytoplasmic membrane (Stout and Gottesman, 1990). The effector is RcsB and its target(s) is the promoter(s) of the *cps* biosynthetic gene cluster (Gottesman *et al.*, 1985; Brill *et al.*, 1988); *cps* transcription is regulated by effector activity. It has been proposed that RcsB is active in its phosphorylated state and that both phosphorylation and dephosphorylation involve RcsC (Gottesman and Stout, 1991). However, phosphorylation and effector-DNA binding have not been shown directly and the prediction is based on protein homologies with other systems where the mechanism is better described. Recent work has implicated another protein, RcsF, as the protein kinase which phosphorylates RcsB, with RcsC serving as an environmentally regulated phosphatase (Gervais and Drapeau,

1992). It has also been proposed that RcsB can be phosphorylated by other sensor proteins, to provide a highly versatile and responsive system (Gervais *et al.*, 1992). RcsB is regulated and autoregulated in a complex fashion and may have multiple cellular roles. For example, RcsB also interacts with FtsZ, a cell division protein (Gervais *et al.*, 1992).

Additional ancillary proteins are also involved in colanic acid regulation. Early studies by Markovitz (reviewed in Markovitz, 1977) showed that *cap*R (now known as *lon*) mutations activated colanic acid expression in *E. coli* K-12. Lon is an ATP-dependent protease involved in UV sensitivity, induction of the SOS response and filamentation. Lon degrades RcsA, an additional positive regulator for colanic acid expression (Stout *et al.*, 1991). It is proposed that RcsA : RcsB dimers provide the functional transcriptional activator for the *cps* system; availability of the effector would therefore be limited by Lon (Gottesman and Stout, 1991). RcsA has a helix-turn-helix DNA-binding motif, although DNA binding has not been demonstrated (Stout *et al.*, 1991).

E. coli K-12 strains are normally non-mucoid but colanic acid synthesis is stimulated by certain growth conditions. These include high phosphate, low nitrogen : carbon ratios or incubation temperatures below 25 °C. *E. coli* strains with group IB and II K antigens also use *rcs* gene products to regulate expression of colanic acid and at 37 °C no significant amounts of colanic acid are produced (Keenleyside *et al.*, 1992, 1993; Jayaratne *et al.*, 1993). The significance of the ability to produce both polymers is unknown; colanic acid has no known role in pathogenicity. Based on structural features, allelic *cps* genes and common regulatory systems, colanic acid and group IA capsules are clearly related, if not part of the same group. The only differentiating property seems to be in the response of the biosynthetic systems to the regulatory *rcs* system. *E. coli* strains with group IA K antigens produce capsule under all growth conditions, including at 37 °C. The *rcs* regulatory system is only required for high levels of group IA K-antigen synthesis (Keenleyside *et al.*, 1992; Jayaratne *et al.*, 1993). The effect on pathogenesis of the regulation of *E. coli* group I K antigens (and colanic acid) is not known and the precise nature of the stimuli which activate expression are key unanswered questions. Interestingly, Rcs homologues control extracellular polysaccharides in diverse pathogenic bacteria, including *Klebsiella* sp., and the Vi antigen in *Salmonella* sp. and *Citrobacter freundii*, as well as plant pathogenic *Erwinia* species (reviewed in Whitfield and Valvano, 1993).

Conclusions

The last 10–15 years have seen significant advances in our understanding of cell surface polysaccharides in *E. coli*. The instrumentation available for rapid determination of polysaccharide structure has facilitated detailed structural analyses and provided a chemical basis for antigenic differences among polysaccharides. This information can now be used to precisely examine the interaction between host cell defences and homogeneous, chemically defined, cell surface components. The application of molecular, genetic and biochemical approaches has identified specific steps in the biosynthesis of cell surface polysaccharides. In addition to providing potential steps for intervention with novel antimicrobial agents, these studies should also provide insight into the evolution of the tremendous antigenic diversity seen in *E. coli* cell surface polysaccharides. Perhaps the most intriguing questions relate to the environmental cues and regulatory mechanisms which modulate expression of cell surface polysaccharides. These mechanisms are crucial to our understanding of the role played by these polysaccharides in pathogenesis.

Acknowledgements

Work on *E. coli* polysaccharides in the authors' laboratory is supported by funding (to C.W.) from the Medical Research Council of Canada.

References

Abe, C., Schmitz, S., Jann, B. and Jann, K. (1988) Monoclonal antibodies against O and K antigens of uropathogenic *Escherichia coli* O4:K12:H$^-$ as opsonins. *Federation of European Microbiological Societies Microbiology Letters* 51, 153–158.

Achtman, M. and Pluschke, G. (1986) Clonal analysis of descent and virulence among selected *Escherichia coli. Annual Reviews in Microbiology* 40, 185–210.

Adlam, C., Knights, J.M., Mugridge, A., Williams, J.M. and Lindon, J.C. (1987) Production of colominic acid by *Pasteurella haemolytica* serotype A2 organisms. *Federation of European Microbiological Societies Microbiology Letters* 42, 23–25.

Barr, K. and Rick, P.D. (1987) Biosynthesis of enterobacterial common antigen in *Escherichia coli. In vitro* synthesis of lipid-linked intermediates. *Journal of Biological Chemistry* 262, 7142–7150.

Barr, K., Nunes-Edwards, P. and Rick, P.D. (1989) *In vitro* synthesis of a lipid-linked trisaccharide involved in synthesis of enterobacterial common antigen. *Journal of Bacteriology* 171, 1326–1332.

Bastin, D.A., Romana, L.K. and Reeves, P.R. (1991) Molecular cloning and expression in *Escherichia coli* K-12 of the *rfb* gene cluster determining the O antigen of an *E. coli* O111 strain. *Molecular Microbiology* 5, 2223–2231.

Bastin, D.A., Stevenson, G., Brown, P.K., Haase, A. and Reeves, P.R. (1993) Repeat unit polysaccharides of bacteria: a model for polymerization resembling that of ribosomes and fatty acid synthetase, with a novel mechanism for determining chain length. *Molecular Microbiology* 7, 725–734.

Batchelor, R.A., Haraguchi, G.E., Hull, R.A. and Hull, S.I. (1991) Regulation by a novel protein of the bimodal distribution of lipopolysaccharide in the outer membrane of *Escherichia coli*. *Journal of Bacteriology* 173, 5699–5704.

Batchelor, R.A., Alifano, P., Biffali, E., Hull, S.I. and Hull, R.A. (1992) Nucleotide sequences of the genes regulating O-polysaccharide chain length (*rol*) from *Escherichia coli* and *Salmonella typhimurium*: protein homology and functional complementation. *Journal of Bacteriology* 174, 5228–5236.

Baumgartner, J.D., Heumann, D., Gerain, J., Weinbreck, P., Grau, G.E. and Glauser, M.P. (1990) Association between protective efficacy of anti-lipopolysaccharide (LPS) antibodies and suppression of LPS-induced tumor necrosis factor α and interleukin 6. Comparison of O side chain-specific antibodies with core LPS antibodies. *Journal of Experimental Medicine* 171, 889–896.

Bazil, V. and Strominger, J.L. (1991) Shedding as a mechanism of down-modulation of CD14 on stimulated human monocytes. *Journal of Immunology* 147, 1567–1574.

Bessin, P., Bonnet, J., Apffel, D., Soulard, C., Desgroux, L., Pelas, I. and Benveniste, J. (1983) Acute circulatory collapse caused by platelet-activating factor (PAF-acether) in dogs. *European Journal of Pharmacology* 86, 403–413.

Beutin, L., Manning, P.A., Achtman, M. and Willetts, N. (1981) *sfr*A and *sfr*B products of *Escherichia coli* are transcriptional control factors. *Journal of Bacteriology* 145, 840–844.

Beutler, B., Mahoney, J., Le Trang, N., Pekala, P. and Cerami, A. (1985a) Purification of cachectin, a lipoprotein lipase-suppressing hormone secreted by endotoxin-induced Raw 264.7 cells. *Journal of Experimental Medicine* 161, 984–995.

Beutler, B.A., Milsark, I.W. and Cerami, A.C. (1985b) Passive immunization against cachectin/tumor necrosis factor protects mice from lethal effect of endotoxin. *Science* 229, 869–871.

Beveridge, T.J. and Graham, L.L. (1991) Surface layers of bacteria. *Microbiological Reviews* 55, 684–705.

Bogard, W.C.J., Dunn, D.L., Abernathy, K., Kilgarriff, C. and Kung, P.C. (1987) Isolation and characterization of murine monoclonal antibodies specific for gram-negative bacterial lipopolysaccharide: association of cross-genus reactivity with lipid A specificity. *Infection and Immunity* 55, 899–908.

Bone, R.C. (1991) The pathogenesis of sepsis. *Annals of Internal Medicine* 115, 457–469.

Bone, R.C. (1993) Gram negative sepsis: a dilemma of modern medicine. *Clinical Microbiology Reviews* 6, 57–68.

Bortolussi, R., Ferrieri, P., Bjorksten, B. and Quie, P.G. (1979) Capsular K1 polysaccharide of *Escherichia coli*: relationship to virulence in newborn rats and resistance to phagocytosis. *Infection and Immunity* 25, 293–298.

Bortolussi, R., Ferrieri, P. and Quie, P.G. (1983) Influence of growth temperature of *Escherichia coli* K1 on capsular antigen production and resistance to opsonization. *Infection and Immunity* 39, 1136–1141.

Boulnois, G.J. and Roberts, I.S. (1990) Genetics of capsular polysaccharide production in bacteria. In: Jann, K. and Jann, B. (eds) *Bacterial Capsules*. Springer-Verlag, New York, pp. 1–18.

Boulnois, G.J., Roberts, I.S., Hodge, R., Hardy, K.R., Jann, K. and Timmis, K.N. (1987) Analysis of the K1 capsule biosynthesis genes of *Escherichia coli*: definition of three functional regions for capsule production. *Molecular and General Genetics* 208, 242–246.

Boulnois, G., Drake, R., Pearce, R. and Roberts, I. (1992) Genome diversity at the *ser*A-linked capsule locus in *Escherichia coli*. *Federation of European Microbiological Societies Microbiology Letters* 100, 121–124.

Bradley, D.E., Anderson, A.N. and Perry, M.B. (1991) Differences between the LPS cores in adherent and non-adherent strains of enteropathogenic *Escherichia coli* O119. *Federation of European Microbiological Societies Microbiology Letters* 80, 13–18.

Brazas, R., Davie, E., Farewell, A. and Rothfield, L.I. (1991) Transcriptional organization of the *rfa*GBIJ locus of *Salmonella typhimurium*. *Journal of Bacteriology* 173, 6168–6173.

Brill, J.A., Quinlan-Walshe, C. and Gottesman, S. (1988) Fine-structure mapping and identification of two regulators of capsule synthesis in *Escherichia coli* K-12. *Journal of Bacteriology* 170, 2599–2611.

Bronner, D., Siebarth, V., Pazzani, C., Roberts, I.S., Boulnois, G.J., Jann, B. and Jann, K. (1993) Expression of the capsular K5 polysaccharide of *Escherichia coli*: biochemical and electron microscopic analysis of mutants with defects in region 1 of the K5 gene cluster. *Journal of Bacteriology* 175, 5984–5992.

Chakraborty, A.K., Friebolin, H. and Stirm, S. (1980) Primary structure of the *Escherichia coli* serotype K30 capsular polysaccharide. *Journal of Bacteriology* 141, 971–972.

Chen, L. and Coleman, W.G.J. (1993) Cloning and characterization of the *Escherichia coli* K-12 *rfa*-2 (*rfa*C) gene, a gene required for lipopolysaccharide inner core synthesis. *Journal of Bacteriology* 175, 2534–2540.

Chen, T.Y., Bright, S.W., Pace, J.L., Russel, S.W. and Morrison, D.C. (1990) Induction of macrophage-mediated tumor cytotoxicity by a hamster monoclonal antibody with specificity for lipopolysaccharide receptor. *Journal of Immunology* 145, 8–12.

Choy, Y.-M. and Dutton, G.G.S. (1973) Structure of the capsular polysaccharide of *Klebsiella* K-type 20. *Canadian Journal of Chemistry* 51, 3015–3020.

Clementz, T. (1992) The gene coding for 3-deoxy-*manno*-octulosonic acid transferase and the *rfa*Q gene are transcribed from divergently arranged promoters in *Escherichia coli*. *Journal of Bacteriology* 174, 7750–7756.

Clementz, T. and Raetz, C.R.H. (1991) A gene coding for 3-deoxy-D-*manno*-octulosonic acid transferase in *Escherichia coli*. Identification, mapping, cloning, and sequencing. *Journal of Biological Chemistry* 266, 9687–9696.

Creeger, E.S. and Rothfield, L.I. (1979) Cloning of genes for bacterial glycosyl transferases. I. Selection of hybrid plasmids carrying genes for two glycosyl transferases. *Journal of Biological Chemistry* 254, 804–810.

Creeger, E.S., Schulte, T. and Rothfield, L.I. (1984) Regulation of membrane glycosyl transferases by the *sfr*B and *rfa*H genes of *E. coli* and *S. typhimurium*. *Journal of Biological Chemistry* 259, 3064–3069.

Cross, A.S. (1990) The biologic significance of bacterial encapsulation. In: Jann,

K. and Jann, B. (eds) *Bacterial Capsules*. Springer-Verlag, New York, pp. 87–95.

Cross, A.S., Gemski, P., Sadoff, J.C., Øskov, F. and Ørskov, I. (1984) The importance of the K1 capsule in invasive infections caused by *Escherichia coli*. *Journal of Infectious Diseases* 149, 184–193.

Cross, A.S., Kim, K.S., Wright, D.C., Sadoff, J.C. and Gemski, P. (1986) Role for lipopolysaccharide and capsule in the serum resistance of bacteremic strains of *Escherichia coli*. *Journal of Infectious Diseases* 154, 497–503.

Cross, A.S., Sadoff, J., Gemski, P. and Kim, K.S. (1988) The relative role of lipopolysaccharide and capsule in the virulence of *E. coli*. In: Cabello, F.C. and Pruzzo, C. (eds) *Bacteria, Complement and the Phagocytic Cell*. Springer Verlag, New York, pp. 319–334.

Crutchley, M.J., Marsh, D.G. and Cameron, J. (1967) Free endotoxin. *Nature (London)* 214, 1052.

Cryz, S.J., Cross, A.S., Sadoff, J.C. and Fürer, E. (1990) Synthesis and characterization of *Escherichia* O18 O-polysaccharide conjugate vaccines. *Infection and Immunity* 58, 373–377.

Cryz, S.J., Cross, A.S., Sadoff, J.C., Wegmann, A., Que, J.U. and Fürer, E. (1991) Safety and immunogenicity of *Escherichia coli* O18 O-specific polysaccharide (O-PS)-toxin A and O-PS-cholera toxin conjugate vaccines in humans. *Journal of Infectious Diseases* 163, 1040–1045.

Devi, S.J.N., Schneerson, R., Egan, W., Vann, W.F., Robbins, J.B. and Shiloach, J. (1991) Identity between the polysaccharide antigens of *Moraxella nonliquefaciens*, group B *Neisseria meningitidis*, and *Escherichia coli* K1 (non-O acetylated). *Infection and Immunity* 59, 732–736.

Ding, M.-J., Svanborg, C., Haraguchi, G.E., Hull, R.A. and Hull, S.I. (1991) Molecular cloning and expression of the O1 *rfb* region from a pyelonephritic *Escherichia coli* O1:H1:K7. *Microbial Pathogenesis* 11, 379–385.

Dodds, K.L., Perry, M.B. and McDonald, I.J. (1987) Alterations in lipopolysaccharide produced by chemostat-grown *Escherichia coli* O157:H7 as a function of growth rate and growth-limiting nutrient. *Canadian Journal of Microbiology* 33, 452–458.

Drach, G.W., Reed, W.P. and Williams, R.C.J. (1971) Antigens common to human and bacterial cells: urinary tract pathogens. *Journal of Laboratory and Clinical Medicine* 78, 725–735.

Dutton, G.G.S. and Parolis, L.A.S. (1989) Polysaccharide antigens of *Escherichia coli*. In: Dea, I.C.M. and Stivola, S.S. (eds) *Recent Developments in Industrial Polysaccharides: Biological and Biotechnological Advances*. Gordon and Breach Science Publishers, New York, pp. 223–240.

Egan, W., Schneerson, R., Warner, K.E. and Zon, G. (1982) Structural studies and chemistry of bacterial capsular polysaccharides. Investigations of phosphodiester-linked capsular polysaccharides isolated from *Haemophilus influenzae* types a, b, c, and f: NMR spectroscopic identification and chemical modification of end groups and the nature of base-catalyzed hydrolytic depolymerization. *Journal of the American Chemical Society* 104, 2898–2910.

Ferrero, E., Jiao, D., Tsuberi, B.Z., Tesio, L., Rong, G.W., Haziot, L. and Goyert, S.M. (1993) Transgenic mice expressing human CD14 are hypersensitive to lipopolysaccharide. *Proceedings of the National Academy of Sciences of the United States of America* 90, 2380–2384.

Finke, A., Jann, B. and Jann, K. (1989a) CMP-KDO-synthetase activity in *Escherichia coli* expressing capsular polysaccharides. *Federation of European Microbiological Societies Microbiology Letters* 69, 129–134.

Finke, A., Roberts, I., Boulnois, G., Pazzani, C. and Jann, K. (1989b) Activity of CMP-2-keto-3-deoxyoctulosonic acid synthetase in *Escherichia coli* strains expressing the capsular K5 polysaccharide: implication for K5 polysaccharide biosynthesis. *Journal of Bacteriology* 171, 3074–3079.

Finke, A., Bronner, D., Nikolaev, A.V., Jann, B. and Jann, K. (1991) Biosynthesis of the *Escherichia coli* K5 polysaccharide, a representative of group II capsular polysaccharides: polymerization *in vitro* and characterization of the product. *Journal of Bacteriology* 173, 4088–4094.

Frank, M.M., Joiner, K. and Hammer, C. (1987) The function of antibody and complement in the lysis of bacteria. *Reviews of Infectious Diseases* 9, S537–S545.

Freudenberg, M.A. and Galanos, C. (1988) Induction of tolerance to lipopolysaccharide (LPS)-D-galactosamine lethality by pretreatment with LPS is mediated by macrophages. *Infection and Immunity* 56, 1352–1357.

Gervais, F.G. and Drapeau, G.R. (1992) Identification, cloning, and characterization of *rcs*F, a new regulator gene for exopolysaccharide synthesis that suppresses the division mutation *fts*Z84 in *Escherichia coli* K-12. *Journal of Bacteriology* 174, 8016–8022.

Gervais, F.G., Phoenix, P. and Drapeau, G.R. (1992) The *rcs*B gene, a positive regulator of colanic acid biosynthesis in *Escherichia coli*, is also an activator of *fts*Z expression. *Journal of Bacteriology* 174, 3964–3971.

Gibb, A.R., Barclay, G.R., Poxton, I.R. and di Padova, F. (1992) Frequencies of lipopolysaccharide core types among clinical isolates of *Escherichia coli* defined with monoclonal antibodies. *Journal of Infectious Diseases* 166, 1051–1057.

Gilbert, R.P. (1960) Mechanisms of hemodynamic effects of endotoxin. *Physiological Reviews* 40, 245–279.

Glode, L.M., Mergenhagen, S.E. and Rosenstreich, D.L. (1976) Significant contribution of spleen cells in mediating the lethal effects of endotoxin *in vivo*. *Infection and Immunity* 14, 626–630.

Glynn, A.A. and Howard, C.J. (1970) The sensitivity to complement of strains of *Escherichia coli* related to their K antigens. *Immunology* 18, 331–346.

Goebel, W.F. (1963) Colanic acid. *Proceedings of the National Academy of Sciences of the United States of America* 49, 464–471.

Goldman, R.C. and Hunt, F. (1990) Mechanism of O-antigen distribution in lipopolysaccharide. *Journal of Bacteriology* 172, 5352–5359.

Goldman, R.C. and Kohlbrenner, W.E. (1985) Molecular cloning of the structural gene coding for CTP:CMP-3-deoxy-*manno*-octulosonate cytidyltransferase from *Escherichia coli* K-12. *Journal of Bacteriology* 163, 256–261.

Goldman, R.C. and Leive, L. (1980) Heterogeneity of antigenic side chain length in lipopolysaccharide from *Escherichia coli* O111 and *Salmonella typhimurium* LT2. *European Journal of Biochemistry* 107, 145–153.

Goldman, R.C., White, D., Ørskov, F., Ørskov, I., Rick, P.D., Lewis, M.S., Bhattacharjee, A.K. and Leive, L. (1982) A surface polysaccharide of *Escherichia coli* O111 contains O-antigen and inhibits agglutination of cells by O-antiserum. *Journal of Bacteriology* 151, 1210–1221.

Goldman, R.C., Joiner, K. and Leive, L. (1984) Serum-resistant mutants of *Escherichia coli* O111 contain increased lipopolysaccharide, lack an O antigen-containing capsule, and cover more of their lipid A-core with O antigen. *Journal of Bacteriology* 159, 877–882.

Goldman, R.C., Kohlbrenner, W.E., Lartey, P. and Pernet, A. (1987) Antibacterial agents specifically inhibiting lipopolysaccharide synthesis. *Nature (London)* 329, 162–164.

Goldman, R.C., Doran, C.L. and Capobianco, J.O. (1988) Analysis of lipopolysaccharide biosynthesis in *Salmonella typhimurium* and *Escherichia coli* by using agents which specifically block incorporation of 3-deoxy-D-*manno*-octulosonate. *Journal of Bacteriology* 170, 2185–2191.

Golenbock, D.T., Hampton, R.Y., Raetz, C.R.H. and Wright, S.D. (1990) Human phagocytes have multiple lipid A-binding sites. *Infection and Immunity* 58, 4069–4075.

Gotschlich, E.C., Fraser, B.A., Nishimura, O., Robbins, J.B. and Liu, T.-Y. (1981) Lipid on capsular polysaccharides of Gram-negative bacteria. *Journal of Biological Chemistry* 256, 8915–8921.

Gottesman, S. and Stout, V. (1991) Regulation of capsular polysaccharide synthesis in *Escherichia coli* K-12. *Molecular Microbiology* 5, 1599–1606.

Gottesman, S., Trisler, P. and Torres-Cabassa, A. (1985) Regulation of capsular polysaccharide synthesis in *Escherichia coli* K-12: characterization of three regulatory genes. *Journal of Bacteriology* 162, 1111–1119.

Greisman, S.E. and Johnston, C.A. (1987) Failure of antisera to J5 and R595 rough mutants to reduce endotoxemic lethality. *Journal of Infectious Diseases* 157, 54–64.

Gupta, D.S., Shashkov, A.S., Jann, B. and Jann, K. (1992) Structures of the O1B and O1C lipopolysaccharide antigens of *Escherichia coli*. *Journal of Bacteriology* 174, 7963–7970.

Haishima, Y., Holst, O. and Brade, H. (1992) Structural investigation of the lipopolysaccharide of *Escherichia coli* rough mutant F653 representing the R3 core type. *European Journal of Biochemistry* 203, 127–134.

Hammond, S.M. (1992) Inhibitors of lipopolysaccharide biosynthesis impair the virulence potential of *Escherichia coli*. *Federation of European Microbiological Societies Microbiology Letters* 100, 293–298.

Hammond, S.M., Claesson, A., Jansson, A.M., Larsson, L.-G., Pring, B.G., Town, C.M., and Ekstrom, B. (1987) A new class of synthetic antibacterials acting on lipopolysaccharide biosynthesis. *Nature (London)* 327, 730–732.

Hampton, R.Y., Golenbock, D.T. and Raetz, C.R.H. (1988) Lipid A binding sites in membranes of macrophage tumor cells. *Journal of Biological Chemistry* 263, 14802–14807.

Haraguchi, G.E., Zähringer, U., Jann, B., Jann, K., Hull, R.I. and Hull, S.I. (1991) Genetic characterization of the O4 polysaccharide gene cluster from *Escherichia coli*. *Microbial Pathogenesis* 10, 351–361.

Heidelberger, M., Jann, K., Jann, B., Ørskov, I. and Ørskov, F. (1968) Relations between structures of three K polysaccharides of *Escherichia coli* and cross reactivity in antipneumococcal sera. *Journal of Bacteriology* 95, 2415–2417.

Heuzenroeder, M.W., Beger, D.W., Thomas, C.J. and Manning, P.A. (1989) Molecular cloning and expression in *Escherichia coli* K-12 of the O101 *rfb* region from *E. coli* B41 (O101:K99/F41) and the genetic relationship to other O101 *rfb* loci. *Molecular Microbiology* 3, 295–302.

Hitchcock, P.J. and Brown, T.M. (1983) Morphological heterogeneity among Salmonella lipopolysaccharide chemotypes in silver-stained polyacrylamide gels. *Journal of Bacteriology* 154, 269–277.

Hogenauer, G. and Waisetschlager, M. (1981) A diazoborane derivative inhibits lipopolysaccharide biosynthesis. *Nature (London)* 293, 662–664.

Holmgren, J., Hanson, L.A., Holm, S.E. and Kaijser, B. (1971) An antigenic relationship between kidney and certain *Escherichia coli* strains. *International Archives of Allergy* 41, 463–474.

Holst, O., Zühringer, U., Brade, H. and Zamojski, A. (1991) Structural analysis of the heptose/hexose region of the lipopolysaccharide from *Escherichia coli* K-12 strain W3100. *Carbohydrate Research* 215, 323–335.

Homonylo, M.K., Wilmot, S.J., Lam, J.S., MacDonald, L.A. and Whitfield, C. (1988) Monoclonal antibodies against the capsular K antigen of *Escherichia coli* (O9:K30:H12): characterization and use in analysis of K antigen organization on the cell surface. *Canadian Journal of Microbiology* 34, 1159–1165.

Horstmann, R.D. (1992) Target recognition failure by the nonspecific defense system: surface constituents of pathogens interfere with the alternative pathway of complement activation. *Infection and Immunity* 60, 721–727.

Horwitz, M.A. (1982) Phagocytosis of microorganisms. *Reviews of Infectious Diseases* 4, 104–123.

Horwitz, M.A. and Silverstein, S.C. (1980) Influence of *Escherichia coli* capsule on complement fixation and on phagocytosis and killing by human phagocytes. *Journal of Clinical Investigation* 65, 82–94.

Hostetter, M.K. (1986) Serotypic variations among virulent pneumococci in deposition and degradation of covalently bound C3b: implications for phagocytosis and antibody production. *Journal of Infectious Diseases* 153, 682–693.

Jann, K. and Jann, B. (1984) Structure and biosynthesis of O-antigens. In: Reitschel, E.T. (ed.) *Handbook of Endotoxin*. Elsevier Science Publishers, Amsterdam, pp. 138–186.

Jann, K. and Jann, B. (1985) Cell surface components and virulence: *Escherichia coli* O and K antigens in relation to virulence and pathogenicity. In: Sussman, M. (ed.) *Virulence of* Escherichia coli*: Reviews and Methods*. Society for General Microbiology, London, pp. 157–176.

Jann, B. and Jann, K. (1990) Structure and biosynthesis of the capsular antigens of *Escherichia coli*. In: Jann, K. and Jann, B. (eds) *Bacterial Capsules*. Springer-Verlag, New York, pp. 19–42.

Jann, K. and Jann, B. (1992) Capsules of *Escherichia coli*, expression and biological significance. *Canadian Journal of Microbiology* 38, 705–710.

Jann, K., Kanegasaki, S., Goldemann, G. and Mäkelä, P.H. (1979) On the effect of *rfe* mutation on the biosynthesis of the O8 and O9 antigens of *E. coli*. *Biochemical and Biophysical Research Communications* 86, 1185–1191.

Jann, K., Goldemann, G., Weisgerber, C., Wolf-Ullisch, C. and Kanegasaki, S. (1982) Biosynthesis of the O9 antigen of *Escherichia coli*. Initial reaction and overall reaction. *European Journal of Biochemistry* 127, 157–164.

Jann, B., Shashkov, A.S., Gupta, D.S., Panasenko, S.M. and Jann, K. (1992a) The O1 antigen of *Escherichia coli*: structural characterization of the O1A/O1A1-specific polysaccharide. *Carbohydrate Polymers* 18, 51–57.

Jann, K., Dengler, T. and Jann, B. (1992b) Core-lipid A on the K40 polysaccharide of *Escherichia coli* O8:K40:H9, a representative of group I capsular polysaccharides. *Zentrablatt für Bakteriologie* 276, 196–204.

Jansson, P.-E., Lindberg, A.A., Lindberg, B. and Wollin, R. (1981) Structural studies on the hexose region of the core in lipopolysaccharides from Enterobacteriaceae. *European Journal of Biochemistry* 115, 571–577.

Jayaratne, P., Keenleyside, W.J., MacLachlan, P.R., Dodgson, C. and Whitfield, C. (1993) Characterization of *rcs*B and *rcs*C from *Escherichia coli* O9:K30:H12 and examination of the role of the *rcs* regulatory system in expression of group I capsular polysaccharides. *Journal of Bacteriology* 175, 5384–5394.

Jayaratne, P., Bronner, D., MacLachlan, R., Dodgson, C., Kido, N. and Whitfield, C. (1994) Cloning and analysis of duplicated *rfbk* and *rfbm* genes involved in formation of GDP-mannose in *Escherichia coli* O9:K30 and participation of *rfb* genes in the synthesis of the group I K30 capsular polysaccharide. *Journal of Bacteriology* 176, 3126–3139.

Johnson, J.G. and Wilson, D.B. (1977) Role of a sugar-lipid intermediate in colanic acid synthesis by *Escherichia coli. Journal of Bacteriology* 129, 225–236.

Joiner, K.A. (1985) Studies on the mechanism of bacterial resistance to complement-mediated killing and the mechanism of action of bactericidal antibody. *Current Topics in Microbiology and Immunology* 121, 99–133.

Joiner, K.A., Goldman, R.C., Hammer, C.H., Lieve, L. and Frank, M.M. (1983) Studies of the mechanism of bacterial resistance to complement-mediated killing. V. IgG and F(ab′)2 mediate killing of *E. coli* O111:B4 by the alternate complement pathway without increasing C5b-9 deposition. *Journal of Immunology* 131, 2563–2569.

Joiner, K.A., Goldman, R., Schmetz, M., Berger, M., Hammer, C.H., Frank, M.M. and Lieve, L. (1984) A quantitative analysis of C3 binding to O-antigen capsule, lipopolysaccharide and outer membrane protein of *E. coli* O111B4. *Journal of Immunology* 132, 369–376.

Joiner, K.A., Schmetz, M.A., Sanders, M.E., Murray, T.G., Hammer, C.H., Dourmashkin, R. and Frank, M.M. (1985) Multimeric complement component C9 is necessary for killing of *Escherichia coli* J5 by terminal attack complex C5b-9. *Proceedings of the National Academy of Sciences of the United States of America* 82, 4808–4812.

Kaufman, B.M., Cross, A.S., Futrovsky, S.L., Sidberry, H.F. and Sadoff, J.C. (1986) Monoclonal antibodies reactive with K1-encapsulated *Escherichia coli* lipopolysaccharide are opsonic and protect mice against lethal challenge. *Infection and Immunity* 52, 617–619.

Keenleyside, W.J., Jayaratne, P., MacLachlan, P.R. and Whitfield, C. (1992) The *rcs*A gene of *Escherichia coli* O9:K30:H12 is involved in the expression of the serotype-specific group I K (capsular) antigen. *Journal of Bacteriology* 174, 8–16.

Keenleyside, W.J., Bronner, D., Jann, K., Jann, B. and Whitfield, C. (1993)

Co-expression of colanic acid and serotype-specific capsular polysaccharides in *Escherichia coli* strains with group II K-antigens. *Journal of Bacteriology* 175, 6725–6730.

Kenne, L. and Lindberg, B. (1983) Bacterial polysaccharides. In: Aspinall, G.O. (ed.) *The Polysaccharides*, Vol. 2. Academic Press, New York, pp. 287–363.

Kido, N., Ohta, M., Iida, K.-I., Hasegawa, T., Ito, H., Arakawa, Y., Komatsu, T. and Kato, N. (1989) Partial deletion of the cloned *rfb* gene of *Escherichia coli* O9 results in synthesis of a new O-antigenic lipopolysaccharide. *Journal of Bacteriology* 171, 3629–3633.

Kim, K.S., Cross, A.S., Zollinger, W. and Sadoff, J. (1985) Prevention and therapy of experimental *Escherichia coli* infection with monoclonal antibody. *Infection and Immunity* 50, 734–737.

Kim, K.S., Kang, J.H. and Cross, A.S. (1986) The role of capsular antigens in serum resistance and *in vivo* virulence of *Escherichia coli. Federation of European Microbiological Societies Microbiology Letters* 35, 275–278.

Kirkland, T.N., Virca, G.D., Kuus-Reichel, T., Multer, F.K., Kim, S.Y., Ulevitch, R.J. and Tobias, P.S. (1990) Identification of lipopolysaccharide-binding proteins in 70Z/3 cells by photoaffinity cross-linking. *Journal of Biological Chemistry* 265, 9520–9525.

Klena, J.D., Ashford, R.S.I. and Schnaitman, C.A. (1992a) Role of *Escherichia coli* K-12 *rfa* genes and the *rfp* gene of *Shigella dysenteriae* 1 in generation of lipopolysaccharide core heterogeneity and attachment of O-antigen. *Journal of Bacteriology* 174, 7297–7307.

Klena, J.D., Pradel, E. and Schnaitman, C.A. (1992b) Comparison of lipopolysaccharide biosynthesis genes *rfa*K, *rfa*L, *rfa*Y, and *rfa*Z of *Escherichia coli* K-12 and *Salmonella typhimurium. Journal of Bacteriology* 174, 4746–4752.

Krönke, K.-D., Boulnois, G., Roberts, I., Bitter-Suermann, D., Golecki, J.R., Jann, B. and Jann, K. (1990a) Expression of the *Escherichia coli* K5 capsular antigen: immunoelectron, microscopic and biochemical studies with recombinant *E. coli. Journal of Bacteriology* 172, 1085–1091.

Krönke, K.-D., Golecki, J.R. and Jann, K. (1990b) Further electron microscopic studies on the expression of *Escherichia coli* group II capsules. *Journal of Bacteriology* 172, 3469–3472.

Kuhn, H.-M., Meier-Dieter, U. and Mayer, H. (1988) ECA, the enterobacterial common antigen. *FEMS Microbiology Reviews* 54, 195–222.

Kundig, F.D., Aminoff, D. and Roseman, S. (1971) The sialic acids. XII. Synthesis of colominic acid by a sialyltransferase from *Escherichia coli* K-235. *Journal of Biological Chemistry* 246, 2543–2550.

Kuo, J.S.-C., Doelling, V.W., Graveline, J.F. and McCoy, D.W. (1985) Evidence for covalent attachment of phospholipid to the capsular polysaccharide of *Haemophilus influenzae* type b. *Journal of Bacteriology* 163, 769–773.

Kusecek, B., Wloch, H., Mercer, A., Vaisänen, V., Pluschke, G., Korhonen, T. and Achtman, M. (1984) Lipopolysaccharide, capsule, and fimbriae as virulence factors among O1, O7, O16, O18, or O75 and K1, K5, or K100 *Escherichia coli. Infection and Immunity* 43, 368–379.

Laakso, D.H., Homonylo, M.K., Wilmot, S.J. and Whitfield, C. (1988) Transfer and expression of the genetic determinants for O and K antigen synthesis in *Escherichia coli* O9:K(A)30:H12 and *Klebsiella* sp. O1:K20, in *Escherichia coli* K-12. *Canadian Journal of Microbiology* 34, 987–992.

Lam, C., Hildenbrandt, J., Schutze, E., Rosenwirth, B., Proctor, R.A. and Stutz, P. (1991) Immunostimulatory, but not antiendotoxin, activity of lipid X is due to small amounts of contaminating N,O-acetylated disaccharide-1-phosphate: *in vitro* and *in vivo* reevaluation of the biological activity of synthetic lipid X. *Infection and Immunity* 59, 2351–2358.

Lauener, R.P., Geha, R.S. and Vercelli, D. (1990) Engagement of the monocyte surface antigen CD14 induces lymphocyte function-associated antigen-1/intercellular adhesion molecule-1-dependent homotypic adhesion. *Journal of Immunology* 145, 1390–1394.

Lee, J.-D., Kato, K., Tobias, P.S., Kirkland, T.N. and Ulevitch, R.J. (1992) Transfection of CD14 into 70Z/3 cells dramatically enhances the sensitivity to complexes of lipopolysaccharide (LPS) and LPS binding protein. *Journal of Experimental Medicine* 175, 1697–1705.

Lefer, A.M., Muller, H.F. and Smith, J.B. (1984) Pathophysiological mechanisms of sudden death induced by platelet activating factor. *British Journal of Pharmacology* 83, 125–130.

Lei, M.-G. and Morrison, D.C. (1988a) Specific endotoxic lipopolysaccharide-binding proteins on murine splenocytes. II. Membrane localization and binding characteristics. *Journal of Immunology* 141, 1006–1011.

Lei, M.-G. and Morrison, D.C. (1988b) Specific endotoxic lipopolysaccharide-binding proteins. I. Detection of lipopolysaccharide-binding sites on splenocytes and splenocyte subpopulations. *Journal of Immunology* 141, 996–1005.

Leying, H., Suerbaum, S., Kroll, H.-P., Stahl, D. and Opferkuch, W. (1990) The capsular polysaccharide is a major determinant of serum resistance in K1-positive blood culture isolates of *Escherichia coli. Infection and Immunity* 58, 222–227.

Lindberg, A.A. and Hellerqvist, C.-G. (1980) Rough mutants of *Salmonella typhimurium*: immunochemical detection and structural analysis of lipopolysaccharides from *rfaH mutants. Journal of General Microbiology* 116, 25–32.

Liu, D. and Reeves, P.R. (1994) *Escherichia coli* K12 regains its O antigen. *Microbiology* 140, 49–57.

MacLachlan, P.R., Keenleyside, W.J., Dodgson, C. and Whitfield, C. (1993) Formation of the K30 (group I) capsule in *Escherichia coli* O9:K30 does not require attachment to lipopolysaccharide lipid A-core. *Journal of Bacteriology* 175, 7515–7522.

Mahoney, J.R.J., Beutler, B.A., Le Trang, N., Vine, W., Ikeda, Y., Kawakami, M. and Cerami, A. (1985) Lipopolysaccharide-treated Raw 264.7 cells produce a mediator that inhibits lipoporotein lipase in 3T3-L1 cells. *Journal of Immunology* 134, 1673–1675.

Mäkelä, P.H. and Stocker, B.A.D. (1984) Genetics of lipopolysaccharide. In: Reitschel, E.T. (ed.) *Handbook of Endotoxin*. Elsevier Science Publishers, Amsterdam, pp. 59–137.

Markovitz, A. (1977) Genetics and regulation of bacterial capsular polysaccharide biosynthesis and radiation sensitivity. In: Sutherland, I.W. (ed.) *Surface Carbohydrates of the Prokaryotic Cell.* Academic Press, New York, pp. 415–462.

Martin, T.R., Mathison, J.C., Tobias, P.S., Leturcq, D.J., Moriarty, A.M.,

Maunder, R.J. and Ulevitch, R.J. (1992) Lipopolysaccharide binding protein enhances the responsiveness of alveolar macrophages to bacterial lipopolysaccharide. *Journal of Clinical Investigation* 90, 2209–2219.

Mathison, J.C. and Ulevitch, R.J. (1979) The clearance, tissue distribution, and cellular localization of intravenously injected lipopolysaccharide in rabbits. *Journal of Immunology* 123, 2133–2143.

Mathison, J.C., Wolfson, E. and Ulevitch, R.J. (1988) Participation of tumor necrosis factor in the mediation of gram-negative bacterial lipopolysaccharide-induced injury in rabbits. *Journal of Clinical Investigation* 81, 1925–1937.

McCabe, W.R., Kaijser, B., Olling, S., Uwaydah, M. and Hanson, L.A. (1978) *Escherichia coli* in bacteremia: K and O antigens and serum sensitivity of strains from adults and neonates. *Journal of Infectious Diseases* 138, 33–41.

McCallum, K.L., Laakso, D.H. and Whitfield, C. (1989) Use of a bacteriophage-encoded glycanase enzyme in the generation of lipopolysaccharide O side chain deficient mutants of *Escherichia coli* O9:K30 and *Klebsiella* O1:K20: role of O and K antigens in resistance to complement-mediated serum killing. *Canadian Journal of Microbiology* 35, 994–999.

McGrath, B.C. and Osborn, M.J. (1991) Localization of terminal steps of O-antigen synthesis in *Salmonella typhimurium*. *Journal of Bacteriology* 173, 649–654.

McGuire, E.J. and Binkley, S.B. (1964) The structure and chemistry of colominic acid. *Biochemistry* 3, 247–251.

Meier, U. and Mayer, H. (1985) Genetic location of genes encoding enterobacterial common antigen. *Journal of Bacteriology* 163, 756–762.

Meier-Dieter, U., Starman, R., Barr, K., Mayer, H. and Rick, P.D. (1990) Biosynthesis of enterobacterial common antigen in *Escherichia coli*. Biochemical characterization of Tn*10* insertion mutants defective in enterobacterial common antigen synthesis. *Journal of Biological Chemistry* 265, 13490–13497.

Meier-Dieter, U., Barr, K., Starman, R., Hatch, L. and Rick, P.D. (1992) Nucleotide sequence of the *Escherichia coli rfe* gene involved in the synthesis of enterobacterial common antigen. *Journal of Biological Chemistry* 267, 746–753.

Michalek, M.T., Mold, C. and Bremer, E.G. (1988) Inhibition of the alternative pathway of human complement by structural analogues of sialic acid. *Journal of Immunology* 140, 1588–1594.

Morrison, D.C. and Ulevitch, R.J. (1978) The effects of bacterial endotoxin on host mediation systems. *American Journal of Pathology* 93, 527–617.

Moxon, E.R. and Kroll, J.S. (1990) The role of bacterial polysaccharide capsules as virulence factors. In: Jann, K. and Jann, B. (eds) *Bacterial Capsules*. Springer Verlag, New York, pp. 65–85.

Munford, R.S., Hall, C.L. and Rick, P.D. (1980) Size heterogeneity of *Salmonella typhimurium* lipopolysaccharides in outer membranes and culture supernatant membrane fragments. *Journal of Bacteriology* 144, 630–640.

Mutharia, L.M., Crockford, G., Bogard, W.C.J. and Hancock, R.E.W. (1984) Monoclonal antibodies specific for *Escherichia coli* J5 lipopolysaccharide: cross-reaction with other gram-negative bacterial species. *Infection and Immunity* 45, 631–636.

Naide, Y., Nikaido, H., Mäkelä, P.H., Wilkinson, R.G. and Stocker, B.A.D.

(1965) Semirough strains of *Salmonella. Proceedings of the National Academy of Sciences of the United States of America* 53, 147–153.

Nawroth, P.P. and Stern, D.M. (1986) Modulation of endothelial cell hemostatic properties by tumor necrosis factor. *Journal of Experimental Medicine* 163, 740–745.

Neal, B.L., Tsiolis, G.C., Heuzenroeder, M.W., Manning, P.A. and Reeves, P.R. (1991) Molecular cloning and expression in *Escherichia coli* K-12 of chromosomal genes determining the O antigen of an *E. coli* O2:K1 strain. *Federation of European Microbiological Societies Microbiology Letters* 82, 345–352.

Nelson, D., Bathgate, A.J. and Poxton, I.R. (1991) Monoclonal antibodies as probes for detecting lipopolysaccharide expression on *Escherichia coli* from different growth conditions. *Journal of General Microbiology* 137, 2741–2751.

Ngeleka, M., Harel, J., Jacques, M. and Fairbrother, J.M. (1992) Characterization of a polysaccharide capsular antigen of septicemic *Escherichia coli* O115:K"V165":F165 and evaluation of its role in pathogenicity. *Infection and Immunity* 60, 5048–5056.

Ohta, M., Ina, K., Kusuzaki, K., Kido, N., Arakawa, Y. and Kato, N. (1991) Cloning and expression of the *rfe-rff* gene cluster of *Escherichia coli. Molecular Microbiology* 5, 1853–1862.

Opal, S., Cross, A. and Gemski, P. (1982) K antigen and serum sensitivity of rough *Escherichia. Infection and Immunity* 37, 956–960.

Oppenheimer, J.J., Kovacs, E.J., Matsushima, K. and Durum, S.K. (1986) There is more than one interleukin 1. *Immunology Today* 7, 45–56.

Ørskov, I. and Nyman, K. (1974) Genetic mapping of the antigenic determinants of two polysaccharide K antigens, K10 and K54, in *Escherichia coli. Journal of Bacteriology* 120, 43–51.

Ørskov, F. and Ørskov, I. (1962) Behaviour of *E. coli* antigens in sexual recombination. *Acta Pathologica et Microbiologica Scandinavica* 55, 99–109.

Ørskov, F. and Ørskov, I. (1992) *Escherichia coli* serotyping and disease in man and animals. *Canadian Journal of Microbiology* 38, 699–704.

Ørskov, F., Ørskov, I., Sutton, A., Schneerson, R., Lin, W., Egan, W., Hoff, G.E. and Robbins, J.B. (1979) Form variation in *Escherichia coli* K1: determined by O-acetylation of the capsular polysaccharide. *Journal of Experimental Medicine* 149, 669–685.

Ørskov, F., Sharma, V. and Ørskov, I. (1984) Influence of growth temperature on the development of *Escherichia coli* polysaccharide K-antigens. *Journal of General Microbiology* 130, 2681–2684.

Ørskov, I., Sharma, V. and Ørskov, F. (1976) Genetic mapping of the K1 and K4 antigens (L) of *Escherichia coli*. Non allelism of K(L) antigens with K antigens of O8:K27(A), O8:K8(L) and O9:K57(B). *Acta Pathologica et Microbiologica Scandinavica Section B* 84, 125–131.

Palva, L. and Mäkelä, P.H. (1980) Lipopolysaccharide heterogeneity in *Salmonella typhimurium* analyzed by sodium dodecyl sulfate/polyacrylamide gel electrophoresis. *European Journal of Biochemistry* 107, 137–143.

Parker, C.T., Kloser, A.W., Schnaitman, C.A., Stein, M.A., Gottesman, S. and Gibson, B.W. (1992) Role of the *rfa*G and *rfa*P genes in determining the lipopolysaccharide core structure and cell surface properties of *Escherichia coli* K-12. *Journal of Bacteriology* 174, 2425–2538.

Pavelka, M.J., Wright, L.F. and Silver, R.P. (1991) Identification of two genes, *kps*M and *kps*T, in region 3 of the polysialic acid gene cluster of *Escherichia coli* K1. *Journal of Bacteriology* 173, 4603–4610.

Pazzani, C., Rosenow, C., Boulnois, G.J., Bronner, D., Jann, K. and Roberts, I.S. (1993) Molecular analysis of region 1 of *Escherichia coli* K5 antigen gene cluster: a region encoding proteins involved in cell surface expression of capsular polysaccharide. *Journal of Bacteriology* 175, 5978–5983.

Pegues, J.C., Chen, L., Gordon, A.W., Ding, L. and Coleman, W.G.J. (1990) Cloning, expression, and characterization of the *Escherichia coli* K-12 *rfa*D gene. *Journal of Bacteriology* 172, 4652–4660.

Peterson, A.A. and McGroarty, E.J. (1985) High-molecular-weight components in lipopolysaccharides of *Salmonella typhimurium*, *Salmonella minnesota*, and *Escherichia coli*. *Journal of Bacteriology* 162, 738–745.

Pluschke, G. and Achtman, M. (1984) Degree of antibody-independent activation of the classical complement pathway by K1 *Escherichia coli* differs with O-antigen type and correlates with virulence of meningitis in newborns. *Infection and Immunity* 43, 684–692.

Pluschke, G. and Achtman, M. (1985) Antibodies to O-antigen of lipopolysaccharide are protective against neonatal infection with *Escherichia coli*. *Infection and Immunity* 49, 365–370.

Pluschke, G., Mercer, A., Kusecek, B., Pohl, A. and Achtman, M. (1983) Induction of bacteremia in newborn rats by *Escherichia coli* K1 is correlated with only certain O (lipopolysaccharide) antigen types. *Infection and Immunity* 39, 599–608.

Porat, R., Johns, M.A. and McCabe, W.R. (1987) Selective pressures and lipopolysaccharide subunits as determinants of resistance of clinical isolates of Gram-negative bacilli to human serum. *Infection and Immunity* 55, 320–328.

Porat, R., Mosseri, R., Kaplan, E., Johns, M.A. and Shibolet, S. (1992) Distribution of polysaccharide side chains of lipopolysaccharide determine resistance of *Escherichia coli* to the bactericidal activity of serum. *Journal of Infectious Diseases* 165, 953–956.

Pradel, E. and Schnaitman, C.A. (1991) Effect of *rfa*H (*sfr*B) and temperature on expression of *rfa* genes of *Escherichia coli* K-12. *Journal of Bacteriology* 173, 6428–6431.

Pradel, E., Parker, C.T. and Schnaitman, C.A. (1992) Structures of the *rfa*B, *rfa*I, *rfa*J, and *rfa*S genes of *Escherichia coli* K-12 and their roles in assembly of the lipopolysaccharide core. *Journal of Bacteriology* 174, 4736–4745.

Proctor, R.A., Will, J.A., El Burhop, K. and Raetz, C.R.H. (1986) Protection of mice against lethal endotoxemia by a lipid A precursor. *Infection and Immunity* 52, 905–907.

Qureshi, N. and Takayama, K. (1990) Structure and function of lipid A. In: Iglewski, B.H. and Clark, V.H. (eds) *Molecular Basis of Bacterial Pathogenesis.* Academic Press, New York, pp. 319–338.

Qureshi, N., Takayama, K. and Kurtz, R. (1991a) Diphosphoryl lipid A obtained from the nontoxic lipopolysaccharide of *Rhodopseudomonas sphaeroides* is an endotoxin antagonist in mice. *Infection and Immunity* 59, 441–444.

Qureshi, N., Takayama, K., Meyer, K.C., Kirkland, T.N., Bush, C.A., Chen, L., Wang, R. and Cotter, R.J. (1991b) Chemical reduction of 3-oxo and unsaturated groups in fatty acids of diphosphoryl lipid A from the lipopolysaccharide of *Rhodopseudomonas sphaeroides*. Comparison of biological properties before and after reduction. *Journal of Biological Chemistry* 257, 6532–6538.

Raetz, C.R.H. (1990) Biochemistry of endotoxins. *Annual Reviews in Biochemistry* 59, 129–170.

Ramadori, G., Meyer zum Buschefelde, K.-H., Tobias, P.S., Mathison, J.C. and Ulevitch, R.J. (1990) Biosynthesis of lipopolysaccharide-binding protein in rabbit hepatocytes. *Pathobiology* 58, 89–94.

Remick, D.G., Kunkel, R.G., Larrick, J.W. and Kunkel, S.L. (1987) Acute *in vivo* effects of human recombinant tumor necrosis factor. *Laboratory Investigation* 56, 583–590.

Robbins, J.B., McCracken, G.H., Gotschlich, E.C., Ørskov, F., Ørskov, I. and Hanson, L.A. (1974) *Escherichia coli* K1 capsular polysaccharide associated with neonatal meningitis. *New England Journal of Medicine* 290, 1216–1221.

Roberts, I., Mountford, R., High, N., Bitter-Suermann, D., Jann, K.K.T. and Boulnois, G. (1986) Molecular cloning and analysis of genes for production of K5, K7, K12, and K92 capsular polysaccharides in *Escherichia coli*. *Journal of Bacteriology* 168, 1228–1233.

Roberts, I.S., Mountford, R., Hodge, R., Jann, K. and Boulnois, G.J. (1988) Common organization of gene clusters for production of different capsular polysaccharides (K antigens) in *Escherichia coli*. *Journal of Bacteriology* 170, 1305–1310.

Rodríguez-Aparicio, L.B., Reglero, A., Ortiz, A.I. and Luengo, J.M. (1988) A protein–sialyl polymer complex involved in colominic acid biosynthesis. *Biochemical Journal* 251, 589–596.

Rohr, T.E. and Troy, F.A. (1980) Structure and biosynthesis of surface polymers containing polysialic acid in *Escherichia coli*. *Journal of Biological Chemistry* 255, 2332–2342.

Roncero, C. and Casadaban, M.J. (1992) Genetic analysis of the genes involved in synthesis of the lipopolysaccharide core in *Escherichia coli* K-12: three operons in the *rfa* locus. *Journal of Bacteriology* 174, 3250–3260.

Schmidt, M.A. and Jann, K. (1982) Phospholipid substitution of capsular (K) polysaccharide antigens from *Escherichia coli* causing extraintestinal infections. *Federation of European Microbiological Societies Microbiology Letters* 14, 69–74.

Schmidt, G., Jann, B. and Jann, K. (1969) Immunochemistry of R lipopolysaccharides of *Escherichia coli*. Different core regions in the lipopolysaccharides of O group 8. *European Journal of Biochemistry* 10, 501–510.

Schmidt, G., Mayer, H. and Mäkelä, P.H. (1976) Presence of *rfe* genes in *Escherichia coli*: their participation in the biosynthesis of O antigen and enterobacterial common antigen. *Journal of Bacteriology* 127, 755–762.

Schmidt, G., Jann, B., Jann, K., Ørskov, I. and Ørskov, F. (1977) Genetic determinants of the synthesis of the polysaccharide capsular antigen K27(A) of *Escherichia coli*. *Journal of General Microbiology* 100, 355–361.

Schnaitman, C.A. and Klena, J.D. (1993) Genetics of lipopolysaccharide biosynthesis in enteric bacteria. *Microbiological reviews* 57, 655–682.

Schumann, R.R., Leong, S.R., Flaggs, G.W., Gray, P.W., Wright, S.D.,

Mathison, J.C., Tobias, P.S. and Ulevitch, R.J. (1990) Structure and function of lipopolysaccharide binding protein. *Science* 249, 1429–1433.

Schütt, C., Schilling, T., Grunwald, U., Schönfeld, W. and Krüger, C. (1992) Endotoxin-neutralizing capacity of soluble CD14. *Research in Immunology* 143, 71–78.

Sherry, B. and Cerami, A. (1988) Cachectin/tumor necrosis factor exerts endocrine, paracrine, and autocrine control of inflammatory responses. *Journal of Cell Biology* 107, 1269–1277.

Silver, R.P. and Vimr, E.R. (1990) Polysialic acid capsules in *Escherchia coli* K1. In: Iglewski, B.H. and Clark, V.L. (eds) *Molecular Basis of Bacterial Pathogenesis.* Academic Press, New York, pp. 39–60.

Silver, R.P., Finn, C.W., Vann, W.F., Aaronson, W., Schneerson, R., Kretschmer, P.J. and Garon, C.F. (1981) Molecular cloning of the K1 capsular polysaccharide genes of *E. coli. Nature (London)* 289, 696–698.

Silver, R.P., Vann, W.F. and Aaronson, W. (1984) Genetic and molecular analyses of *Escherichia* K1 antigen genes. *Journal of Bacteriology* 157, 568–575.

Silver, R.P., Aaronson, W. and Vann, W.F. (1987) Translocation of capsular polysaccharides in pathogenic strains of *Escherichia coli* requires a 60-kilodalton periplasmic protein. *Journal of Bacteriology* 169, 5489–5495.

Smith, A.N., Boulnois, G.J. and Roberts, I.S. (1990) Molecular analysis of the *Escherichia coli* K5 *kps* locus: identification and characterization of an inner-membrane capsular polysaccharide transport system. *Molecular Microbiology* 4, 1863–1869.

Stawski, G., Nielsen, L., Ørskov, F. and Ørskov, I. (1990) Serum sensitivity of a diversity of *Escherichia* antigenic reference strains. Correlation with an LPS variation phenomenon. *Acta Pathologica Microbiologica et Immunologica Scandinavica* 98, 828–838.

Steenbergen, S.M. and Vimr, E.R. (1990) Mechanism of polysialic acid chain elongation in *Escherichia coli* K1. *Molecular Microbiology* 4, 603–611.

Steenbergen, S.M., Wrona, T.J. and Vimr, E.R. (1992) Functional analysis of the sialyltransferase complexes in *Escherichia coli* K1 and K92. *Journal of Bacteriology* 174, 1099–1108.

Stendahl, O. and Edebo, L. (1972) Phagocytosis of mutants of *Salmonella typhimurium* by rabbit polymorphonuclear cells. *Acta Pathologica et Microbiologica Scandinavica Section B* 80, 481–488.

Stephens, K.E., Ishikaza, A., Larrick, J.W. and Raffin, T.A. (1988) Tumor necrosis factor causes pulmonary permeability and edema. *American Review of Respiratory Diseases* 137, 1364–1370.

Stevens, P., Huang, S.N.-Y., Welch, W.D. and Young, L.S. (1978) Restricted complement activation by *Escherichia coli* with the K1 capsular serotype: a possible role in pathogenicity. *Journal of Immunology* 121, 2174–2180.

Stevens, P., Young, S. and Adamu, Ṣ. (1983) Opsonization of various capsular (K) *E. coli* by the alternative complement pathway. *Immunology* 50, 497–502.

Stout, V. and Gottesman, S. (1990) RcsB and RcsC: a two-component regulator of capsule synthesis in *Escherichia coli* K-12. *Journal of Bacteriology* 172, 659–669.

Stout, V., Torres-Cabassa, A., Maurizi, M.R., Gutnick, D. and Gottesman, S. (1991) RcsA, an unstable positive regulator of capsular polysaccharide synthesis. *Journal of Bacteriology* 173, 1738–1747.

Sutherland, I.W. and Norval, M. (1970) The synthesis of exopolysaccharide by *Klebsiella aerogenes* membrane preparations and the involvement of lipid intermediates. *Biochemical Journal* 120, 567–576.

Takayama, K., Qureshi, N., Beutler, B. and Kirkland, T.N. (1989) Diphosphoryl lipid A from *Rhodobacter sphaeroides* ATCC 17023 blocks induction of cachectin in macrophages by lipopolysaccharide. *Infection and Immunity* 57, 1336–1338.

Taylor, P.W. (1983) Bactericidal and bacteriolytic activity of serum against gram-negative bacteria. *Microbiological Reviews* 47, 46–83.

Taylor, P.W. and Robinson, M.K. (1980) Determinants that increase the serum resistance of *Escherichia coli. Infection and Immunity* 29, 278–280.

Teng, N.N.H., Kaplan, H.S., Hebert, J.M., Moore, C., Douglas, H., Wunderlich, A. and Braude, A.I. (1985) Protection against gram-negative bacteremia and endotoxemia with human monoclonal IgM antibodies. *Proceedings of the National Academy of Sciences of the United States of America* 82, 1790–1794.

Tobias, P.S., McAdam, K.P.W.J., Soldau, K. and Ulevitch, R.J. (1985) Control of lipopolysaccharide–high density lipoprotein interactions by an acute-phase reactant in human serum. *Infection and Immunity* 50, 73–76.

Tobias, P.S., Soldau, K. and Ulevitch, R.J. (1986) Isolation of a lipopolysaccharide-binding acute phase reactant from rabbit serum. *Journal of Experimental Medicine* 164, 777–793.

Tobias, P.S., Soldau, K. and Ulevitch, R.J. (1989) Identification of a lipid A binding site in the acute phase reactant lipopolysaccharide binding protein. *Journal of Biological Chemistry* 264, 10867–10871.

Tomás, J.M., Ciurana, B., Benedí, V.J. and Juarez, A. (1988) Role of lipopolysaccharide and complement in susceptibility of *Escherichia coli* and *Salmonella typhimurium* to non-immune serum. *Journal of General Microbiology* 134, 1009–1016.

Tracey, K.J., Beutler, B., Lowry, S.F., Merryweather, J., Wolpe, S., Milsark, I.W., Hariri, R.J., Fahey, T.J.I., Zentella, A., Albert, J.D. *et al.* (1986) Shock and tissue injury induced by recombinant human cachetin. *Science* 234, 470–474.

Tracey, K.J., Fong, Y., Hesse, D.G., Manogue, K.R., Lee, A.T. and Kuo, G.C. (1987a) Anti-cachetin/TNF monoclonal antibodies prevent septic shock during lethal bacteraemia. *Nature (London)* 330, 662–664.

Tracey, K.J., Lowry, S.F., Fahey, T.J.I., Albert, J.D., Fong, Y., Hesse, D., Beutler, B., Manogur, K.R., Calvano, S., Wei, H. *et al.* (1987b) Cachetin/tumor necrosis factor induces lethal shock and stress hormone responses in the dog. *Surgery, Gynaecology and Obstetrics* 164, 415–422.

Treon, S.P., Thomas, P. and Broitman, S.A. (1993) Lipopolysaccharide (LPS) processing by Kupffer cells releases a modified LPS with increased hepatocyte binding and decreased tumor necrosis factor-α stimulatory capacity. *Proceedings of the Society for Experimental Biology and Medicine* 202, 153–158.

Trisler, P. and Gottesman, S. (1984) *lon* transcriptional regulation of genes necessary for capsular polysaccharide synthesis in *Escherichia coli* K-12. *Journal of Bacteriology* 160, 184–191.

Troy, F.A. (1992) Polysialylation: from bacteria to brains. *Glycobiology* 2, 5–23.

Troy, F.A. and McCloskey, M.A. (1979) Role of a membranous sialyltransferase complex in the synthesis of surface polymers containing polysialic acid in *Escherichia coli.* Temperature-induced alteration in the assembly process. *Journal of Biological Chemistry* 254, 7377–7387.

Troy, F.A., Frerman, F.E. and Heath, E.C. (1971) The biosynthesis of capsular polysaccharide in *Klebsiella aerogenes. Journal of Biological Chemistry* 246, 118–133.

Troy, F.A., Vijay, I.K. and Tesche, N. (1975) Role of undecaprenol phosphate in synthesis of polymers containing sialic acid in *Escherichia coli. Journal of Biological Chemistry* 250, 156–163.

Valvano, M.A. (1992) Pathogenicity and molecular genetics of O-specific side-chain lipopolysaccharides of *Escherichia coli. Canadian Journal of Microbiology* 38, 711–719.

Van Dijk, W.C., Verbrugh, H.A., van der Tol, M.E., Peters, R. and Verhoef, J. (1979) Role of *Escherichia coli* K capsular antigens during complement activation, C3 fixation, and opsonization. *Infection and Immunity* 25, 603–609.

Vermeulen, C., Cross, A., Byrne, W.R. and Zollinger, W. (1988) Quantitative relationship between capsular content and killing of K1-encapsulated *Escherichia coli. Infection and Immunity* 56, 2723–2730.

Vimr, E.R. (1991) Map position and genomic organization of the *kps* cluster for polysialic acid synthesis in *Escherichia coli* K1. *Journal of Bacteriology* 173, 1335–1338.

Vimr, E.R., Bergstrom, R., Steenbergen, S.M., Boulnois, G. and Roberts, I. (1992) Homology among *Escherichia coli* K1 and K92 polysialyltransferases. *Journal of Bacteriology* 174, 5127–5131.

Weisgerber, C. and Jann, K. (1982) Glucosyldiphosphoundecaprenol, the mannose acceptor in the synthesis of the O9 antigen of *Escherichia coli.* Biosynthesis and characterization. *European Journal of Biochemistry* 127, 165–168.

Weisgerber, C. and Troy, F.A. (1990) Biosynthesis of the polysialic acid capsule in *Escherichia coli* K1. The endogenous acceptor of polysialic acid is a membrane protein of 20 kDa. *Journal of Biological Chemistry* 265, 1578–1587.

Weisgerber, C., Jann, B. and Jann, K. (1984) Biosynthesis of the O9 antigen of *Escherichia coli.* Core structure of *rfe* mutant as indication of assembly mechanism. *European Journal of Biochemistry* 140, 553–556.

Weiss, J., Beckerdite-Quagliata, S. and Elsbach, P. (1980) Resistance of Gram-negative bacteria to purified bactericidal leukocyte proteins. Relation to binding and bacterial lipopolysaccharide structure. *Journal of Clinical Investigation* 65, 619–628.

Weiss, J., Hutzler, M. and Kao, L. (1986) Environmental modulation of lipopolysaccharide chain length alters the sensitivity of *Escherichia coli* to the neutrophil bactericidal/permeability-increasing protein. *Infection and Immunity* 51, 594–599.

Whitfield, C. and Valvano, M.A. (1993) Biosynthesis and expression of cell surface polysaccharides in gram-negative bacteria. *Advances in Microbial Physiology* 35, 135–246.

Whitfield, C., Schoenhals, G. and Graham, L. (1989) Mutants of *Escherichia coli* O9:K30 with altered synthesis and expression of the capsular K antigen. *Journal of General Microbiology* 135, 2589–2599.

Woisetschläger, M. and Högenauer, G. (1987) The *kds*A gene coding for 3-deoxy-D-manno-octulosonic acid 8-phosphate synthetase is part of an operon in *Escherichia coli. Molecular and General Genetics* 207, 369–373.

Wright, S.D., Tobias, P.S., Ulevitch, R.J. and Ramos, R.A. (1989) Lipopolysaccharide (LPS) binding protein opsonizes LPS-bearing particles for recognition by a novel receptor on macrophages. *Journal of Experimental Medicine* 170, 1231–1241.

Wright, S.D., Ramso, R.A., Tobias, P.S., Ulevitch, R.J. and Mathison, J.C. (1990) CD14, a receptor for complexes of lipopolysaccharide (LPS) and LPS binding protein. *Science* 249, 1431–1433.

Ziegler, E.J., McCutchan, J.A., Fierer, J., Glauser, M.P., Sadoff, J.C., Douglas, H. and Braude, A.I. (1982) Treatment of gram-negative bacteremia and shock with human antiserum to a mutant *Escherichia coli. New England Journal of Medicine* 307, 1225–1230.

Ziegler, E.J., Fischer, C.J. Jr, Sprung, C.L. Straube, R.C., Sadoff, J.C., Foulke, G.E., Wortel, C.H., Fink. M.P., Dellinger, R.P., Teng, N.N.H., Allen, I.E., Berger, H.J., Knatterud, G.L., LoBuglio, A.F., Smith, C.R. and the HA-1A Sepsis Study Group (1991) Treatment of gram-negative bacteremia and septic shock with HA-1A human monoclonal antibody against endotoxin. *New England Journal of Medicine* 324, 429–436.

Zuckerman, S.H. and Qureshi, N. (1992) *In vivo* inhibition of lipopolysaccharide-induced lethality and tumor necrosis factor synthesis by *Rhodobacter sphaeroides* diphosphoryl lipid A is dependent on corticosteroid induction. *Infection and Immunity* 60, 2581–2587.

Outer Membrane Proteins 18

R.E.W. Hancock and K. Piers
Department of Microbiology and Immunology, University of British Columbia, Vancouver, BC, Canada V6T 1W5

Introduction

The outer membranes of Gram-negative bacteria are intimately involved in the lifestyles of these organisms, including their lifestyle within a human or animal host. Although outer membranes are not often named as virulence determinants, they have several roles that merit such a designation including those in exclusion of bile salts, resistance to proteases and other enzymes, resistance to serum bactericidal killing, excretion of other bacterial virulence factors, limitation of antibiotic uptake, uptake of important nutrients in short supply in the host, endotoxicity, and anchoring of adhesins and flagella (Nikaido and Vaara, 1985; Inouye, 1987; Hancock and Bell, 1989; Hancock, 1991). In this chapter we will summarize the properties of the outer membrane proteins of *E. coli* with special attention to those important in virulence and/or growth *in vivo*. Only a limited discussion of regulation or mechanisms of secretion will be included and the readers are referred to more detailed reviews on these subjects (Igo *et al.*, 1990; Mizuno and Mizushima, 1990; Pugsley, 1993). *E. coli* was the prototype for the first investigations on outer membranes and is by far the best studied of all organisms. For detailed discussion of outer membranes in other organisms three recent reviews may be consulted (Nikaido and Vaara, 1985; Hancock, 1991; Hancock *et al.*, 1993).

Outer Membrane Structure

The *E. coli* outer membrane constitutes a typical asymmetrical bilayer studded with proteins (Fig. 18.1; Hancock *et al.*, 1993). The outer

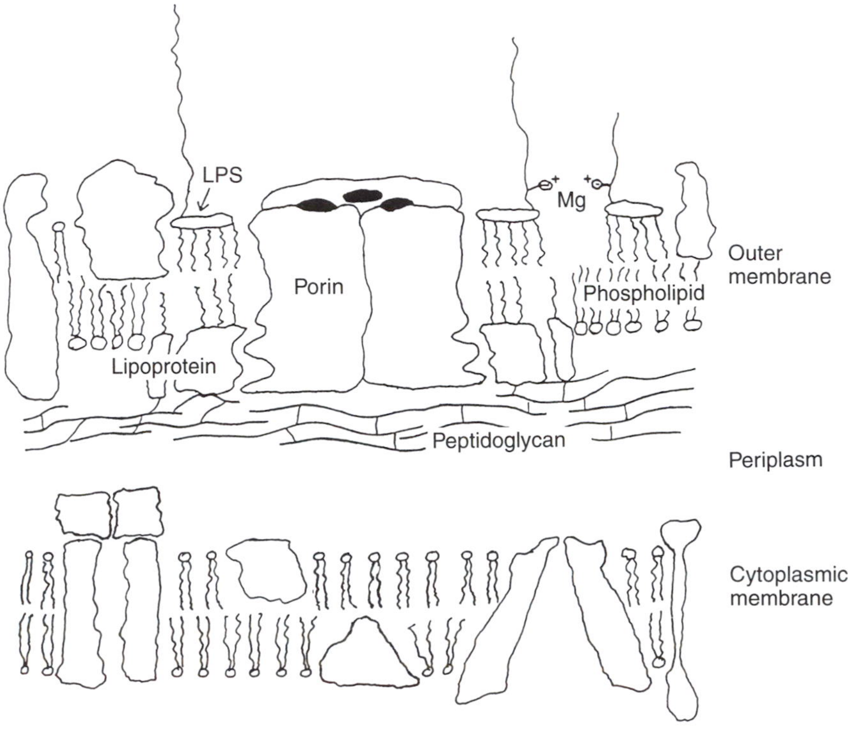

Fig. 18.1. Schematic diagram of the Gram-negative outer membrane.

monolayer of this asymmetrical bilayer contains the glycolipid molecule lipopolysaccharide (LPS) (discussed in Chapter 17), while the inner monolayer contains phospholipids, primarily phosphatidyl ethanolamine, phosphatidyl glycerol and cardiolipin (Cronan, 1979). This partitioning of lipidic species is almost complete as demonstrated by chemical and enzyme accessibility studies, immuno-electron microscopy, and freeze fracture studies (Avrameas, 1969; Funahara and Nikaido, 1980). The negatively charged LPS in the outer monolayer and its tight non-covalent association with itself via divalent cation crossbridging and with proteins via hydrophilic, charge-charge and hydrophobic forces (Nikaido and Vaara, 1985; Hancock, 1991; Hancock *et al.*, 1993), confer several important properties on the outer membrane. These include exclusion of many hydrophobic substances, such as dyes, detergents and bile salts, and resistance to attack by phospholipases and other enzymes. In addition, the uptake of cationic substances including antibiotics, such as polymyxins, aminoglycosides and azithromycin, and antibacterial peptides, such as defensins and bactenicins, involves a self-promoted uptake pathway that is initiated by initial interaction of these cationic peptides at the divalent cation crossbridging sites on LPS (reviewed in Hancock and Bell, 1989; Hancock, 1991).

Proteins constitute nearly 60% by weight of the *E. coli* outer membrane. The predominant protein species are present at a copy number of 5×10^4 to 2×10^5 polypeptides per cell and are termed 'major' outer membrane proteins (Lugtenberg *et al.*, 1975). The major outer membrane proteins of *E. coli* cells grown on rich broth are OmpF, OmpC, OmpA and Lpp. However other proteins can become predominant under specific growth conditions or when *E. coli* harbours phages or plasmids that encode these proteins (see below). In addition to the major proteins, 50 or more other polypeptides can be observed in lower copy number on two-dimensional sodium dodecyl sulfate polyacrylamide gel electrophoresis (SDS-PAGE). Many of these proteins are exposed on the surface of the outer membrane as judged by their function as phage or colicin receptors (Table 18.1), or their reactivity in intact cells with antibodies. However, this must be qualified since such assessments of surface localization are usually performed in *E. coli* K-12, which is a rough, LPS O-antigen-deficient variant, and such variants are rarely found *in vivo*. *E. coli* strains derived from infections, containing smooth LPS and/or capsules, fail to react with a variety of phages, colicins or protein-specific antibodies (see below).

Table 18.1. Functions of *E. coli* outer membrane proteins.

Function	Major components
Non-specific passage of small hydrophilic compounds	OmpF, OmpC
Specific uptake of hydrophilic substances	FepA, FecA, Fiu, FhuA, BtuB, LamB, Tsx
Uptake of fatty acids	FadL
Structural role	OmpA, Lpp, ExcC, OmpH
Protein excretion	TolC
Export and anchoring of surface appendages	FimD, FlgH
Enzymes	OmpT, PldA
Receptors for phages	FhuA, BtuB, LamB, FadL, OmpC, OmpF, OmpA, Tsx
Receptors for colicins	FepA, FhuA, Cir, BtuB, OmpF, Tsx
F pilus mating aggregate stabilization	OmpA

Outer Membrane Protein Functions

Outer membrane proteins have a variety of known functions, as summarized in Table 18.1. The first functions described were receptor functions for phages and bacteriocins (Konisky, 1979). However, since such functions would result in eventual cell death, it seemed unlikely that these were the major roles of the outer membrane proteins. Indeed, each of these receptors has now been ascribed an alternative function. For example, the receptors for phages T6 (Tsx) and λ (LamB) function in nucleoside and maltose/maltodextrin uptake, respectively, whilst the receptors for colicins B and E1 function in ferri-enterobactin and vitamin B_{12} uptake, respectively. In general, *E. coli* outer membrane proteins serve the following functions: the general porins mediate passage of hydrophilic solutes in a size-dependent fashion; the substrate-specific porins have a binding site within their channels that imparts selectivity for a given substrate; they may have roles in cell shape and structural stability; and specific proteins possess enzymatic activities, are involved in secretion and/or anchoring of surface appendages, or mediate excretion of haemolysin into the environment (Table 18.2). In addition, outer membrane proteins expressed from plasmid or lysogenic phage genes can have functions of importance in pathogenesis, including adherence and complement resistance (Table 18.3).

Outer Membrane Proteins

E. coli K-12 has by far the best characterized outer membrane of any organism, with 25 chromosomally encoded proteins for which the genes have been cloned and sequenced, and two other genetically defined proteins (Table 18.2). This section discusses the known properties of these proteins.

General porins

Porins represent a ubiquitous class of outer membrane proteins that form channels across the outer membrane (Hancock, 1986; Benz *et al.*, 1988). They are highly conserved in both general structure and function, although their primary sequences vary substantially from organism to organism (Jeanteur *et al.*, 1993). Porins are characterized as outer membrane proteins that are capable of forming channels when reconstituted into model membrane systems (Table 18.4). These proteins have a number of properties in common:

1. They all contain substantial β-sheet structure.
2. They have similar molecular weights (31 000–48 000).

Table 18.2. Chromosomally encoded outer membrane proteins of *E. coli*.

Name	Mol. wt	DNA seq acc^{N} no.	Map position	Function	Regulation	Other[a]
Eae	102,000	Z11541	—	Attachment and effacement of epithelial layers	By plasmid pMAR5	MW94
FimD	97,260	X51655	98.1′	Required for surface localization of type 1 fimbriae	Fim B/E; phase variation	—
Fiu	83,000	—	18′	Ferric iron uptake – scavenger pathway	Low iron derepressible (*fur*)	MW83
FecA	81,718	M20981	93′	Ferric citrate uptake (*fur*), citrate inducible	Low iron derepressible	MW80.5
FepA	79,908	J04216	13.6′	Ferric-enterobactin receptor/ permeation; colicins B,D receptor; gated porin	Low iron derepressible (*fur*)	MW81
FhuA	78,992	XO5810 M12486	3.7′	Ferri-ferrichrome receptor/ permeation; phages T1, ϕ80, T5 receptor; colicin M receptor	Low iron derepressible (*fur*)	MW78
FhuE	77,453	X17615	24.7′	Ferri-coprogen, ferri-rhodoturulic acid, ferrioxamine B receptor/ permeation	Low iron derepressible (*fur*)	MW76
Cir	67,179	J04229	46.4′	Ferric iron uptake-savenger pathway; colicin Ia, Ib receptor	Low iron derepressible (*fur*)	MW74

Table 18.2. *continued*

Name	Mol. wt	DNA seq acc[N] no.	Map position	Function	Regulation	Other[a]
BtuB	66,412	M10112	89.7′	Vitamin B12 receptor/ permeation; phage BF23 receptor; colicins E1, E2, E3 receptor	—	MW60
TolC	66,000	X54049	66.4′	Required for haemolysin secretion	Constitutive minor protein	MW66, TRI
Hag	51,172	M14358	42.4′	Flagellin subunit	Constitutive	MW55; HM
LamB	47,932	V00298	91.5′	Maltodextrin-specific porin; phages λ, K10 receptor	Maltose induced (malT) PG	MW55, TRI, PG
FadL	45,969	M37714	50.6′	Fatty acid binding/ permeation; phage T2 receptor	Fatty acid induced, glucose repressed	MW43, HM
K	40,000	—	—	General porin	Found in encapsulated strains	MW40, TRI, PG
NmpC	39,500	M13457	12.6′	General porin (defective Tsr′ encoded)	Normally inactivated by IS5 insertion	MW39.5, TRI, PG
OmpC	38,307	K00541	47.7′	General porin, Phage Tulb receptor, Phage K20, K21, K22 receptor	High salt induced (*envZ*, *OmpR*); acid pH	MW37, TRI, PG
OmpG (CE1248)	37,000	—	29′	General porin – weakly expressed	*Cog*	MW37, TRI, PG
PhoE	36,782	X00786	5.7′	General porin – anion selective (*phoB*, *phoR*, *phoM*)	Low phosphate induced	MW38, TRI, PG

OmpF	35,705	J01655	20.7′	General porin, colicin N receptor, phage Tul receptor temperature induced (*mic* F)	Low salt induced (*envZ*, *OmpR*); high growth	MW36, TRI, PG
OmpT	35,567	X06903	12.9′	Endoprotease	Constitutive	MW37
OmpA	35,159	J01654	21.7′	Porin; structural role – cell shape, stability; Phage K3, Tull receptor; stabilizes F pilus mating aggregates	Constitutive	MW33, HM, PG (TRI)
Tsx	31,418	M57685	9′	Nucleoside-specific porin; albicidin uptake; phage T6 receptor, colicin K receptor	Dual promoters: (1) cAMP + CAP induced; *cytR* repressed; (2) *desR* repressed	MW28
PldA	30,809	X00780 X02143	86.1′	Phospholipase A	Constitutive low level	MW27
FlgH	27,000	—	24′	Flagella L-ring	—	MW27
Pal	18,748	X65796	17′ (*excC*)	Outer membrane stability	Constitutive	MW17, PG, LP
OmpH (HlpA)	15,692	M21118	38′	LPS binding protein – possible structural role	Constitutive	MW17
Lpp	6,961	J01645	36.7′	Structure, osmotic stability	Constitutive	MW9, LP
OmsB	6,949	M22859	28.0′	Unknown	High osmolarity inducible	MW8, LP

[a] Code for other:

MW33 = apparent mol. wt = 33 K after boiling prior to SDS-PAGE;
TRI = trimers observed when run on SDS-PAGE;
(TRI) = evidence of native trimers but not observed on SDS-PAGE;
HM = heat modifiable (moves from low apparent molecular weight position to high apparent molecular weight position upon heating);
PG = peptidoglycan associated;
LP = lipoprotein.

Table 18.3. Plasmid and phage encoded outer membrane proteins of *E. coli.*

Name	Mol. wt	DNA seq acc^{N} no.	Encoded by	Function	Regulation	Other[a]
FanD	84,500	X13560	pK99	Export/expression of pK99 functions	—	—
FaeD	82,100	X56003	pK88ab	Export of K88ab fimbrial subunits	—	—
PapC	81,000	X61239	pF13	Export/expression of P fimbriae	—	—
lutA	74,000	X05814	pColV	Ferric aerobactin receptor/ permeation (*fur*)	Low iron derepressible	MW74
ScrY	55,408	S44133	pUR400	Sucrose/maltodextrin specific porin; general porin	Sucrose induced (*scR*)	MW55, TRI
TraB	55,000	—	F	F pilus assembly/biosynthesis	—	—
Lc(HK253)	39,000	—	ΦHK253	General porin; lambdoid phage receptor	Growth temperature	MW39, TRI
Lc(PA102)	36,500	JO2580	ΦPA102	General porin	—	MW36.5 TRI, PG

TraT	25,000	JO1769	pR100	Complement resistance; surface exclusion	—	LP
	25,000	X52553	pR6–5	Surface exclusion	—	LP
	25,000	M13465	pED208	Surface exclusion	—	LP
	26,017	X14566	F	Complement resistance; surface exclusion	—	LP
TraF	25,000	M20787	F	F pilus assembly/biosynthesis	—	—
TraK	24,000	X54458 X54459[b]	F	F pilus assembly/biosynthesis	—	—
TraP	23,500	—	F	Function unknown	—	—
TraL	10,350	K01147	F	F pilus assembly/biosynthesis	—	—
BRP	2,900	X04466	pCloDF13 (geneH)	Bacteriocin release protein	—	LP
		J01566	pColE1 (*kil*)	Bacteriocin release protein	—	LP
		M29885	pColE2 (*cel*B)	Bacteriocin release protein	—	LP
		J01574	pColE3 (*hic*)	Bacteriocin release protein	—	LP
		Xo2391	pColA (*cal*)	Bacteriocin release protein	—	LP

[a] See Table 18.2 for codes.
[b] Genes from related plasmids.

3. They form native trimers in the outer membrane as assessed by cross-linking studies or crystallography.
4. All contain channels that allow the passage of ions.

The two possible exceptions to these rules are an as yet uncharacterized voltage-sensitive channel (Buechner *et al.*, 1990) and the Tsx protein (Bremer *et al.*, 1990), both of which have rather unusual properties.

The general porins lack known substrate specificity (Hancock, 1986; Nikaido, 1992). Five of these have had their sequences defined genetically, namely OmpF, OmpC, PhoE, NmpC and Lc(PA-2) (Tables 18.2 and 18.3). This group of proteins shares the following structural properties: they have sequence similarity with about 56% identical amino acids, they are immunologically cross-reactive, they have very similar molecular weights of 35 000–40 000, and they form trimers that are resistant to denaturation by the detergent SDS. In addition, their functional properties are quite analogous. Model membrane studies have indicated that they have similar channels, with single channel conductances ranging from 1.5 to 2 nS in 1 M KCl solution, and weak ion selectivity (Table 18.4),

Table 18.4. Conductance characteristics of *E. coli* porins.

Porin	Growth conditions favouring production	Single channel conductance in 1 M KCl (n^S)	Selectivity (pK^+/pCl^-)	Binding
OmpF	Low salt	~ 1.9	Cation (3.7)	—[a]
OmpC	High salt	1.5	Cation (26)	—
PhoE	Low phosphate	1.8	Anion (0.33)	—
OmpG (CE1248)	Cog mutation	2.5	Cation (12.5)	—
NmpC	IS5B deletion	1.8	Anion (0.27)	—
OmpA	Constitutive	0.7	Anion (0.7)	—
LamB	Maltose	0.16	Cation	Maltose/ maltodextrins
Tsx	Various	0.01	Cation (4.2)	Bases/ nucleosides
Voltage sensitive	—[b]	0.6	Cation	—
Lc(PA-2)	Lysogeny	~ 2.0	Cation (6.5)	—
Lc(HK253)	Lysogeny	2.5	Cation (12)	—
K	Plasmid	1.8	ND	—
ScrY	Plasmid	1.4	Cation (8.6)	Sucrose maltodextrins

[a] No specific binding site.
[b] Actual protein has not been isolated.

indicating that all form large water-filled channels. Other porins, OmpG, protein K and Lc (HK253) share similar properties and may thus be related (Table 18.4).

The porins that have been investigated in the greatest detail are OmpF, OmpC and PhoE. OmpF and OmpC can be observed in the outer membranes of *E. coli* grown *in vitro* on many laboratory media. However, their production is influenced by medium constituents. The best studied of these is the medium osmolarity; high osmolarity favours OmpC production, whereas low osmolarity favours OmpF production. Osmolarity is sensed by the transmembrane sensor EnvZ which phosphorylates the OmpR activator, causing it to bind to the OmpC promotor and stimulate transcription (Igo *et al.*, 1990; Mizuno and Mizushima, 1990). Other regulatory elements include the micF antisense RNA which is transcribed from the upstream sequences of the *ompC* gene, and which down-regulates OmpF production when OmpC production is stimulated by high osmolarity or by changes in other environmental conditions (Andersen *et al.*, 1989). This inverse regulation is important since the high osmolarity found *in vivo* has been proposed to result in almost exclusive synthesis of OmpC (Nikaido and Vaara, 1985). Since OmpC has a smaller channel than OmpF (Nikaido and Rosenberg, 1983; Benz *et al.*, 1985) it has been proposed that this would restrict uptake of antibiotics, rendering *E. coli* more antibiotic resistant *in vivo* than *in vitro*.

PhoE which is highly similar to both OmpF and OmpC (they share >85% identical amino acids) is not found under most growth conditions and is absent *in vivo* (Robledo *et al.*, 1990). It is part of the phosphate-starvation-inducible Pho regulon (Tommassen *et al.*, 1987), and is activated upon growth in phosphate-deficient medium. However although anion selectivity of its channel favours uptake of anions, it does not contain a binding site for phosphates or polyphosphates (Darveau *et al.*, 1984; Bauer *et al.*, 1989).

Recently the crystal structures of OmpF and PhoE were published (Cowan *et al.*, 1992). They demonstrated remarkable similarity to the structure of the general porin from *Rhodobacter capsulatus* (Weiss *et al.*, 1991), despite the almost complete lack of sequence homology (n.b. it must be noted, however, that use of a refined amphipathicity prediction has permitted conceptual alignment of these sequences (Jeanteur *et al.*, 1993)). The general structure of the OmpF porin is shown in Fig. 18.2. Both OmpF and PhoE consist of 16 β-strands tilted at an angle of 35–50° and arranged in an ordered antiparallel fashion. The β-strands form a β-barrel structure that circles the central channel. Between these β-strands are eight short β-turns of two to three residues on the periplasmic side and eight longer loops on the outer surface side of the barrel. The loops are tightly packed and one long loop, L3, enters the channel to create the most constricted part of the channel and thus contribute to the channel's

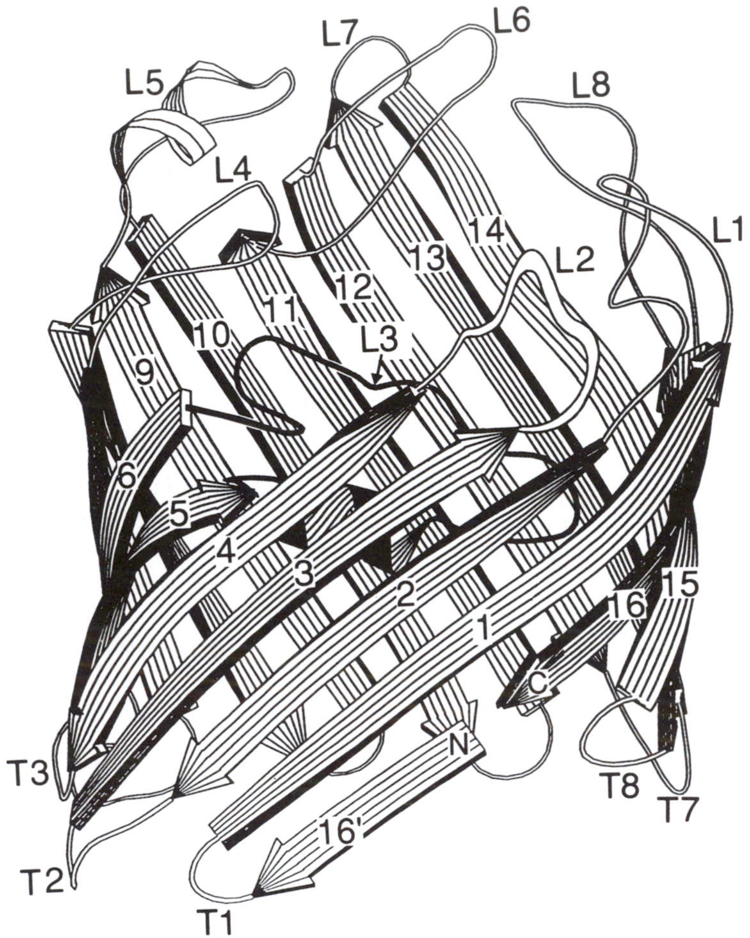

Fig. 18.2. General structure of the OmpF porin. Arrows represent β-strands and are labelled 1–16 starting from the strand after the first short turn. The long loops are denoted L1–L8 while the short turns at the other end are called T1–T8. Loop L2 protrudes to the viewer and is believed to be involved in monomer association, while L3 folds back into the barrel and is believed to contribute to the porin size. (Reproduced with permission from Cowan *et al.*, 1992.)

exclusion limit and ion selectivity (through charged amino acids in the loop). For example, the replacement in loop L3 of Gly-131 of OmpF with Lys-131 in PhoE, leading to an added positive charge at the channel constriction, explains the anion selectivity of PhoE, compared with OmpF (Table 18.3). Three monomeric subunits as described above are packed into a native trimer with strong hydrophobic interactions involving many residues of the subunits. This tight packing of monomers to form the native trimer probably explains the resistance of porins to denaturation, whereas the tight packing of the loop regions may explain the resistance of porins to proteolysis.

The other five general porins mentioned above are difficult to rationalize. Only one, OmpG, is found in wild-type *E. coli* K-12 strains. Misra and Benson (1989) observed a porin-like protein, OmpG, in *E. coli* cells that had acquired the ability to grow on large oligosaccharides in the absence of the specific porin LamB. Subsequently, Hancock *et al.* (1992) found a porin, which they called CE1248 porin, which was made in low levels in porin-deficient *E. coli* mutants. The large single channel conductance of this porin indicates that it should permit passage of larger sugars than OmpF or OmpC, and thus we hypothesize that this porin is OmpG, and is responsible for trans-outermembrane permeation of hydrophilic substances in the absence of OmpF or OmpC. Two other general porins, L_c (HK253) and L_c (PA-2), are encoded by lysogenic phages (Blasband *et al.*, 1986; Verhoef *et al.*, 1987), whereas the porin NmpC is encoded by the defective lambdoid prophage *Tsr*, but is inactivated in wild-type *E. coli* by insertion of IS5B (Blasband *et al.*, 1986). NmpC was found in pseudorevertants of porin-deficient *E. coli* strains which had spontaneously excised this insertion element. Protein K on the other hand is found almost exclusively in encapsulated *E. coli* strains (Sutcliffe *et al.*, 1983; Whitfield *et al.*, 1983). Although clearly related to OmpF, its regulation and genetics have not been well studied.

One other general porin that is clearly unrelated to the OmpF family has recently come to light, namely OmpA. It was assumed for many years that OmpA lacked porin activity, but the strong homology of this protein to the well-characterized porin OprF of *P. aeruginosa* (Woodruff and Hancock, 1989) caused a re-examination of this assumption. OmpA was demonstrated to form channels in two different model systems (Sugawara and Nikaido, 1992; Saint *et al.*, 1993). These channels appear to be quite large but to have low permeability, an apparent contradiction that has been reconciled by proposing that the channel contains a bend which increases frictional interactions within the channel. OmpA seems to be a member of a family of proteins with homology in their C-terminal 150 amino acids (Woodruff and Hancock, 1989; Gentry-Weeks *et al.*, 1992) and due to its role in cell structure will be discussed in more detail below. It is worth noting that OmpA has many structural similarities to the OmpF family, including high content of β-sheet structure, native trimer configuration, similar monomer size, association with the peptidoglycan and LPS, and lack of long stretches of hydrophobic amino acids (see Hancock, 1986; Woodruff and Hancock, 1989).

Substrate specific porins

Nikaido (1992) argued that outer membrane channel-forming proteins that contain, within their channels, a specific binding site, should be termed specific channels due to their fundamental differences in physiological behaviour. However these proteins retain many of the distinguishing features of porins including trimeric association, high content of β-sheet, association with the peptidoglycan and LPS and significant permeability to ions. Thus while the maltodextrin-specific channel-forming LamB protein has a rather distant evolutionary relationship to the OmpF-like porins or the OmpA family (Jeanteur *et al.*, 1993), we utilize the term substrate-specific porins here to reflect these structural similarities since it is often difficult to discriminate these families. For example the major porin of *Bordetella pertussis* is anion specific but related to the non-specific porins of *Neisseria* spp. (Li *et al.*, 1991). The plasmid encoded ScrY porin of *E. coli* on the other hand has the permeability characteristics of both specific and non-specific porins (Table 18.4).

Only three substrate-specific porins are known in *E. coli* (Table 18.4). An earlier conclusion that PhoE was phosphate and/or polyphosphate selective (Overbeeke and Lugtenberg, 1982; Dargent *et al.*, 1986) was in error (Darveau *et al.*, 1984; Bauer *et al.*, 1989), although PhoE, by virtue of its anion selectivity, demonstrates relatively high intrinsic permeability to large anions.

The best characterized substrate-specific porin is LamB, which is named for its role as the cellular receptor for bacteriophage λ. It is present in low amounts in cells growing on rich medium but is maltose inducible by a process that involves the *malT* apoactivator and maltose as a coactivator (Smelcman and Hofnung, 1975). Genetic studies including linker insertion mutagenesis, insertion of foreign epitopes, and sequencing of mutants that affect phage or antibody binding, have resulted in a sophisticated two-dimensional folding model for LamB (Saurin *et al.*, 1989). Cells deficient in LamB can still grow on maltose, since at high concentrations of external maltose, uptake through the general porins is sufficient to permit transit of maltose across the outer membrane. However LamB is obligately required (Smelcman and Hofnung, 1975) for growth on larger malto-oligo-saccharides (maltodextrins).

Model membrane studies have confirmed that LamB channels contain a binding site for maltose and maltodextrins. For example, in planar lipid bilayer experiments, these sugars block the conductance of ions through the channel, by binding to sites within the channel. As the size of the maltodextrin increases, the binding affinity (concentration of sugar leading to a 50% decrease in ion conductance) increases, up to maltopentose ($K_s = 59\,\mu M$) and stays high for larger sugars (Benz *et al.*, 1987). The existence of such binding sites has been confirmed by starch binding (Francis *et al.*, 1991a, b) and equilibrium flow dialysis (Gehring *et al.*, 1991) experiments. The latter have confirmed the existence of three independent binding sites, presumably one per monomer in the LamB trimer, and two-dimensional crystal reconstruction studies (Lepault *et al.*, 1988) have indicated an analogous structure (i.e. three independent channels) to that observed for OmpF (Fig. 18.2). Molecular genetic studies have identified specific amino acids that are involved in maltodextrin binding including residues 8–18, 74–82, 118–121, 152–154 and 360, suggesting that several regions of the polypeptide must collaborate in forming the binding site(s) (Dargent *et al.*, 1988; Heine *et al.*, 1988; Francis *et al.*, 1991a, b; Benz *et al.*, 1992; Chan and Ferenci, 1993). As discussed by Benz and colleagues (Benz *et al.*, 1987, 1992), the higher affinity of the channel for maltodextrins with four or more glucose residues implies that the channel may have a series of binding sites spaced in such a way that they can bind to more than one residue of the maltodextrin simultaneously.

The plasmid-encoded ScrY porin is involved in sucrose utilization by cells containing the sucrose regulon of plasmid pUR400 (Schmid *et al.*, 1988; Hardesty *et al.*, 1991). ScrY shows 23% amino acid identity with LamB. As mentioned above, the general permeation properties of Scr Y are similar to OmpF in that it forms large water-filled channels (Schülein *et al.*, 1991). However it is also similar to Lam B in having a maltodextrin binding site(s) for which binding affinity is a function of size of the maltodextrin.

The Tsx protein was originally characterized as the receptor for colicin K and bacteriophage T6. Hantke (1976) demonstrated that cells lacking Tsx had decreased rates of uptake of nucleosides and deoxynucleosides when these substrates were present at low (nM) extracellular concentrations. Model membrane channel studies (Benz *et al.*, 1988; Maier and Bremer, 1988) indicated that Tsx had limited permeability for ions, with a single channel conductance nearly 200-fold lower than that of OmpF. However this low conductance could be blocked by a variety of nucleosides and deoxynucleosides with a binding constant (K_s) as low as $50\,\mu M$. Despite these similarities to LamB, Tsx is unusual in that is quite susceptible to detergent denaturation (Bremer *et al.*, 1990) in contrast to all other porins. As befits a nucleoside channel, it is regulated by two repressors, DeoR and CytR (acting at separate, tandem promoters), which also control nucleoside transport/catabolism. Tsx is also involved in uptake of a plant-derived antibiotic albicidin which has no close resemblance to a nucleoside, but is a DNA synthesis inhibitor (Birch *et al.*, 1990).

The FadL protein is known to be involved in uptake of long-chain fatty acids from the medium (Black *et al.*, 1987). It is as yet unknown whether it functions as a substrate-specific porin or through another mechanism, although its role in outer membrane translocation has been definitively demonstrated and it binds fatty acids with very high affinity (K_d = 6.3 nM) (Black *et al.*, 1987; Mangroo and Gerber, 1992)). Unlike the porins, its sequence demonstrates an abundance of hydrophobic residues (Black, 1991). Nevertheless, it is heat modifiable on SDS-PAGE gels (Black *et al.*, 1987), a result consistent with its high content of β-sheet, while its molecular weight is similar to that of the substrate-specific porin LamB (Table 18.2). FadL is induced by the presence of fatty acids in the medium. Interestingly it demonstrates 42% identity with protein P1 from *Haemophilus influenzae* (Black, 1991).

Iron regulated outer membrane proteins

Iron is an essential nutrient of most bacteria and is available in limited amounts under most environmental conditions and *in vivo* (Braun *et al.*, 1976a). When *E. coli* cells are grown under conditions of low iron, they synthesize an enzyme system that produces, from shikimic acid, the siderophore enterobactin, a cyclic trimer of dihydroxybenzoylserine. In addition, five iron-regulated outer membrane proteins of apparent molecular weights 83 K (Fiu), 81 K (FepA), 78 K (FhuA and FhuE) and 74 K (Cir) are synthesized (Braun *et al.*, 1976a; Hancock *et al.*, 1976). The biosynthetic and outer membrane protein genes constitute a regulon which is repressed by the Fur repressor which binds to a consensus Fur-box nucleotide sequence present in the upstream region of each of the operons involved (Hantke, 1982). It has been proposed that iron is a corepressor such that iron deficiency causes the Fur repressor to dissociate from the Fur-box permitting transcription of all of the coregulated operons (Bagg and Neilands, 1987a, b). In addition to the above iron-regulated outer membrane proteins, the FecA protein is Fur-regulated and depressed by growth on low iron, providing citrate is present (Pressler *et al.*, 1988), whereas the col V-plasmid-encoded outer membrane protein Iut and the biosynthetic genes for the siderophore aerobactin are also iron regulated in *E. coli* cells harbouring this plasmid (de Lorenzo *et al.*, 1986).

Siderophores bind iron with high affinity, and when released into the medium, can capture iron from other weaker iron binding systems such as the human serum protein transferrin. Subsequently, the iron–siderophore complex binds to a specific outer membrane protein and this triggers translocation across the outer membrane. Of the *E. coli* proteins mentioned above, FepA binds the complex of iron with enterobactin (Braun *et al.*, 1976a; Armstrong *et al.*, 1990), whereas FecA binds ferric–citrate complexes (Pressler *et al.*, 1988) and Iut binds ferric–aerobactin complexes (Bagg and Neilands, 1987b). The proteins Fiu and Cir apparently have quite loose specificity and bind complexes of iron with enterobactin breakdown products (Nikaido and Rosenberg, 1990) as well as complexes of iron with a variety of catechol-containing β-lactams (Curtis *et al.*, 1988; Nikaido and Rosenberg, 1990; Critchley *et al.*, 1991), and have thus been proposed to serve as scavenger systems to enhance iron influx. However the two other iron-regulated outer membrane proteins, FhuE and FhuA, function strictly as agents of parasitism since they demonstrate specificity for the ferrated siderophores of fungi (Sauer *et al.*, 1990; Killmann and Braun, 1992).

The translocation of iron across the outer membrane depends in all cases on a protein called TonB (Postle, 1990). It was proposed, based on the influence of *tonB* mutations on the energized, irreversible binding of bacteriophages T1 and ϕ80 to FhuA (formerly called TonA) that TonB serves to couple the proton motive force to this outer membrane protein (Hancock and Braun, 1976). Subsequently this proposal was extended to the translocation of siderophore–iron complexes and vitamin B_{12} (via BtuB) across the outer membrane (Schöffler and Braun, 1989; Hannavy *et al.*, 1990; Kadner, 1990). It was demonstrated that TonB is a cytoplasmic membrane protein anchored by a single N-terminal hydrophobic anchor (Postle, 1990). However, it was proposed that an unusual segment of X-Pro dipeptide repeats served to span the periplasm and contact the iron-regulated outer membrane proteins and BtuB, permitting the transmission of 'protein conformational changes from the cytoplasmic membrane across the periplasm' as a means of coupling the proton motive force to outer membrane transport (Hannavy *et al.*, 1990). Consistent with this, it was previously demonstrated that point mutations in the TonB boxes of specific iron-regulated outer membrane proteins and BtuB could suppress point mutations in the *tonB* gene which otherwise inactivated TonB (Gudmundsdottir *et al.*, 1989) and vice versa (Bell *et al.*, 1990).

Recently evidence was presented that FepA might function as a gated porin, in which TonB would serve in a gatekeeper role (Rutz *et al.*, 1992). Thus deletion of those cell surface loops that were involved in binding of ferric enterobactin resulted in mutant proteins that were incapable of high affinity uptake. Instead these mutant FepA derivatives formed non-specific diffusion channels indicating that the parent channel might be a gated channel.

FepA, FhuA and the related TonB-dependent outer membrane vitamin B_{12} translocator BtuB, have been subjected to genetic manipulations designed at mapping the transmembrane and surface topology of these proteins (Maier and Bremer, 1988; Murphy and Klebba, 1989; Armstrong *et al.*, 1990; Carmel *et al.*, 1990; Murphy *et al.*, 1990; Koebnik and Braun, 1993). Each protein has been confirmed as having similarities to the two-dimensional maps of the porins with antiparallel β-sheet regions separated by loop regions. However, they are proposed to contain 29–32 membrane-spanning β-chains (Murphy *et al.*, 1990; Koebnik and Braun, 1993). Ligand, monoclonal antibody and bacteriocin binding domains have been localized on the two-dimensional maps.

Detailed studies have been performed on the events that occur subsequent to translocation across the outer membrane (see Postle, 1990), but are not within the scope of this chapter. However it is worth noting that two proteins, ExbB and TolQ, have been proposed to potentially be involved in translocation of specific siderophore–iron complexes across the outer membrane (Postle, 1990).

Structural proteins

Deletion of both outer membrane proteins, OmpA and Lpp, resulted in cells that adopted a rounded morphology and were unable to grow in medium with low divalent cation concentrations (Sonntag *et al.*, 1978). This suggested a structural role for both sets of proteins.

Subsequently it was demonstrated that OmpA is a multifunctional outer membrane protein that serves as the parent of a family of proteins in other bacteria with related carboxy-terminal sequences (Gentry-Weeks *et al.*, 1992), one of which, *P. aeruginosa* OprF, has a similar structural role to that proposed for OmpA (Woodruff and Hancock, 1989). Interestingly, studies with deletion variants of OprF have indicated that the sequences required to complement the structural consequences of the lack of OprF in *P. aeruginosa* OprF:Ω mutants, reside within the OmpA homologous carboxy-terminal region (E. Rawling and R.E.W. Hancock, unpublished). The way in which OmpA serves such a structural role in shape determination is unknown, but apparently does not involve a loss of the other known shape-determining protein of *E. coli*, namely penicillin-binding protein 2 (Sonntag *et al.*, 1978). Nevertheless, since the peptidoglycan is involved in shape maintenance, it is possible that the tight association of OmpA with the underlying peptidoglycan (Endermann *et al.*, 1978) may be of some importance. In addition to this structural role, OmpA serves as a porin (Sugawara and Nikaido, 1992; Saint *et al.*, 1993), as a phage receptor (Skurray *et al.*, 1974), is involved in stabilization of mating aggregates between F-plasmid containing donors and plasmidless recipients (Skurray *et al.*, 1974; Ried and Henning, 1987), and plays a role in pathogenesis (see below).

The N-terminal portion of OmpA is arranged as a porin-like sequence of eight antiparallel β-strands separated by small periplasmic or larger external loop regions. However the proposed periplasmic localization of the carboxy-terminal region of OmpA (Morona *et al.*, 1985) should be re-examined based on its high content of β-sheet and the demonstration that the homologous region of OprF contains at least four surface-localized epitopes (Finnen *et al.*, 1992), whereas the homologous region of *Neisseria* protein PIII is partly involved in the serum blocking activity of this protein (Virji and Heckels, 1989), a function shared by OmpA (see below).

The other protein involved in cell structure is Lpp, otherwise known as the Braun lipoprotein. Lpp is a 58 amino acid protein containing three covalently bound fatty acids at the N-terminal cysteine. It is present in *E. coli* in high copy number (7×10^5 copies per cell) with one-third of Lpp molecules being covalently linked by the ε-amino group of its C-terminal lysine to the carboxyl group of diaminopimelate of the peptidoglycan; the other two thirds are not covalently linked to the peptidoglycan (Inouye *et al.*, 1972; Braun, 1975). Both forms of Lpp are largely organized in alpha-helices (Braun *et al.*, 1976b) and are probably associated with the outer membrane primarily via insertion of the fatty acids into the inner monolayer of the outer membrane. Loss of lipoprotein causes cells to become leaky (Suzuki *et al.*, 1978), consistent with the structural role mentioned above, in *lpp ompA* double mutants (Sonntag *et al.*, 1978). Again the association of lipoprotein with the peptidoglycan seems to be of importance in this structural role, and it seems likely that the covalently bound form is most important in this regard (Fung *et al.*, 1978; Woodruff and Hancock, 1989). Another small lipoprotein found in the *E. coli* outer membrane is OsmB (Jung *et al.*, 1989). Although osmotically inducible, its precise function is at present unknown.

In addition to these two structural proteins, *E. coli* also contains an outer membrane protein, the peptidoglycan associated lipoprotein (PAL), which is part of a family of related higher-molecular-weight lipoproteins that are non-covalently peptidoglycan associated (Mizuno, 1979; Chen and Henning, 1987). Mutants (*exc*C) lacking this protein demonstrate leakage of several periplasmic enzymes and increased sensitivity to deoxycholate and other compounds (Lazzaroni and Portalier, 1992). Use of Tn*phoA* fusion techniques demonstrated that the N-terminal portion is associated with the outer membrane, whereas the carboxy-terminal portion is necessary for interaction with the peptidoglycan. Of great interest is the recent observation that the carboxy terminus of PAL can be partially aligned with that of OmpA (Gentry-Weeks *et al.*, 1992) (Fig. 18.3).

A protein previously termed histone-like protein I (HLP-I) was found to have 91% identical amino acids to the OmpH outer membrane protein of *S. typhimurium*, suggesting it may be an outer membrane protein (Hirvas *et al.*, 1990). Its high basicity (pI >10) indicates a potential structural role in binding to negatively charged LPS. The protein, termed Protein III by Hindennach and Henning (1975), may possibly be OmpH, but confirmation of this and its possible function awaits the isolation of mutants lacking OmpH.

```
OmpA    apkdntwytgaklgwsqyhdtgfinnngpthenqlgagafggyqvnpyvgfemgydwlgr   60
OprF    qgqnsveieafgkryftdsvrnmknadlyggsigyfltddvelalsygeyhdvrgtyetg   60
PAL     cssnknasndgsegmlgagtgmdanggngnmsseeqar----------------------   38
PIII    geasvqgytvsgqsneivrnnygecwknayfdkasqgrvecgdavavpepepapvavveq   60

OmpA    mpykgsvengaykaqgvqltaklgypitddldiytrlggmvwradtksnvygknhdtgvs  120
OprF    nkkvhgnltsldaiyhfgtpgvglrpyvsaglahqnitninsdsqgrqqmtmanigaglk  120
PAL     ------------------------------------------------------------   38
PIII    apq---------------------------------------------------------   63

OmpA    pvfaggveyaitpeiatrleyqwtnnigdahtigtrpdngmlslgvsyrfgqgeaapvva  180
OprF    yyftenffakasldgqyglekrdnghqgewmaglgvgfnfggskaapapepvadvcsdsd  180
PAL     ------------------------------------------------------------   38
PIII    ------------------------------------------------------------   63

OmpA    papapape------------------VQTKHFTLKSDVLFNFNKATLKPEGQAALDQLYS  222
OprF    ndgvcdnvdkcpdtpanvtvdangcpAVAEVVRVQLDVKFDFDKSKVKENSYADIKNLAD  240
PAL     --------------------------LQMQQLQQNNIVYFDLDKYDIRSDFAQMLDAHAN   72
PIII    --------------------------YVDETISLSAKTLFGFDKDSLRAEAQDNLKVLAQ   97

OmpA    QLSnldpkdgSVVVLGYTDRIGSDAYNQGLSERRAQSVVDYLISK-GIPADKISARGMGE  281
OprF    FMKqypst--STTVEGHTDSVGTDAYNQKLSERRANAVRDVLVNEyGVEGGRVNAVGYGE  298
PAL     FLRsnpsy--KVTVEGHADERGTPEYNISLGERRANAVKMYLQGK-GVSADQISIVSYGK  129
PIII    RLSrtnvq--SVRVEGHTDFMGSEKYNQALSERRAYVVANNLVSN-GVPASRISAVGLGE  154

OmpA    SNPVTGNTcdnvkqraalidclapdrrveievkgikdvvtqpqa----------------  325
OprF    SRPVADNAtaegrainrrveaeveaeak--------------------------------  326
PAL     EKPAVLGHdeaaysknrravlvy-------------------------------------  152
PIII    SQAQMTQVcqaevaklgakaskakkrealiaciepdrrvdvkirsivtrqvvparnhhgh  214
```

Fig. 18.3. Sequence alignment of OmpA, PIII, OprF and PAL amino acid sequences. The signal sequence has been removed to simplify the alignment. Upper case letters represent blocks of homology as defined by the program MACAW, version 1.06 (Schuler *et al.*, 1991).

Enzymes

Only two well-characterized enzymes (PldA and OmpT) are known to be associated with the outer membrane of *E. coli*. PldA is the so-called detergent-resistant phospholipase A of *E. coli* (Homma *et al.*, 1984). OmpT is identical to protease VII from *E. coli* (Grodberg *et al.*, 1988; Sugimura, 1988), and is well known for its role in degradation of secreted recombinant proteins (Baneyx and Georgiou, 1990). However, neither enzyme has been definitively identified as having a physiological function.

Appendages

Most *E. coli* cells contain flagella which are involved in directed movement (chemotaxis) towards attractant chemicals (McNab, 1987a, b). The structural protein of flagella, flagellin (FliC), may often be observed in outer membranes as a doublet of approximately 52,000 molecular weight, although strictly speaking it is not an outer membrane protein. The flagellin traverses the outer membrane through the outer membrane ring protein, FlaY, which has been proposed to form a tight greaseless bearing that permits flagella rotation without disrupting the outer membrane (McNab, 1987a, b).

About 70% of wild-type *E. coli* strains contain type 1 or common fimbriae that mediate mannose-inhibitable binding to eukaryotic cells (Pallesen *et al.*, 1989). The structural subunit of type 1 fimbriae, FimA, is apparently assembled by the outer membrane FimD protein (Klemm, 1985). FimD has general homology to the PapC protein which is part of the operon for expression of P (pyelonephritis associated) pili and to FaeD and FanD which are involved in expression of K88 and K99 pili, respectively (Krogfelt, 1991). The best studied of these proteins, PapC, has been proposed to function as an outer membrane usher that releases the pilin structural subunit from the PapD protein (the PapD protein serves to 'chaperone' the pilin subunit across the periplasm), and then orchestrates an ordered progression of pilin subunits into the growing pilus (Jones *et al.*, 1992). Another outer membrane protein, PapH, which is associated with the synthesis of P fimbriae, has been proposed to serve as an outer membrane anchor for the pilus. Given the general homology of the pilus expression systems in *E. coli*, we assume that analogous proteins are present for other pili. While the type 1 fimbriae are by far the most common, other chromosomally encoded pili operons have been found in *E. coli* (including the P-pili mentioned above) and as many as three separate operons have been demonstrated in a single uropathogenic *E. coli* strain (Rhen *et al.*, 1983).

Many *E. coli* contain the F plasmid. This plasmid encodes as many as eight different Tra proteins which reside in the outer membrane and have general functions in pilus assembly or surface exclusion (Willetts and Skurray, 1987).

Protein export

There are few proteins that are exported across the outer membrane of *E. coli*, other than the appendage proteins discussed above. In the case of fimbriae, there are specific proteins involved in the translocation across the outer membrane and assembly of these fimbriae as discussed above. However the haemolysin of *E. coli* is secreted from cells by an independent pathway. In this case, it is thought that the minor outer membrane protein TolC is involved in secretion in some as-yet undetermined fashion (Wandersman and Delepelaire, 1990). Interestingly, recent data has suggested that TolC may be a peptide-specific porin (R. Benz, unpublished results).

Role of Outer Membrane Proteins in Pathogenesis

The functions served by outer membrane proteins during growth of cells *in vitro* may also be of some importance during growth in a host. For example the regulation and pore functions of porins play a role in antibiotic susceptibility *in vivo*, the export of pilin and flagellin is important in the adhesive and motility functions of these appendages, and the excretion of haemolysin provides *E. coli* with its only excreted virulence factor. In addition to these general functions, there is a variety of functions more specifically associated with pathogenesis.

Attachment and effacement

In most cases, the adherence of *E. coli* to eukaryotic cells is mediated by a minor protein subunit that is attached as part of a complex to the tip of pili (Chapter 16). For example, the adhesin for type 1 pili is actually the FimH protein (Krogfelt *et al.*, 1990), whereas the adhesin for P fimbriae is the PapG protein (Jones *et al.*, 1992). In the latter case, it has been demonstrated that transposon mutants lacking the actual fimbrial subunit PapA, can still adhere (Jones *et al.*, 1992). Under such circumstances, the PapG adhesin subunit would be in close juxtaposition to the outer membrane, and it would be difficult to prove definitively whether such an adhesin were an outer membrane protein or not.

There is strong evidence that a specific outer membrane protein is involved in a process known as attachment and effacement (Chapter 20). This process involves a 94-kDa outer membrane protein (Eae or intimin), which is the product of the chromosomal *eaeA* gene, and a plasmid-encoded regulator called Per (Jerse and Kaper, 1991). The Eae protein may be involved in the more intimate adherence of *E. coli* with epithelial cells that causes cytoskeletal rearrangements but it is uncertain whether this protein is an actual adhesin, or whether it acts indirectly in this process. The *eaeA* gene has been cloned and sequenced from both enteropathogenic and enterohaemorrhagic *E. coli* and has substantial homology to *Yersinia* proteins called invasins that are involved in invasion (Isberg *et al.*, 1987). Interestingly, an outer membrane protein of similar molecular weight has been proposed to function in epithelial cell invasion by enterotoxigenic *E. coli* (Elsinghorst, 1992), suggesting quite broad distribution of this outer membrane function in pathogens.

Serum resistance

E. coli cells harbouring F plasmid or F-like plasmids are more resistant to the bactericidal action of serum. One of these F-like plasmids, Col V, is strongly associated with virulence (Binns *et al.*, 1979). This serum (complement) resistance is mediated by a plasmid-encoded protein TraT (Moll *et al.*, 1980), an oligomeric lipoprotein that is exposed on the surface of the outer membrane (Sukupolvi and O'Connor, 1990). Colony hybridization studies using gene probes have shown that as many as 70% of strains from patients with bacteraemia, septicaemia, or enteric infections contain a homologue of TraT, whereas only 20–40% of *E. coli* strains from normal faeces gave positive hybridization signals (Montenegro *et al.*, 1985). The natural function of TraT in F-plasmid biology is to mediate surface exclusion, which inhibits DNA transfer from cells harbouring a closely related plasmid (Harrison *et al.*, 1992). This property is independent of serum resistance per se, since F-like plasmids fall into surface exclusion specificity groups that appear to depend on differences in a 5-amino acid region of TraT (Harrison *et al.*, 1992).

The molecular mechanism whereby TraT mediates resistance to serum is unclear, although it has been suggested that TraT influences the correct functioning or assembly of the membrane attack complex (components C5–9) (Moll *et al.*, 1980; Ogata *et al.*, 1982). One possible mechanism could be the blocking of specific LPS divalent cation binding sites which have been proposed to be involved in complement insertion into outer membranes (Hancock, 1984). Alternatively, TraT could support the role of OmpA in serum resistance (see below), since Riede and Eschbach (1986) have demonstrated that TraT is capable of interacting with OmpA.

Recently, Weiser and Gotschlich (1991) demonstrated that OmpA-deficient mutants of an *E. coli* K-1 strain demonstrated a substantially increased susceptibility to killing via the classical pathway of complement killing. Coincident with this, the OmpA-deficient strain demonstrated a significantly reduced ability to cause chick embryo lethality and bacteraemia in neonatal rats. Thus OmpA has a clear role in serum resistance. Interestingly, OmpA shows substantial carboxy-terminal sequence homology to protein pIII from *Neisseria gonorrhoeae* which mediates resistance to complement-mediated killing (Virji and Heckels, 1989). Indeed protein pIII has been termed the serum-blocking protein since specific IgG antibodies to pIII block the bactericidal action of even immune serum (Rice *et al.*, 1986). Preliminary data suggest this is also true for OmpA (Weiser *et al.*, 1992).

In vivo *expression/antigenicity*

Many studies have examined heterogeneity in the SDS-PAGE profiles of *E. coli* isolates from normal faeces (Hofstra and Dankert, 1980; Jann and Jann, 1980), neonatal meningitis (van Alphen *et al.*, 1983), urinary tract (Jann and Jann, 1980; Achtman *et al.*, 1983, 1986), intestinal disease (Jann and Jann, 1980; Chart *et al.*, 1988) and septicaemia (Kapur *et al.*, 1992). In every case substantial variability was observed in the apparent molecular weights and amounts of the major outer membrane proteins. This was evident for outer membrane proteins, identified by immunological methods or from the influence of solubilization temperature on the electrophoretic mobilities, including OmpA, the porins (Hofstra and Dankert, 1980; van Alphen *et al.*, 1983) and the iron-regulated outer membrane proteins (Chart *et al.*, 1988). Although this has been suggested to indicate a clonal relationship for similar isolates (Achtman *et al.*, 1983), no unique relationship between such clonal groups and virulence or disease specificity has been identified. In addition there is no obvious utility of clonal subgrouping by outer membrane protein patterns, in direct contrast to results for other bacteria.

E. coli have been isolated directly from animal models (Griffiths *et al.*, 1983; Sciortino and Finkelstein, 1983) and from infected human urine (Lam *et al.*, 1984; Robledo *et al.*, 1990) and characterized without subculturing. With one major exception, their outer membrane profiles demonstrate a similar complement of proteins to those observed in cells grown *in vitro* in rich broth. Iron-regulated outer membrane proteins are highly induced, indicating that bacteria grow *in vivo* under iron-deficient conditions, at least when growing at the densities required to permit subsequent analysis. Another consequence of *in vivo* growth is apparently down-regulation of OmpF, as indicated by the phenotype of a β-lactam-resistant isolate obtained from an infected patient (Medeiros *et al.*, 1987) and by the outer membrane protein profiles of bacteria obtained directly from the urine of bacteriuric patients (Robledo *et al.*, 1990).

The expression of outer membrane proteins *in vivo* is also revealed by the immune response to surface antigens. Taplits and Michael (1979) suggested that the immune response to the surface proteins of *E. coli* B, a rough non-encapsulated bacterium, was dominant. Proteins recognized include OmpA (Puohiniemi *et al.*, 1990), the porins, Pal and Lpp (Nicolle *et al.*, 1988; Henriksen and Maeland, 1990). Extensive investigations have demonstrated strong conservation of most outer membrane protein epitopes, including those of OmpF, OmpC (Hofstra and Dankert, 1980; Bentley and Klebba, 1988), PhoE (van der Ley *et al.*, 1986a), Pal, Lpp (Henriksen *et al.*, 1989), FepA (Rutz *et al.*, 1991), OmpA (Hofstra and Dankert, 1980; Overbeeke and Lugtenberg, 1980), TraT (Bitter-Suermann *et al.*, 1984), Fiu and Cir (Chart *et al.*, 1988). Nevertheless, with few exceptions, outer membrane proteins usually make poor vaccines (Bolin and Jensen, 1987; Vuopio-Varkila *et al.*, 1988). Moreover, it appears that antigenic epitopes on the surface of outer membrane proteins are weakly or not-at-all accessible to antibodies (Hofstra *et al.*, 1979; van der Ley *et al.*, 1986b; Gómez-Miguel *et al.*, 1987; Bentley and Klebba, 1988), high-molecular-weight substrates (Ferenci and Lee, 1986) and phages (van der Ley *et al.*, 1986a) due to shielding by LPS O-side-chains, and furthermore, the most surface-exposed epitopes have undergone the greatest antigenic variation (Pagès *et al.*, 1988; Rutz *et al.*, 1991).

Endotoxin-associated proteins

Almost all outer membrane proteins, when extracted, remain non-covalently associated with LPS (e.g. Yamada and Mizushima, 1980) and this interaction appears to be tight and specific (Datta *et al.*, 1977; Schweizer *et al.*, 1978; Parr *et al.*, 1986). Lipopolysaccharide isolated by various techniques (Strittmatter and Galanos, 1987) often contains outer membrane proteins. Likewise LPS (and its Lipid A portion, endotoxin) may be released together with proteins *in vivo* (Leive *et al.*, 1968). Although this association can modulate the effects of endotoxin, it is still uncertain as to whether it is physiologically important.

Other roles

A variety of other roles in pathogenesis have been ascribed to outer membrane proteins, based largely on *in vitro* assays. However it is not known whether these functions have any *in vivo* significance. For example, reactive arthritis is caused, in patients with the HLA-B27 type, by a variety of Gram-negative bacteria, but not *E. coli*. This is thought to be due to molecular mimicry in which a bacterial surface antigen induces self antibodies directed against HLA-B27. It is of interest that antisera specific for HLA-B27 reacts with two *E. coli* outer membrane proteins of apparent molecular weights 35,000 and 23,000. The former is OmpA (Zhang *et al.*, 1989) and the specific epitopes have been shown to comprise two peptide regions, both of which contain two consecutive arginine residues (Yu *et al.*, 1991).

Outer membrane proteins are capable of interacting directly with B lymphocytes as judged by their ability to stimulate B cell replication (mitogenicity). *E. coli* proteins that have been ascribed this function are OmpF, OmpA (Bessler and Henning, 1979), Lpp (Melchers *et al.*, 1975) and endotoxin protein (Sultzer and Goodman, 1976). Evidence has also been presented that porins can specifically bind Clq and activate antibody-independent killing via the classical complement pathway (Loos and Clas, 1987).

Use as vaccines and carriers of epitopes

As discussed above, outer membrane proteins have demonstrated limited promise as vaccines against heterologous bacteria. However a variety of *E. coli* outer membrane proteins including LamB, TraT, PhoE and OmpA, have been shown to be able to accept extra amino acids without compromising expression or correct assembly into the outer membrane (see Hofnung, 1991 for review). Comparisons of the PhoE sites accepting extra amino acids (which are introduced as oligonucleotides into the corresponding location in the gene) with the three-dimensional structure have demonstrated that it is the surface loops connecting adjacent antiparallel β-strands which exclusively accept insertion of epitopes (Cowan *et al.*, 1992). A wide variety of foreign epitopes have been expressed in outer membrane proteins and, when the resultant recombinant antigens are used as vaccines, specific protective antibodies can be elicited in animals (Hofnung, 1991).

Future Perspectives

We are approaching a time when every single outer membrane protein in *E. coli* will have been characterized. For example, more than 25% of the *E. coli* K-12 genome has been sequenced (Médigue *et al.*, 1991). However while we now understand how many individual outer membrane proteins function, we still have an inadequate understanding of the interactions between components of the outer membrane, and the way outer membranes are functionally integrated with other cell compartments. It is in this area that we expect the majority of work will concentrate in the next decade.

Acknowledgements

The financial assistance of the Medical Research Council of Canada and Canadian Bacterial Diseases Network in the author's own research is gratefully acknowledged.

References

Achtman, M., Mercer, A., Kusecek, B., Pohl, B., Heuzenroeder, M., Aaronson, W., Sutton, A. and Silver, R.P. (1983) Six widespread bacterial clones among *Escherichia coli* K1 isolates. *Infection and Immunity* 39, 315–335.

Achtman, M., Heuzenroeder, M., Kusecek, B., Ochman, H., Cougant, D., Väisanen-Rhen, V., Korhonen, T., Stuart, S., Ørskov, F. and Ørskov, I. (1986) Clonal analysis of *Escherichia coli* O2:K1 isolated from diseased humans and animals. *Infection and Immunity* 51, 268–276.

Andersen, J., Forst, S.A., Zhao, K., Inouye, M. and Delihas, N. (1989) The function of *micF* RNA. *Journal of Biological Chemistry* 264, 17961–17970.

Armstrong, S.K., Francis, C.L. and McIntosh, M.A. (1990) Molecular analysis of the *Escherichia coli* ferric enterobactin receptor FepA. *Journal of Biological Chemistry* 265, 14536–14543.

Avrameas, S. (1969) Indirect immunoenzyme techniques for the intracellular detection of antigens. *Immunochemistry* 6, 825–831.

Bagg, A. and Neilands, J.B. (1987a) Ferric uptake regulation protein acts as a repressor, employing iron(II) as a cofactor to bind the operator of an iron transport operon in *Escherichia coli. Biochemistry* 26, 5471–5477.

Bagg, A. and Neilands, J.B. (1987b) Molecular mechanism of regulation of siderophore-mediated iron assimilation. *Microbiological Reviews* 51, 509–518.

Baneyx, F. and Georgiou, G. (1990) *In vivo* degradation of secreted fusion proteins by the *Escherichia coli* outer membrane protease OmpT. *Journal of Bacteriology* 172, 491–494.

Bauer, K., Struyvé, M., Bosch, D., Benz, R. and Tommassen, J. (1989) One single lysine residue is responsible for the special interaction between polyphosphate and the outer membrane porin PhoE of *Escherichia coli. Journal of Biological Chemistry* 264, 16393–16398.

Bell, P.E., Nau, C.D., Brown, J.T., Konisky, J. and Kadner, R.J. (1990) Genetic suppression demonstrates interaction of TonB protein with outer membrane transport proteins in *Escherichia coli. Journal of Bacteriology* 172, 3826–3829.

Bentley, A.T. and Klebba, P.E. (1988) Effect of lipopolysaccharide structure on reactivity of antiporin monoclonal antibodies with the bacterial cell surface. *Journal of Bacteriology* 170, 1063–1068.

Benz, R., Schmid, A. and Hancock, R.E.W. (1985) Ion selectivity of Gram-negative bacterial porins. *Journal of Bacteriology* 162, 722–727.

Benz, R., Schmid, A. and Vos-Scheperkeuter, G.H. (1987) Mechanism of sugar transport through the sugar-specific LamB channel of *Escherichia coli* outer membrane. *Journal of Membrane Biology* 100, 21–29.

Benz, R., Schmid, A., Maier, C. and Bremer, E. (1988) Characterization of the nucleoside-binding site inside the Tsx channel of *Escherichia coli* outer membrane. *European Journal of Biochemistry* 176, 699–705.

Benz, R., Francis, G., Nakae, T. and Ferenci, T. (1992) Investigation of the selectivity of maltoporin channels using mutant LamB proteins: mutations changing the maltodextrin binding site. *Biochimica et Biophysica Acta* 1104, 299–307.

Bessler, W. and Henning, U. (1979) Protein I and protein II from the outer membrane of *Escherichia coli* are mouse B-lymphocyte mitogens. *Zeitschrift für Immunitätsforschung* 155, 398.

Binns, M.M., Davies, D.L. and Hardy, K.G. (1979) Cloned fragments of the plasmid ColV, I-K94 specifying virulence and serum resistance. *Nature (London)* 279, 778–781.

Birch, R.G., Pemberton, J.M. and Basnayake, W.V.S. (1990) Stable albicidin resistance in *Escherichia coli* involves an altered outer-membrane nucleoside uptake system. *Journal of General Microbiology* 136, 51–58.

Bitter-Suermann, D., Peters, H., Jürs, M., Nehrbass, R., Montenegro, M. and Timmis, K. (1984) Monoclonal antibody detection of IncF group plasmid-encoded TraT protein in clinical isolates of *Escherichia coli. Infection and Immunity* 46, 308–313.

Black, P.N. (1991) Primary sequence of the *Escherichia coli fadL* gene encoding an outer membrane protein required for long-chain fatty acid transport. *Journal of Bacteriology* 173, 435–442.

Black, P.N., Said, B., Ghosn, C.R., Beach, J.V. and Nunn, W.D. (1987) Purification and characterization of an outer membrane-bound protein involved in long-chain fatty acid transport in *Escherichia coli. Journal of Biological Chemistry* 262, 1412–1419.

Blasband, A.J., Marcotte Jr, W.R. and Schnaitman, C.A. (1986) Structure of the *lc* and *nmpC* outer membrane porin protein genes of lambdoid bacteriophage. *Journal of Biological Chemistry* 261, 12723–12732.

Bolin, C.A. and Jensen, A.E. (1987) Passive immunization with antibodies against iron-regulated outer membrane proteins protects turkeys from *Escherichia coli* septicemia. *Infection and Immunity* 55, 1239–1242.

Braun, V. (1975) Covalent lipoprotein from the outer membrane of *Escherichia coli. Biochimica et Biophysica Acta* 415, 335–377.

Braun, V., Hancock, R.E.W., Hantke, K. and Hartmann, A. (1976a) Functional organization of the outer membrane of *Escherichia coli*: phage and colicin receptors as components of iron uptake systems. *Journal of Supramolecular Structure* 5, 37–58.

Braun, V., Rotering, H., Ohms, J.-P. and Hagenmeier, H. (1976b) Conformational studies on murien-lipoprotein from the outer membrane of *Escherichia coli. European Journal of Biochemistry* 70, 601–610.

Bremer, E., Middendorf, A., Martinussen, J. and Valentin-Hansen, P. (1990) Analysis of the *tsx* gene, which encodes a nucleoside-specific channel-forming protein (Tsx) in the outer membrane of *Escherichia coli. Gene* 96, 59–65.

Buechner, M., Delcour, A.H., Martinac, B., Adler, J. and Kung, C. (1990) Ion channel activities in the *Escherichia coli* outer membrane. *Biochimica et Biophysica Acta* 1024, 111–121.

Carmel, G., Hellstern, D., Henning, D. and Coulton, J.W. (1990) Insertion mutagenesis of the gene encoding the ferrichrome-iron receptor of *Escherichia coli* K-12. *Journal of Bacteriology* 172, 1861–1869.

Chan, W.C. and Ferenci, T. (1993) Combinatorial mutagenesis of the *lamB* gene: residues 41 through 43, which are conserved in *Escherichia coli* outer membrane proteins, are informationally important in maltoporin structure and function. *Journal of Bacteriology* 175, 858–865.

Chart, H., Stevenson, P. and Griffiths, E. (1988) Iron-regulated outer membrane proteins of *Escherichia coli* strains associated with enteric or extraintestinal diseases of man and animals. *Journal of General Microbiology* 134, 1549–1559.

Chen, R. and Henning, U. (1987) Nucleotide sequence of the gene for the peptidoglycan-associated lipoprotein of *Escherichia coli* K12. *European Journal of Biochemistry* 163, 73–77.

Cowan, S.W., Schirmer, T., Rummel, G., Steiert, M., Ghosh, R., Pauptit, R.A., Jansonius, J.N. and Rosenbusch, J.P. (1992) Crystal structures explain function properties of two *Escherichia coli* porins. *Nature* 358, 727–733.

Critchley, I.A., Basker, M.J., Edmondson, R.A. and Knott, S.J. (1991) Uptake of a catecholic cephalosporin by the iron transport system of *Escherichia coli. Journal of Antimicrobial Chemotherapy (London)* 28, 377–388.

Cronan, J.E. (1979) Phospholipid synthesis and assembly. In: Inouye, M. (ed.)

Bacterial Outer Membranes. John Wiley & Sons, New York, pp. 35–65.
Curtis, N.A.C., Eisenstadt, R.L., East, S.J., Cornford, R.J., Walker, L.A. and White, A.J. (1988) Iron-regulated outer membrane proteins of *Escherichia coli* K-12 and mechanism of action of catechol-substituted cephalosporins. *Antimicrobial Agents and Chemotherapy* 32, 1879–1886.
Dargent, B., Hofmann, W., Pattus, F. and Rosenbusch, J.P. (1986) The selectivity filter of voltage-dependent channels formed by phosphoporin (PhoE protein) from *Escherichia coli. European Molecular Biology Organization Journal* 5, 773–778.
Dargent, B., Charbit, A., Hofnung, M. and Pattus, F. (1988) Effect of point mutations on the *in-vitro* pore properties of maltoporin, a protein of *Escherichia coli* outer membrane. *Journal of Molecular Biology* 201, 497–506.
Darveau, R.P., Hancock, R.E.W. and Benz, R. (1984) Chemical modification of the anion selectivity of the PhoE porin from the *E. coli* outer membrane. *Biochimica et Biophysica Acta* 774, 69–74.
Datta, D.B., Arden, B. and Henning, U. (1977) Major proteins of the *Escherichia coli* outer cell envelope membrane as bacteriophage receptors. *Journal of Bacteriology* 131, 821–829.
de Lorenzo, V., Bindereif, A., Paw, B.H. and Neilands, J.B. (1986) Aerobactin biosynthesis and transport genes of plasmid ColV-K30 in *Escherichia coli* K-12. *Journal of Bacteriology* 165, 570–578.
Elsinghorst, E.A. (1992) Epithelial cell invasion by the enterotoxigenic *E. coli tib* locus is associated with a 118 kDa outer membrane protein. In: *Abstracts of the 92nd Annual Meeting of the American Society for Microbiology, 1992.* American Society for Microbiology, Washington, DC, Abstr. B-181, p. 56.
Endermann, R., Krämer, C. and Henning, U. (1978) Major outer membrane proteins of *Escherichia coli* K-12: evidence for protein II being a transmembrane protein. *Federation of European Biochemical Societies Letters* 86, 21–24.
Ferenci, T. and Lee, K.-S. (1986) Exclusion of high-molecular-weight maltosaccharides by lipopolysaccharide O-antigen of *Escherichia coli* and *Salmonella typhimurium. Journal of Bacteriology* 167, 1081–1082.
Finnen, R.L., Martin, N.L., Seihnel, R.J., Woodruff, W.A., Rosok, M. and Hancock, R.E.W. (1992) Analysis of the *Pseudomonas aeruginosa* major outer membrane protein OprF by use of truncated OprF derivatives and monoclonal antibodies. *Journal of Bacteriology* 174, 4977–4985.
Francis, G., Brennan, L. and Ferenci, T. (1991a) Affinity-chromatographic purification of sixteen cysteine-substituted maltoporin variants: thiol reactivity and cross-linking in an outer membrane protein of *Escherichia coli. Biochimica et Biophysica Acta* 1067, 89–96.
Francis, G., Brennan, L., Stretton, S. and Ferenci, T. (1991b) Genetic mapping of starch- and Lambda-receptor sites in maltoporin: identification of substitutions causing direct and indirect effects on binding sites by cysteine mutagenesis. *Molecular Microbiology* 5, 2293–2301.
Funahara, Y. and Nikaido, H. (1980) Asymmetric localization of lipopolysaccharides on the outer membrane of *Salmonella typhimurium. Journal of Bacteriology* 141, 1463–1465.
Fung, J., MacAlister, T.J. and Rothfield, L.I. (1978) Role of murein lipoprotein in morphogenesis of the bacterial division septum: phenotypic similarity of

*iky*D and *lpo* mutants. *Journal of Bacteriology* 133, 1467–1471.
Gehring, K., Cheng, C.-H., Nikaido, H. and Jap, B.K. (1991) Stoichiometry of maltodextrin-binding sites in LamB, an outer membrane protein from *Escherichia coli. Journal of Bacteriology* 173, 1873–1878.
Gentry-Weeks, C.R., Hultsch, A.-L., Kelly, S.M., Keith, J.M. and Curtiss III, R. (1992) Cloning and sequencing of a gene encoding a 21-kilodalton outer membrane protein from *Bordetella avium* and expression of the gene in *Salmonella typhimurium. Journal of Bacteriology* 174, 7729–7742.
Gómez-Miguel, M.J., Moriyón, I. and López, J. (1987) *Brucella* outer membrane lipoprotein shares antigenic determinants with *Escherichia coli* Braun lipoprotein and is exposed on the cell surface. *Infection and Immunity* 55, 258–262.
Griffiths, E., Stevenson, P. and Joyce, P. (1983) Pathogenic *Escherichia coli* express new outer membrane proteins when grown *in vivo. Federation of European Microbiological Societies Microbiology Letters* 16, 95–99.
Grodberg, J., Lundrigan, M.D., Toledo, D.L., Mangel, W.F. and Dunn, J.J. (1988) Complete nucleotide sequence and deduced amino acid sequence of the *omp*T gene of *Escherichia coli* K-12. *Nucleic Acids Research* 16, 1209.
Gudmundsdottir, A., Bell, P.E., Lundrigan, M.D., Bradbeer, C. and Kadner, R.J. (1989) Point mutations in a conserved region (TonB box) of *Escherichia coli* outer membrane protein BtuB affect Vitamin B_{12} transport. *Journal of Bacteriology* 171, 6526–6533.
Hancock, R.E.W. (1984) Alterations in outer membrane permeability. *Annual Review of Microbiology* 38, 237–264.
Hancock, R.E.W. (1986) Model membrane studies of porin function. In: Inouye, M. (ed.) *Bacterial Outer Membranes as Model Systems*. John Wiley & Sons, New York, pp. 187–225.
Hancock, R.E.W. (1991) Bacterial outer membranes: evolving concepts. *American Society for Microbiology News* 57, 175–182.
Hancock, R.E.W. and Bell, A. (1989) Antibiotic uptake into Gram negative bacteria. In: Jackson, G.G., Schlumberger, H.D. and Zeiler, H.J. (eds) *Perspectives in Anti-Infective Therapy*. Vieweg and Sohn, Braunshcweig, pp. 21–28.
Hancock, R.E.W. and Braun, V. (1976) Nature of the energy requirement for the irreversible adsorption of bacteriophages T1 and d80 to *Escherichia coli* K-12. *Journal of Bacteriology* 12, 409–415.
Hancock, R.E.W., Hantke, K. and Braun, V. (1976) Iron transport in *Escherichia coli* K-12: involvement of the colicin B receptor and of a citrate-inducible protein. *Journal of Bacteriology* 127, 1370–1375.
Hancock, R.E.W., Egli, C., Benz, R. and Siehnel, R.J. (1992) Overexpression in *Escherichia coli* and functional analysis of a novel PP_i-selective porin, OprO, from *Pseudomonas aeruginosa. Journal of Bacteriology* 174, 471–476.
Hancock, R.E.W., Karunaratne, D.N. and Bernegger-Egli, C. (1993) Molecular organization and structural role of outer membrane macromolecules. In: Ghuysen, J.-M. and Hakenbach, R. (eds) *Bacterial Cell Wall*. Elsevier Science Publishers, Amsterdam (in press).
Hannavy, K., Barr, G.C., Dorman, C.J., Adamson, J., Mazengera, L.R., Gallagher, M.P., Evans, J.S., Levine, B.A., Trayer, I.P. and Higgins, C.F.

(1990) TonB protein of *Salmonella typhimurium* – a model for signal transduction between membranes. *Journal of Molecular Biology* 216, 897–910.

Hantke, K. (1976) Phage T6-colicin K receptor and nucleoside transport in *Escherichia coli. Federation of European Biochemical Societies Letters* 70, 109–112.

Hantke, K. (1982) Negative control of iron uptake systems in *Escherichia coli. Federation of European Microbiological Societies Microbiology Letters* 15, 83–86.

Hardesty, C., Ferran, C. and DiRienzo, J.M. (1991) Plasmid-mediated sucrose metabolism in *Escherichia coli*: characterization of *scr*Y, the structural gene for a phosphoenolpyruvate-dependent sucrose phosphotransferase system outer membrane porin. *Journal of Bacteriology* 173, 449–456.

Harrison, J.L., Taylor, I.M., Platt, K. and O'Connor, C.D. (1992) Surface exclusion specificity of the TraT lipoprotein is determined by single alterations in a five-amino-acid region of the protein. *Molecular Microbiology* 6, 2825–2832.

Heine, H.-G., Francis, G., Lee, K.-S. and Ferenci, T. (1988) Genetic analysis of sequences in maltoporin that contribute to binding domains and pore structure. *Journal of Bacteriology* 170, 1730–1738.

Henriksen, A.Z. and Maeland, J.A. (1990) Antibody response to defined domains on enterobacterial outer membrane proteins in healthy persons and patients with bacteraemia. *Acta Pathologica Microbiologica et Immunologica Scandinavica* 98, 163–172.

Henriksen, A.Z., Maeland, J.A. and Brakstad, O.G. (1989) Monoclonal antibodies against three different enterobacterial outer membrane proteins. Characterization, cross-reactivity, and binding to bacteria. *Acta Pathologica Microbiologica et Immunologica Scandinavica* 97, 559–568.

Hindennach, I. and Henning, U. (1975) The major proteins of the *Escherichia coli* outer cell envelope membrane. *European Journal of Biochemistry* 59, 207–213.

Hirvas, L., Coleman, J., Koshi, P.K. and Vaara, M. (1990) Bacterial 'histone-like protein I' (HLP-I) is an outer membrane constituent. *Federation of European Biochemical Societies* 262, 123–126.

Hofnung, M. (1991) Expression of foreign polypeptides at the *Escherichia coli* cell surface. *Methods in Cell Biology* 34, 77–105.

Hofstra, H. and Dankert, J. (1980) Major outer membrane proteins: common antigens in Enterobacteriaceae species. *Journal of General Microbiology* 119, 123–131.

Hofstra, H., Van Tol, M.J.D. and Dankert, J. (1979) Immunofluorescent detection of the major outer membrane protein II in *Escherichia coli* O26 : K60. *Federation of European Microbiological Societies Microbiology Letters* 6, 147–150.

Homma, H., Kobayashi, T., Chiba, N., Karasawa, K., Mizushima, H., Kudo, I., Inoue, K., Ikeda, H., Sekiguchi, M. and Nojima, S. (1984) The DNA sequence encoding *pldA* gene, the structural gene for detergent-resistant phospholipase A of *Escherichia coli. Journal of Biochemistry* 96, 1655–1664.

Igo, M.M., Slauch, J.M. and Silhavy, T.J. (1990) Signal transduction in bacteria: kinases that control gene expression. *New Biologist* 2, 5–9.

Inouye, M. (ed.) (1987) *Bacterial Outer Membranes as Model Systems*. John Wiley & Sons, New York.

Inouye, M., Shaw, J. and Shen, C. (1972) The assembly of a structural lipoprotein in the envelope of *Escherichia coli*. *Journal of Biological Chemistry* 247, 8154–8159.

Isberg, R.R., Voorhis, D.L. and Falkow, S. (1987) Identification of invasin: a protein that allows enteric bacteria to penetrate cultured mammalian cells. *Cell* 50, 769–778.

Jann, B. and Jann, K. (1980) SDS polyacrylamide gel electrophoresis patterns of the outer membrane proteins from *E. coli* strains of different pathogenic origin. *Federation of European Microbiological Societies Microbiology Letters* 7, 19–22.

Jeanteur, D., Lakey, J.H. and Pattus, F. (1993) The porin superfamily: diversity and common features. In: Ghuysen, J.-M. and Hakenbach, R. (eds) *Bacterial Cell Wall*. Elsevier Science Publishers, Amsterdam (in press).

Jerse, A.E. and Kaper, J.B. (1991) The *eae* gene of enteropathogenic *Escherichia coli* encodes a 94-kilodalton membrane protein, the expression of which is influenced by the EAF plasmid. *Infection and Immunity* 59, 4302–4309.

Jones, C.H., Jacob-Dubuisson, F., Kuehn, D.M., Slonim, L., Striker, R. and Hultgren, S.J. (1992) Adhesin presentation in bacteria requires molecular chaperones and ushers. *Infection and Immunity* 60, 4445–4451.

Jung, J.U., Gutierrez, C. and Villarejo, M.R. (1989) Sequence of an osmotically inducible lipoprotein gene. *Journal of Bacteriology* 171, 511–520.

Kadner, R.J. (1990) Vitamin B_{12} transport in *Escherichia coli*: energy coupling between membranes. *Molecular Microbiology* 4, 2027–2033.

Kapur, V., White, D.G., Wilson, R.A. and Whittam, T.S. (1992) Outer membrane protein patterns mark clones of *Escherichia coli* O2 and O78 strains that cause avian septicemia. *Infection and Immunity* 60, 1687–1691.

Killmann, H. and Braun, V. (1992) An aspartate deletion mutation defines a binding site of the multifunctional FhuA outer membrane receptor of *Escherichia coli* K-12. *Journal of Bacteriology* 174, 3479–3486.

Klemm, P. (1985) Fimbrial adhesins of *Escherichia coli*. *Reviews of Infectious Diseases* 7, 321–340.

Koebnik, R. and Braun, V. (1993) Insertion derivatives containing segments of up to 16 amino acids identify surface- and periplasm-exposed regions of the FhuA outer membrane receptor of *Escherichia coli* K-12. *Journal of Bacteriology* 175, 826–839.

Konisky, J. (1979) Specific transport systems and receptor for colicins and phages. In: Inouye, M. (ed.) *Bacterial Outer Membranes*. John Wiley & Sons, New York, pp. 319–359.

Krogfelt, K.A. (1991) Bacterial adhesion: genetics, biogenesis, and role in pathogenesis of fimbrial adhesins of *Escherichia coli*. *Reviews of Infectious Diseases* 13, 721–735.

Krogfelt, K.A., Bergmans, H. and Klemm, P. (1990) Direct evidence that the FimH protein is the mannose-specific adhesin of *Escherichia coli* Type 1 fimbriae. *Infection and Immunity* 58, 1995–1998.

Lam, C., Turnowsky, F., Schwarzinger, E. and Neruda, W. (1984) Bacteria recovered without subculture from infected human urines expressed iron-regulated outer membrane proteins. *Federation of European Microbiological Societies Microbiology Letters* 24, 255–259.

Lazzaroni, J.-C. and Portalier, R. (1992) The *excC* gene of *Escherichia coli* K-12 required for cell envelope integrity encodes the peptidoglycan-associated lipoprotein (PAL). *Molecular Microbiology* 6, 735–742.

Leive, L., Shovlin, V.K. and Mergenhagen, S.E. (1968) Physical, chemical, and immunological properties of lipopolysaccharide released from *Escherichia coli* by ethylenediaminetetraacetate. *Journal of Biological Chemistry* 243, 6384–6391.

Lepault, J., Dargent, B., Tichelaar, W., Rosenbusch, J.P., Leonard, K. and Pattus, F. (1988) Three-dimensional reconstruction of maltoporin from electron microscopy and image processing. *European Molecular Biology Organization Journal* 7, 261–268.

Li, Z.M., Hannah, J.H., Stibitz, S., Nguyen, N.Y., Manclark, C.R. and Brennan, M.J. (1991) Cloning and sequencing of the structural gene for the porin protein of *Bordetella pertussis. Molecular Microbiology* 5, 1649–1656.

Loos, M. and Clas, F. (1987) Antibody-independent killing of Gram-negative bacteria via the classical pathway of complement. *Immunology Letters* 14, 203–208.

Lugtenberg, B., Meijers, J., Peters, R. and van der Hoeck, P. (1975) Electrophoretic resolution of the major outer membrane protein of *Escherichia coli* K-12 into four bands. *Federation of European Biochemical Societies Letters* 58, 254–258.

Maier, C. and Bremer, E. (1988) Pore-forming activity of the Tsx protein from the outer membrane of *Escherichia coli. Journal of Biological Chemistry* 263, 2493–2499.

Mangroo, D. and Gerber, G.E. (1992) Photoaffinity labeling of fatty acid-binding proteins involved in long chain fatty acid transport in *Escherichia coli. Journal of Biological Chemistry* 267, 17095–17101.

McNab, R.M. (1987a) Flagella. In: Neidhardt, F.C., Ingraham, J.L., Low, K.B. Magasanik, B., Schaechter, M. and Umbarger, H.E. (eds) Escherichia coli *and* Salmonella typhimurium: *Cellular and Molecular Biology*. American Society for Microbiology, Washington, DC, pp. 70–83.

McNab, R.M. (1987b) Motility and chemotaxis. In: Neidhardt, F.C., Ingraham, J.L., Low, K.B., Magasanik, B., Schaechter, M. and Umbarger, H.E. (eds) Escherichia coli *and* Salmonella typhimurium: *Cellular and Molecular Biology*. American Society for Microbiology, Washington, DC, pp. 732–759.

Medeiros, A.A., O'Brien, T.F., Rosenberg, E.Y. and Nikaido, H. (1987) Loss of OmpC porin in a strain of *Salmonella typhimurium* causes increased resistance to cephalosporins during therapy. *Journal of Infectious Diseases* 156, 751–757.

Médigue, C., Viari, A., Hénaut, A. and Danchin, A. (1991) *Escherichia coli* molecular genetic map (1500 kbp): update II. *Molecular Microbiology* 5, 2629–2640.

Melchers, F., Braun, V. and Galanos, C. (1975) The lipoprotein of the outer membrane of *Escherichia coli*: a B-lymphocyte mitogen. *Journal of Experimental Medicine* 142, 473–482.

Misra, R. and Benson, S.A. (1989) A novel mutation, cog, which results in production of a new porin protein (OmpG) of *Escherichia coli* K-12. *Journal of Bacteriology* 171, 4105–4111.

Mizuno, T. (1979) A novel peptidoglycan-associated lipoprotein found in the cell envelope of *Pseudomonas aeruginosa* and *Escherichia coli*. *Journal of Biochemistry* 86, 991–1000.

Mizuno, T. and Mizushima, S. (1990) Signal transduction and gene regulation through the phosphorylation of two regulatory components: the molecular basis for the osmotic regulation of the porin genes. *Molecular Microbiology* 4, 1077–1082.

Moll, A., Manning, P.A. and Timmis, K.N. (1980) Plasmid-determined resistance to serum bactericidal activity: a major outer membrane protein, the *tra*T gene product, is responsible for plasmid-specified serum resistance in *Escherichia coli*. *Infection and Immunity* 28, 359–367.

Montenegro, M.A., Bitter-Suermann, D., Timmis, J.K., Agero, M.E., Cabello, F.C., Sanyal, S.C. and Timmis, K.N. (1985) *traT* gene sequences, serum resistance and pathogenicity-related factors in clinical isolates of *Escherichia coli* and other Gram-negative bacteria. *Journal of General Microbiology* 131, 1511–1521.

Morona, R., Krämer, C. and Henning, U. (1985) Bacteriophage receptor area of outer membrane protein OmpA of *Escherichia coli* K-12. *Journal of Bacteriology* 164, 539–543.

Murphy, C.K. and Klebba, P.E. (1989) Export of FepA : PhoA fusion proteins to the outer membrane of *Escherichia coli* K-12. *Journal of Bacteriology* 171, 5894–5900.

Murphy, C.K., Kalve, V.I. and Klebba, P.E. (1990) Surface topology of the *Escherichia coli* K-12 ferric enterobactin receptor. *Journal of Bacteriology* 172, 2736–2746.

Nicolle, L.E., Ujak, E., Brunka, J. and Bryan, L.E. (1988) Immunoblot analysis of serologic response to outer membrane proteins of *Escherichia coli* in elderly individuals with urinary tract infections. *Journal of Clinical Microbiology* 26, 2087–2091.

Nikaido, H. (1992) Porins and specific channels of bacterial outer membranes. *Molecular Microbiology* 6, 435–442.

Nikaido, H. and Rosenberg, E.Y. (1983) Porin channels in *Escherichia coli*: studies with liposomes reconstituted from purified proteins. *Journal of Bacteriology* 153, 241–252.

Nikaido, H. and Rosenberg, E.Y. (1990) Cir and Fiu proteins in the outer membrane of *Escherichia coli* catalyze transport of monomeric catechols: study with β-lactam antibiotics containing catechol and analogous groups. *Journal of Bacteriology* 172, 1361–1367.

Nikaido, H. and Vaara, M. (1985) Molecular basis of bacterial outer membrane permeability. *Microbiological Reviews* 49, 1–32.

Ogata, R.T., Winters, C. and Levine, R.P. (1982) Nucleotide sequence analysis of the complement resistance gene from plasmid R100. *Journal of Bacteriology* 151, 819–827.

Overbeeke, N. and Lugtenberg, B. (1980) Major outer membrane proteins of *Escherichia coli* strains of human origin. *Journal of General Microbiology* 121, 373–380.

Overbeeke, N. and Lugtenberg, B. (1982) Recognition site for phosphorus-containing compounds and other negatively charged solutes on the PhoE protein pore of the outer membrane of *Escherichia coli* K12. *European Journal of Biochemistry* 126, 113–118.

Pagès, J.M., Pagès, C., Bernadac, A. and Prince, P. (1988) Immunological evidence for differences in the exposed regions of OmpF porins from *Escherichia coli* B and K-12. *Molecular Immunology* 25, 555–563.

Pallesen, L., Madsen, O. and Klemm, P. (1989) Regulation of the phase switch controlling expression of type 1 fimbriae in *Escherichia coli. Molecular Microbiology* 3, 925–931.

Parr, T.R., Poole, K., Crockford, G.W.K. and Hancock, R.E.W. (1986) Lipopolysaccharide-free *Escherichia coli* OmpF and *Pseudomonas aeruginosa* protein P porins are functionally active in lipid bilayer membranes. *Journal of Bacteriology* 165, 523–526.

Postle, K. (1990) TonB and the Gram-negative dilemma. *Molecular Microbiology* 4, 2019–2025.

Pressler, U., Staudenmaier, H., Zimmermann, L. and Braun, V. (1988) Genetics of the iron dicitrate transport system of *Escherichia coli. Journal of Bacteriology* 170, 2716–2724.

Pugsley, A.P. (1993) The complete general secretory pathway in Gram-negative bacteria. *Microbiological Reviews* 57, 50–108.

Puohiniemi, R., Karvonen, M., Vuopio-Varkila, J., Muotiala, A., Helander, I.M. and Sarvas, M. (1990) A strong antibody response to the periplasmic C-terminal domain of the OmpA protein of *Escherichia coli* is produced by immunization with purified OmpA or with whole *E. coli* or *Salmonella typhimurium* bacteria. *Infection and Immunity* 58, 1691–1696.

Rhen, M., Mäkelä, P.H. and Korhonen, T.K. (1983) P-fimbriae of *Escherichia coli* are subject to phase variation. *Federation of European Microbiological Societies Microbiology Letters* 19, 267–271.

Rice, P.A., Vayo, H.E., Tam, M.R. and Blake, M.S. (1986) Immunoglobulin G antibodies directed against protein III block killing of serum resistant *Neisseria gonorrhoeae* by immune sera. *Journal of Experimental Medicine* 164, 1735–1748.

Ried, G. and Henning, U. (1987) A unique amino acid substitution in the outer membrane protein OmpA causes conjugation deficiency in *Escherichia coli* K-12. *Federation of European Biochemical Societies Letters* 223, 387–390.

Riede, I. and Eschbach, M.-L. (1986) Evidence that TraT interacts with OmpA of *Escherichia coli. Federation of European Biochemical Societies Letters* 205, 241–245.

Robledo, J.A., Serrano, A. and Domingue, G.J. (1990) Outer membrane proteins of *E. coli* in the host–pathogen interaction in urinary tract infection. *Journal of Urology* 143, 386–391.

Rutz, J.M., Abdullah, T., Singh, S.P., Kalve, V.I. and Klebba, P.E. (1991) Evolution of the ferric enterobactin receptor in Gram-negative bacteria. *Journal of Bacteriology* 173, 5964–5974.

Rutz, J.M., Liu, J., Lyons, J.A., Goranson, J., Armstrong, S.K., McIntosh, M.A., Feix, J.B. and Klebba, P.E. (1992) Formation of a gated channel by a ligand-specific transport protein in the bacterial outer membrane. *Science* 258, 471–475.

Saint, N., De, E., Julien, S., Orange, N. and Molle, G. (1993) Ionophore properties of OmpA of *Escherichia coli. Biochimica et Biophysica Acta* 1145, 119–123.

Sauer, M., Hantke, K. and Braun, V. (1990) Sequence of the *fhuE* outer-membrane receptor gene of *Escherichia coli* K12 and properties of mutants. *Molecular Microbiology* 4, 427–437.

Saurin, W., Francoz, E., Martineau, P., Charbit, A., Dassa, E., Duplay, P., Gilson, E., Molla, A., Ronco, G., Szmelcman, S. and Hofnung, M. (1989) Periplasmic binding protein dependent transport system for maltose and maltodextrins: some recent studies. *Federation of European Microbiological Societies Microbiology Reviews* 63, 53–60.

Schmid, K., Ebner, R., Altenbuchner, J., Schmitt, R. and Lengeler, J.W. (1988) Plasmid-mediated sucrose metabolism in *Escherichia coli* K12: mapping of the *scr* genes of pUR400. *Molecular Microbiology* 2, 1–8.

Schöffler, H. and Braun, V. (1989) Transport across the outer membrane of *Escherichia coli* K12 via the FhuA receptor is regulated by the TonB protein of the cytoplasmic membrane. *Molecular and General Genetics* 217, 378–383.

Schülein, K., Schmid, K. and Benzl, R. (1991) The sugar-specific outer membrane channel ScrY contains functional characteristics of general diffusion pores and substrate-specific porins. *Molecular Microbiology* 5, 2233–2241.

Schuler, G.D., Altschul, S.F. and Lipman, D.J. (1991) A workbench for multiple alignment construction and analysis. *Proteins: Structure, Function, and Genetics* 9, 180–190.

Schweizer, M., Hindennach, I., Garten, W. and Henning, U. (1978) Major proteins of the *Escherichia coli* outer cell envelope membrane interaction of protein II with lipopolysaccharide. *European Journal of Biochemistry* 82, 211–217.

Sciortino, C.V. and Finkelstein, R.A. (1983) *Vibrio cholerae* expresses iron-regulated outer membrane proteins *in vivo. Infection and Immunity* 42, 990–996.

Skurray, R.A., Hancock, R.E.W. and Reeves, P. (1974) Con-mutants: class of mutants in *Escherichia coli* K-12 lacking a major cell wall protein and defective in conjugation and adsorption of a bacteriophage. *Journal of Bacteriology* 119, 726–735.

Smelcman, S. and Hofnung, M. (1975) Maltose transport in *Escherichia coli* K-12: involvement of the bacteriophage lambda receptor. *Journal of Bacteriology* 124, 112–118.

Sonntag, I., Schwarz, H., Hirota, Y. and Henning, U. (1978) Cell envelope and shape of *Escherichia coli*: multiple mutants missing the outer membrane lipoprotein and other major outer membrane proteins. *Journal of Bacteriology* 136, 280–285.

Strittmatter, W. and Galanos, C. (1987) Characterization of protein co-extracted together with LPS in *Escherichia coli*, *Salmonella minnesota* and *Yersinia enterocolitica. Microbial Pathogenesis* 2, 29–36.

Sugawara, E. and Nikaido, H. (1992) Pore-forming activity of OmpA protein of *Escherichia coli. Journal of Biological Chemistry* 267, 2507–2511.

Sugimura, K. (1988) Mutant isolation and cloning of the gene encoding protease VII from *Escherichia coli*. *Biochemical and Biophysical Research Communications* 153, 753–759.

Sukupolvi, S. and O'Connor, C.D. (1990) TraT lipoprotein, a plasmid-specified mediator of interactions between Gram-negative bacteria and their environment. *Microbiological Reviews* 54, 331–341.

Sultzer, B.M. and Goodman, G.W. (1976) Endotoxin protein: a B-cell mitogen and polyclonal activator of C3H/HeJ lymphocytes. *Journal of Experimental Medicine* 144, 821–827.

Sutcliffe, J., Blumenthal, R., Walter, A. and Foulds, J. (1983) *Escherichia coli* outer membrane protein K is a porin. *Journal of Bacteriology* 156, 867–872.

Suzuki, H., Nishimura, Y., Yasuda, S., Nishimura, M., Yamada, M. and Hirota, Y. (1978) Murein-lipoprotein of *Escherichia coli*: a protein involved in the stabilization of bacterial cell envelope. *Molecular and General Genetics* 167, 1–9.

Taplits, M. and Michael, J.G. (1979) Immune response to *Escherichia coli* B surface antigens. *Infection and Immunity* 25, 943–945.

Tommassen, J., Koster, M. and Overduin, P. (1987) Molecular analysis of the promoter region of the *Escherichia coli* K-12 *phoE* gene. Identification of an element, upstream from the promoter, required for efficient expression of PhoE protein. *Journal of Molecular Biology* 198, 633–641.

van Alphen, L., van Kempen-De Troye, F. and Zanen, H.C. (1983) Characterization of cell envelope proteins and lipopolysaccharides of *Escherichia coli* isolates from patients with neonatal meningitis. *Federation of European Microbiological Societies Microbiology Letters* 16, 261–267.

van der Ley, P., de Graaff, P. and Tommassen, J. (1986a) Shielding of *Escherichia coli* outer membrane proteins as receptors for bacteriophages and colicins by O-antigenic chains of lipopolysaccharide. *Journal of Bacteriology* 168, 449–451.

van der Ley, P., Kuipers, O., Tommassen, J. and Lugtenberg, B. (1986b) O-antigenic chains of lipopolysaccharide prevent binding of antibody molecules to an outer membrane pore protein in Enterobacteriaceae. *Microbial Pathogenesis* 1, 43–49.

Verhoef, C., Benz, R., Poon, A.P.W. and Tommassen, J. (1987) New pore protein produced in cells lysogenic for *Escherichia coli* phage HK253*hrk*. *European Journal of Biochemistry* 164, 141–145.

Virji, M. and Heckels, J.E. (1989) Location of a blocking epitope on outer-membrane protein III of *Neisseria gonorrhoeae* by synthetic peptide analysis. *Journal of General Microbiology* 135, 1895–1899.

Vuopio-Varkila, J., Karvonen, M. and Saxon, H. (1988) Protective capacity of antibodies to outer-membrane components of *Escherichia coli* in a systemic mouse peritonitis model. *Journal of Medical Microbiology* 25, 77–84.

Wandersman, C. and Delepelaire, P. (1990) TolC, an *Escherichia coli* outer membrane protein required for hemolysin secretion. *Proceedings of the National Academy of Sciences of the United States of America* 87, 4776–4780.

Weiser, J.N. and Gotschlich, E.C. (1991) Outer membrane protein A (OmpA) contributes to serum resistance and pathogenicity of *Escherichia coli* K-1. *Infection and Immunity* 59, 2252–2258.

Weiser, J.N., Blake, M.S. and Gotschlich, E.C. (1992) Antibodies to outer membrane protein A (OmpA) block bactericidal killing of *Escherichia coli*. In: *Abstracts of the 92nd Annual Meeting of the American Society for Microbiology*. American Society for Microbiology, Washington, DC, Abstr. B-175, p. 55.

Weiss, M.S., Abele, U., Weckesser, J., Welte, W., Schiltz, E. and Schulz, G.E. (1991) Molecular architecture and electrostatic properties of a bacterial porin. *Science* 254, 1627–1630.

Whitfield, C., Hancock, R.E.W. and Costerton, J.W. (1983) Outer membrane protein K of *Escherichia coli*: purification and pore-forming properties in lipid bilayer membranes. *Journal of Bacteriology* 156, 873–879.

Willetts, N. and Skurray, R. (1987) Structure and function of the F factor and mechanism of conjugation. In: Neidhardt, F.C., Ingraham, J.L., Low, K.B., Magasanik, B., Schaechter, M. and Umbarger, H.E. (eds) Escherichia coli *and* Salmonella typhimurium: *Cellular and Molecular Biology*. American Society for Microbiology, Washington, DC, pp. 1110–1133.

Woodruff, W.A. and Hancock, R.E.W. (1989) *Pseudomonas aeruginosa* outer membrane protein F: structural role and relationship to the *Escherichia coli* OmpA protein. *Journal of Bacteriology* 171, 3304–3309.

Yamada, H. and Mizushima, S. (1980) Interaction between major outer membrane protein (0–8) and lipopolysaccharide in *Escherichia coli* K12. *European Journal of Biochemistry* 103, 209–218.

Yu, D.T., Hamachi, T., Hamachi, M. and Tribbick, G. (1991) Analysis of the molecular mimicry between HLA-B27 and a bacterial OmpA protein using synthetic peptides. *Clinical and Experimental Immunology* 85, 510–514.

Zhang, J.-J., Hamachi, M., Hamachi, T., Zhao, Y.-P. and Yu, D.T.Y. (1989) The bacterial outer membrane protein that reacts with anti-HLA-B27 antibodies is the OmpA protein. *Journal of Immunology* 143, 2955–2960.

Iron Acquisition Systems in *Escherichia coli*

19

E. Griffiths
National Institute for Biological Standards and Control, Blanche Lane, South Mimms, Potters Bar, Hertfordshire EN6 3QG, UK

Iron and Bacterial Virulence

Spectacular advances in biochemistry, molecular biology and immunology over the past decade, together with the advent of recombinant DNA technology, have yielded powerful new techniques for studying bacterial pathogens and the diseases they cause. Although several approaches are currently being used, most investigations into bacterial virulence have been carried out with organisms grown *in vitro* under conditions that do not necessarily reflect microbial behaviour *in vivo*. That this is likely to give at best only a partial picture of bacterial characteristics associated with virulence is now increasingly recognized and more and more attention is being given to the environmentally regulated properties of bacterial pathogens (Griffiths, 1991).

One of the best understood properties of the environment encountered by pathogens in host tissues, and of its effects on bacterial characteristics and growth, concerns the availability of iron. Our understanding of the way the host normally restricts the availability of the metal has increased enormously in recent years and a considerable literature has developed on the relationship between iron and pathogenicity (Bullen and Griffiths, 1987; Crosa, 1989; Weinberg, 1989; Martinez *et al.*, 1990; Williams and Griffiths, 1992; Wooldridge and Williams, 1993). Iron is now recognized as playing a crucial role in infection. Its importance lies in the strictly limited availability of the metal in living tissues and progress made in understanding the strategies used by pathogens for acquiring iron *in vivo*, and their responses to iron restriction has provided a fresh insight into microbial pathogenicity. Much of this new understanding of what is happening as pathogenic bacteria adapt to and grow in the iron-restricted extracellular environment of the host has come from studies with Gram-negative organisms, especially *E. coli*. This is because *E. coli* provided an ideal experimental model; a great deal was already known about its biochemistry and genetics and it also causes important infections in both man and animals. Work with *E. coli* established the principle that pathogenic bacteria undergo considerable phenotypic changes both in their metabolism and in the composition of their outer membranes when growing *in vitro* under iron restriction and *in vivo* during infection, and this information has served as a guideline for the often more difficult investigations of other pathogens.

Availability of Iron *in vivo*

The amount of free iron which might be available to bacteria invading the body fluids of humans and animals is normally extremely small even though the actual quantity of iron present may be considerable. The reason for this is that the iron present is held primarily inside cells as haem or in the iron-storage protein ferritin, and that which is extracellular in plasma or other body fluids is attached to high-affinity iron binding glycoproteins, transferrin and lactoferrin, which are often present in significant quantities (up to 4–5 mg ml^{-1}). A related protein called ovotransferrin is found in avian egg white. These iron-binding proteins have molecular masses of about 80 kDa and they consist of two similar but not identical half molecules, disposed in space as two distinct lobes, each of which contains a single iron-binding site. Each protein molecule is therefore capable of reversibly binding two atoms of ferric iron, a process which requires the presence of an anion, usually bicarbonate, on a 1 : 1 molar basis. Since these proteins have association constants for iron of about 10^{36} and bind iron very tightly, and are normally only partially saturated with Fe^{3+}, the amount of free iron in equilibrium with an iron-binding protein at neutral pH is of the order of 10^{-18}M, which is far too low to support bacterial growth. In the case of transferrin, the iron-binding affinity is diminished below pH 6, but lactoferrin retains its iron-binding properties under more acidic conditions, such as those which often prevail at sites of inflammation where lactoferrin can accumulate (McClelland and van Furth, 1976; Ainscough *et al.*, 1980; Crichton and Ward, 1992). In addition, during infection the host reduces the total amount of iron bound to serum transferrin. This is called the hypoferraemia of infection, a process which can be reproduced experimentally by injecting small amounts of endotoxin (Kluger and Bullen, 1987; Konijn and Hershko, 1989). Since virtually all known bacterial pathogens need iron to multiply, then clearly only those organisms that can adapt to this severely iron-restricted environment and produce mechanisms for assimilating protein-bound iron, or can acquire it from some other source, such as liberated haem, will be able to multiply successfully in normal body fluids to establish extracellular infections.

Little is known about the availability of iron inside cells, although it seems that in some cells at least iron is readily available to support bacterial growth (Lawlor *et al.*, 1987, Nassif *et al.*, 1987; Byrd and Horwitz, 1989). The nature of this 'available pool' of iron is unknown although it is probably composed of iron complexed to relatively low molecular weight chelators. This is likely to represent only a very small amount of cellular iron in view of the toxicity of the loosely bound metal (Griffiths, 1987a). It is not known whether ferritin can act directly as an iron source for bacterial pathogens.

Siderophore-mediated Iron Uptake

Four possible mechanisms have been considered which might enable invading organisms to assimilate ferric (Fe^{3+}) iron bound to the high affinity iron-binding glycoproteins of the host (Table 19.1). Little is known about mechanisms 1 and 2 (Table 19.1), although much progress is now being made in understanding the direct receptor-mediated systems (number 3) which involve bacterial transferrin- and lactoferrin-receptors (Williams and Griffiths, 1992). *E. coli* does not have receptors for the iron-binding proteins, nor does it appear to have an extracellular iron reductase system (Table 19.1, mechanism 2), but it can utilize ferrous (Fe^{2+}) iron when available, for example during anaerobiosis (Hantke, 1987a). At present, the best understood systems used by pathogenic bacteria to acquire iron from host iron-binding proteins are those which depend on the production of low-molecular-weight high-affinity iron-chelating compounds called siderophores and several reviews on the topic have been published (Griffiths, 1987b; Crosa, 1989; Weinberg, 1989; Neilands,

Table 19.1. Possible mechanisms used by pathogenic bacteria for assimilating iron bound to host iron-binding proteins.

1. Proteolytic cleavage of the iron-binding protein disrupting the iron-binding site and releasing iron.

2. Reduction of the Fe^{3+}–protein complex to Fe^{2+}–protein complex with the consequent release and uptake of ferrous iron.

3. Direct interaction between the bacterial cell surface and the Fe^{3+}–protein complex in a manner analogous to the interaction between transferrin and the mammalian transferrin-receptor.

4. Production of low-molecular-weight iron-chelating compounds, called siderophores, that remove iron from the Fe^{3+}–protein complex and deliver it to the bacterial cell via specific ferric-siderophore receptors.

1990; Wooldridge and Williams, 1993). Perhaps the best characterized of these systems are those used by the enteric bacteria and in particular *E. coli*.

Enterobactin

E. coli, as well as *Salmonella typhimurium* and *Klebsiella pneumoniae*, produce the phenolate iron chelator enterobactin (also called enterochelin) under conditions of iron restriction *in vitro* (O'Brien and Gibson, 1970; Pollack and Neilands, 1970; Rogers, 1973; Rogers *et al.*, 1977). This compound is the cyclic triester of 2,3-dihydroxy-*N*-benzoyl-L-serine (Fig. 19.1) and, like most siderophores, it is synthesized only during iron-restricted growth. Enterobactin efficiently removes iron from iron-binding proteins and transports it into the bacterial cell; the process is represented diagrammatically in Fig. 19.2. This chelator acts as a hexadentate chelating agent through its three catechol groups and, when coordinating with ferric iron, it acts as a six-proton acid; at neutral pH, therefore, the hexa coordinate complex carries three negative charges $[Fe\ (ent)]^{3-}$ (Harris *et al.*, 1979c).

The single most outstanding feature of siderophores is their extremely high affinity for ferric iron. The formation constant for ferric enterobactin was, until very recently, the highest ever recorded for a ferric iron chelator, being near 10^{52} at neutral pH (Harris *et al.*, 1979a, c). A siderophore from a marine bacterium has now been discovered with a reported affinity for iron resembling that of enterobactin (Reid *et al.*, 1993). Organisms using enterobactin-mediated iron transport are, therefore, able to compete effectively for iron complexed to iron-binding proteins. The fact that an enterobactin-producing strain of *Salmonella* obtained iron from transferrin when the protein was inside a dialysis bag shows that contact between the

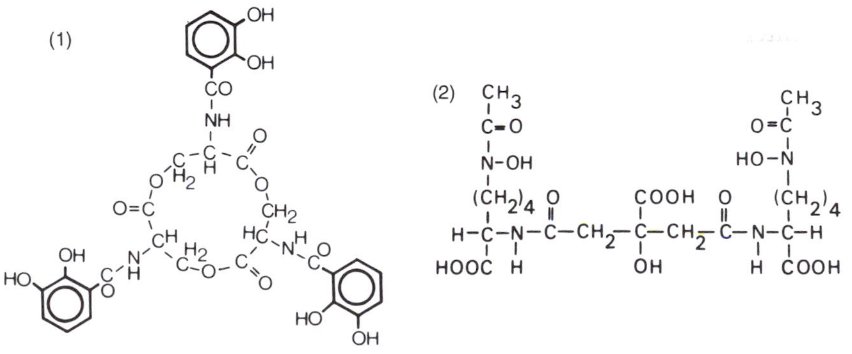

Fig. 19.1. Structural formula: 1, enterobactin; 2, aerobactin.

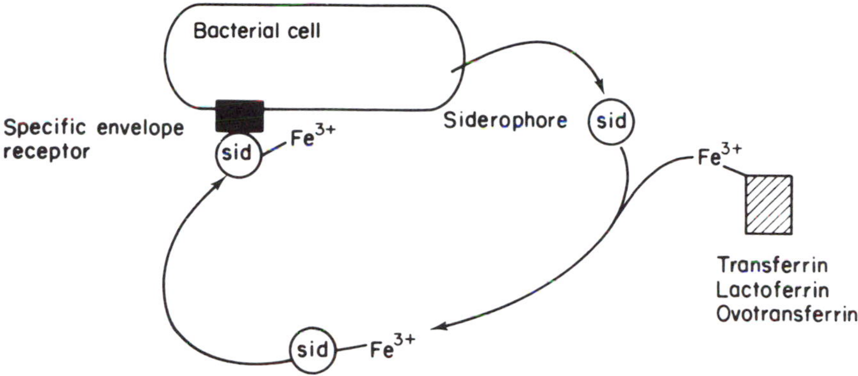

Fig. 19.2. Schematic representation of siderophore-mediated iron uptake in *E. coli*.

transferrin and the bacterial cell surface is not required for siderophore-mediated removal of iron (Tidmarsh and Rosenberg, 1981). This is in contrast to receptor-mediated mechanisms where direct interaction between a bacterial receptor and the iron-binding protein is essential for iron uptake (Williams and Griffiths, 1992).

Enterobactin synthesis in *E. coli* involves the products of seven genes, *ent* A to G, located in the enterobactin gene cluster at 13 minutes on the *E. coli* chromosome (Young *et al.*, 1971; Greenwood and Luke, 1976; Fleming *et al.*, 1985; Earhart, 1987; Liu *et al.*, 1989; Nahlik *et al.*, 1989; Ozenberger *et al.*, 1989). Synthesis begins with the conversion of chorismic acid, a central precursor of the aromatic amino acid biosynthetic pathway, via isochorismate, into 2,3-dihydroxybenzoic acid (Liu *et al.*, 1990; Rusnak *et al.*, 1990). The final assembly of 2,3-dihydroxybenzoic acid and L-serine into enterobactin is an adenosine triphosphate (ATP) requiring process carried out by the products of genes *ent* D, *ent* E, *ent* F and *ent* G which appear to work as a multienzyme complex (Armstrong *et al.*, 1989).

Although *E. coli* can use enterobactin to obtain iron complexed to transferrin, lactoferrin or ovotransferrin, using this chelator is an energetically expensive process. Enterobactin requires ATP for its synthesis and it is used only once for transporting iron into the bacterial cell. This is because the cyclic triester linkages of the Fe^{3+}-enterobactin are cleaved by a specific esterase when the iron-loaded molecule enters the cell, ultimately producing 2,3-dihydroxybenzoylserine which is then discarded (Rosenberg and Young, 1974; Greenwood and Luke, 1978). It has been proposed that hydrolysis of the bonds is necessary to release the iron because the ferric ester has too low a reduction potential to enable enterobactin reduction to release the metal (Cooper *et al.*, 1978; Harris *et al.*, 1979c; Raymond and Carrano, 1979). However, a carbocyclic analogue of enterobactin, which lacks ester bonds, effectively supplies iron to an enterobactin-deficient strain of *E. coli* and this raised questions about the exact role of the esterase. These questions have not yet been fully answered (Hollifield and Neilands, 1978). A ferrous–enterobactin complex has been identified and it has been suggested that this might play a part in translocating iron across the cytoplasmic membrane (Hider *et al.*, 1979). The metal is held much less tightly in ferrous–enterobactin than in the usual ferri-form and this could donate the iron readily to other coordinating ligands within the cell. Nevertheless, whatever the function of the esterase, *E. coli fes* mutants, which lack esterase activity, are unable to use the ferric complex of enterobactin (Langman *et al.*, 1972; Rosenberg and Young, 1974). Recently, the esterase of *E. coli* has been overexpressed and purified (Brickman and McIntosh, 1992) and there is a suggestion that reduction of iron from the ferric to the ferrous state in enterobactin may depend upon and be subsequent to esterase activity. However, the hydrolysis of the cyclic platform of enterobactin seems to be independent of any reduction of the complexed metal.

Studies on enterobactin-dependent iron uptake have mainly been carried out *in vitro* using the laboratory strain *E. coli* K12. However, pathogenic strains of *E. coli* also produce this chelator; indeed, virtually all wild-type and clinical isolates of *E. coli* produce enterobactin (Griffiths, 1987b). Furthermore, it is known to be produced *in vivo* during infection (Griffiths and Humphreys, 1980). Enterobactin and its degradation products were detected in the peritoneal washings from guinea-pigs infected with *E. coli* O111, a finding which supports the idea that the presence of iron-binding proteins in body fluids maintain an iron-restricted environment *in vivo*.

Aerobactin

In addition to producing the phenolate-based siderophore enterobactin under conditions of iron restriction, several clinical isolates of *E. coli*, as well as *Klebsiella* and certain strains of *Salmonella*, also synthesize and secrete into the surrounding medium a second high-affinity hydroxamate type iron chelator called aerobactin (Fig. 19.1). In particular, many *E. coli* strains which cause systemic or other extraintestinal infections produce aerobactin (Williams, 1979; Valvano *et al.*, 1986; Griffiths, 1987b; Lafonte *et al.*, 1987; Jacobson *et al.*, 1988; de Lorenzo and Martinez, 1988; Zingler *et al.*, 1988; Gadó *et al.*, 1989; Opal *et al.*, 1990). Unlike the case of enterobactin, where the biosynthetic genes are always chromosomal, those for aerobactin synthesis can be located in the chromosome or on a plasmid. For example, *E. coli* strains which cause sepsis in man and animals carry the aerobactin synthetic genes on the Colicin V plasmid [p Col V] as well as non Col V plasmids (Williams, 1979; Williams and Warner, 1980; Griffiths, 1987b; Gonzalo *et al.*, 1988; Crosa, 1989). Enteroinvasive strains of *E. coli* and *Shigella flexneri*, which also produce aerobactin (Payne *et al.*, 1983; Griffiths *et al.*, 1985b), have their aerobactin genes in the chromosome (Marolda *et al.*, 1987). The widespread distribution of the aerobactin-mediated iron uptake system genes suggested that the aerobactin operon may be genetically mobile and there is some evidence (de Lorenzo *et al.*, 1988a) to support this view, although for a number of reasons (Waters and Crosa, 1986) it is doubtful whether the 18-kb fragment between the two IS1 elements in p Col V-K30, which contains the aerobactin genes, constitutes a true transposon.

Aerobactin is a member of the hydroxamic acid–citrate family of siderophores and was originally isolated from *Aerobacter aerogenes* (Gibson and Magrath, 1969). It is a conjugate of 6-(*N*-acetyl-*N*-hydroxylamine)-2-aminohexanoic acid and citric acid and it has been shown to form an octahedral complex with ferric iron using the two bidentate hydroxamate groups, the central carboxylate and probably the citrate hydroxyl group (Harris *et al.*, 1979b). The biosynthesis of aerobactin involves the conversion of L-lysine to N^6-hydroxylysine, catalysed by the oxygenase IucD, followed by acetylation, catalysed by IucB, and the condensation of N^6-acetyl-N^6-hydroxylysine with citric acid, a reaction catalysed by IucA; the resulting N^2-citryl-N^6-acetyl-N^6-hydroxylysine then condenses with a further molecule of N^6-acetyl-N^6-hydroxylysine, by the action of Iuc C, to produce aerobactin (Neilands, 1991). The nomenclature Iuc, for *i*ron *u*ptake *c*helate, was coined by Williams and Warner (1980), the four enzymes being encoded by four genes *iuc*A, *iuc*B, *iuc*C and *iuc*D.

Although epidemiological data suggest that the presence of an aerobactin iron-uptake system promotes the ability of the pathogen to cause septicaemia and meningitis, not all pathogens which produce aerobactin cause septicaemia. Both enteroinvasive *E. coli* and *S. flexneri* produce aerobactin but do not cause septicaemia (Griffiths *et al.*, 1985b; Payne, 1989). The aerobactin iron uptake system has also been detected in some enteropathogenic strains of *E. coli* (Roberts *et al.*, 1986). It is still not clear why acquiring the ability to make a second siderophore confers a selective advantage on bacteria that can already make enterobactin. However, there have been a number of hypotheses (Griffiths, 1987b; de Lorenzo and Martinez, 1988; Crosa, 1989).

Kinetically, hydroxamate-based iron chelators like aerobactin seem inferior to catecholate-based siderophores in removing iron from transferrin (Carrano and Raymond, 1979). However, the presence of other factors in body fluids could well influence the overall effectiveness of different siderophores *in vivo*, and care must be taken in extrapolating data obtained *in vitro* to the situation *in vivo* during infection. Pollack *et al.* (1976) and

Konopka *et al.* (1982) have shown that the kinetic barrier to efficient hydroxamate-mediated, especially aerobactin-mediated, removal of iron from transferrin can be partially overcome by adding other anions to the system. Another important difference between the mode of action of these two chelators is that aerobactin is recycled whereas enterobactin is only used once for transporting iron into the bacterial cell (Raymond and Carrano, 1979; Braun *et al.*, 1984). Furthermore, serum albumin has been reported to bind enterobactin, but not aerobactin, decreasing its effective concentration in serum and possibly impeding enterobactin-mediated mobilization of transferrin iron (Konopka and Neilands, 1984). Anti-enterobactin antibodies (Moore *et al.*, 1980; Moore and Earhart, 1981), as well as anti 'O'-polysaccharide antibodies which interfere with enterobactin secretion (Fitzgerald and Rogers, 1980), have been detected in sera and these could further inhibit enterobactin-mediated iron uptake.

For various reasons, therefore, the growth of *E. coli* strains which rely entirely on enterobactin for acquiring iron might be expected to be restricted compared to those which produce aerobactin. The fact that higher dose levels of aerobactin negative (Col V^-) *E. coli* O18:K1:H7 grew as well as the aerobactin positive Col V^+ strain in host tissues suggests that the enterobactin-mediated iron-uptake mechanism can function *in vivo* but that the aerobactin iron-uptake systems may be important at low infective doses (Smith and Huggins, 1980). Roberts *et al.* (1989) have shown that the aerobactin-mediated iron-uptake system of plasmid Col V-K30, genetically isolated from other plasmid determinants by molecular cloning, is sufficient to restore to full virulence, in a mouse peritonitis model, a clinical *E. coli* isolate whose resident aerobactin-encoding Col V plasmid had been lost by curing. However, it is not known whether both enterobactin and aerobactin are required for full virulence. So far no well-characterized Ent^- Aer^+ strains of *E. coli* have been reported amongst clinical isolates from septicaemic disease, although most strains of *S. flexneri* produce only aerobactin. Interestingly, the failure of *S. flexneri* to produce enterobactin is due not to lack of genes involved in the production of the siderophore but to a defect in their expression (Schmitt and Payne, 1988; Crosa, 1989; Payne, 1989).

Other siderophores

An increasingly reported phenomenon is the ability of bacteria to use siderophores produced by other microorganisms, but which they themselves are unable to synthesize (West and Sparling, 1987; Williams *et al.*, 1990). *E. coli* is capable of using the fungal hydroxamate-type chelators ferrichrome, coprogen and rhodotorulic acid (Leong and Neilands, 1976; Hantke 1983). Like aerobactin, and unlike enterobactin, ferrichrome is not destroyed when transporting iron into *E. coli* (Leong and Neilands, 1976) but it is acetylated on one of the hydroxyl-amino oxygens after reductive separation of Fe^{3+} (Hartmann and Braun, 1980). This seems to be an essential step in the ferrichrome-mediated iron-transport system. Some *E. coli* strains also appear to be able to use ferrioxamine B as a source of iron (Nelson *et al.*, 1992); this is a hydroxamate siderophore made by certain strains of *Streptomyces*. A previous report by Rabsch and Reissbrodt (1988) suggested that *E. coli* was unable to take iron from ferrioxamine B and further work will be needed to see if this discrepancy is due to strain differences or to the level of chelator used. In addition, citrate can supply iron to *E. coli*, although the affinity of this substance for iron does not approach that of the true siderophores. The citrate-mediated iron-transport system is induced when the bacteria are grown in an iron-limited medium containing citrate (Woodrow *et al.*, 1978; Hussain *et al.*, 1981; Zimmermann *et al.*, 1984). It is not know how widely this system is distributed in pathogenic strains of *E. coli*, nor whether the iron–dicitrate transport system can function *in vivo* during infection. Citrate seems not to be used as a carbon source by most *E. coli*, although *E. coli* containing HI plasmids have been reported to use it as the sole source of energy (Smith *et al.*, 1978). Dihydroxybenzoylserine, a breakdown product of enterobactin, can also stimulate the growth of *E. coli* under iron-limiting conditions by acting like a siderophore (Hantke, 1990).

Iron-regulated Outer Membrane Proteins

An integral part of siderophore-mediated iron-uptake systems is the production of outer-membrane proteins which act as receptors for ferric-siderophores, as well as mechanisms for the release of chelator-bound iron (Neilands, 1982; Griffiths, 1987b). The need for specific receptors is due, in part, to the fact that the molecular weights of some siderophores exceed the diffusion limit (about 600) of the small water-filled pores of the outer membrane (Nikaido, 1979; Braun *et al.*, 1991). However, the molecular mass of the iron–dicitrate complex ($Fe(Cit)_2$) is probably no greater than 443. The fact that there is a specific receptor for this iron complex too suggests that the iron requirements of the cell can best be satisfied by an initial adsorption of the iron-loaded siderophore to the surface receptors where iron can be accumulated relative to its concentration in the growth environment. The strict requirement for a receptor for siderophore-mediated iron uptake is demonstrated by the fact that strains lacking such proteins in their outer membrane, or which have receptor proteins altered by insertion mutagenesis, are devoid of transport activity (Grewal *et al.*, 1982; Carmel *et al.*, 1990). Such mutants can be obtained relatively easily in *E. coli* since most of the siderophore receptors also function as receptors for bacteriophages and/or colicins (Table 19.2).

Table 19.2. Functions of iron-regulated outer membrane proteins in *E. coli*.

Receptor	Apparent molecular mass	Phage/colicin binding	Function
Cir	74 kDa	Colicin I	Catecholate-mediated iron uptake
Iut A	74 kDa	Cloacin DF13	Uptake of Fe^{3+}-aerobactin
Fhu	78 kDa	Phages T1, T5 and ϕ 80, Colicin M	Uptake of ferrichrome
Fec A	80.5 kDa	—	Uptake of Fe^{3+}-citrate
Fep A	81 kDa	Colicin B	Uptake of Fe^{3+}-enterobactin
Fhu E	76 kDa	—	Uptake of Fe^{3+}-coprogen and Fe^{3+}-rhodotorulic acid
Fox B	66 kDa + 26 kDa	—	Uptake of ferrioxamine B
Fiu	83 kDa	—	Catecholate-mediated iron uptake
76 kDa	76 kDa	Cloacin DF13	Uptake of Fe^{3+}-aerobactin in enteroinvasive strains and *S. flexneri*

E. coli produce several new outer membrane proteins under iron-restricted growth conditions and some of these have been identified as ferric siderophore receptors (Table 19.2). An 81-kDa protein (FepA) acts as the receptor for ferric enterobactin. This protein is the product of the *fep*A gene which maps along with *ent* and *fes* genes in a cluster at about 13 minutes on the *E. coli* chromosome (Neilands, 1982). Together these genes are responsible for the biosynthesis, transport and hydrolysis of enterobactin and their expression is regulated by iron. A 78-kDa protein (FhuA) (for *f*erric *h*ydroxamate *u*ptake), an iron-regulated protein encoded by the *fhu*A gene located at 3.5 minutes on the chromosome of *E. coli*, functions as the receptor for ferrichrome (Neilands, 1982; Coulton *et al.*, 1983; Carmel *et al.*, 1990; Braun *et al.*, 1991). Ferric coprogen and ferric rhodotorulic acid also have their own receptor protein, FhuE (Braun *et al.*, 1991), as does ferrioxamine B, FoxB (Nelson *et al.*, 1992). The Col V-plasmid encoded 74-kDa protein (IutA) functions as the receptor for the other major hydroxamate-type siderophore, aerobactin, in *E. coli* harbouring this plasmid (Bindereif *et al.*, 1982; Grewal *et al.*, 1982).

Two other well-characterized *E. coli* iron-regulated proteins, the 83-kDa protein (Fiu protein) and another 74-kDa protein (Cir) have been known for a long time but until recently no specific function had been assigned to them, although it was suspected that they might act as receptors for some as yet undiscovered siderophore (Hantke, 1983). Recently, a novel group of β-lactam antibiotics substituted with catechols, and which exhibit a 100-fold higher antibiotic activity than classical cephalosporins against *E. coli* and other Gram-negative bacteria, have been shown to have enhanced uptake into the bacterial cells via Cir and Fiu, suggesting that both these receptors played a part in the uptake of some natural catecholate-type siderophore (Watanabe *et al.*, 1987; Curtis *et al.*, 1988). In 1990, Hantke showed that 2,3-dihydroxybenzoylserine, a degradation product of enterobactin, can also act as a siderophore for *E. coli* and that this is taken up by the bacterial cell via Fiu and Cir, and less effectively by FepA. The strains of *E. coli* which can use ferric dicitrate as an iron source produce an outer membrane protein with an apparent molecular mass of about 81 kDa, the FecA protein, when growing in iron-restricted media containing citrate (Frost and Rosenberg, 1973; Hancock *et al.*, 1976; Wagegg and Braun, 1981). This protein is part of the citrate-mediated iron transport system and is induced by iron restriction but only in the presence of citrate (Hussein *et al.*, 1981; Wagegg and Braun, 1981; Zimmermann *et al.*, 1984; Pressler *et al.*, 1988).

All of the above-mentioned outer membrane receptor proteins require additional proteins to complete the process of transporting iron into the bacterial cell. For example, all of the hydroxamate siderophores require not only outer membrane siderophore-specific receptors like FhuA, FhuE or Iut, but also common transport functions specified by genetically defined loci including *fhu*C, *fhu*D, *fhu*B and *exb*B (Hantke and Zimmermann, 1981; Coulton *et al.*, 1987; Köster and Braun, 1989, 1990a, b; Köster and Böhm, 1992). Siderophore-mediated iron-uptake mechanisms differ from porin-mediated diffusion of solutes across the outer membrane because of their substrate specificities and their requirement for energy. Energy-coupled transport processes across the outer membrane depend crucially on the TonB protein and the complex mechanisms involved in the transport of iron across the outer membrane are well described by Braun *et al.* (1991) and by Köster (1991). The TonB protein, which is involved not only with all high-affinity iron transport processes but also with the utilization of certain other nutrients like vitamin B_{12}, functions by coupling the energy providing metabolism of the inner cytoplasmic membrane to outer membrane receptor activity. TonB is anchored in the cytoplasmic membrane but mostly exposed to the periplasmic space (Postle and Skare, 1988; Hannavy *et al.*, 1990) and believed to interact directly with the periplasmic portion of the outer membrane protein receptors (Brewer *et al.*, 1990). For the interaction between the TonB protein and the various receptors to take place it might be expected that there would be a common structure in the outer membrane proteins which is recognized by TonB. Such structures have now been identified in many of the proteins thought to interact with TonB; they are located close to the N-termini of these proteins and called the 'TonB box' (Braun *et al.*, 1991), although it seems this peptide sequence is not sufficient to mediate specific interactions with TonB (Brewer *et al.*, 1990; Hannavy *et al.*, 1990). By binding to the receptor protein, TonB is believed to induce conformational changes in the receptor which allow the ferric siderophore to enter the periplasmic space.

Recent studies on FepA have led to the novel idea that all of the outer membrane receptors may be 'gated porins' (Rutz *et al.*, 1992). FepA is a 723-amino-acid protein with three distinct parts: a β-barrel domain located in the membrane bilayer, which could act as a non-specific channel through the membrane; a surface exposed region, which binds ferric enterobactin; and a 'TonB-box' within the periplasmic end of the molecule which can interact with TonB. Deletion of the cell-surface ligand binding peptides generated mutant FepA proteins that were incapable of high-affinity uptake of enterobactin but, instead, surprisingly formed non-specific, passive channels in the outer membrane which allowed enterobactin through the membrane; these pores acted independently of TonB (Rutz *et al.*, 1992). In normal FepA protein the channel would be closed at the cell surface by loops of hydrophilic peptides that selectively bind enterobactin. Once activated by TonB, the 'gate' is opened by conformational alterations in FepA and allows ferric-enterobactin into the channel and through into the periplasm. Such a mechanism preserves the permeability of the outer membrane but operates in response to the interaction of FepA with ferric-enterobactin and with TonB.

The extensive sequence homology among the TonB-dependent receptors of *E. coli* suggests that the other receptors may transport their siderophores by this 'gated' porin mechanism, the TonB protein itself acting as a sort of 'molecular gatekeeper'. Once in the periplasm the various siderophores bind to other components of the system located in the cytoplasmic membrane and the ferric siderophore, or the iron, is then translocated across the membrane into the cell by another energy-dependent process.

Most of the work on iron transport in *E. coli* has been carried out with laboratory strains, such as *E. coli* K12. From the point of view of infection it is understanding what goes on in pathogenic strains that is important, the nature of the outer membrane siderophore receptors being of particular interest since the bacterial cell surface interacts directly with the host. Pathogenic strains of *E. coli* produce new proteins similar to those of *E. coli* K12 when grown *in vitro* in the presence of iron-binding proteins (Griffiths *et al.*, 1983, 1985a, b). However, the relative abundance of the 83-kDa, 81-kDa, 78-kDa and 74-kDa proteins expressed in different pathogenic strains of *E. coli* under the same iron-restricted growth conditions varies considerably and some strains produce additional iron-regulated outer membrane proteins not usually seen in *E. coli* K12. Quite apart from Iut A, the 74-kDa aerobactin receptor which is normally produced by pathogenic *E. coli* strains carrying the Col V-plasmid, enteroinvasive strains of *E. coli* produce aerobactin and a 76-kDa protein which acts as the aerobactin receptor (Griffiths *et al.*, 1985b). These organisms produce shigellosis-like illnesses in humans and exhibit an iron-regulated outer membrane protein profile identical to that seen with laboratory constructed *E. coli* K12–*S. flexneri* hybrids under the same growth conditions (Griffiths *et al.*, 1985b). The *S. flexneri* parent strain used in these constructions also produces a 76-kDa protein during iron restriction and this is believed to be the aerobactin receptor in this organism.

By analysing over 70 strains of *E. coli* from various human and animal infections, Chart *et al.* (1988) found considerable qualitative and quantitative differences between the sodium dodecyl sulfate-polyacrylamide gel electrophoresis (SDS-PAGE) patterns obtained for the iron-regulated outer membrane proteins of different strains. Nevertheless, three distinct and characteristic profiles, based on the most prominent bands expressed, could be identified, although not all isolates produced patterns which matched exactly with one of these (Fig. 19.3). Only isolates giving rise to patterns seen in Fig. 19.3, lanes 2 and 3, seem to be associated with extraintestinal infections in humans. These two patterns were not observed in *E. coli* strains isolated from cases of human enteric diseases or animal septicaemia or enteric diseases. The animal isolates examined gave an iron-regulated outer membrane protein profile similar to that seen in Fig. 19.3, lane 1. The human enteroinvasive strains exhibited a profile like the other human

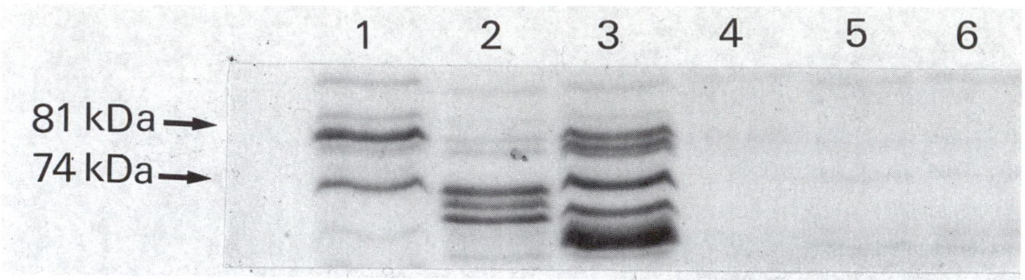

Fig. 19.3. Representatives of three characteristic SDS-PAGE profiles consistently distinguished amongst the iron-regulated outer membrane proteins of *E. coli* (lanes 1–3); only the relevant portion of the gel is shown. The same portion of the gel after SDS-PAGE of the outer membrane proteins from the same organisms grown under iron-replete conditions is shown in lanes 4–6. Lanes 1 and 4, *E. coli* O25:H$^-$(enterotoxigenic strain); lanes 2 and 5, *E. coli* O1:K1 (from human urinary tract infection); lanes 3 and 6, *E. coli* O18:K1 (from meningitis in human newborn). Each strain carried 25 μg protein. (From Chart, *et al.*, 1988. Reproduced by permission of the Society for General Microbiology.)

enteric strains except that they produced the additional 76-kDa protein, the aerobactin receptor. None of these differences between strains are evident in the iron replete organisms (Fig. 19.3).

In the laboratory, the iron-regulated proteins discussed above can be induced in pathogens by growing them in the presence of iron-binding proteins or by adding iron-chelating agents such as α, α′-dipyridyl, ethylenediamine-di-(*o*-hydroxyphenylacetic acid) (EDDA) or desferrioxamine (Desferal, Ciba-Geigy Corp) to growth media. Although the latter reagents are convenient and economical to use, the pattern of bacterial iron-regulated proteins obtained is not always identical to that obtained by using the naturally occurring iron-binding protein (Chart *et al.*, 1986). Caution should therefore be exercised when interpreting data concerning the nature of iron-regulated proteins produced by different strains when the data are obtained with such systems. That some of these iron-regulated proteins are indeed expressed *in vivo* during infection has been clearly demonstrated. Griffiths *et al.* (1983) showed that the iron-regulated outer membrane proteins of *E. coli* O111 recovered without subculture from the peritoneal cavities of infected guinea-pigs were major components of the outer membrane and were present in amounts equal to or slightly greater than the so-called major outer membrane proteins with apparent molecular masses of 30–40 kDa. Unlike *E. coli* O111, which showed the same pattern of iron-regulated outer membrane proteins when grown *in vivo* during infection as when grown *in vitro* in the presence of ovotransferrin, *E. coli* O18:K1:H7, a pathogenic strain carrying a Col V plasmid, produced not only the iron-regulated proteins seen *in vitro* but an extra new protein during growth *in vivo* (Griffiths *et al.*, 1985a). This protein had a molecular weight of about 68 kDa and is not associated with the presence of the Col V plasmid. Interesting differences in the pattern of the major outer membrane proteins of *E. coli* O18 were also noted in cells grown *in vivo*; these changes may well reflect other environmental changes experienced by the bacteria, such as changes in osmotic pressure (Griffiths, 1991).

Since it was first shown that *E. coli* isolated from experimental infections were growing under iron-restricted conditions (Griffiths *et al.*, 1978, 1983; Griffiths and Humphreys, 1980), others have shown that *E. coli* and other pathogens isolated directly from human infections are also expressing the iron-regulated proteins and thus growing under conditions of iron restriction during natural infection of the human host (Table 19.3). Antibodies which react with some of the iron-regulated proteins of *E. coli* and other pathogens have also been detected (Griffiths *et al.*, 1985a; Shand *et al.*, 1985; Fernandez-Beros *et al.*, 1989; Todhunter *et al.*, 1991). Whether such antibodies play any part in protecting the host against infection, possibly by interfering with siderophore-mediated iron uptake, is unclear. As part of an investigation into the possible protective role of anti-receptor antibodies, Chart and Griffiths (1985 and unpublished data) examined the antigenic homology of Fep A, the enterobactin receptor, in different strains of *E. coli* by using polyclonal and monoclonal antibodies. Results showed that the molecular weight and some of the antigenic properties of the enterobactin receptor were highly conserved. However, antibodies raised to the purified and denatured Fep A not surprisingly

Table 19.3. Pathogenic bacteria shown to express iron-regulated membrane proteins *in vivo* during infection.

Organism	Source	Host
E. coli	Peritoneum	Guinea pig[a]
E. coli	Urine	Human with urinary tract infection[b]
Klebsiella pneumoniae	Urine	Human with urinary tract infection[b, c]
Proteus mirabilis	Urine	Human with urinary tract infection[b]
Pseudomonas aeruginosa	Lung	Human with cystic fibrosis[d]
Salmonella enteritidis	Peritoneum	Chicken[e]
Vibrio cholerae	Intestines	Rabbits[f]

[a] Griffiths *et al.* (1983).
[b] Lam *et al.* (1984).
[c] Shand *et al.* (1985).
[d] Brown *et al.* (1984).
[e] Chart *et al.* (1993).
[f] Sciortino and Finkelstein (1983).

failed to react with the protein *in situ* on the surface of the *E. coli* strain tested, and had no effect on bacterial multiplication. However, specific antibodies raised in rabbits to the Fhu A (78-kDa) protein of *E. coli* have been reported to partially inhibit ferrichrome-mediated iron transport and also to block the adsorption of phage T5 onto the 78-kDa receptor (Coulton, 1982). Likewise, polyclonal antibodies against the Col V plasmid-encoded aerobactin receptor inhibited the binding of siderophore to membranes containing the Iut A protein and to *E. coli*-K12 strains expressing Iut A (Roberts *et al.*, 1989).

It must be borne in mind, however, that even if antibodies do recognize the appropriate epitopes on a bacterial cell's surface receptor, they may not always be able to interact with the receptor *in situ* in all strains of *E. coli.* In some cases the lipopolysaccharide is likely to interfere with antibody–antigen interaction by masking the receptor protein, just as lipopolysaccharide can interfere with the interaction of cloacin with its receptor Iut A (Derbyshire *et al.*, 1989). Thus, the polyclonal antibodies to the Iut A which reacted with the receptor in *E. coli* K12 failed to inhibit the binding of aerobactin to clinical isolates of *E. coli* expressing Iut A (Roberts *et al.*, 1989). Nevertheless, Bolin and Jensen (1987) have reported that turkeys passively immunized with antibodies against the iron-regulated outer membrane proteins of *E. coli* O78:K80:H9 were protected against experimental colisepticaemia. However, the actual mechanisms involved in this particular protection have never been shown to be clearly due to antibodies blocking receptor activity.

Acquisition of Iron from Haem Compound

In addition to obtaining iron from iron-binding proteins, *E. coli* may also under certain circumstances obtain sufficient iron for multiplication *in vivo* from cell-free haemoglobin or haem. Haem and haemoglobin can act as an alternative source of iron for a number of pathogens, including *Neisseria gonorrhoeae*, *N. meningitidis*, *Vibrio cholerae*, *V. vulnificus*, *Plesiomonas shigelloides*, *Streptococcus pneumoniae*, *Yersiniae enterocolitica*, *S. flexneri* and *Haemophilus influenzae* (Coulton and Pang, 1983: Helms *et al.*, 1984; Dyer *et al.*, 1987; Stull, 1987; Stoebner and Payne, 1988; Williams *et al.*, 1990; Daskaleros *et al.*, 1991; Stojiljkovic and Hantke, 1992; Tai *et al.*, 1993). In the case of *E. coli*, it has been known for a long time that both haem and haemoglobin can greatly enhance the susceptibility of animals and humans to *E. coli* infections (Davis and Yull, 1964; Bornside *et al.*, 1968; Bullen *et al.*, 1968, 1991), and that it is the iron component of these molecules which is the important factor (Lee *et al.*, 1979). However, although much work has been directed towards understanding siderophore-mediated iron transport systems in *E. coli*, much less attention has been given to the mechanisms used by *E. coli* to obtain iron from haem and haemoglobin. Therefore, at present, little is known about these systems even though haem-binding proteins have been found in a number of other organisms (Hanson *et al.*, 1992; Lee, 1992; Bramanti and Holt, 1993).

Law *et al.* (1992) have shown that the iron in haemoglobin is used in preference to that in ovotransferrin when both iron sources are present. The uptake of ovotransferrin-bound iron only took place upon the exhaustion of haemoglobin-derived iron. In these experiments, the growth rate of *E. coli* was related to the haemoglobin concentration and was much higher than that of the same strain growing in the same medium without haemoglobin. During periods of haemoglobin-stimulated growth of *E. coli*, the enterobactin-mediated iron-uptake system was found to be expressed and Law *et al.* (1992) suggest that it may be involved in the transport of haemoglobin-derived iron into the bacterial cell although it is not clear how this might be achieved.

Even though *E. coli* and other pathogens can use the iron in haemoglobin and haem, there is normally only a trace of these molecules free in plasma. In plasma, tetrameric haemoglobin liberated by haemolysis or tissue damage dissociates into dimers which are then bound by haptoglobin and usually taken up into liver parenchymal cells via receptor-mediated endocytosis and both haemoglobin and haptoglobin molecules are then catabolized (Hershko, 1975; Kino *et al.*, 1980). Free haemoglobin is not present until the binding capacity of circulating haptoglobin has been saturated. Unlike haptoglobin-bound haemoglobin, free haemoglobin is unstable and is readily oxidized to methaemoglobin, the ferrous haem of haemoglobin being converted to ferric-haem of methaemoglobin. Ferrihaem dissociates readily from methaemoglobin and the free haem is bound by haemopexin and albumin (Hershko, 1975; Smith, 1990); haem bound to haemopexin is delivered to hepatic cells by receptor-mediated endocytosis and catabolized. Thus, if bacteria are to use this source of iron, there must be sufficient free haemoglobin or haem present in the blood stream to overwhelm the binding proteins, or the pathogens must acquire it from these protein complexes.

Some organisms, like *E. coli* (Eaton *et al.*, 1982), are unable to use haemoglobin bound to haptoglobin as a source of iron and such work has suggested the possible use of haptoglobin in treating potentially fatal haemoglobin-mediated bacterial infections. However, this may not apply in all cases, and other pathogens like *V. vulnificus* can utilize haemoglobin in the haemoglobin–haptoglobin complex (Helms *et al.*, 1984). Meningococci are also able to use bound haemoglobin but not haem bound to haemopexin (Dyer *et al.*, 1987). On the other hand, *H. influenzae* is able to use the haem–haemopexin complex and recently an iron-regulated haemopexin receptor has been identified in this organism (Wong *et al.*,

1994). Although Eaton *et al.* (1982) showed that some *E. coli* strains are unable to use haemoglobin bound to haptoglobin, those strains were not well characterized and there is no information as to whether other strains of *E. coli* might be able to do so.

It has been suggested that increasing the level of cell-free haem or haemoglobin by haemolysin-induced haemolysis of erythrocytes is a way of increasing the available iron pool *in vivo* (Linggood and Ingram, 1982). Haemolysins are known virulence determinants of *E. coli* as well as of other pathogens (Martinez *et al.*, 1990); *E. coli* strains which cause extraintestinal infections, in particular, produce haemolysins (Opal *et al.*, 1990) and these seem to be derepressed under conditions of iron limitation (Lebek and Grünig, 1985; Grünig *et al.*, 1987). Haemolysin production in *V. cholerae*, *Serratia marcescens* and *V. parahaemolyticus* has also been shown to be iron regulated (Poole and Braun, 1988; Stoebner and Payne, 1988; Dai *et al.*, 1992). Of course, haemolysins not only lyse erythrocytes but other mammalian cells as well (Bhakdi *et al.*, 1990; Suttorp *et al.*, 1990) and no doubt this also contributes to their role in pathogenesis.

Molecular Mechanisms of Regulation by Iron

As might be expected, considerable progress has been made over the past few years in understanding the molecular mechanisms by which iron regulates iron uptake systems in *E. coli.* Most of the genes involved in the biosynthesis and transport of siderophores in *E. coli* are negatively regulated in a coordinated manner by iron via a transcriptional repressor called Fur, which uses ferrous (Fe^{2+}) iron as the corepressor. Mn^{2+} can also act as a corepressor in the Fur system (Bagg and Neilands, 1987a, 1987b; O'Halloran, 1993). Fur, a small polypeptide of 148 amino acids (17 kDa) (Schaffer *et al.*, 1985), is the product of the regulatory gene *fur*, located at about 15.5 minutes on the *E. coli* chromosome. Mutations in *fur* result in mutants which are constitutively derepressed for iron assimilation systems (Hantke, 1981), including the uptake of uncomplexed Fe^{2+} (Hantke, 1987a). Binding sites for the active Fe^{2+}-Fur repressor protein, called the 'iron-box', have been identified in several iron-regulated promoters in *E. coli* (Bagg and Neilands, 1987a, 1987b; Elkins and Earhart, 1989; Griggs and Konisky, 1989; Postle, 1990; Niederhoffer *et al.*, 1990). These DNA sequences consist of a highly A- and T-rich palindrome and deletions that disrupt the palindromic structure make the promoter unresponsive to regulation by iron (Calderwood and Mekalanos, 1988). It has also been shown that the presence of a consensus 'iron-box' sequence, 5′-GATAATGATAATCATTATC, is sufficient in itself to allow *fur*-mediated iron regulation of a gene to occur (Calderwood and Mekalanos, 1988).

The general mode of action of Fur involves the binding of the Fur protein–Fe^{2+} complex to the operator when iron supply is plentiful, the Fur protein binding to DNA as a dimer. This blocks transcription of relevant mRNA species and results in low levels of synthesis of iron-regulated enzymes and proteins. As the internal iron levels fall in the bacterial cell during iron restriction in the medium, less Fe^{2+} is available for binding to the Fur protein; the Fur protein in its metal free state binds poorly or not at all to the 'iron-box' and this leads to derepression of iron-regulated operons and to increased synthesis of iron-related functions. In addition, at least two *E. coli* genes seem to be positively regulated, either directly or indirectly by Fur (Hantke, 1987b; Niederhoffer *et al.*, 1990). The expression of the citrate-mediated iron transport system is also controlled by iron via the Fur repressor. However, here control is complicated by the fact that regulation also involves induction by Fe^{3+}-dicitrate itself, although citrate does not enter the bacterial cell (Hussein *et al.*, 1981; Zimmerman *et al.*, 1984). In this case regulation is believed to involve, in addition to Fur, two other regulatory proteins called FecR and FecI, which are responsible for monitoring Fe^{3+}-dicitrate levels in the periplasm and in gene induction respectively (van Hove *et al.*, 1990).

The coordinated response of *E. coli* to low levels of iron involves not only the expression of the high-affinity iron-acquisition systems, the siderophores and siderophore receptors, but also the synthesis of a number of factors seemingly not directly related to iron metabolism, like toxins. Thus, the phage-encoded genes for Shiga-like toxin type 1 (*slt* genes) of *E. coli* are regulated by iron via Fur (Calderwood and Mekalanos, 1987); the structural genes for this toxin, *slt*A and *slt*B, are transcribed as an operon from a promoter upstream of *slt*A which contains an 'iron-box'. Other *E. coli* genes under iron and Fur control include the superoxide dismutase genes, *sod*A and *sodB, the ton*B gene, the haemolytic activity encoded by certain Hly plasmids and *fur* itself (Grünig *et al.*, 1987; de Lorenzo *et al.*, 1988b; Niederhoffer *et al.*, 1990; Postle, 1990; Fee, 1991). However, in contrast to the fairly simple general on–off regulation by iron and Fur, control of the *fur* gene is more complicated. This gene is not only negatively autoregulated by Fur and Fe^{2+}, but also positively regulated through the cyclic AMP-CAP system (catabolite-activator protein) (de Lorenzo *et al.*, 1988b). It is suggested that this type of regulation may establish a link between the modulation of iron metabolism and the metabolic status of the cell (de Lorenzo *et al.*, 1988b). An apparent role for cAMP-CAP control operating in conjunction with Fur has also been found in the *cir* gene, which has long been known to be under iron regulation (Griggs *et al.*, 1990).

In addition to regulation through the Fur system, a global response to iron limitation has been observed at the level of tRNA modification (Griffiths, 1987b; Persson, 1993). *E. coli* growing under iron-restricted conditions produce tRNA species for phenylalanine, tyrosine, tryptophan, serine, cysteine and leucine which lack a methylthio group (ms^2) which is present on the isopentenyl-adenosine (i^6A) located next to the anticodon (A37) of tRNAs from the iron-replete bacteria (Griffiths and Humphreys, 1978; Buck and Griffiths, 1981, 1982). These tRNAs isolated from *E. coli* grown *in vivo* during infection likewise lack the ms^2 group (Griffiths *et al.*, 1978). Indeed this discovery provided the first positive proof that bacteria growing *in vivo* during infection were growing under iron-restricted conditions. Similar tRNA changes have been observed in *S. typhimurium* growing under iron restriction (Buck and Ames, 1984). Such under modification of tRNAs has been shown to induce pleiotropic effects on bacterial physiology, in some instances by effects on the translational efficiency of the tRNAs, in others by altering codon context effects and in others by unknown mechanisms (Buck and Griffiths, 1981, 1982; Bouadloun *et al.*, 1986; Ericson and Björk, 1986; Petrullo and Elseviers, 1986; Blum, 1988). For example, the failure to methylthiolate tRNA due to iron restriction decreases the translational efficiencies of the tRNAs affected, which in turn, through attenuation mechanisms, leads to increased synthesis of aromatic amino acids, as well as to increased transport of aromatic amino acids into the cell (Buck and Griffiths, 1981, 1982). It is thought that such regulatory features may be involved with adapting *E. coli* for growth in iron-restricted environments (Buck and Griffiths, 1982).

Since enterobactin is synthesized from chorismic acid by way of a branch of the aromatic amino acid biosynthetic pathway, derepression of the enterobactin system will require adjustments to the whole aromatic pathway to ensure production of aromatic amino acids, if needed, and other essential aromatic compounds. Such regulation could provide the cell with considerable regulatory flexibility which may be important for growth under iron restriction. There is also evidence that the lack of modification of A37 located next to the anticodon of certain tRNAs leads to an increased frequency in spontaneous mutations when the cell needs to adapt to environmental stress (Connolly and Winkler, 1989, 1991).

Concluding Comments

Although considerable progress has been made over the past few years in our understanding of the role of iron in infection, much of the pioneering work having been undertaken with *E. coli*, some aspects remain unclear. Only in some instances has the role of a siderophore-mediated iron uptake system been clearly shown to be essential for virulence. Highly virulent strains of *V. anguillarum*, for example, which are responsible for a devastating septicaemia in fish, carry a plasmid encoding a siderophore-dependent iron-transport system that allows the organisms to grow under iron-restricted conditions. On losing the plasmid, *V. anguillarum* loses both its ability to grow under such conditions and its virulence (Crosa, 1989). In the case of *E. coli*, the contribution of enterobactin to virulence is less obvious, although it seems that aerobactin production and utilization is associated with an ability to cause infection at a lower infective dose. However, no studies have been carried out with pathogenic strains of *E. coli* to show conclusively that one or both of these siderophores are essential for virulence; strains could be engineered to be deficient in both the aerobactin and enterobactin iron uptake systems. Traces of haem or haemoglobin could serve as iron sources for *E. coli in vivo*, but whether the ability to use exogenous siderophores plays any part in natural infection is unknown. Recently, interest has arisen in the additional contribution siderophores might make to the pathogenesis of infection by suppressing host immune responses (Autenrieth *et al.*, 1991) and by promoting inflammation and tissue damage at sites of infection through siderophore-induced free radical formation (Coffman *et al.*, 1990). Depending on their biochemical properties, siderophores behave differently in such systems and this may lead to different clinical consequences.

The recognition that the restricted availability of iron in tissue fluids not only presents *E. coli* and other microbial pathogens with the problem of acquiring sufficient metal for multiplication *in vivo*, but also constitutes a major environmental signal which acts alone, or in conjunction with other controls, to regulate the expression of a number of virulence and metabolic genes has been a significant development (Griffiths, 1987b; Mekalanos, 1992). Analysis of pathogens grown under specific environmental conditions, such as iron restriction, is now leading to a clearer picture of the characteristics associated with virulence, since some crucial determinants are not produced by organisms grown in rich broth media and thus have been missed by investigators. For example, a new iron-regulated enterotoxin has recently been discovered in enteroinvasive *E. coli* which is distinct from the known cytotoxins (Fasano *et al.*, 1990). This information is crucial for understanding microbial pathogenicity and has important consequences for vaccine design (Griffiths, 1991).

Whilst considerable advances have been made in understanding the molecular basis of iron-related virulence processes, less progress has been made in understanding the consequences of increased iron availability on clinical infections and this continues to be a controversial topic (Hershko *et al.*, 1988; Bullen *et al.*, 1991). The abnormal presence of freely available iron *in vivo* would be expected to increase the rate of bacterial multiplication and to tip the balance in favour of the invading pathogen. For example, certain strains of *E. coli* have a doubling time of about 35 minutes when growing in the presence of an iron-binding protein but this is reduced to approximately 25 minutes when iron is freely available in the medium (Griffiths and Humphreys, 1978). Even a modest reduction in the rate of bacterial growth can make a big difference to the size of a bacterial population over a matter of hours and this might be crucial in deciding the outcome of an infection. Some authors (Bullen *et al.*, 1991) cite clinical situations to support the importance of iron availability in determining infection whereas others remain sceptical (Hershko *et al.*, 1988). In reality, the factors that decide the outcome of infections are numerous and complex, and it is not surprising that it is often difficult to establish their relative contribution in clinical settings.

There is no doubt that an increased availability of iron can in some circumstances be crucial to the clinical outcome of infection. Freely available haem or haemoglobin clearly promotes infection and the catastrophic combination of haemoglobin and *E. coli* in the peritoneal cavity in man has long been known (Kluger and Bullen, 1987). Proposals to use cross-linked haemoglobins as red-cell substitutes in transfusion medicine should therefore be very carefully evaluated. Any advantages these products might have over whole blood could be outweighed by the promotion of bacterial proliferation *in vivo* and an increase in the susceptibility of recipients to infection. However, further research is required into the effect of changes in host iron metabolism and transferrin saturation levels on the susceptibility of compromised individuals to infections by *E. coli* and other pathogens.

References

Ainscough, E.W., Brodie, A.M., Plowman, J.E., Bloor, S.J., Loehr, J.S. and Loehr, T.M. (1980) Studies on human lactoferrin by electron paramagnetic resonance, fluorescence and resonance Raman spectroscopy. *Biochemistry* 19, 4072–4079.

Armstrong, S.K., Pettis, G.S., Forrester, L.J. and McIntosh, M.A. (1989) The *Escherichia coli* enterobactin biosynthesis gene, *ent*D: nucleotide sequence and membrane localization of its protein product. *Molecular Microbiology* 3, 757–766.

Autenrieth, I., Hantke, K. and Heesemann, J. (1991) Immunosuppression of the host and delivery of iron to the pathogen: a possible dual role of siderophores in the pathogenesis of microbial infections? *Medical Microbiology and Immunology* 180, 135–141.

Bagg, A. and Neilands, J.B. (1987a) Molecular mechanism of regulation of siderophore-mediated iron assimilation. *Microbiological Reviews* 51, 509–518.

Bagg, A. and Neilands, J.B. (1987b) Ferric uptake regulation protein acts as a repressor, employing iron (II) as a co-factor to bind the operator of an iron transport operon in *Escherichia coli*. *Biochemistry* 26, 5471–5477.

Bhakdi, S., Muhly, M., Korom, S. and Schmidt, G. (1990) Effects of *Escherichia coli* hemolysin on human monocytes. *Journal Clinical Investigation* 85, 1746–1753.

Bindereif, A., Braun, V. and Hantke, K. (1982) The cloacin receptor of Col

V-bearing *Escherichia coli* is part of the Fe^{3+}-aerobactin transport system. *Journal of Bacteriology* 150, 1472–1475.

Blum, P.H. (1988) Reduced *leu* operon expression in a *mia A* mutant of *Salmonella typhimurium. Journal of Bacteriology* 170, 5125–5133.

Bolin, C.A. and Jensen, A.E. (1987) Passive immunization with antibodies against iron-regulated outer membrane proteins protects turkeys from *Escherichia coli* septicaemia. *Infection and Immunity* 55, 1239–1242.

Bornside, G.H., Bouis, P.J. and Cohn, I. (1968) Haemoglobin and *Escherichia coli*, a lethal intraperitoneal combination. *Journal of Bacteriology* 95, 1567–1571.

Bouadloun, F., Srichaiyo, T., Isaksson, L.A. and Björk, G.R. (1986) Influence of modification next to the anticodon in tRNA on codon context sensitivity of translational suppression and accuracy. *Journal of Bacteriology* 166, 1022–1027.

Bramanti, T.E. and Holt, S.C. (1993) Hemin uptake in *Porphyromonas gingivalis*: Omp 26 is a hemin-binding surface protein. *Journal of Bacteriology* 175, 7413–7420.

Braun, V., Brazel-Faisst, C. and Schneider, R. (1984) Growth stimulation of *Escherichia coli* in serum by iron(III)-aerobactin: recycling of aerobactin. *Federation of European Microbiological Societies Microbiology Letters* 21, 99–103.

Braun, V., Günter, K. and Hantke, K. (1991) Transport of iron across the outer membrane. *Biology of Metals* 4, 14–22.

Brewer, S., Tolley, M., Trayer, I.P., Barr, G.C., Dorman, C.J., Hannavy, K., Higgins, C.F., Evans, J.S., Levin, B.A. and Wormald, M.R. (1990) Structure and function of X-Pro dipeptide repeats in the Ton B proteins of *Salmonella typhimurium* and *Escherichia coli. Journal of Molecular Biology* 216, 883–895.

Brickman, T.J. and McIntosh, M.A. (1992) Overexpression and purification of ferric enterobactin esterase from *Escherichia coli*: demonstration of enzymatic hydrolysis of enterobactin and its iron complex. *Journal of Biological Chemistry* 267, 12350–12355.

Brown, M.R.W., Anwar, H. and Lambert, P.A. (1984) Evidence that mucoid *Pseudomonas aeruginosa* in the cystic fibrosis lung grows under iron-restricted conditions. *Federation of European Microbiological Societies Microbiology Letters* 21, 113–117.

Buck, M. and Ames, B.N. (1984) A modified nucleotide in tRNA as a possible regulator of anaerobiosis: synthesis of *cis*-2-methylthio-ribosylzeatin in the tRNA of *Salmonella. Cell* 36, 523–531.

Buck, M. and Griffiths, E. (1981) Regulation of aromatic amino acid transport by tRNA: role of 2-methylthio-N^6-(Δ^2-isopentenyl) adenosine. *Nucleic Acids Research* 9, 401–414.

Buck, M. and Griffiths, E. (1982) Iron-mediated methylthiolation of tRNA as a regulator of operon expression in *Escherichia coli. Nucleic Acids Research* 10, 2609–2624.

Bullen, J.J. and Griffiths, E. (eds) (1987) *Iron and Infection: Molecular, Physiological and Clinical Aspects.* John Wiley & Sons, Chichester.

Bullen, J.J., Leigh, L.C. and Rogers, H.J. (1968) The effect of iron compounds on the virulence of *Escherichia coli* for guinea pigs. *Immunology* 15, 581–588.

Bullen, J.J., Ward, C.G. and Rogers, H.J. (1991) The critical role of iron in some clinical infections. *European Journal of Clinical Microbiology and Infectious Diseases* 10, 613–617.

Byrd, T.F. and Horwitz, M.A. (1989) Interferon gamma-activated human monocytes down-regulate transferrin receptors and inhibit the intracellular multiplication of *Legionella pneumophila* by limiting the availability of iron. *Journal of Clinical Investigation* 83, 1457–1465.

Calderwood, S.B. and Mekalanos, J.J. (1987) Iron regulation of Shiga-like toxin expression in *Escherichia coli* is mediated by the *fur* locus. *Journal of Bacteriology* 169, 4759–4764.

Calderwood, S.B. and Mekalanos, J.J. (1988) Confirmation of the Fur operator site by insertion of a synthetic oligonucleotide into an operon fusion plasmid. *Journal of Bacteriology* 170, 1015–1017.

Carmel, G., Hellstren, D., Henning, D. and Coulton, J.W. (1990) Insertion mutagenesis of the gene encoding the ferrichrome-iron receptor of *Escherichia coli* K12. *Journal of Bacteriology* 172, 1861–1869.

Carrano, C.J. and Raymond, K.N. (1979) Ferric iron sequestering agents: 2. Kinetics and mechanisms of iron removal from transferrin by enterochelin and synthetic tricatechols. *Journal of the American Chemical Society* 101, 5401–5404.

Chart, H. and Griffiths, E. (1985) Antigenic and molecular homology of the ferric-enterobactin receptor protein of *Escherichia coli*. *Journal of General Microbiology* 131, 1503–1509.

Chart, H., Buck, M., Stevenson, P. and Griffiths, E. (1986) Iron regulated outer membrane proteins of *Escherichia coli*: variations in expression due to the chelator used to restrict the availability of iron. *Journal of General Microbiology* 132, 1373–1378.

Chart, H., Stevenson, P. and Griffiths, E. (1988) Iron-regulated outer-membrane proteins of *Escherichia coli* strains associated with enteric or extraintestinal diseases of man and animals. *Journal of General Microbiology* 134, 1549–1559.

Chart, H., Conway, D. and Rowe, B. (1993) Outer membrane characteristics of *Salmonella enteritidis* phage type 4 growing in chickens. *Epidemiology and Infection* 111, 449–454.

Coffman, T.J., Cox, C.D., Edeker, B.L. and Britigan, B.E. (1990) Possible role of bacterial siderophores in inflammation: iron bound to the *Pseudomonas* siderophore pyochelin can function as a hydroxyl radical catalyst. *Journal of Clinical Investigation* 86, 1030–1037.

Connolly, D.M. and Winkler, M.E. (1989) Genetic and physiological relationships among the *mia*A gene, 2-methylthio-N^6-(Δ^2-isopentenyl)-adenosine tRNA modification and spontaneous mutagenesis in *Escherichia coli* K12. *Journal of Bacteriology* 171, 3233–3246.

Connolly, D.M. and Winkler, M.E. (1991) Structure of *Escherichia coli* K12 *mia*A and characterization of the mutator phenotype caused by *mia*A insertion mutations. *Journal of Bacteriology* 173, 1711–1721.

Cooper, S.R., McArdle, J.V. and Raymond, K.N. (1978) Siderophore electrochemistry: relation to intracellular release mechanism. *Proceedings of the*

National Academy of Sciences of the United States of America 75, 3551–3554.

Coulton, J.W. (1982) The ferrichrome-iron receptor of *Escherichia coli* K12: antigenicity of the Fhu A protein. *Biochimica et Biophysica Acta* 717, 154–162.

Coulton, J.W. and Pang, J.C.S. (1983) Transport of hemin by *Haemophilus influenzae* type b. *Current Microbiology* 9, 93–98.

Coulton, J.W., Mason, P. and DuBow, M.S. (1983) Molecular cloning of the ferrichrome-iron receptor of *Escherichia coli* K12. *Journal of Bacteriology* 156, 1315–1321.

Coulton, J.W., Mason, P. and Allatt, D.D. (1987) *fhu*C and *fhu*D genes for iron (III)–ferrichrome transport into *Escherichia coli* K12. *Journal of Bacteriology* 169, 3844–3849.

Crichton, R.R. and Ward, R.J. (1992) Structure and molecular biology of iron binding proteins and the regulation of 'free' iron pools. In Lauffer, R.B. (ed.), *Iron and Human Disease.* CRC Press, Boca Raton, Florida, pp. 23–75.

Crosa, J.H. (1989) Genetics and molecular biology of siderophore-mediated iron transport in bacteria. *Microbiology Reviews* 53, 517–530.

Curtis, N.A.C., Eisenstadt, R.L., East, S.J., Cornford, R.J., Walker, L.A. and White, A.J. (1988) Iron-regulated outer membrane proteins of *Escherichia coli* K12 and mechanism of action of catechol substituted cephalosporins. *Antimicrobial Agents and Chemotherapy* 32, 1879–1886.

Dai, J.H., Lee, Y.S. and Wong, H.C. (1992) Effects of iron limitation on production of a siderophore, outer membrane proteins and haemolysin and on hydrophobicity, cell adherence and lethality for mice of *Vibrio parahemolyticus. Infection and Immunity* 60, 2952–2956.

Daskaleros, P.A., Stoebner, J.A. and Payne, S.M. (1991) Iron uptake in *Plesiomonas shigelloides*: cloning of the genes for the heme-iron uptake system. *Infection and Immunity* 59, 2706–2711.

Davis, J.H. and Yull, A.B. (1964) A toxic factor in abdominal injury II. The role of the red cell component. *Journal of Trauma* 4, 84–87.

de Lorenzo, V. and Martinez, J.L. (1988) Aerobactin production as a virulence factor: a re-evaluation. *European Journal of Clinical Microbiology and Infectious Diseases* 7, 621–629.

de Lorenzo, V., Herrero, M. and Neilands, J.B. (1988a) IS1-mediated mobility of the aerobactin system of p Col V-K30 in *Escherichia coli. Molecular and General Genetics* 213, 487–490.

de Lorenzo, V., Herrero, M., Giovannini, F. and Neilands, J.B. (1988b) Fur (ferric uptake regulation) protein and CAP (catabolite activator protein) modulate transcription of *fur* gene in *Escherichia coli. European Journal of Biochemistry* 173, 537–546.

Derbyshire, P., Baldwin, T., Stevenson, P., Griffiths, E., Roberts, M., Williams, P., Hall, T.L. and Formal, S.B. (1989) Expression in *Escherichia coli* K12 of the 76000-dalton iron-regulated outer membrane protein of *Shigella flexneri* confers sensitivity to Cloacin DF13 in the absence of *Shigella* O antigen. *Infection and Immunity* 57, 2794–2798.

Dyer, D.W., West, E.P. and Sparling, P.F. (1987) Effects of serum carrier proteins on the growth of pathogenic Neisseriae with heme-bound iron. *Infection and Immunity* 55, 2171–2175.

Earhart, C.F. (1987) Ferri-enterobactin transport in *Escherichia coli*. In: Winkelmann, G., van der Helm, D. and Neilands, J.B. (eds), *Iron Transport in Microbes, Plants and Animals*. VCH Publishers, Weinheim, Germany, pp. 67–84.

Eaton, J.W., Brandt, P., Mahoney, J.R. and Lee, J.T. (1982) Haptoglobin: a natural bacteriostat. *Science* 215, 691–693.

Elkins, M.F. and Earhart, C.F. (1989) Nucleotide sequence and regulation of the *Escherichia coli* gene for ferrienterobactin transport protein Fep B. *Journal of Bacteriology* 171, 5443–5451.

Ericson, J.U. and Björk, G.R. (1986) Pleiotropic effects induced by modification deficiency next to the anticodon of tRNA from *Salmonella typhimurium* LT2. *Journal of Bacteriology* 166, 1013–1021.

Fasano, A., Kay, B.A., Russell, R.G., Maneval, D.R., Jr, and Levine, M.M. (1990) Enterotoxin and cytotoxin production by enteroinvasive *Escherichia coli*. *Infection and Immunity* 58, 3717–3723.

Fee, J.A. (1991) Regulation of *sod* genes in *Escherichia coli*: relevance to superoxide dismutase function. *Molecular Microbiology* 5, 2599–2610.

Fernandez-Beros, M.E., Gonzalez, C., McIntosh, M.A. and Cabello, F.C. (1989) Immune response to the iron-deprivation-induced proteins of *Salmonella typhi* in typhoid fever. *Infection and Immunity* 57, 1271–1275.

Fitzgerald, S.P. and Rogers, H.J. (1980) Bacteriostatic effect of serum: role of antibody to lipopolysaccharide. *Infection and Immunity* 27, 302–308.

Fleming, T.P., Nahlik, M.S., Neilands, J.B. and McIntosh, M.A. (1985) Physical and genetic characterization of cloned enterobactin genomic sequences from *Escherichia coli*. *Gene* 34, 47–54.

Frost, G. and Rosenberg, H. (1973) The inducible citrate-dependent iron transport system in *Escherichia coli* K12. *Biochimica et Biophysica Acta* 330, 90–101.

Gadó, I., Milch, H., Czirók, E. and Herpay, M. (1989) The frequency of aerobactin production and its effect on the pathogenicity of human *Escherichia coli* strains. *Acta Microbiologica Hungarica* 36, 51–60.

Gibson, F. and Magrath, D.I. (1969) The isolation and characterization of a hydroxamic acid (aerobactin) formed by *Aerobacter aerogenes* 62-1. *Biochimica et Biophysica Acta* 192, 175–184.

Gonzalo, M.P., Martinez, J.L., Baguero, F., Gómez-Lus, R. and Pérez-Diaz, J.C. (1988) Aerobactin production linked to transferable antibiotic resistance in *Escherichia coli* strains isolated from sewage. *Federation of European Microbiological Societies Microbiology Letters* 50, 57–59.

Greenwood, K.T. and Luke, R.K.J. (1976) Studies on the enzymatic synthesis of enterochelin in *Escherichia coli* K12: four polypeptides involved in the conversion of 2,3-dihydroxybenzoate to enterochelin. *Biochimica et Biophysica Acta* 454, 285–297.

Greenwood, K.T. and Luke, R.K.J. (1978) Enzymic hydrolysis of enterochelin and its iron complex in *Escherichia coli* K12. *Biochimica et Biophysica Acta* 525, 209–218.

Grewal, K.K., Warner, P.J. and Williams, P.H. (1982) An inducible outer membrane protein involved in aerobactin mediated iron transport by Col V strains of *Escherichia coli*. *Federation of European Biochemical Societies Letters* 140, 27–30.

Griffiths, E. (1987a) Iron in biological systems. In: Bullen J.J. and Griffiths E. (eds) *Iron and Infection: Molecular, Physiological and Clinical Aspects.* John Wiley & Sons, Chichester, pp. 1–25.

Griffiths, E. (1987b) The iron-uptake systems of pathogenic bacteria. In: Bullen J.J. and Griffiths E. (eds) *Iron and Infection: Molecular, Physiological and Clinical Aspects.* John Wiley & Sons, Chichester, pp. 69–137.

Griffiths, E. (1991) Environmental regulation of bacterial virulence – implications for vaccine design and production. *Trends in Biotechnology* 9, 309–315.

Griffiths, E. and Humphreys, J. (1978) Alterations in tRNAs containing 2-methylthio-N^6-(Δ^2-isopentenyl)-adenosine during growth of enteropathogenic *Escherichia coli* in the presence of iron-binding proteins. *European Journal of Biochemistry* 82, 503–513.

Griffiths, E. and Humphreys, J. (1980) Isolation of enterochelin from the peritoneal washings of guinea-pigs lethally infected with *Escherichia coli. Infection and Immunity* 28, 286–289.

Griffiths, E., Humphreys, J., Leach, A. and Scanlon, L. (1978) Alterations in the tRNAs of *Escherichia coli* recovered from lethally infected animals. *Infection and Immunity* 22, 312–317.

Griffiths, E., Stevenson, P. and Joyce, P. (1983) Pathogenic *Escherichia coli* express new outer membrane proteins when growing *in vivo. Federation of European Microbiological Societies Microbiology Letters* 16, 95–99.

Griffiths, E., Stevenson, P., Thorpe, R. and Chart, H. (1985a) Naturally occurring antibodies in human sera that react with the iron-regulated outer membrane proteins of *Escherichia coli. Infection and Immunity* 47, 808–813.

Griffiths, E., Stevenson, P., Hale, T.L. and Formal, S.B. (1985b) The synthesis of aerobactin and a 76000 dalton iron-regulated outer membrane protein by *Escherichia coli* K12–*Shigella* hybrids and by enteroinvasive strains of *Escherichia coli. Infection and Immunity* 49, 67–71.

Griggs, D.W. and Konisky, J. (1989) Mechanism for iron-regulated transcription of the *Escherichia coli cir* gene: metal-dependent binding of Fur protein to the promoters. *Journal of Bacteriology* 171, 1048–1054.

Griggs, D.W., Kafka, K., Nau, C.D. and Konisky, J. (1990) Activation of expression of the *Escherichia coli cir* gene by an iron-independent regulatory mechanism involving cyclic AMP–cyclic AMP receptor protein complex. *Journal of Bacteriology* 172, 3529–3533.

Grünig, H.M., Rutschi, D., Schoch, C. and Lebek, G. (1987) The chromosomal *fur* gene regulates the extracellular haemolytic activity encoded by certain Hly plasmids. *Zentralblatt für Bakteriologie, Mikrobiologie und Hygiene* 266, 231–238.

Hancock, R.E.W., Hantke, K. and Braun, V. (1976) Iron transport in *Escherichia coli* K12: involvement of the colicin B receptor and of a citrate-inducible protein. *Journal of Bacteriology* 127, 1370–1375.

Hannavy, K., Barr, G.C., Dorman, C.J., Adamson, J., Mazengera, L.M., Gallagher, M.P., Evans, J.S., Levin, B.A., Trayer, I.P. and Higgins, C.F. (1990) Ton B protein of *Salmonella typhimurium*: a model for signal transduction between membranes. *Journal of Molecular Biology* 216, 897–910.

Hanson, M.S., Slaughter, C. and Hansen, E.J. (1992) The *hbp* A gene of *Haemophilus influenzae* type b encodes a heme-binding lipoprotein conserved among heme-dependent *Haemophilus* species. *Infection and Immunity* 60, 2257–2266.

Hantke, K. (1981) Regulation of ferric ion transport in *E. coli.* Isolation of a constitutive mutant. *Molecular and General Genetics* 182, 288–292.

Hantke, K. (1983) Identification of an iron uptake system specific for coprogen and rhodotorulic acid in *Escherichia coli* K12. *Molecular and General Genetics* 191, 301–306.

Hantke, K. (1987a) Ferrous iron transport mutants in *Escherichia coli* K12. *Federation of European Microbiological Societies Microbiology Letters* 44, 53–57.

Hantke, K. (1987b) Selection procedure for deregulated iron transport mutants (fur) in *Escherichia coli* K12: *fur* not only affects iron metabolism. *Molecular and General Genetics* 210, 135–139.

Hantke, K. (1990) Dihydroxybenzoylserine – a siderophore for *E. coli. Federation of European Microbiological Societies Microbiology Letters* 67, 5–8.

Hantke, K. and Zimmermann, L. (1981) The importance of the *exb*B gene for vitamin B_{12} and ferric iron transport. *Federation of European Microbiological Societies Microbiology Letters* 12, 31–35.

Harris, W.R., Carrano, C.J. and Raymond, K.N. (1979a) Spectrophotometric determination of the proton dependent stability constant of ferric enterochelin. *Journal of the American Chemical Society* 101, 2213–2214.

Harris, W.R., Carrano, C.J. and Raymond, K.N. (1979b) Co-ordination chemistry of microbial iron transport compounds: 16: isolation, characterization and formation constants of ferric aerobactin. *Journal of the American Chemical Society* 101, 2722–2727.

Harris, W.R., Carrano, C.J., Cooper, S.R., Sofen, S.R., Avdeef, A.E., McArdle, J.V. and Raymond, K.N. (1979c) Co-ordination chemistry of microbial iron transport compounds: 19: stability constants and electrochemical behaviour of ferric enterobactin and model complexes. *Journal of the American Chemical Society* 101, 6097–6104.

Hartmann, A. and Braun, V. (1980) Iron transport in *Escherichia coli*: uptake and modification of ferrichrome. *Journal of Bacteriology* 143, 246–255.

Helms, S.D., Oliver, J.D. and Travis, J.C. (1984) Role of heme compounds and haptoglobin in *Vibrio vulnificus* pathogenicity. *Infection and Immunity* 45, 345–349.

Hershko, C. (1975) The fate of circulating haemoglobin. *British Journal of Haematology* 29, 199–204.

Hershko, C., Peto, T.E.A. and Weatherall, D.J. (1988) Iron and infection. *British Medical Journal* 296, 660–664.

Hider, R.C., Silver, J., Neilands, J.B., Morrison, I.E.G. and Rees, L.V.C. (1979) Identification of iron (II)–enterobactin and its possible role in *Escherichia coli* iron transport. *Federation of European Biochemical Societies Letters* 102, 325–328.

Hollifield Jr, W.C. and Neilands, J.B. (1978) Ferric enterobactin transport system of *Escherichia coli* K12: extraction, assay and specificity of the outer membrane receptor. *Biochemistry* 17, 1922–1928.

Hussain, S., Hantke, K. and Braun, V. (1981) Citrate-dependent iron transport system in *Escherichia coli* K12. *European Journal of Biochemistry* 117, 431–437.

Jacobson, S.H., Tullus, K., Wretlind, B. and Brauner, A. (1988) Aerobactin-mediated uptake of iron by strains of *Escherichia coli* causing pyelonephritis and bacteraemia. *Journal of Infection* 16, 147–152.

Kino, K., Tsunoo, H., Higa, Y., Takami, M., Hamaguchi, H. and Nakajima, H. (1980) Hemoglobin–haptoglobin receptor in rat liver plasma membrane. *Journal of Biological Chemistry* 255, 9616–9620.

Kluger, M.J. and Bullen, J.J. (1987) Clinical and physiological aspects. In: Bullen J.J. and Griffiths E. (eds) *Iron and Infection: Molecular, Physiological and Clinical Aspects.* John Wiley & Sons, Chichester, pp. 243–282.

Konijn, A.M. and Hershko, C. (1989) The anaemia of inflammation and chronic disease. In: de Sousa M. and Brock, J.H. (eds) *Iron in Immunity, Cancer and Inflammation*. John Wiley & Sons, Chichester, pp. 111–143.

Konopka, K. and Neilands, J.B. (1984) Effect of serum albumin on siderophore-mediated utilization of transferrin iron. *Biochemistry* 23, 2122–2127.

Konopka, K., Bindereif, A. and Neilands, J.B. (1982) Aerobactin-mediated utilization of transferrin iron. *Biochemistry* 21, 6503–6508.

Köster, W. (1991) Iron (III) hydroxamate transport across the cytoplasmic membrane of *Escherichia coli. Biology of Metals* 4, 23–32.

Köster, W. and Böhm, B. (1992) Point mutations in two conserved glycine residues within the integral membrane protein Fhu B affect iron (III) hydroxamate transport. *Molecular and General Genetics* 232, 399–407.

Köster, W. and Braun, V. (1989) Iron-hydroxamate transport into *Escherichia coli* K12: localization of Fhu D in the periplasm and of Fhu B in the cytoplasmic membrane. *Molecular and General Genetics* 217, 233–239.

Köster, W. and Braun, V. (1990a) Iron (III) hydroxamate transport in *Escherichia coli*: substrate binding to the periplasmic Fhu D protein. *Journal of Biological Chemistry* 265, 21407–21410.

Köster, W. and Braun, V. (1990b) Iron III-hydroxamate transport of *Escherichia coli*: restoration of iron supply by coexpression of the N- and C-terminal halves of the cytoplasmic membrane protein Fhu B cloned on separate plasmids. *Molecular and General Genetics* 223, 379–384.

Lafonte, J.P., Dho, M., D'Hauteville, H.M., Bree, A. and Sansonetti, P.J. (1987) Presence and expression of aerobactin genes in virulent avian strains of *Escherichia coli. Infection and Immunity* 55, 193–197.

Lam, C., Turnowsky, F., Schwarzinger, E. and Neruda, W. (1984) Bacteria recovered without subculture from infected human urines expressed iron regulated outer membrane proteins. *Federation of European Microbiological Societies Microbiology Letters* 24, 255–259.

Langman, L., Young, I.G., Frost, G., Rosenberg, H. and Gibson, F. (1972) Enterochelin system of iron transport in *Escherichia coli*: mutations affecting ferric-enterochelin esterase. *Journal of Bacteriology* 112, 1142–1149.

Law, D., Wilkie, K.M., Freeman, R. and Gould, F.K. (1992) The iron uptake mechanisms of enteropathogenic *Escherichia coli*: the use of haem and haemoglobin during growth in an iron-limited environment. *Journal of Medical Microbiology* 37, 15–21.

Lawlor, K.M., Daskaleros, P.A., Robinson R.E. and Payne, S.M. (1987) Virulence of iron-transport mutants of *Shigella flexneri* and utilization of host iron compounds. *Infection and Immunity* 55, 594–599.

Lebek, G. and Grünig, H.M. (1985) Relation between the hemolytic property and iron metabolism in *Escherichia coli. Infection and Immunity* 50, 23–30.

Lee, B.C. (1992) Isolation of haemin-binding proteins of *Neisseria gonorrhoeae. Journal of Medical Microbiology* 36, 121–127.

Lee, J.T., Arenholz, D.A., Nelson, R.D. and Simmonds, R.L. (1979) Mechanism of the adjuvant effect of haemoglobin in experimental peritonitis V. The significance of the co-ordinated iron component. *Surgery* 86, 41–47.

Leong, J. and Neilands, J.B. (1976) Mechanisms of siderophore iron transport in enteric bacteria. *Journal of Bacteriology* 126, 823–830.

Linggood, M.A. and Ingram, P.L. (1982) The role of alpha haemolysin in the virulence of *Escherichia coli* for mice. *Journal of Medical Microbiology* 15, 23–30.

Liu, J., Duncan, K. and Walsh, C.T. (1989) Nucleotide sequence of a cluster of *Escherichia coli* biosynthesis genes: identification of *ent*A and purification of its product 2,3-dihydro-2,3-dihydroxybenzoate dehydrogenase. *Journal of Bacteriology* 171, 791–798.

Liu, J., Quinn, N., Berchtold, G.A. and Walsh, C.T. (1990) Overexpression, purification and characterization of isochorismate synthetase (Ent C), the first enzyme in the biosynthesis of enterobactin from chorismate. *Biochemistry* 29, 1417–1425.

Marolda, C.L., Valvano, M.A., Lawlor, K.M., Payne, S.M. and Crosa, J.H. (1987) Flanking and internal regions of chromosomal genes mediating aerobactin iron uptake systems in enteroinvasive *Escherichia coli* and *Shigella flexneri. Journal of General Microbiology* 133, 2269–2278.

Martinez, J.L., Delgado-Iribarren, A. and Baquero, F. (1990) Mechanisms of iron acquisition and bacterial virulence. *Federation of European Microbiological Societies Microbiology Reviews* 75, 45–56.

McClelland, D.B.L. and van Furth, R. (1976) Antimicrobial factors in the exudates of skin windows in human subjects. *Clinical and Experimental Immunology* 25, 442–448.

Mekalanos, J.J. (1992) Environmental signals controlling expression of virulence determinants in bacteria. *Journal of Bacteriology* 174, 1–7.

Moore, D.G. and Earhart, C.F. (1981) Specific inhibition of *Escherichia coli* ferrienterochelin uptake by a normal human serum immunoglobulin. *Infection and Immunity* 31, 631–635.

Moore, D.G., Yancey, R.J., Lankford, C.E. and Earhart, C.F. (1980) Bacteriostatic enterochelin-specific immunoglobulin from normal human serum. *Infection and Immunity* 27, 418–423.

Nahlik, M.S., Brickman, T.J., Ozenberg, B.A. and McIntosh, M.A. (1989) Nucleotide sequence and transcriptional organization of the *Escherichia coli* enterobactin biosynthesis cistrons *ent*B and *ent*A. *Journal of Bacteriology* 171, 784–790.

Nassif, X., Mazert, M.C., Mournier, J. and Sansonetti, P.J. (1987) Evaluation with *iuc*: Tn*10* mutant of the role of aerobactin production in the virulence of *Shigella flexneri. Infection and Immunity* 55, 1963–1969.

Neilands, J.B. (1982) Microbial envelope proteins related to iron. *Annual Review of Microbiology* 36, 285–309.

Neilands, J.B. (1990) Molecular biology and regulation of iron acquisition by

Escherichia coli K12. In: Iglewski, B.H. and Clark, V.L. (eds) *The Bacteria, Vol. I.* Academic Press, New York, pp. 205–223.

Neilands, J.B. (1991) Mechanism and regulation of synthesis of aerobactin in *Escherichia coli* K12 (p Col V–K30). *Canadian Journal of Microbiology* 38, 728–733.

Nelson, M., Carrano, C.J. and Szaniszlo, P.J. (1992) Identification of the ferrioxamine B receptor, Fox B, in *Escherichia coli* K12. *BioMetals* 5, 37–46.

Niederhoffer, E.C., Naranjo, C.M., Bradley, K.L. and Fee, J.A. (1990) Control of *Escherichia coli* superoxide dismutase (*sod*A and *sod*B) genes by the ferric uptake regulation (*fur*) locus. *Journal of Bacteriology* 172, 1930–1938.

Nikaido, H. (1979) Non specific transport through the outer membrane. In: Inoue, M. (ed.) *Bacterial Outer Membranes: Biogenesis and Functions.* John Wiley & Sons, New York., pp. 361–407.

O'Brien, I.G. and Gibson, F. (1970) The structure of enterochelin and related 2,3-dihydroxy-*N*-benzoylserine conjugates from *Escherichia coli. Biochimica et Biophysica Acta* 215, 393–402.

O'Halloran, T.V. (1993) Transition metals in control of gene expression. *Science* 261, 715–725.

Opal, S.M., Cross, A.S., Gemski, P. and Lyhte, L.W. (1990) Aerobactin and α-hemolysin as virulence determinants in *Escherichia coli* isolated from human blood, urine and stool. *Journal of Infectious Diseases* 161, 794–796.

Ozenberger, B.A., Brickman, T.J. and McIntosh, M.A. (1989) Nucleotide sequence of the *Escherichia coli* isochorismate synthetase gene *ent*C and evolutionary relationship of isochorismate synthetase and other chorismate-utilizing enzymes. *Journal of Bacteriology* 171, 775–783.

Payne, S.M. (1989) Iron and virulence in *Shigella. Molecular Microbiology* 3, 1301–1306.

Payne, S.M., Niesel, D.W., Peixotto, S.S. and Lawlor, K.M. (1983) Expression of hydroxamate and phenolate siderophores by *Shigella flexneri. Journal of Bacteriology* 155, 949–955.

Persson, B.C. (1993) Modification of tRNA as a regulatory device. *Molecular Microbiology* 8, 1011–1016.

Petrullo, L.A. and Elseviers, D. (1986) Effect of a 2-methylthio-N^6-isopentenyladenosine deficiency on peptidyl-tRNA release in *Escherichia coli. Journal of Bacteriology* 165, 608–611.

Pollack, J.R. and Neilands, J.B. (1970) Enterobactin, an iron transport compound from *Salmonella typhimurium. Biochemical and Biophysical Research Communications* 38, 989–992.

Pollack, S., Aisen, P., Lasky, F.D. and Vanderhoff, G. (1976) Chelate mediated transfer of iron from transferrin to desferrioxime. *British Journal of Haematology* 34, 231–235.

Poole, K. and Braun, V. (1988) Iron regulation of *Serratia marcescens* hemolysin gene expression. *Infection and Immunity* 56, 2967–2971.

Postle, K. (1990) Aerobic regulation of the *Escherichia coli ton* B gene by changes in iron availability and the *fur* locus. *Journal of Bacteriology* 172, 2287–2293.

Postle, K. and Skare, J.T. (1988) *Escherichia coli* Ton B protein is exported from the cytoplasm without proteolytic cleavage of its amino terminus. *Journal of Biological Chemistry* 262, 11000–11007.

Pressler, U., Staudenmaier, H., Zimmermann, L. and Braun, V. (1988) Genetics of the iron dicitrate transport system in *Escherichia coli. Journal of Bacteriology* 170, 2716–2724.

Rabsch, R. and Reissbrodt, W. (1988) Further differentiation of Enterobacteriaceae by means of siderophore pattern analysis. *Zentralblatt für Bakteriologie Mikrobiologie und Hygiene* 268, 306–317.

Raymond, K.N. and Carrano, C.J. (1979) Co-ordination chemistry of microbial iron transport. *Accounts of Chemical Research* 12, 183–190.

Reid, R.T., Live, D.H., Faulkner, D.J. and Butler, A. (1993) A siderophore from a marine bacterium with an exceptional ferric ion affinity constant. *Nature (London)* 366, 455–458.

Roberts, M., Partha Sarathy, S., Lam-Po-Tang, M.K.L. and Williams, P.H. (1986) The aerobactin iron uptake system in enteropathogenic *Escherichia coli*: evidence for an extinct transposon. *Federation of European Microbiological Societies Microbiology Letters* 37, 215–219.

Roberts, M., Wooldridge, K.G., Garine, H., Kuswandi, S.I. and Williams, P.H. (1989) Inhibition of biological activities of the aerobactin receptor protein in rough strains of *Escherichia coli* by polyclonal antiserum raised against native protein. *Journal of General Microbiology* 135, 2387–2398.

Rogers, H.J. (1973) Iron-binding catechols and virulence in *Escherichia coli. Infection and Immunity* 7, 445–456.

Rogers, H.J., Synge, C., Kimber, B. and Bayley, P.M. (1977) Production of enterochelin by *Escherichia coli* O111. *Biochimica et Biophysica Acta* 497, 548–557.

Rosenberg, H. and Young, I.G. (1974) Iron transport in the enteric bacteria, In: Neilands, J.B. (ed.) *Microbial Iron Metabolism.* Academic Press, New York, pp. 67–82.

Rusnak, F., Liu, J., Quinn, N., Berchtold, G.A. and Walsh, C.T. (1990) Subcloning of the enterobactin biosynthetic gene *ent*B: expression, purification, characterization and substrate specificity of isochorismatase. *Biochemistry* 29, 1425–1435.

Rutz, J.M., Liu, J., Lyons, J.A., Goranson, J., Armstrong, S.K., McIntosh, M.A., Feix, J.B. and Klebba, P.E. (1992) Formation of a gated channel by a ligand-specific transport protein in the bacterial outer membrane. *Science* 258, 471–475.

Schaffer, S., Hantke, K. and Braun, V. (1985) Nucleotide sequence of the iron regulatory gene *fur. Molecular and General Genetics* 201, 204–212.

Schmitt, M.P. and Payne, S.M. (1988) Genetics and regulation of enterobactin genes in *Shigella flexneri. Journal of Bacteriology* 170, 5579–5587.

Sciortino, C.V. and Finkelstein, R.A. (1983) *Vibrio cholerae* expresses iron-regulated outer membrane proteins *in vivo. Infection and Immunity* 42, 990–996.

Shand, G.H., Anwar, H., Kadurugamuwa, J., Brown, M.R.W., Silverman, S.H. and Melling, J. (1985) *In vivo* evidence that bacteria in urinary tract infection grow under iron-restricted conditions. *Infection and Immunity* 48, 35–39.

Smith, A. (1990) Transport of tetrapyrroles: mechanisms and biological and regulatory consequences. In: Dailey, H.A. (ed.) *Biosynthesis and Metabolism of Heme and Chlorophyll.* McGraw-Hill, New York, pp. 435–489.

Smith, H.W. and Huggins, M.B. (1980) The association of the O18:K1 and H7 antigens and the Col V plasmid of a strain of *Escherichia coli* with its virulence and immunogenicity. *Journal of General Microbiology* 121, 387–400.

Smith, H.W., Parsell, Z. and Green, P. (1978) Thermosensitive H1 plasmids determining citrate utilization. *Journal of General Microbiology* 109, 305–311.

Stoebner, J.A. and Payne, S.M. (1988) Iron-regulated hemolysin production and utilization of heme and hemoglobin by *Vibrio cholerae. Infection and Immunity* 56, 2891–2895.

Stojiljkovic, I. and Hantke, K. (1992) Hemin uptake system of *Yersinia enterocolitica*: similarities with other Ton B-dependent systems in Gram-negative bacteria. *European Molecular Biology Organization Journal* 11, 4359–4367.

Stull, T.L. (1987) Protein sources of heme for *Haemophilus influenzae. Infection and Immunity* 55, 148–153.

Suttrop, N., Flöer, B., Schnittler, H., Seeger, W. and Bhakdi, S. (1990) Effects of *Escherichia coli* hemolysin on endothelial cell function. *Infection and Immunity* 58, 3796–3801.

Tai, S.S., Lee, C.-J. and Winter, R.E. (1993) Hemin utilization is related to virulence of *Streptococcus pneumoniae. Infection and Immunity* 61, 5401–5405.

Tidmarsh, G.F. and Rosenberg, L.T. (1981) Acquisition of iron from transferrin by *Salmonella paratyphi* B. *Current Microbiology* 6, 217–220.

Todhunter, D.A., Smith, K.L. and Hogan, J.S. (1991) Antibodies to iron-regulated outer membrane proteins of coliform bacteria isolated from bovine intramammary infections. *Veterinary Immunology and Immunopathology* 28, 107–115.

Valvano, M.A., Silver, R.P. and Crosa, J.H. (1986) Occurrence of chromosome- or plasmid-mediated aerobactin iron transport systems and hemolysin production among clonal groups of human invasive strains of *Escherichia coli* K1. *Infection and Immunity* 52, 192–199.

Van Hove, B., Staudenmaier, H. and Braun, V. (1990) Novel two-component transmembrane transcription control: regulation of iron dicitrate transport in *Escherichia coli* K12. *Journal of Bacteriology* 172, 6749–6758.

Wagegg, W. and Braun, V. (1981) Ferric citrate transport in *Escherichia coli* requires outer membrane receptor protein Fec A. *Journal of Bacteriology* 145, 156–163.

Watanabe, N.A., Nagasu, T., Katsu, K. and Kitoh, K. (1987) E-0702, a new cephalosporin, is incorporated into *Escherichia coli* cells via the *ton* B-dependent iron transport system. *Antimicrobial Agents and Chemotherapy* 31, 497–504.

Waters, V.L. and Crosa, J.H. (1986) DNA environment of the aerobactin iron uptake system genes in prototypic Col V plasmids. *Journal of Bacteriology* 167, 647–654.

Weinberg, E.D. (1989) Cellular regulation of iron assimilation. *Quarterly Review of Biology* 64, 261–290.

West, S.H. and Sparling, P.F. (1987) Aerobactin utilization by *Neisseria gonorrhoeae* and cloning of a genomic DNA fragment that complements *Escherichia coli fhu*B mutations. *Journal of Bacteriology* 169, 3414–3421.

Williams, P. and Griffiths, E. (1992) Bacterial transferrin receptors – structure, function and contribution to virulence. *Medical Microbiology and Immunology* 181, 301–322.

Williams, P.H. (1979) Novel iron uptake system specified by Col V plasmids: an important component in the virulence of invasive strains of *Escherichia coli*. *Infection and Immunity* 26, 925–932.

Williams, P.H. and Warner, P.J. (1980) Col V-plasmid-mediated, Colicin V-independent iron uptake system of invasive strains of *Escherichia coli*. *Infection and Immunity* 29, 411–416.

Williams, P., Morton, D.J., Towner, K.J., Stevenson, P. and Griffiths, E. (1990) Utilization of enterobactin and other exogenous iron sources by *Haemophilus influenzae*, *H. parainfluenzae* and *H. paraphrophilus*. *Journal of General Microbiology* 136, 2343–2350.

Wong, J.C.Y., Holland, J., Parsons, T., Smith, A. and Williams, P. (1994) Identification and characterization of an iron-regulated hemopexin receptor in *Haemophilus influenzae* type b. *Infection and Immunity* 62, 48–59.

Woodrow, G.C., Langman, L., Young, I.G. and Gibson, F. (1978) Mutations affecting the citrate-dependent iron uptake systems in *Escherichia coli*. *Journal of Bacteriology* 133, 1524–1526.

Wooldridge, K.G. and Williams, P.H. (1993) Iron uptake mechanisms of pathogenic bacteria. *Federation of European Microbiological Societies Microbiology Reviews* 12, 325–348.

Young, I.G., Langman, L., Luke, R.K.J. and Gibson, F. (1971) Biosynthesis of the iron transport compound enterochelin: mutants of *Escherichia coli* unable to synthesize 2,3-dihydroxy-benzoate. *Journal of Bacteriology* 106, 51–57.

Zimmermann, L., Hantke, K. and Braun, V. (1984) Exogenous induction of the iron dicitrate transport system of *Escherichia coli* K12. *Journal of Bacteriology* 159, 271–277.

Zingler, G., Nimmick, W., Naumann, G., Ratasch, W. and Reissbrodt, R. (1988) Aerobactin production and dulcitol fermentation in clonal groups of *Escherichia coli* O1:K1 strains from urinary tract infections. *Federation of European Microbiological Societies Microbiology Letters* 49, 489–491.

20 Attaching and Effacing *Escherichia coli*

S. Knutton
Institute of Child Health, University of Birmingham, The Nuffield Building, Francis Road, Birmingham B16 8ET, UK

Introduction

'Attaching and effacing' (AE) is the term first used by Moon *et al.* (1983) to describe an intestinal lesion associated with adherent *E. coli*. Attaching because of the intimate attachment of bacteria, effacing because of the localized effacement of brush border microvilli. This brush border membrane lesion was first reported by Staley *et al.* (1969) in newborn pigs and later by others in rabbits (Polotsky *et al.*, 1977; Takeuchi *et al.*, 1978) and in humans (Ulshen and Rollo, 1980; Clausen and Christie, 1982; Rothbaum *et al.*, 1982) where it was shown to be a feature of intestinal colonization by enteropathogenic *E. coli* (EPEC) strains. This was a milestone in research into this important class of human enteric pathogen because, for the first time since their description in the 1940s and 1950s, it defined a basis for their virulence. AE activity is now also recognized as a property of human enterohaemorrhagic *E. coli* (EHEC), another important class of diarrhoeagenic *E. coli* in humans, and also of EPEC-like and EHEC-like *E. coli* found in a variety of animals including pigs, calves, lambs, rabbits and dogs. Collectively, *E. coli* possessing AE activity are termed attaching and effacing *E. coli* (AEEC). This property is not unique to *E. coli* however, as recent reports have described similar effects produced by *Hafnia alvei* (Albert *et al.*, 1991) and *Citrobacter freundii* (Schauer and Falkow, 1993).

Although an understanding of the virulence of AEEC initially lagged behind that of some other categories of diarrhoeagenic *E. coli*, the last few years have seen major advances in our understanding of the AE activity of *E. coli* in both EPEC and EHEC of human and animal origin. The major advances have come from studies of the clinically and commercially most important AEEC. Consequently this chapter will focus on AE activity associated with human EPEC and EHEC, and EPEC-like and EHEC-like *E. coli* in pigs and calves.

AE Activity of Enteropathogenic *E. coli*

Enteropathogenic *E. coli* (EPEC) is the term used by Neter *et al.* (1955) to describe a limited number of O:H serotypes of *E. coli* that were epidemiologically associated with outbreaks of infantile summer diarrhoea in the 1940s and 1950s. Traditionally, EPEC have been defined on the basis of these classical O:H serotypes (Robins-Browne, 1987), but as our understanding of EPEC pathogenicity has improved it is becoming clear that EPEC strains are better described on the basis of specific virulence characteristics. EPEC do not possess any of the well-defined virulence characteristics of other diarrhoea-causing *E. coli* such as enterotoxins or *Shigella*-like epithelial cell invasiveness (Levine, 1987) but in the late 1970s and early 1980s several reports showed that EPEC strains were capable of adhering to the small and large intestine and producing the striking and characteristic pathognomonic AE lesion (Ulshen and Rollo, 1980; Clausen and Christie, 1982; Rothbaum *et al.*, 1982). Since that time the importance of AE activity in EPEC virulence has consistently been confirmed in animal models of EPEC infection (Moon *et al.*, 1983; Tzipori *et al.*, 1985, 1989) and in human volunteer challenge studies (Levine *et al.*, 1985).

Structural features of the AE lesion

The AE lesion visualized by electron microscopy in infected intestinal tissue is characterized by localized destruction of brush border microvilli, intimate (<10 nm) attachment of bacteria to the apical enterocyte membrane, often in a raised cup-like pedestal structure, and by a dense plaque of cytoskeletal filaments in the apical cytoplasm beneath adherent bacteria (Ulshen and Rollo, 1980; Rothbaum *et al.*, 1982) (Fig. 20.1).

Intermediate stages during lesion formation, which might shed some light on the pathogenic mechanisms involved, were not readily available from analysis of patient biopsies. However, *in vitro* studies using cultured human intestinal mucosa infected with EPEC did allow such stages during AE lesion formation to be observed (Knutton *et al.*, 1987a). Initial non-intimate attachment of bacteria to the intact brush border surface was followed, paradoxically, by localized elongation of brush border microvilli and then by disruption of brush border microvilli by a process of membrane vesiculation. The final stage involved intimate attachment of bacteria to enterocyte surface devoid of microvilli and accumulation of cytoskeletal elements beneath adherent bacteria. Cell swelling and intimate bacterial

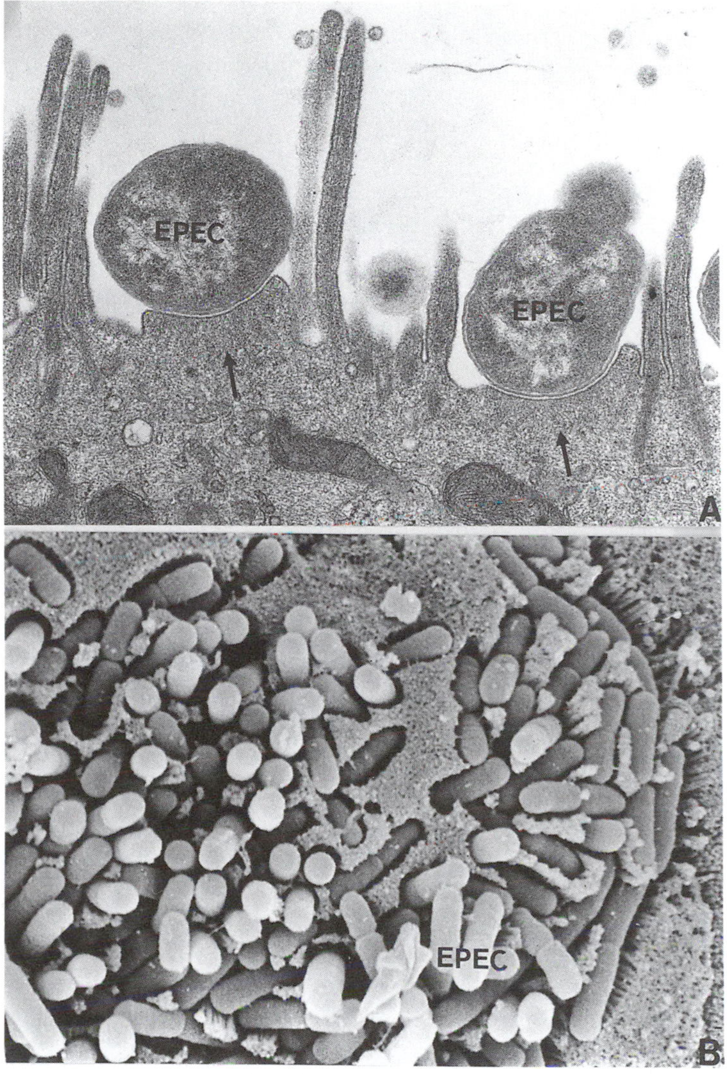

Fig. 20.1. Transmission electron micrograph of EPEC-infected human intestinal mucosa showing the characteristic AE lesion with localized destruction of microvilli, intimate attachment of bacteria on raised pedestal-like structures, and actin accumulation beneath attached bacteria (arrows) (A). Intimate bacterial attachment and localized destruction of microvilli are also clearly seen by scanning electron microscopy (B). Magnification: panel A, × 27,000; panel B, × 480. (Reproduced with permission from Knutton *et al.*, 1987a.)

attachment appeared to produce the pedestal-like structures upon which bacteria appear to sit (Fig. 20.1).

Cravioto *et al.* (1979) showed that EPEC, unlike many other *E. coli* strains, adhere to epithelial cells *in vitro*. EPEC adhere to cultured mammalian cell lines, such as HeLa and HEp-2 cells, in distinct localized microcolonies, a pattern that has been termed localized adherence (LA) (Scaletsky *et al.*, 1984). When EPEC adhere to cultured cells they produce a lesion in the cell membrane morphologically identical to that seen in infected intestinal epithelial cells; bacteria are seen intimately attached to the apical cell surface frequently on pedestal-like structures with a dense plaque of cytoskeletal filaments beneath attached bacteria (Fig. 20.2A) (Knutton *et al.*, 1987b).

Breakdown of the brush border cytoskeleton and accumulation of cytoskeletal filaments beneath AE bacteria suggested that the filaments were probably composed of actin. This was confirmed by staining filamentous actin with fluorescein isothiocyanate (FITC)-conjugated phalloidin. Intense spots of fluorescence were seen at sites which corresponded exactly with the position of each AE bacterium (Fig. 20.2B and C). Such a pattern

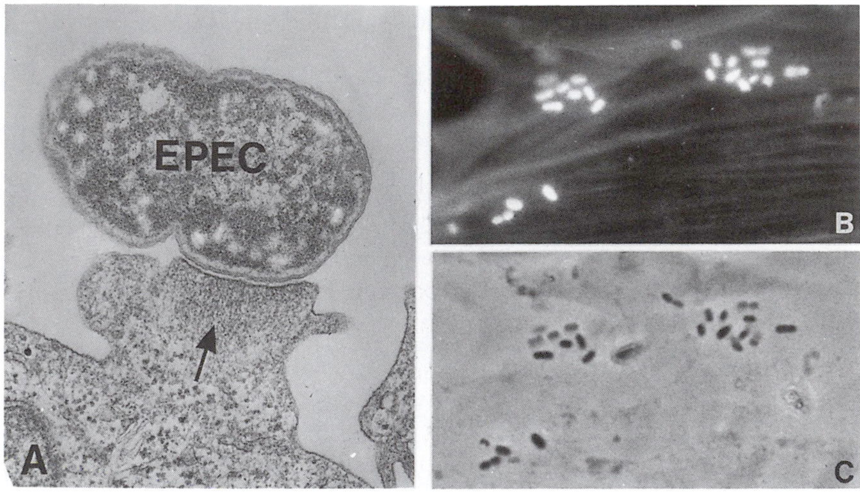

Fig. 20.2. Electron micrograph showing a typical AE lesion produced by EPEC in cultured HEp-2 cells including a dense plaque of cytoskeletal filaments beneath the attached bacterium (A, arrow). Fluorescence actin staining (B) and the corresponding phase contrast micrograph showing bacteria (C) confirm that the filamentous plaque is composed primarily of actin. Magnification: panel A, × 36,000; panels B,C, × 630. (Reproduced with permission from Knutton *et al.*, 1987b, and Knutton *et al.*, 1989.)

of actin accumulation is unique to AE bacteria and led to the development of a highly specific fluorescence actin staining (FAS) test for identifying bacteria possessing AE activity (Knutton *et al.*, 1989).

Genetics of AE activity

In tissue culture cell adhesion assays EPEC display LA and AE activity. LA is associated with a high-molecular-weight (55–70 MDa) 'EPEC Adherence Factor' (EAF) plasmid which is found in most classical EPEC strains (Baldini *et al.*, 1983). However, comparison of the adherence and AE properties of EPEC strain E2348 (O127:H6) isolated from an outbreak of infant diarrhoea in the UK, a plasmid-cured derivative of E2348 and a laboratory *E. coli* transformant possessing pMAR2, the 60-MDa E2348 EAF plasmid, showed that genes encoding AE activity were encoded on the bacterial chromosome (Knutton *et al.*, 1987b). Plasmid-cured E2348, although only very weakly adherent to HEp-2 cells and human intestinal mucosa, retained AE activity as assessed by the FAS assay (Knutton *et al.*, 1989) and by electron microscopy (Knutton *et al.*, 1987a), whereas the plasmid transformant showed LA but was FAS test negative and did not exhibit intimate attachment (Knutton *et al.*, 1987b).

EAF plasmids must nevertheless be important in EPEC pathogenesis because plasmid-cured E2348 is significantly less pathogenic in human volunteers than is the parental E2348 strain (Levine *et al.*, 1985). A DNA probe (EAF probe) developed from an uncharacterized region of an EAF plasmid correlates well with LA and has been used extensively in epidemiological studies (Nataro *et al.*, 1985; Levine *et al.*, 1988). Two important functions of the plasmid have been indicated:

1. EAF genes enhance expression of chromosomal genes associated with AE activity (Jerse and Kaper, 1991) (see below).
2. EAF genes encode an adhesin responsible for LA and whose role *in vivo* is possibly to promote the initial brush border adhesion of EPEC.

However, the identity of a plasmid-encoded adhesin has remained elusive. Of particular current interest is a bundle-forming pilus (BFP) (Girón *et al.*, 1991). These rope-like bundles of fimbriae have not previously been seen because they require media containing blood or tissue culture media containing serum for their expression *in vitro* (Vuopio-Varkila and Schoolnik, 1991). However, while there is good correlation between expression of BFP and the LA phenotype (Girón *et al.*, 1991), it remains to be demonstrated that BFP is also an adhesin which promotes cell attachment.

Attaching and effacing genes

Investigators have used transposon insertion mutagenesis to characterize genes involved in AE activity. Jerse *et al.* (1990) used Tn*phoA* to mutagenize a plasmid-cured derivative of EPEC strain E2348 and screened the mutants for loss of fluorescence in the FAS assay. One mutant negative in the assay was unable to adhere intimately to epithelial cells. An oligonucleotide probe derived from the nucleotide sequence adjacent to the transposon insertion was then used to select a hybridizing clone from a cosmid gene bank. The chromosomal gene interrupted by Tn*phoA* was called *eae* for E. *coli* *a*ttaching and *e*ffacing. Its role in EPEC pathogenesis was confirmed in volunteers who received either the wild-type E2348 strain or an isogenic mutant deleted of the *eae* gene (Donnenberg and Kaper, 1991). Diarrhoea developed in 11 of 11 volunteers who received E2348 but in only 4 of 11 who received the deletion mutant (Donnenberg and Kaper, 1992). However, occurrence of diarrhoea in some volunteers given the deletion mutant indicates that there are other determinants of EPEC diarrhoea.

The cloned *eae* gene has been sequenced and a gene probe (*eae* probe) containing an internal 1-kb fragment of the *eae* gene found to be highly sensitive (100%) and specific (98%) for detecting AE EPEC strains (Jerse *et al.*, 1990). The predicted gene product shows homology (one-third identical and one-half similar amino acids) with the invasins of *Yersinia pseudotuberculosis* and *Yersinia enterocolitica*. Invasins bind to integrin receptors on epithelial cells and promote invasion of *Yersinia* (Isberg and Leong, 1990) which suggests a possible role for intimin, the 94-kDa outer membrane protein product of the *eae* gene (Jerse and Kaper, 1991) in intimate adherence to epithelial cells. This is supported by the observation that the *eae* deletion mutant adheres but does not give a positive FAS test or show intimate adhesion to epithelial cells (Donnenberg and Kaper, 1991). Adhesion does cause some degree of actin condensation however, because the mutant produces what has been termed a 'shadow' phenotype in the FAS assay (Donnenberg *et al.*, 1990). Reintroduction of the *eae* gene on a plasmid into the deletion mutant restored a positive FAS assay and AE activity (Donnenberg and Kaper, 1991). Thus, intimin is necessary but, by itself, not sufficient to produce full AE activity.

eae, recently renamed *eae*A (Donnenberg and Kaper, 1992), appears to be just one gene in a cluster of genes (*eae* gene cluster) involved in intimate adherence since Tn*phoA* mutants downstream of *eae*A are unable to attach intimately to epithelial cells even though they produce intimin and export it to the outer membrane. Loss of AE activity in such mutants can be restored by reintroducing cloned regions 3′ of *eae*A on plasmids. Other genes of the *eae* cluster have yet to be characterized. Expression of *eae*A has also been shown to be influenced by genes of the EAF plasmid

(Jerse and Kaper, 1991) which may explain the weak adherence properties of plasmid-cured strains and their low levels of virulence (Levine *et al.*, 1985).

Mechanism of AE lesion formation

EPEC bind to the brush border surface, destroy microvilli and cause an accumulation of cytoskeletal elements beneath themselves. For an extracellular bacterium to induce such gross intracellular cytoskeletal changes there must be some signal transduction mechanism following initial binding of EPEC. Several recent studies have investigated second messenger production and other intracellular events involved in lesion formation. There is no evidence for elevation in cyclic nucleotide levels following EPEC infection (Long-Krug *et al.*, 1984), but the observation that treatments which perturb the calcium balance of cells caused ultrastructural changes similar to those seen in EPEC-infected cells, led Baldwin *et al.* (1991) to examine intracellular calcium levels. The observed elevation in intracellular calcium levels (Baldwin *et al.*, 1991), together with inhibition of lesion formation by buffering intracellular calcium (Baldwin *et al.*, 1993), suggested a molecular basis for microvillous breakdown since increased intracellular calcium levels have been shown to activate villin, a calcium-dependent brush border microvillous actin severing protein, causing fragmentation of the microvillous actin cytoskeleton with resultant vesiculation of the microvillous membrane (Matsudaira and Burgess, 1982). Intracellular calcium increase was inhibited by dantrolene suggesting calcium release from intracellular stores (Baldwin *et al.*, 1991). Unfortunately, calcium imaging studies which could demonstrate the predicted localized elevation in calcium levels at sites of bacterial adhesion have yet to be performed. A gradient of calcium concentration as calcium returns to basal levels might also explain the observed elongation of brush border microvilli prior to their breakdown and vesiculation (Knutton *et al.*, 1987a).

Calcium is a well-known second messenger regulator in a number of signal transduction pathways and functions through activation of specific protein kinases. Host cell proteins that become phosphorylated during EPEC infection *in vitro* have been identified. Baldwin *et al.* (1990) reported phosphorylation of several proteins after EPEC infection of HEp-2 cells, the most prominent of which had molecular weights of 21 and 29 kDa. These same proteins were phosphorylated in infected Caco-2 and human intestinal epithelial cells (Manjarrez-Hernandez *et al.*, 1992). The 21-kDa protein was purified and shown to be myosin light chain (MLC) (Manjarrez-Hernandez *et al.*, 1991). Phosphoamino acid analysis and comparison with known protein kinase activators and inhibitors indicated phosphorylation by both protein kinase C (PKC) and MLC kinase (Baldwin *et al.*, 1990; Manjarrez-Hernandez *et al.*, 1992). MLC associated with the cytoskeleton was predominantly phosphorylated by MLC kinase; in contrast MLC phosphorylated by PKC was predominantly in the supernatant. Evidence for the involvement of myosin in lesion formation, is the observation that myosin, like actin, becomes accumulated in the AE lesion (Manjarrez-Hernandez *et al.*, 1992). In addition to actin and myosin, α-actinin, ezrin and talin have been identified in the filamentous plaque beneath AE bacteria (Finlay *et al.*, 1992). These cytoskeletal proteins may be important because of their roles as actin binding proteins linking actin to transmembrane protein receptors.

Tyrosine phosphorylation following EPEC infection has also been reported. Using a phosphotyrosine monoclonal antibody, Rosenshine *et al.* (1992) identified a 90-kDa HeLa cell protein that becomes phosphorylated. The same antibody used for fluorescence microscopy gave an appearance very similar to the FAS assay and showed that EPEC bacteria become surrounded by tyrosine phosphorylated proteins (Rosenshine *et al.*, 1992). eaeA mutants retain their ability to induce tyrosine phosphorylation but other Tn*phoA* mutants with Tn*phoA* insertions at chromosomal loci distinct from the *eae* gene cluster which fail to induce tyrosine phosphorylation have been identified (Rosenshine *et al.*, 1992). Such mutants exhibit LA and intimate adhesion but do not induce actin accumulation and do not show disruption of the cell cytoskeleton by electron microscopy. Thus the *eae* genes appear to be necessary for intimate adhesion but only augment cytoskeletal changes induced by other, as yet uncharacterized, chromosomal genes.

The separation of plasmid encoded LA from chromosomally encoded AE activity initially led to the proposal of a two-stage model of EPEC infection (Knutton *et al.*, 1987a). The more recent genetic analysis now indicates that AE activity can be dissected into cytoskeletal disruption and intimate adhesion events and this has led Donnenberg and Kaper (1992) to propose a three-stage model (Fig. 20.3). Initially bacteria adhere to cells by plasmid-encoded adhesins, possibly by BFP pili (Fig. 20.3A). Signal transduction events leading to protein tyrosine phosphorylation, elevation of intracellular calcium levels and effacement of microvilli occur in stage two (Fig. 20.3B). In stage three intimin allows bacteria to become intimately bound to the epithelial cell membrane and accumulation of actin and other cytoskeletal proteins to occur (Fig. 20.3C).

Importance of AE activity in EPEC disease

Infant diarrhoea due to EPEC is now rare in developed countries but it remains important in the developing world where it is sometimes the principal cause of diarrhoea (Gomes *et al.*, 1989; Cravioto *et al.*, 1991). Outbreaks of EPEC diarrhoea have generally been associated with classical EAF^+ AE EPEC serotypes but it is now becoming clear that EPEC

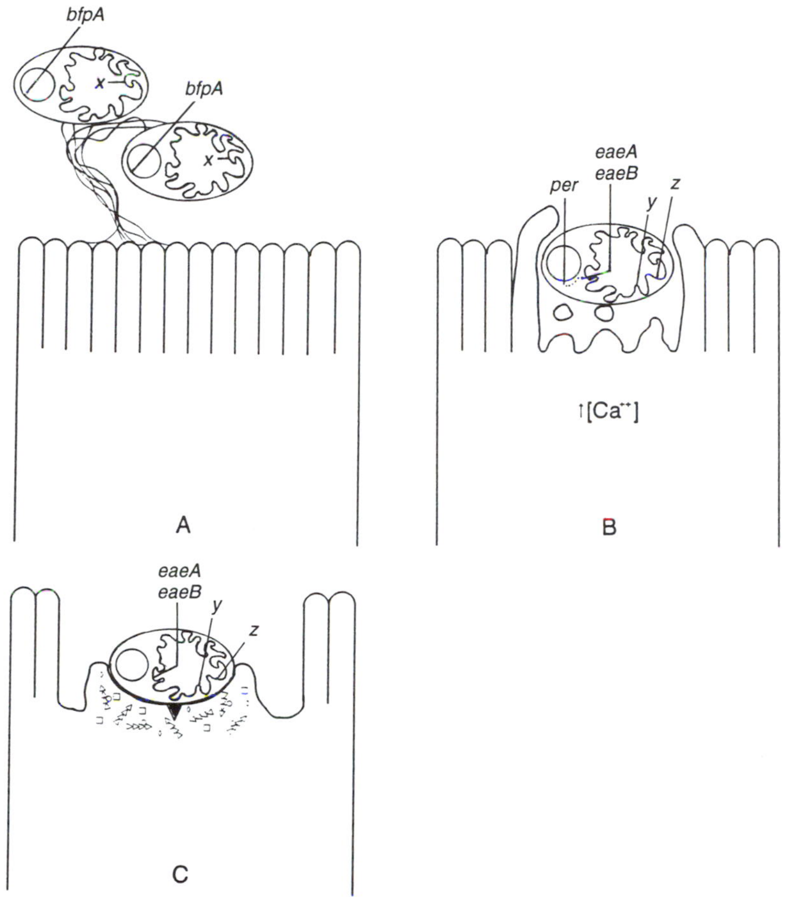

Fig. 20.3. Three-stage model of EPEC pathogenesis. Localized adherence (A), the initial interaction between the bacterium and the epithelial cell, is mediated by BFPs but involves additional chromosomal (gene x) and plasmid loci. In the second stage of infection (B), chromosomal genes (y and z) initiate a signal transduction event that results in increased intracellular calcium levels and effacement of microvilli. Simultaneously, the *eae* gene cluster is activated by the product of the plasmid *per* locus. The third stage of infection (C) results when intimin (solid triangle), the product of the *eae*A locus, and other products of the *eae* gene cluster mediate close attachment to the epithelial cell. From this proximity, effects on the epithelial cell are amplified with accumulation of filamentous actin and other cytoskeletal proteins (geometric shapes). (Reproduced with permission from Donnenberg and Kaper, 1992.)

belonging to serotypes not normally classed as EPEC and EAF$^-$ AE EPEC may be isolated from patients with diarrhoea (Knutton *et al.*, 1991; Scotland *et al.*, 1991; Pedroso *et al.*, 1993). EPEC generally cause disease in the very young (<1 year) still with high mortality and it is frequently associated with chronic illness (Ulshen and Rollo, 1980; Rothbaum *et al.*, 1982).

In spite of all the recent advances in our understanding of EPEC, the pathophysiology that leads to fluid secretion and diarrhoea remains to be elucidated. There is no doubt that the AE activity of EPEC is important in pathogenicity because human volunteer and animal model studies have consistently shown that full virulence is associated with production of the AE lesion. However, this may simply reflect its importance in mucosal adhesion and intestinal colonization; other epithelial cell responses triggered by EPEC may be responsible for the diarrhoeal symptoms. Loss of absorptive surface resulting from AE EPEC adhesion is likely to contribute to diarrhoea but this alone is unlikely to explain the rapid onset of diarrhoea seen in some human EPEC infections (Levine *et al.*, 1985). In addition to any role in AE lesion formation, EPEC-induced phosphorylation of cytoskeletal proteins may influence intestinal transport by affecting tight junction permeability (Madara, 1989). In animals, stimulators of protein kinase activity produce a similar degree of hypersecretion to that caused by cholera toxin (Fondacaro *et al.*, 1985). EPEC-induced phosphorylation of proteins other than cytoskeletal proteins, for example those involved in ion transport, could be important in the mechanism of secretory EPEC diarrhoea.

EPEC infection of cultured epithelial cells results in loss of cell viability, an effect that can be delayed by chelating intracellular calcium (Baldwin *et al.*, 1993). A further consequence of prolonged elevation in calcium levels in EPEC-infected cells, therefore, may be loss of cell viability resulting ultimately in villous atrophy and gross intestinal damage that has been reported in direct histopathological studies (Rothbaum *et al.*, 1982). This may explain the marked persistence of diarrhoea caused by EPEC in some infants.

AE Activity of Enterohaemorrhagic *E. coli*

Enterohaemorrhagic *E. coli* (EHEC) are a recently recognized class of enteric pathogens responsible for outbreaks and sporadic cases of bloody diarrhoea and colitis (Riley *et al.*, 1983). The clinical syndrome of haemorrhagic colitis (HC) differs from classical dysentery due to *Shigella* and enteroinvasive *E. coli* in that the diarrhoea is bloody and copious and is unaccompanied by faecal leucocytes. In addition to HC, EHEC are associated with the subsequent development of serious and sometimes life-threatening complications, particularly haemolytic uraemic syndrome (HUS) and thrombotic thrombocytopenic purpura (Karmali *et al.*, 1985; Kovacs *et al.*, 1990). HC occurs most frequently in developed countries and is primarily associated with ingestion of contaminated meat and dairy products, particularly unpasteurized milk and undercooked ground beef.

The first report of two outbreaks of HC which occurred in 1982 identified the causative organisms as *E. coli* O157 : H7, a serotype not previously recognized as a cause of diarrhoea in humans (Riley *et al.*, 1983). *E. coli* O157 : H7 remains the most frequent EHEC isolate although several other serotypes including O157 : H− , O26 : H− , O26 : H11 also belong to this group.

EHEC, like EPEC, do not produce heat-labile or heat-stable enterotoxins or show shigella-like invasiveness (Levine *et al.*, 1987) but they do share with EPEC the capacity to produce AE intestinal lesions. In addition EHEC produce bacteriophage-encoded cytotoxins which are highly related to Shiga toxin (a virulence factor of *Shigella dysenteriae* type 1) and so have been called Shiga-like toxins (SLTs) (Strockbine *et al.*, 1986). They are also called verotoxins (VTs) because of their cytotoxic effect on Vero cells (Konowalchuk *et al.*, 1977). Shiga-like toxins are potent inhibitors of protein synthesis (O'Brien and Holmes, 1987).

AE activity of EHEC

Attaching and effacing activity has been demonstrated in several animal models of EHEC infection including gnotobiotic piglets (Francis *et al.*, 1986; Tzipori *et al.*, 1986, 1987, 1989), infant rabbits (Potter *et al.*, 1985; Pai *et al.*, 1986; Sherman *et al.*, 1988) and chickens (Beery *et al.*, 1985) and also in *in vitro* mammalian cell models (Knutton *et al.*, 1989). In contrast to EPEC, which colonize the proximal small bowel and large bowel, EHEC produce characteristic lesions mainly in the surface and glandular epithelium of the caecum, colon and, to a lesser extent, the terminal ileum. EHEC lesions are morphologically identical to EPEC lesions and are characterized by intimate bacterial attachment with effacement of brush border microvilli, pedestal-like membrane structures and accumulation of cytoskeletal filaments (Fig. 20.4A). Although EPEC and EHEC AE lesions are morphologically similar, in gnotobiotic piglets EPEC and EHEC infections can be distinguished both by anatomical site of infection, severity of the lesions and degree of polymorph infiltration. EPEC colonize the entire intestine of piglets whereas EHEC only colonize the caecum and colon. EPEC lesions tend to be less severe than with EHEC and there is usually some leucocyte infiltration which is not seen with EHEC. Similar AE lesions have not been demonstrated in human disease because, assuming similar intestinal colonization of EHEC to that seen in animal models, it would

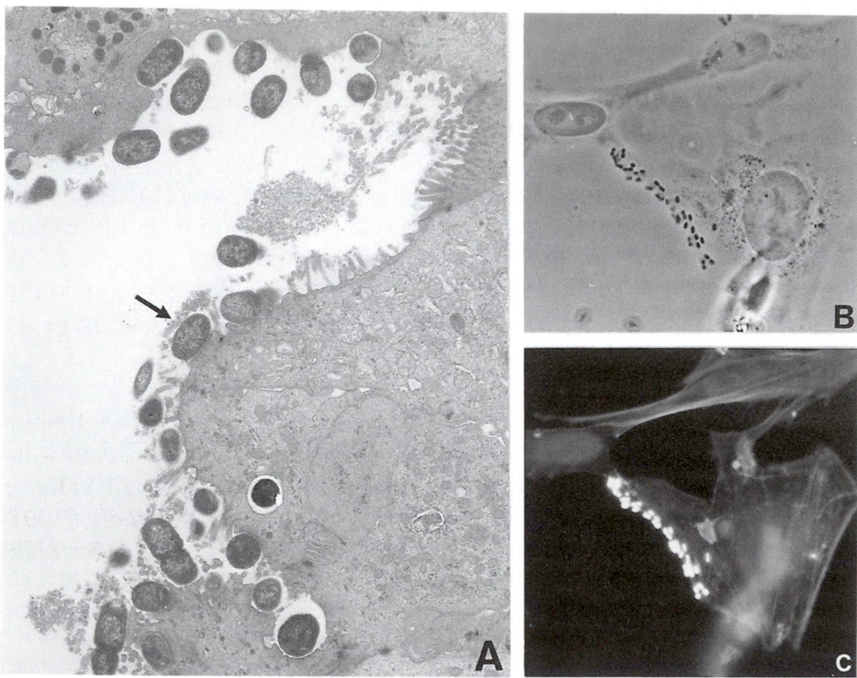

Fig. 20.4. Electron micrograph showing typical AE adherence of bacteria to colonic mucosa in the infant rabbit model of EHEC infection with effacement of microvilli, cupping, pedestals (arrow) and intimate bacterial adhesion (A). EHEC adhere in localized aggregates to tissue culture cells (B) and produce AE lesions demonstrated by fluorescent actin staining (C). Magnification: panel A, × 5600; panels B,C, × 525. (Reproduced with permission from Dr Phil Sherman (A) and from Knutton *et al.*, 1989 (B), (C).)

require biopsies to be taken from the ileocaecal region during acute infection (Kelly, 1987).

AE activity of EHEC has also been demonstrated in *in vitro* models. EHEC adhere to cultured mammalian cells such as HEp-2 cells in localized microcolonies and display AE activity as indicated by actin accumulation in the FAS test (Fig. 20.4B and C) (Knutton *et al.*, 1989).

Genetics of EHEC AE activity

The gene probe containing an internal 1-kb fragment of the EPEC *eae*A gene (*eae* probe) that is 100% sensitive and 98% specific for EPEC strains showing AE activity also recognized 24 of 25 EHEC strains (Jerse *et al.*, 1990). In each case the probe recognized chromosomal genes (Jerse *et al.*,

1991). Two groups have now cloned and sequenced *eae*A genes from EHEC strains and shown that EPEC and EHEC *eae*A genes are strikingly similar. One study reported an EHEC *eae*A homologue that was 86% and 83% identical to the EPEC locus at the nucleotide and predicted amino acid sequence levels, respectively (Yu and Kaper, 1992); the other study showed an EHEC *eae*A sequence 97% homologous to the EPEC *eae*A gene for the first 2200 base pairs and 59% over the last 800 base pairs (Beebakhee *et al.*, 1992). It is interesting that the amino acid sequence divergence is at the C terminal end of *eae*A because the receptor-binding domain of the homologous *Yersinia* invasin gene product is reported to be near the C-terminus (Leong *et al.*, 1990). If the intimins are a family of adhesins, different receptor specificities could be a major factor in the different sites of intestinal colonization by EPEC and EHEC.

Intimin, the product of the EPEC *eae*A gene, is a 94-kDa OMP (Jerse and Kaper, 1991). EHEC also produce a 94 kDa OMP, antibodies to which block EHEC adhesion to epithelial cells and block the ability of EHEC to induce actin accumulation in the FAS assay (Sherman *et al.*, 1991). However, it has yet to be demonstrated that this 94-kDa OMP is an EHEC intimin encoded by the EHEC *eae*A gene.

Plasmid-encoded genes are essential for EPEC virulence because they encode:

1. An adhesin essential for mucosal colonization.
2. Genes which regulate expression of intimin.

EHEC plasmids are much less well characterized although several studies have investigated the role of a large (60 MDa) plasmid common to most EHEC strains. A DNA probe prepared from an uncharacterized part of the 60-MDa plasmid of an O157:H7 EHEC strain (CVD419 probe) was found to be highly sensitive and extremely specific in identifying O157:H7 strains and a good method for identifying other EHEC serotypes (Levine *et al.*, 1987). EHEC do not possess EAF plasmids or BFP. Karch *et al.* (1987) showed that the 60-MDa plasmid in one EHEC strain encoded a rod-like fimbrial antigen important in mediating attachment to Henle 407 human intestinal but not to HEp-2 cells. Toth *et al.* (1990) reported a similar type of adhesion to both Henle 407 and HEp-2 cells that was reduced in a plasmid-cured derivative and was fully restored when the plasmid was reintroduced. Ultrastructural studies, however, indicated adherence by structures other than fimbriae that have yet to be characterized. When examining strains using the FAS test, Knutton *et al.* (1989) showed that EHEC, like EPEC, adhered to HEp-2 cells in localized microcolonies, a pattern very different to the weak diffuse adherence reported in the other studies. Clearly, the role of plasmids in EHEC adhesion to cultured cells needs further clarification.

In gnotobiotic piglets the presence or absence of the 60-MDa plasmid of one EHEC strain did not appear to be of major importance in intestinal colonization (Tzipori *et al.*, 1987). Similarly, in a mouse model both EHEC and a plasmid-cured derivative stably colonized the intestine (Wadolkowski *et al.*, 1990). However, when both strains were fed to streptomycin-treated mice simultaneously the plasmid-cured derivative was generally unable to co-colonize the intestinal tract, suggesting that the plasmid may encode factors important in establishing colonization.

Importance of AE activity in EHEC disease

Putative virulence characteristics of EHEC are production of one or more Shiga-like toxins, plasmid-encoded adhesins and AE activity. Their importance in human disease has not been assessed; one can only extrapolate from the animal studies as to their likely importance. In gnotobiotic piglets AE activity was the most important virulence factor and the 60-MDa plasmid or the capacity to produce SLT were not essential for expression of virulence (Tzipori *et al.*, 1987). In contrast, SLT appeared to play a major role in the pathogenesis of diarrhoea caused by EHEC in infant rabbits (Pai *et al.*, 1986). Most likely, AE activity of EHEC is essential as the mechanism of intestinal colonization. Diarrhoea, which develops after 3–4 days, probably occurs by reduced absorbtion and loss of fluid and electrolytes secondary to mucosal damage produced in the large bowel. SLTs probably act to exacerbate damage to the colonic epithelium and damage mesenteric blood vessels resulting in the bloody, oedematous lesions which are pathognomonic for HC (Tesh and O'Brien, 1991).

Porcine Enteropathogenic *E. coli*

As a result of increasing intensification of farrowing management, diarrhoea has become an economically important disease in pigs. *E. coli* is the most important aetiological agent of neonatal and postweaning diarrhoea and, in most cases, the diarrhoea can be attributed to enterotoxigenic *E. coli*. Lesions suggesting AEEC infections have only recently been demonstrated in natural cases of porcine diarrhoea (Janke *et al.*, 1989). *E. coli* belonging to serogroup O45:K'E65', which have been associated with oedema disease and postweaning diarrhoea but shown not to produce enterotoxins or Shiga-like toxins, have recently been associated with AE activity (Helie *et al.*, 1991).

In natural AEEC infections a multifocal colonization of the brush border of mature enterocytes by bacteria with effacement of microvilli, enterocyte degeneration, and light to moderate inflammation in the lamina propria was observed, mostly in the ileum of infected pigs (Janke *et al.*, 1989). AE activity of porcine isolates belonging to serogroup

O45:K'E65' has been confirmed in experimental infections of newborn pigs (Helie *et al.*, 1991). Typical AE lesions characterized by intimate bacterial adhesion to mature enterocyte brush borders with effacement of microvilli was observed by light and electron microscopy (Fig. 20.5). Bacteria were also seen in intracytoplasmic vacuoles of mature enterocytes and, in areas of heavier colonization, in the lamina propria of the intestinal mucosa. A moderate inflammatory response with mild focal ulceration of the intestinal mucosa was also observed. In a sequential study AE lesions were established in the duodenum, jejunum and ileum at 12 hours but did not develop in the caecum and colon until 24–48 hours postinoculation. Thus, porcine AEEC cause AE lesions and colonize the gut in a manner very similar to human EPEC strains.

Ultrastructural features of early stages of lesion formation in pigs suggested tight adherence of irregularly disposed bacteria with only subsequent

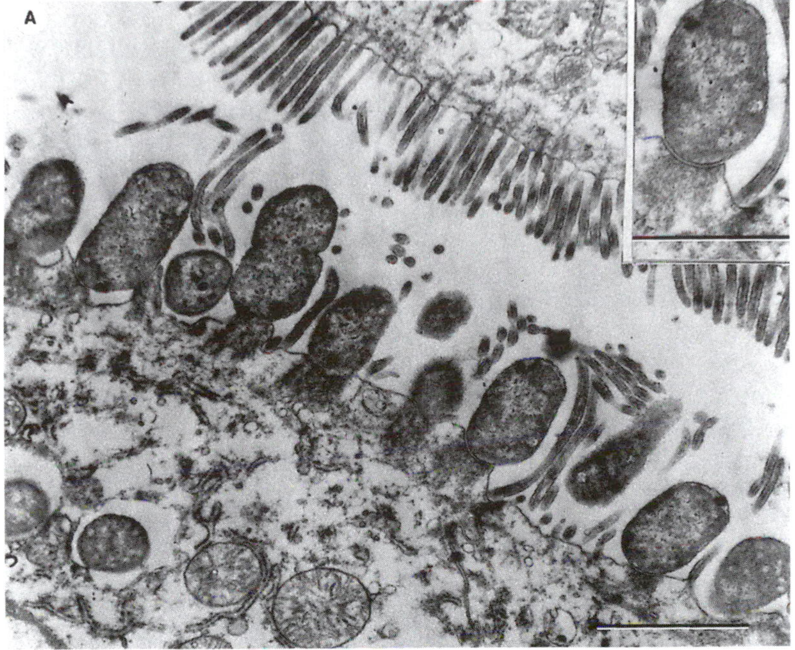

Fig. 20.5. Electron micrograph showing ileal epithelial cells of a pig experimentally infected with porcine EPEC. Characteristic AE lesions with effacement of microvilli, pedestal-like structures, and dense plaques of cytoskeletal filaments beneath attached bacteria are clearly seen. Magnification: × 21,000; inset × 31,000. (Reproduced with permission from Helie *et al.*, 1991.)

development of the characteristic ~10-nm gap separating bacterial and enterocyte surfaces. Strains of serotype O45:K'E65' do not hybridize with probes for EAF or BFP (Bosse *et al.*, 1992) and so it may be that porcine EPEC differ from human EPEC in their mechanism of initial attachment.

In the absence of specific probes for porcine AEEC, *E. coli* isolated from pigs with postweaning diarrhoea have been screened with probes developed for human EPEC. Bosse *et al.* (1992) screened isolates for EAF and *eae* factors and these were found in 12% and 7% of all isolates respectively although they were only identified together in one strain. EAF was found most frequently in serogroups O26:K60, O138:K81 and O141:K85ac whereas *eae* was most frequent in serogroups O45:K'E65' and O108:KV189. The *eae* probe recognizes homologous AE genes in human EHEC and rabbit EPEC strains; it presumably recognizes homologous genes in porcine EPEC. The role or importance of EAF in porcine strains is not clear.

Significance of AE activity in porcine EPEC disease

At the present time AEEC only represent a small proportion of diarrhoeagenic porcine *E. coli* (Bosse *et al.*, 1992). The mechanisms by which they cause diarrhoea are not yet known. However, the similarity to human EPEC both in terms of the pattern of intestinal colonization, type of lesion produced and positivity with the *eae* probe strongly suggests that porcine and human EPEC will have similar pathogenic mechanisms.

AE Activity of Bovine Enterohaemorrhagic *E. coli*

Natural AEEC infections have been described in humans, calves, pigs, lambs, dogs, cats and rabbits. In most cases AEEC infections in animals produce EPEC-like lesions, the exception being in calves where lesions similar to those produced by EHEC strains in humans are produced. In the original description (Chanter *et al.*, 1984) an atypical *E. coli* strain S102–9 ($O5:K^-:H^-$) isolated from calves with 'dysentery' was strongly associated with intestinal colonization, colonic lesions and bloody diarrhoea when fed to gnotobiotic piglets (Chanter *et al.*, 1985). A subsequent study described diarrhoea with copious volumes of blood in the faeces indicative of a haemorrhagic colitis type syndrome (Hall *et al.*, 1985). This type of bloody diarrhoea was seen in both natural infections of young calves and experimental infection of gnotobiotic calves where bacterial colonization was most pronounced in the colon of both farm and gnotobiotic calves although the ileum was also infected. The duodenum and jejunum were not affected. The pathology included thickened colon and rectal walls and reddened mucosa covered by an exudate that contained blood and mucus.

By electron microscopy, bacteria were seen closely adherent to the luminal surface of enterocytes, often in cup-shaped depressions or on cytoplasmic pedestals and microvilli were either distorted, disoriented or absent (Fig. 20.6). Bacteria were not seen within enterocytes. There was exfoliation of infected enterocytes and a mild acute inflammation of the underlying lamina. The lack of staining of some bacteria with an antibody raised against strain S102–9 suggested that AEEC of different serotypes may also have been involved. Strain S102–9 and other *E. coli* belonging to the same somatic O serogroup (O5) and isolated from calves with bloody diarrhoea did not produce enterotoxins but did produce a cytotoxin cytopathic for Vero cells (Chanter *et al.*, 1986). Similar observations were reported from North America following experimental infection of gnotobiotic calves with a verotoxin producing *E. coli* O5:K4:H– isolated from a 2-day-old calf (Moxley and Francis, 1986) and infection of a colostrum-deprived 4-day-old calf with a VT producing *E. coli* O111:H– (Schoonderwoerd *et al.*, 1988),

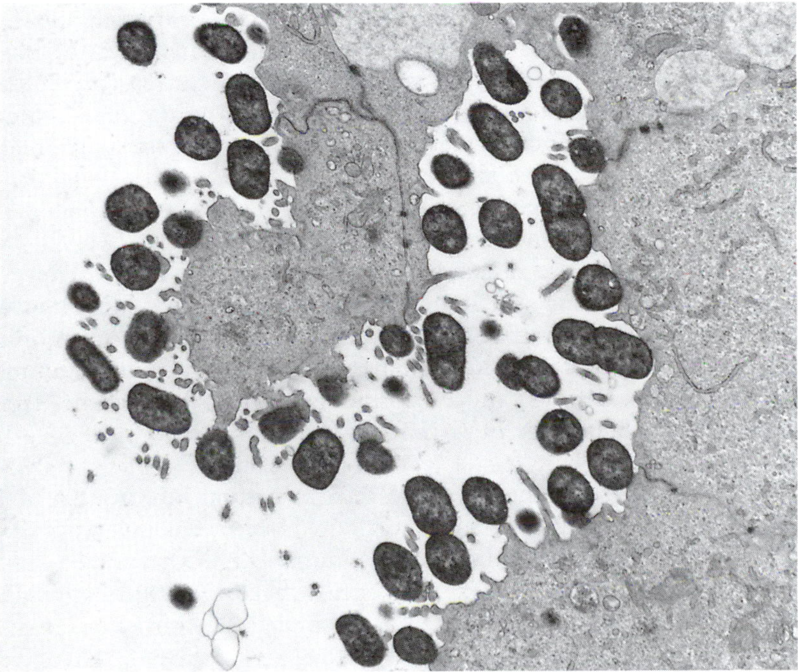

Fig. 20.6. Electron micrograph showing colon of a calf experimentally infected with bovine EHEC. Typical AE lesions with effacement of microvilli, cupping, pedestals and intimate bacterial attachment are seen. Magnification: × 8500. (Reproduced with permission from Hall *et al.*, 1985.)

thus confirming that calves naturally contract infections very similar to those caused by human EHEC. Verotoxin-producing *E. coli* serotype O26:H− has also been associated with AE infection and diarrhoea in young calves (Janke *et al.*, 1990).

The role of SLTs (VTs) was assessed in a comparative study in which gnotobiotic piglets infected with strain S109–2 and a non-VT producing AEEC X114/83 (O101:K$^-$) isolated from bovine gut (Hall *et al.*, 1988) and also in calves experimentally infected with VT1 and VT2 producing AEEC (Wray *et al.*, 1989). These studies showed that VT is not involved in the pathogenesis of AE lesions, that VT1 and VT2 produce similar clinical features and that VT is probably associated with production of diarrhoea in gnotobiotic pigs.

Strain S102–9 adheres in a localized manner (LA) to HEp-2 and Henle 407 cells but does not hybridize with the EAF probe. However, it does hybridize with the CVD419 probe developed to identify human EHEC strains (Hall *et al.*, 1990). Loss of the 46-MDa plasmid in strain S102–9 that hybridizes with the CVD419 probe did not cause a decrease in adhesion, indicating that the CVD419 probe is not specific for genes conferring the ability to adhere to cultured cells in this strain. Fimbriae and non-fimbrial haemagglutinins, which could be involved in cell adhesion of strain S102–9, have been reported but have yet to be further characterized (Chanter *et al.*, 1986). Actin accumulation detected in the FAS test confirmed the AE activity of tissue culture cell adherent strain S102–9 (Hall *et al.*, 1990; Meyer *et al.*, 1992).

Because of their production of VT in large amounts, their AE colonization of the large bowel and their association with haemorrhagic colitis, most bovine AEEC appear to be animal equivalents of human EHEC. However, non-verotoxin producing AEEC identified in the small and large intestine of calves with watery diarrhoea suggest that natural EPEC-like as well as EHEC-like infections also occur in calves (Pearson *et al.*, 1989).

Significance of AE activity in bovine EHEC-like disease

AE colonization of the large intestine seen in natural infections confirms the essential role of bovine AE activity in intestinal colonization. The similarity of the clinical syndrome with human EHEC suggests a similar role of AE activity and SLTs in damaging the colonic epithelium and mesenteric blood vessels resulting in a haemorrhagic colitis.

Conclusions

AEEC are now recognized as important causes of diarrhoea in both humans and animals. From the original ultrastructural observations it was clear that the interaction of these organisms with the host intestinal mucosal surface was complex. This complexity, which requires coordinated expression of multiple structural and regulatory genes on both plasmids and the chromosome, is slowly being unravelled to reveal a successful group of enteric pathogens that have learnt to utilize host signal transduction pathways and subvert the host cytoskeletal system in their endeavour to stably and efficiently colonize the gut. Other epithelial cell responses and virulence determinants (e.g. cytotoxins produced by EHEC) contribute to pathophysiologies that lead to the different diarrhoeal syndromes characteristic of AEEC.

References

Albert, M.J., Alam, K., Islam, M., Montanaro, J., Rahman, A.S.M.H., Haider, K., Hossain, M.A., Kibriya, A.K.M.G. and Tzipori, S. (1991) *Hafnia alvei*, a probable cause of diarrhoea in humans. *Infection and Immunity* 59, 1507–1513.

Baldini, M.M., Kaper, J.B., Levine, M.M., Candy, D.C. and Moon, H.W. (1983) Plasmid-mediated adhesion in enteropathogenic *Escherichia coli*. *Journal of Pediatric Gastroenterology and Nutrition* 2, 534–538.

Baldwin, T.J., Brooks, S.F., Knutton, S., Manjarrez-Hernandez, H.A., Aitken, A. and Williams, P.H. (1990) Protein phosphorylation by protein kinase C in HEp-2 cells infected with enteropathogenic *Escherichia coli*. *Infection and Immunity* 58, 761–765.

Baldwin, T.J., Ward, W., Aitken, A., Knutton, S. and Williams, P.H. (1991) Elevation of intracellular free calcium levels in HEp-2 cells infected with enteropathogenic *Escherichia coli*. *Infection and Immunity* 59, 1599–1604.

Baldwin, T.J., Lee-Delauney, M.B., Knutton, S. and Williams, P.H. (1993) Calcium-calmodulin dependence of actin accretion and lethality in cultured HEp-2 cells infected with enteropathogenic *Escherichia coli*. *Infection and Immunity* 61, 76–763.

Beebakhee, G., Louie, M., De Azavedo, J. and Brunton, J. (1992) Cloning and nucleotide sequence of the *eae* homologue from enterohemorrhagic *Escherichia coli* serotype O157 : H7. *Federation of European Microbiological Societies Microbiological Letters* 91, 63–68.

Beery, J.T., Doyle, M.P. and Schoeni, J.L. (1985) Colonization of chicken cecae by *Escherichia coli* associated with hemorrhagic colitis. *Applied and Environmental Microbiology* 49, 310–315.

Bosse, M., Fairbrother, J.M., Harel, J. and Desautels, C. (1992) Detection of genes for EAF and *eae* in *Escherichia coli* isolated from pigs with postweaning diarrhoea using colony hybridization. *Abstracts of the 92nd General Meeting of the American Society for Microbiology, 1992*. American Society for Microbiology, Washington, DC, Abstract B-66, p. 37.

Chanter, N., Morgan, J.H., Bridger, J.C., Hall, G.A. and Reynolds, D.R. (1984) Dysentery in gnotobiotic calves caused by atypical *Escherichia coli*. *Veterinary Record* 114, 71.

Chanter, N., Hall, G.A., Bland, A.P., Hayle, A.J. and Parsons, K.R. (1986) Dysentery in calves caused by an atypical strain of *Escherichia coli* (S102–9). *Veterinary Microbiology* 12, 241–253.

Clausen, C.R. and Christie, D.L. (1982) Chronic diarrhea in infants caused by adherent enteropathogenic *Escherichia coli. Journal of Pediatrics* 100, 358–361.

Cravioto, A., Gross, R.J., Scotland, S.M. and Rowe, B. (1979) An adhesive factor found in strains of *Escherichia coli* belonging to the traditional infantile enteropathogenic serogroups. *Current Microbiology* 3, 95–99.

Cravioto, A., Tello, A., Navarro, A., Ruiz, J., Vill-fan, A., Uribe, F. and Eslava, C. (1991) Association of *Escherichia coli* HEp-2 adherence patterns with type and duration of diarrhoea. *Lancet* 337, 262–264.

Donnenberg, M.S. and Kaper, J.B. (1991) Construction of an *eae* deletion mutant of enteropathogenic *Escherichia coli* by using a positive-selection suicide vector. *Infection and Immunity* 59, 4310–4317.

Donnenberg, M.S. and Kaper, J.B. (1992) Enteropathogenic *Escherichia coli. Infection and Immunity* 60, 3953–3961.

Donnenberg, M.S., Calderwood, S.B., Donohue-Rolfe, A., Keusch, G.T. and Kaper, J.B. (1990) Construction and analysis of Tn*phoA* mutants of enteropathogenic *Escherichia coli* unable to invade HEp-2 cells. *Infection and Immunity* 58, 1565–1571.

Finlay, B.B., Rosenshine, I., Donnenberg, M.S. and Kaper, J.B. (1992) Cytoskeletal composition of attaching and effacing lesions associated with enteropathogenic *Escherichia coli* adherence to HeLa cells. *Infection and Immunity* 60, 2541–2543.

Fondacaro, J.D. and Henderson, L.S. (1985) Evidence for protein kinase C as a regulator of intestinal electrolyte transport. *American Journal of Physiology* 249, G422–G426.

Francis, D.H., Collins, J.E. and Duimstra, J.R. (1986) Infection of gnotobiotic pigs with an *Escherichia coli* O157 : H7 strain associated with an outbreak of hemorrhagic colitis. *Infection and Immunity* 51, 953–956.

Girón, J.A., Ho, S.Y. and Schoolnik, G.K. (1991) An inducible bundle-forming pilus of enteropathogenic *Escherichia coli. Science* 254, 710–713.

Gomes, T.A.T., Blake, P.A. and Trabulsi, L.R. (1989) Prevalence of *Escherichia coli* strains with localised, diffuse, and aggregative adherence to HeLa cells in infants with diarrhea and matched controls. *Journal of Clinical Microbiology* 27, 266–269.

Hall, G.A., Reynolds, D.J., Chanter, N., Morgan, J.H., Parsons, K.R., Debney, T.G., Bland, A.P. and Bridger, J.C. (1985) Dysentery caused by *Escherichia coli* (S102–9) in calves: natural and experimental disease. *Veterinary Pathology* 22, 156–163.

Hall, G.A., Chanter, N. and Bland, A.P. (1988) Comparison in gnotobiotic pigs of lesions caused by verotoxigenic and non-verotoxigenic *Escherichia coli. Veterinary Pathology* 25, 205–210.

Hall, G.A., Dorn, C.R., Chanter, N., Scotland, S.M., Smith, H.R. and Rowe, B. (1990) Attaching and effacing lesions *in vivo* and adhesion of tissue culture cells of verocytotoxin-producing *Escherichia coli* belonging to serogroup O5 and O103. *Journal of General Microbiology* 136, 779–786.

Helie, P., Morin, M., Jacques, M. and Fairbrother, J.M. (1991) Experimental infection of newborn pigs with an attaching and effacing *Escherichia coli* O45:K'E65' strain. *Infection and Immunity* 59, 814–821.

Isberg, R.R. and Leong, J.M. (1990) Multiple β_1, chain integrins are receptors for invasin, a protein that promotes bacterial penetration into mammalian cells. *Cell* 60, 861–871.

Janke, B.H., Francis, D.H., Collins, J.E., Libal, M.C., Zeman, D.H. and Johnson, D.D. (1989) Attaching and effacing *Escherichia coli* infections in calves, pigs, lambs, and dogs. *Journal of Veterinary Diagnostic Investigations* 1, 6–11.

Janke, B.H., Francis, D.H., Collins, J.E., Libal, M.C., Zeman, D.H., Johnson, D.D. and Neiger, R.D. (1990) Attaching and effacing *Escherichia coli* infection as a cause of diarrhoea in young calves. *Journal of the American Veterinary Medical Association* 196, 897–901.

Jerse, A.E. and Kaper, J.B. (1991) The *eae* gene of enteropathogenic *Escherichia coli* encodes a 94-kilodalton membrane protein, the expression of which is influenced by the EAF plasmid. *Infection and Immunity* 59, 4302–4309.

Jerse, A.E., Yu, J., Tall, B.D. and Kaper, J.B. (1990) A genetic locus of enteropathogenic *Escherichia coli* necessary for the production of attaching and effacing lesions on tissue culture cells. *Proceedings of the National Academy of Sciences of the United States of America* 87, 7839–7843.

Jerse, A.E., Gicquelais, K.G. and Kaper, J.B. (1991) Plasmid and chromosomal elements involved in the pathogenesis of attaching and effacing *Escherichia coli. Infection and Immunity* 59, 3869–3875.

Karch, H., Heesemann, J., Laufs, R., O'Brien, A.D., Tacket, C.O. and Levine, M.M. (1987) A plasmid of enterohemorrhagic *Escherichia coli* O157:H7 is required for expression of a new fimbrial antigen and for adhesion to epithelial cells. *Infection and Immunity* 55, 455–461.

Karmali, M.A., Petric, M., Corazon, L., Fleming, P.C., Arbus, G.S. and Lior, H. (1985) The association between haemolytic uraemic syndrome and infection by verotoxin producing *E. coli. Journal of Infectious Diseases* 55, 775–782.

Kelly, J.K., Pai, C.H., Jadusingh, I.H., MacInnis, M.L., Shaffer, E.A. and Hershfield, N.B. (1987) The histopathology of rectosigmoid biopsies from adults with bloody diarrhoea due to verotoxin-producing *Escherichia coli. American Journal of Clinical Pathology* 88, 78–82.

Knutton, S., Lloyd, D.R. and McNeish, A.S. (1987a) Adhesion of enteropathogenic *Escherichia coli* to human intestinal enterocytes and cultured human intestinal mucosa. *Infection and Immunity* 55, 69–77.

Knutton, S., Baldini, M.M., Kaper, J.B. and McNeish, A.S. (1987b) Role of plasmid-encoded adherence factors in adhesion of enteropathogenic *Escherichia coli* to HEp-2 cells. *Infection and Immunity* 55, 78–85.

Knutton, S., Baldwin, T., Williams, P.H. and McNeish, A.S. (1989) Actin accumulation at sites of bacterial adhesion to tissue culture cells: basis of a new diagnostic test for enteropathogenic and enterohemorrhagic *Escherichia coli. Infection and Immunity* 57, 1290–1298.

Knutton, S., Phillips, A.D., Smith, H.R., Gross, R.J., Shaw, R., Watson, P. and Price, E. (1991) Screening of enteropathogenic *Escherichia coli* in infants with diarrhea by the fluorescent actin staining test. *Infection and Immunity* 59, 365–371.

Konowalchuk, J., Speirs, J.I. and Stavric, S. (1977) Vero response to a cytotoxin from *Escherichia coli. Infection and Immunity* 18, 775–779.

Kovacs, M.J., Roddy, J., Gregoire, S., Cameron, W., Eidus, L. and Drouin, J. (1990) Thrombotic thrombocytopenic purpura following haemorrhagic colitis due to *Escherichia coli* O157:H7. *American Journal of Medicine* 88, 177–179.

Leong, J.M., Fournier, R.S. and Isberg, R.R. (1990) Identification of the integrin binding domain of the *Yersinia tuberculosis* invasin protein. *European Molecular Biology Organization Journal* 9, 1979–1989.

Levine, M.M. (1987) *Escherichia coli* that cause diarrhea: enterotoxigenic, enteropathogenic, enteroinvasive, enterohemorrhagic and enteroadherent. *Journal of Infectious Diseases* 155, 377–389.

Levine, M.M., Nataro, J.P., Karch, H., Baldini, M.M., Kaper, J.B., Black, R.E., Clements, M.L. and O'Brien, A.D. (1985) The diarrheal response of humans to some classic serotypes of enteropathogenic *Escherichia coli* is dependent on a plasmid encoding an enteroadhesiveness factor. *Journal of Infectious Diseases* 152, 550–559.

Levine, M.M., Xu, J., Kaper, J.B., Lior, H., Prado, V., Tall, B., Nataro, J., Karch, H. and Wachsmuth, K. (1987) A DNA probe to identify enterohemorrhagic *Escherichia coli* of O157:H7 and other serotypes that cause hemorrhagic colitis and hemolytic uremic syndrome. *Journal of Infectious Diseases* 156, 175–182.

Levine, M.M., Prado, V., Robins-Browne, R., Lior, H., Kaper, J.B., Moseley, S.L., Gicquelais, K., Nataro, J.P., Vial, P. and Tall, B. (1988) Use of DNA probes and HEp-2 cell adherence assay to detect diarrheagenic *Escherichia coli. Journal of Infectious Diseases* 158, 224–228.

Long-Krug, S.A., Weikel, C.S., Tiemens, K.T., Hewlett, E.L., Levine, M.M. and Guerrant, R.L. (1984) Do enteropathogenic *Escherichia coli* produce heat-labile enterotoxin, heat-stable enterotoxins a or b, or cholera toxin A subunits? *Infection and Immunity* 46, 612–614.

Madara, J.L. (1989) Loosening tight junctions: lessons from the intestine. *Journal of Clinical Investigation* 83, 1089–1094.

Manjarrez-Hernandez, H.A., Amess, B., Sellars, L., Baldwin, T.J., Knutton, S., Williams, P.H. and Aitken, A. (1991) Purification of a 20 kDa phosphoprotein from epithelial cells and identification as a myosin light chain: phosphorylation induced by enteropathogenic *Escherichia coli* and phorbol ester. *Federation of European Microbiological Societies Microbiological Letters* 292, 121–127.

Manjarrez-Hernandez, H.A., Baldwin, T.J., Aitken, A., Knutton, S. and Williams, P.H. (1992) Intestinal epithelial cell protein phosphorylation in enteropathogenic *Escherichia coli* diarrhoea. *Lancet* 339, 521–523.

Matsudaira, P.T. and Burgess, D.R. (1982) Partial reconstruction of the microvillus core bundle: characterization of villin as a Ca^{++}-dependent, actin-bundling/depolymerizing protein. *Journal of Cell Biology* 92, 648–656.

Meyer, A., Corboz, L., Straumann-Kunz, U. and Pospischil, A. (1992) Interactions with enteropathogenic *Escherichia coli* (EPEC) in cattle. 1. Comparison of different animal models and a cell culture system for the establishment of a detection system for 'attaching and effacing' (AE) lesions. *Zentralblatt fur Veterinarmedizin – Reihe B* 39, 575–584.

Moon, H.W., Whipp, S.C., Argenzio, R.A., Levine, M.M. and Gianella, R.A. (1983) Attaching and effacing activities of rabbit and human enteropathogenic *Escherichia coli* in pig and rabbit intestines. *Infection and Immunity* 41, 1340–1351.

Moxley, R.A. and Francis, D.H. (1986) Natural and experimental infection with an attaching and effacing strain of *Escherichia coli* in calves. *Infection and Immunity* 53, 339–346.

Nataro, J.P., Scaletsky, C.A., Kaper, J. B., Levine, M.M. and Trabulsi, L.R. (1985) Plasmid-mediated factors conferring diffuse and localised adherence of enteropathogenic *Escherichia coli. Infection and Immunity* 48, 373–383.

Neter, E., Westphal, O., Lüderitz, O., Gino, R.M., Gorzynski, E.A. (1955) Demonstration of antibodies against enteropathogenic *Escherichia coli* in sera of children of various ages. *Pediatrics* 16, 801–808.

O'Brien, A.D. and Holmes, R.K. (1987) Shiga and shiga-like toxins. *Microbiological Reviews* 51, 206–220.

Pai, C.H., Kelly, J.K. and Meyers, G.L. (1986) Experimental infection of infant rabbits with verotoxin-producing *Escherichia coli. Infection and Immunity* 51, 16–23.

Pearson, G.R., Watson, C.A., Hall, G.A. and Wray, C. (1989) Natural infections with an attaching and effacing *Escherichia coli* in the small and large intestines of a calf with diarrhoea. *Veterinary Record* 124, 297–299.

Pedroso, M.Z., Freymuller, E., Trabulsi, L.R. and Gomes, T.A.T. (1993) Attaching–effacing lesions and intracellular penetration in HeLa cells and human duodenal mucosa by two *Escherichia coli* strains not belonging to classical enteropathogenic *E. coli* serogroups. *Infection and Immunity* 61, 1152–1156.

Polotsky, Y.E., Dragunskaya, E.M., Seliverstova, V.G., Avdeeva, T.A., Chakhutinskaya, M.G., Kétyi, I., Vertényi, A., Ralovich, B., Emódy, L., Malovics, I., Safonova, N.V., Snigirevskaya, E.S. and Karyagina, E.I. (1977) Pathogenic effect of enterotoxigenic *Escherichia coli* and *Escherichia coli* causing infantile diarrhoea. *Acta Microbiology Academy Sciences Hungary* 24, 221–236.

Potter, M.E., Kaufmann, A.F., Thomason, B.M., Blake, P.A. and Farmer, J.J. (1985) Diarrhea due to *Escherichia coli* O157 : H7 in the infant rabbit. *Journal of Infectious Diseases* 152, 1341–1343.

Riley, L.W., Remis, R.S., Helgerson, S.D., McGee, H.B., Wells, J.G., Davis, B.R., Herbert, R.J., Olcott, E.S., Johnson, L.M., Hargrett, N.T., Blake, P.A. and Cohen, M.L. (1983) Haemorrhagic colitis associated with a rare *Escherichia coli* serotype. *New England Journal of Medicine* 308, 681–685.

Robins-Browne, R.M. (1987) Traditional enteropathogenic *Escherichia coli* of infantile diarrhea. *Reviews of Infectious Diseases* 9, 28–53.

Rosenshine, I., Donnenberg, M.S., Kaper, J.B. and Finlay, B.B. (1992) Signal transduction between enteropathogenic *Escherichia coli* (EPEC) and epithelial cells: EPEC induces tyrosine phosphorylation of host cell proteins to initiate cytoskeletal rearrangement and bacterial uptake. *European Molecular Biology Organization Journal* 11, 3551–3560.

Rothbaum, R., McAdams, A.J., Gianella, R. and Partin, J.C. (1982) A clinicopathological study of enterocyte-adherent *Escherichia coli*: a cause of protracted diarrhea in infants. *Gastroenterology* 83, 441–454.

Scaletsky, I.C.A., Silva, M.L.M. and Trabulsi, L.R. (1984) Distinctive patterns of adherence of enteropathogenic *Escherichia coli* to HeLa cells. *Infection and Immunity* 45, 534–536.

Schauer, D.B. and Falkow, S. (1993) Attaching and effacing locus of a *Citrobacter freundii* biotype that causes transmissible murine colonic hyperplasia. *Infection and Immunity* 61, 2486–2492.

Schoonderwoerd, M., Clarke, R.C., van Dreumel, A.A. and Rawluk, S.A. (1988) Colitis in calves: natural and experimental infection with a verotoxin-producing strain of *Escherichia coli* O111:NM. *Canadian Journal of Veterinary Research* 52, 484–487.

Scotland, S.M., Smith, H.R. and Rowe, B. (1991) *Escherichia coli* O128 strains from infants with diarrhea commonly show localized adhesion and positivity in the fluorescent-actin staining test but do not hybridize with an enteropathogenic *E. coli* adherence factor probe. *Infection and Immunity* 59, 1569–1571.

Sherman, P., Soni, R. and Karmali, M. (1988) Attaching and effacing adherence of vero cytotoxin-producing *Escherichia coli* to rabbit intestinal epithelium *in vivo*. *Infection and Immunity* 56, 756–761.

Sherman, P., Cockerill, F., Soni, R. and Brunton, J. (1991) Outer membranes are competitive inhibitors of *Escherichia coli* O157:H7 adherence to epithelial cells. *Infection and Immunity* 59, 890–899.

Staley, T.E., Jones, E.W. and Corley, L.D. (1969) Attachment and penetration of *Escherichia coli* into intestinal epithelium of the ileum in newborn pigs. *American Journal of Pathology* 56, 371–392.

Strockbine, N.A., Marques, L.R.M., Newland, J.W., Smith, H.W., Holmes, R.K. and O'Brien, A.D. (1986) Two toxin-converting phages from *Escherichia coli* O157:H7 strain 933 encode antigenically distinct toxins with similar biologic activities. *Infection and Immunity* 53, 135–140.

Takeuchi, A., Inman, L.R., O'Hanley, P.D., Cantey, J.R. and Lushbaugh, W.B. (1978) Scanning and transmission electron microscopic study of *Escherichia coli* O15 (RDEC-1) enteric infection in rabbits. *Infection and Immunity* 19, 686–694.

Tesh, V.L. and O'Brien, A.D. (1991) The pathogenic mechanisms of Shiga and Shiga-like toxins. *Molecular Microbiology* 5, 1817–1822.

Toth, I., Cohen, M.L., Rumschlag, H.S., Riley, L.W., Whire, E.H., Carr, J.H., Bond, W.W. and Wachsmuth, I.K. (1990) Influence of the 60-megadalton plasmid on adherence of *Escherichia coli* O157:H7 and genetic derivatives. *Infection and Immunity* 58, 1223–1231.

Tzipori, S., Robins-Browne, R.M., Gonis, G., Hayes, J., Withers, M. and McCartney, E. (1985) Enteropathogenic *Escherichia coli* enteritis: evaluation of the gnotobiotic piglet as a model of human infection. *Gut* 26, 570–578.

Tzipori, S., Wachsmuth, I.K., Chapman, C., Birner, R., Brittingham, J., Jackson C. and Hogg, J. (1986) The pathogenesis of haemorrhagic colitis caused by *Escherichia coli* O157:H7 in gnotobiotic piglets. *Journal of Infectious Diseases* 154, 712–716.

Tzipori, S., Karch, H., Wachsmuth, I.K., Robins-Browne, R.M., O'Brien, A.L., Lior, H., Cohen, M.L., Smithers, J. and Levine, M.M. (1987) Role of a 60-megadalton plasmid and shiga-like toxins in the pathogenesis of infection caused by enterohemorrhagic *Escherichia coli* O157 : H7 in gnotobiotic piglets. *Infection and Immunity* 55, 3117–3125.

Tzipori, S., Gibson, R. and Montanaro, J. (1989) Nature and distribution of mucosal lesions associated with enteropathogenic and enterohemorrhagic *Escherichia coli* in piglets and the role of plasmid-mediated factors. *Infection and Immunity* 57, 1142–1150.

Ulshen, M.H. and Rollo, J.L. (1980) Pathogenesis of *Escherichia coli* gastroenteritis in man – another mechanism. *New England Journal of Medicine* 302, 99–101.

Vuopio-Varkila, J. and Schoolnik, G.K. (1991) Localized adherence by enteropathogenic *Escherichia coli* is an inducible phenotype associated with the expression of new outer membrane proteins. *Journal of Experimental Medicine* 174, 1167–1177.

Wadolkowski, A.E., Burris, J.A. and O'Brien, A.D. (1990) Mouse model for colonization and disease caused by enterohemorrhagic *Escherichia coli* O157 : H7. *Infection and Immunity* 58, 2438–2445.

Wray, C., McLaren, I. and Pearson, G.R. (1989) Occurrence of 'attaching and effacing' lesions in the small intestine of calves experimentally infected with bovine isolates of verotoxic *E. coli*. *Veterinary Record* 125, 365–368.

Yu, J. and Kaper, J.B. (1992) Cloning and characterization of the *eae* gene of enterohemorrhagic *Escherichia coli* O157:H7. *Molecular Microbiology* 6, 411–417.

IV

Diagnosis and Prevention of Diseases Caused by *Escherichia coli*

Laboratory Diagnosis of *Escherichia coli* Infections **21**

C. Wray and M.J. Woodward
Bacteriology Department, Central Veterinary Laboratory, Woodham Lane, New Haw, Addlestone, Surrey KT15 3NB, UK

Introduction

E. coli, a normal inhabitant of the intestinal tract, is associated with both enteric and extraintestinal infections in animals. In the case of enteric infections, the challenge for the laboratory is to determine whether an isolate is normal flora or an agent of disease. In extraintestinal infections, isolation of *E. coli* from a suitable sample is often all that is required, but quantitative culture is sometimes used to guide in assessing significance of the isolate.

The development of serological methods and the association of specific serotypes of *E. coli* with enteric disease in various species were the mainstay of laboratory diagnosis. However, detection of virulence determinants is now the major method. Thus, identification of fimbrial adhesins and/or enterotoxins is the preferred method for determining whether an enteric isolate from a diseased animal is a pathogen.

This chapter aims to review the various tests that are used to identify pathogenic *E. coli*. Some of the methodology is only appropriate to a reference or research laboratory, but smaller diagnostic laboratories should be able to use many of the techniques.

Serotyping of *E. coli*

Somatic O antigens

The specificity of the numerous O antigens is determined by the chemical structure of the polysaccharides. The antigens are thermostable, resist alcohol, dilute acid and heating at 100°C for 2.5 hours. Somatic antigens are not single antigens but are composed of several antigenic components and are consequently called O-group antigens. Different O groups may share antigenic components, giving rise to cross antigenicity. Somatic antigens are subject to smooth (S) to rough (R) variation when the organism becomes auto-agglutinable in normal saline and loses its serological specificity. Some O antigens are also subject to lysogenic conversion. Currently, 173 O groups are recognized, some of which have minor antigenic differences within the group.

Capsular K antigens

The term capsular or envelope K antigen was originally used for surface antigens that caused O inagglutinability. This is a phenomenon in which the agglutination of living organisms in an O antiserum prepared against the heat-treated homologous strain is inhibited or blocked by the K antigen. The K antigens were originally divided into three classes (L, A and B) according to the effect of heat on agglutinability, antigenicity and antibody-binding power of the strains. The L type of K antigen is heat-labile. After heating at 100°C for 1 hour cultures with the L type of K antigen are agglutinated by O antiserum but not K antiserum and lose their ability to bind K antibody. The A type of K antigen is inactivated by heating at 121°C for 2.5 hours; the heat-treated culture becomes agglutinable in O antiserum but not K antiserum, but retains the ability to bind antibody. There is less evidence for existence of the B type of K antigen, which differs from the L type in retaining agglutinin-binding power after heating.

The A type of K antigen is always found in strains belonging to O groups 8, 9, 20 and 101, whereas the L type is associated with many different O groups. The term L antigen has been retained for certain fimbrial antigens such as the K88 and K99 antigens, which are associated with some enterotoxigenic *E. coli* (ETEC) strains from pigs and cattle. These antigens possess many of the characteristics of the L antigens but are now known to be fimbriae. K88 and K99 antigens are now called F4 and F5, respectively, to denote their fimbrial nature. Currently, 80 K antigens have been described and are found in many combinations with O and H antigens.

Flagella (H) antigens

These are thermolabile protein antigens contained in the flagella of the bacteria. Some *E. coli* do not possess flagella and are non-motile. Because most strains are poorly motile on first isolation, it is usually necessary to passage them through semisolid agar or other motility media. Some cultures may be more motile at room temperature than at 35–37°C and incubation at room temperature may be preferred. The H antigens are numbered from H1 to H49 and H51 to H56, the H50 antigen having been deleted.

Serotyping Procedures

O antigen identification

For a fuller description of the various procedures readers are referred to publications by Sojka (1965), Gross and Rowe (1985) and Ewing (1986). Full serological identification of *E. coli* isolates can only be undertaken in a few established reference laboratories. However, only a small number of O groups are associated with ETEC from piglets, calves and lambs, and a diagnostic laboratory can use OK or fimbrial typing sera to obtain a presumptive diagnosis (Sojka, 1971).

Preparation of 'O' typing serum

Known O antigen is prepared by inoculating agar slopes with smooth colonies and incubating overnight at 37°C and then making a dense suspension in saline. To inactivate K antigens of the L (or B) variety the suspension is heated at 100°C for 2.5 hours, while strains with the A type K antigen are heated at 121°C for 2.5 hours. Only suspensions that are homogeneous and not autoagglutinating upon heating are used to inoculate rabbits. After the appropriate immunization course, the serum is harvested and tested against the antigen suspension in tube agglutination tests, which involve incubation in a waterbath at 50°C overnight when granular aggregates develop. Somatic antisera should be checked for specificity by testing against all known O antigens. Monospecific sera may be prepared by removing non-specific reactions by absorption with heterologous antigen(s).

Serotyping

The O antisera, at the appropriate dilutions, are divided into pools, according to their major antigenic relationships. An 'O' antigen suspension of an unknown strain is prepared as above and tested against each pool. If no agglutination occurs then a saline suspension from an overnight agar slope or broth culture is autoclaved at 121°C for 2.5 hours and the suspension retested. The suspension is then tested against the individual 'O' antisera contained in the pools in which agglutination occurred.

K antisera preparation and identification

Unheated living or formalin-killed cells are used to prepare OK antisera in rabbits. Slide agglutination tests using O antisera, if available, may be used to determine when the organism is 'O inagglutinable'. The titre is determined using a formalin–broth culture; the tests, preferably in a WHO plate, are incubated for 2 hours at 37°C, and overnight at 4°C. Typical K agglutination is indicated by the formation of a disc or pellicle. For routine purposes antisera may be used in slide agglutination tests. Monospecific sera may be prepared by absorbing the antiserum with, preferably, unheated K^- colonies, or in the case of the L type K antigen it may be possible to use a heated suspension of K^+ colonies.

A simple electrophoretic method (CIE) which is suitable for the identification of acidic polysaccharide K antigens has been described by Semjen *et al.* (1977). In most cases only a single line corresponding to the K antigen results, although a few strains with anodic O antigens may also give a line corresponding to this.

Flagella H antisera preparation and identification

Flagella (H) antigens for the production of antisera are prepared from highly motile cultures which have been selected by passage through semisolid agar (0.1–0.4% agar). When shown to be highly motile, the organism is subcultured into nutrient broth which is incubated overnight at 37°C and then formalinized (0.5%) and inoculated into rabbits using an appropriate schedule. Tests for H agglutination are incubated in a waterbath at 50°C and read after 2 hours. The agglutination is very loose and resembles cotton wool.

Diagnosis of Infections Caused by Enterotoxigenic *E. coli*

Although the determination of somatic or fimbrial antigen may allow a presumptive identification of ETEC, it is desirable to confirm the identification by determining the ability to produce enterotoxin(s) and adhesive antigens. Heat-labile enterotoxins (LT) and heat-stable enterotoxins (STa and STb) are discussed in Chapter 14 and fimbrial adhesins are discussed in Chapter 16. This section will discuss methods for their detection.

Heat-labile enterotoxin (LT)

LT occurs most frequently in human and porcine strains of ETEC and is only rarely associated with bovine isolates. There appears to be one type of porcine LT, whereas two types of human LT have been recognized

(Pickett *et al.*, 1986). Several tests for detection of LT are based on biological properties of the toxin or antigenicity of the molecule. The following are tests that can be used.

Ligated intestine test

LT's ability to induce accumulation of fluid in ligated segments of small intestine in rabbits or pigs may be used as a means of detecting the toxin. This test may be necessary in investigations of enterotoxicity of bacterial products, but there can be no justification for its use in the diagnostic laboratory.

Tissue culture assays

LT causes morphological changes in certain cell cultures such as mouse adrenal tumour Yl cells, African green monkey kidney cells (Vero) and Chinese hamster ovary cells. In the first two cell lines, LT causes rounding of the cells and in the latter it causes elongation. Vero cells are the cell-line of choice. A polymyxin B extract of *E. coli* is added to the Vero cells, which are then examined at 24 and 48 hours. A more detailed protocol is described later in the section on verocytotoxin (VT) producing *E. coli*.

Latex particle agglutination test

Several immunoassays have been developed and some are commercially available. Tests for detection of LT-I producing *E. coli* isolates from humans can be used for porcine LT producing strains because of the close relationship between the two toxins. One such test is the reversed passive latex agglutination test which is designed to detect LT in culture fluid. Latex particles are sensitized with purified polyclonal antiserum raised in rabbits immunized with purified cholera toxin. These latex particles agglutinate in the presence of LT.

Heat-stable enterotoxin STa

Suckling mouse test

STa may be detected by the suckling mouse test (SMT) which was originally described by Dean *et al.* (1972) and standardized by Gianella (1976). The principle of the test is that the injection of an STa preparation into the stomach of 2–4-day-old suckling mice causes fluid accumulation in the intestine. The mice are injected intragastrically with 0.1 ml of STa preparation stained with Evans blue. Each strain is tested in three to four mice which are maintained at 30 °C before euthanasia 3–4 hours later. The entire intestine, excluding the stomach, is removed and weighed, and the ratio of the pooled gut weight to the combined weight of the remaining carcasses is calculated. A ratio >0.9 indicates a positive result.

Immunological procedures

Although STs are not immunogenic, antibodies have been raised to them by coupling to a protein carrier such as bovine IgG, bovine serum albumin or haemocyanin. This allowed the development of radioimmunoassays for the detection of ST (Frantz and Robertson, 1981; Gianella *et al.*, 1981) and more recently enzyme-linked immunosorbent assays (ELISAs). A competitive enzyme immunoassay is commercially available (Carroll *et al.*, 1990) for the detection of STa in culture fluid. This test uses a synthetic peptide STa analogue to coat the wells and a monoclonal antibody–enzyme conjugate. The antibody binds specifically to the solid-phase toxin or to the toxin, if present, in the culture filtrate. This results in reduced binding of the conjugate to the solid phase and a reduced colour intensity when compared to the negative toxin control.

Heat-stable enterotoxin STb

Although this toxin is prevalent in porcine *E. coli* isolates, simple laboratory assays are not available. Animal inoculation and immunological procedures have been described, but the use of gene probes probably offers the easiest way for its detection (see later).

Animal inoculation

Although the toxin is inactive in the SMT, it evokes a positive response in the ligated gut test in weaned pigs and rabbits. Since STb is sensitive to trypsin degradation, blocking of endogenous protease enhances its stability (Whipp, 1990). Either rats or mice may be used for STb assays. Rats (250–350 g) are anaesthetized with pentobarbital and the intestine is rinsed twice with saline containing 1 mg soyabean trypsin inhibitor (TI). Intestinal loops (5–6 cm) beginning about 5 cm distal to the ligament of Treitz are injected with 0.5 ml of toxin solution containing 2 mg TI per ml. The rats are euthanized 2.5 hours later and the volume of fluid per centimetre of intestine is determined. Tests in mice are conducted as for STa except that 2 mg TI is added for each millilitre of inoculum. However, the infant mice are much less sensitive than the rats.

Hitotsubashi *et al.* (1992) anaesthetized 30–35 g mice with sodium pentobarbital and washed the intestinal lumen three times with saline containing a protease inhibitor (aprotinin at 100 units ml^{-1}). One or two 4-cm loops were tied off in the small intestine with the most proximal loop

4 cm posterior to the ligament of Treitz. A 0.2-ml volume of toxin preparation was injected and the mice were euthanized 3 hours later. Activity was expressed as grams of loop tissue and contents per centimetre of loop.

Immunological procedures

An ELISA was developed by Urban *et al.* (1990) for the detection of STb produced by *E. coli* strains. Based on an antigenic profile of STb, a peptide was synthesized, coupled to keyhole limpet haemocyanin and used to immunize rabbits. Purified antibodies were then used to develop a direct-binding STb ELISA, which could detect 1–2 ng of toxin in crude culture filtrates.

Diagnosis of Infections Due to Verocytotoxigenic *E. coli*

Laboratory diagnosis of infections due to verotoxigenic *E. coli* (VTEC) is dependent on demonstration of VT, without regard for the type(s) of VT produced by the isolate. Histological examination of the intestine may show attaching and effacing (AE) lesions characteristic of some VTEC infections. However, intestine is not always available; some VTEC (such as oedema disease strains of *E. coli*) do not induce AE lesions, and some AE lesions are not associated with VTEC.

A major problem in isolating VTEC from infected animals is that there may be relatively low numbers of these organisms among the faecal *E. coli*. This may be due to a long incubation period for VTEC-mediated diseases. In human infections, sorbitol MacConkey agar is often used to facilitate detection of the predominantly sorbitol-negative O157:H7, but no comparable media are available for animal infections. The Vero cell assay or immunological procedures may be used to detect production of VT by isolated *E. coli* or by VTEC in mixed culture. By reading the test at different times and observing the kind of changes in the cells, VT and other *E. coli* toxins may be detected with Vero cell cultures.

Vero cell tests for detection of VT and other E. coli *toxins*

Vero cell monolayers

The cells should be within 3 days of passage, when they are harvested and resuspended in Hank's or Eagle's medium after Versenes treatment to give 2×10^5 cells ml^{-1}. A 96-well tissue culture tray is seeded with 200 μl of the cell suspension and incubated at 37°C in 5% carbon dioxide and raised humidity for 18–20 hours. This should yield semiconfluent growth. The outer rows of wells are not used and every other well can be left as a negative control for ease of comparison, when 10 μl of the supernatant are added to test wells. The plates are covered and then returned to the incubator.

Preparation of the culture supernatant

Single colonies are subcultured on blood agar which is incubated overnight at 37°C. Alternatively, colony sweeps from a large number of *E. coli* colonies on the initial culture plate may be subcultured. Subcultures into Mundell's broth (Mundell *et al.*, 1976) or trypticase soya broth are incubated overnight at 37°C. Polymyxin B (10,000 units ml^{-1}) is added and the broth incubated for a further 4 hours on an orbital shaker. The culture is then centrifuged (17,000 × **g** for 30 minutes) and the supernatant filtered using a pore size of 0.22 μm. Alternatively, the broth culture may be subjected to sonication.

Verocytotoxin in faeces

Verocytotoxin present in faeces can be detected directly by its cytotoxic effect on Vero cells (Karmali *et al.*, 1983). Faeces (1 g) are mixed with phosphate-buffered saline on a vortex mixer until the suspension is homogeneous. The suspension is centrifuged and filtered through a 0.2 μm membrane filter. The sterile supernatant is serially diluted and 100 μl of each dilution added in duplicate to a Vero cell monolayer. The wells are examined for 2–3 days to detect Vero cell death.

Reading of test results

The cytopathic effect of the different toxins varies and occurs at different stages. The test for LT is read at 24 hours, for cytotoxic nectrotizing factor (CNF) at 48 hours and for VT at 72 hours. In practice, the test for VT is often read at 120 hours.

1. **LT.** Changes occur within 18–24 hours when the cells lose their elongated appearance and tend to become round or globular. Sometimes the cells are globular with ‘tails or tendrils’.

2. **CNF.** Changes occur at 24–48 hours when the affected cells appear enlarged and multinucleate, and the cell sheet resembles a mosaic.

3. **VT.** Affected cells have a shrivelled appearance and detach from the well.

The specificity of the tests is confirmed by neutralization with specific antiserum. In the case of VT, activity is confirmed by neutralization with VT1 and VT2 antisera.

Immunological procedures

Monoclonal antibodies to verocytotoxin were developed by Strockbine *et al.* (1985), who showed that the monoclonals neutralized cytotoxicity and immunoprecipitated labelled VTs in the presence of protein A. Using these monoclonal antibodies a colony blot assay was developed, in which the suspect colonies were grown on agar for 18–24 hours and then transferred to a nitrocellulose membrane. After release with polymyxin B, the crude VT was detected by staining with VT-specific conjugated monoclonal antibody. Karch *et al.* (1986) used agar containing subinhibitory concentrations of trimethoprim-sulfamethoxazole to enhance toxin production and thereby improve the effectiveness of the test.

ELISA tests for the detection of VT-producing cultures or for direct detection of VTEC in faeces or foods have been developed by a number of workers. Downes *et al.* (1989) used a sandwich ELISA with a monoclonal antibody for specific toxin capture and a conjugated rabbit polyclonal second antibody for detection. They reported that although their tests could detect 200 pg VT1 and 75 pg VT2 they were not as sensitive as the Vero cells for detection of faecal toxin.

The receptor for VT1 and VT2 is globotriosyl ceramide (Gb3) which occurs in hydatid cyst fluid. Porcine VT2e, in contrast, binds to globotetraosyl ceramide (Gb4). Consequently, ELISAs using hydatid cyst fluid to coat the plate and bind the toxin have been developed (Acheson *et al.*, 1990). Conjugated polyclonal or monoclonal antibodies may then be used to indicate the presence of toxin. The sensitivity of such assays for the detection of VTEC in faeces can be increased by treating the faecal culture with mitomycin (Law *et al.*, 1992).

E. coli which Produce Cytotoxic Necrotizing Factor

The cytotoxic necrotizing factor (CNF) toxins have been discussed in Chapter 15. Both CNF1 and CNF2 cause multinucleation and giant cell formation in Vero cells, HeLa cells and Chinese hamster ovary cells and this property may be used for their detection. Most CNF-positive *E. coli* belong to a small range of O groups which include O groups 2, 4, 6, 22, 32, 75, 83 and 88 (Holland, 1990). However, these *E. coli* have been isolated from a wide range of clinical conditions in man and animals and their significance in disease has not been established (McLaren and Wray, 1986; Pohl *et al.*, 1992). The procedure for detection of CNF is described in the preceding section on Vero cell tests for detection of VT and other cytotoxins.

Fimbrial Antigens

Fimbrial antigens which confer colonizing ability on ETEC are convenient targets for detection of ETEC. However, their identification may be complicated by the presence of other fimbriae on ETEC and by difficulties in getting them to be expressed *in vitro*. For example, most *E. coli*, whether they are pathogenic or not, produce type 1 pili which are expressed at both 37°C and 18°C and mediate adherence to a variety of surfaces including human type A and guinea-pig erythrocytes. Type 1 fimbriae-mediated adhesion to erythrocytes is inhibited by D-mannose and is therefore called mannose-sensitive haemagglutination (MSHA).

Several of the fimbrial antigens which mediate attachment of pathogenic *E. coli* to host cells cause attachment to erythrocytes and/or epithelial cells that is not impaired by D-mannose (mannose-resistant haemagglutination). Fimbrial antigens are associated not only with ETEC, but also with VTEC and *E. coli* implicated in extraintestinal infections such as bacteraemia and urinary tract infection. Some such as F4 (K88), F5 (K99) and F6 (987P) have been recognized for many years but others have been identified more recently (Table 21.1).

The specific tests that are used for identification of fimbriae vary considerably. The conditions for the test need to recognize that expression is often temperature and growth medium dependent. Also, some adhesins, such as the F6 antigen may show phase variation and not be expressed in culture. Similarly, the recently described F107 antigen (Bertschinger *et al.*, 1990) is expressed *in vivo* but strains expressing this antigen *in vitro* are uncommon. Electron microscopy and immuno-electron microscopy are useful for visualization of the fimbriae. Simple immunological tests are in common use and are very good, provided specific antisera are available. These include slide agglutination, latex particle agglutination, ELISA, haemagglutination, and *in vitro* attachment to intestinal villi.

Techniques for the identification of E. coli *adhesins*

Slide agglutination tests

These are used in many laboratories for the identification of F4, F5 and F6 adhesins. The procedure for the preparation of OK antisera is employed and when the titre is sufficient the serum can be absorbed with the homologous culture grown at 20°C, at which temperature the F antigen is not expressed. Monoclonal antibodies are available and may also be used in slide agglutinations.

Table 21.1. Recently described putative adhesive fimbrial antigens.

Antigen designation	O group	*E. coli* type/disease syndrome	Reference
F42	8	Porcine ETEC	Yano *et al.* (1986)
F17	8, 9, 15, 78, 86, 101	Bovine ETEC, septicaemic *E. coli*	Girardeau *et al.* (1980) (FY)
			Pohl *et al.* (1982) (Att 25)
F107	138, 139	Oedema disease, PWD[a]	Bertschinger *et al.* (1990)
F107 variants	141	PWD	Nagy *et al.* (1992)
	141	PWD	Kennan and Monckton (1990)
F165	9, 15, 78, 101, 115	Septicaemia in pigs	Fairbrother *et al.* (1986)
	4, 7, 8, 117, 149	Septicaemia in calves	
CS31A	9, 17, 18, 23, 78, 87, 117, 134, 161, 157	Septicaemia in calves	Girardeau *et al.* (1988)
M326	65	Porcine VTEC	Aning *et al.* (1983)
8813	25, 108, 138, 141, 147, 157	Porcine ETEC	Salajka *et al.* (1992)
C1213	9, 20, 78, 153	Calf diarrhoea	Varga (1991)
F11	1, 2, 78	Poultry septicaemia	van den Bosch *et al.* (1993)

[a] PWD, postweaning diarrhoea in pigs.

Latex particle agglutination tests

Monoclonal antibodies coupled to latex particles to form stable agglutination reagents have been used for detection of the F4, F5, F6 and F41 fimbrial adhesins on cultured *E. coli* (Thorns *et al.*, 1989). These are now commercially available.

ELISA based systems

ELISA have been developed for the detection of the F4 and other antigens in animal faeces (van der Heijden, 1981; Mills *et al.*, 1983). Various modifications have been reported subsequently which involve the use of monoclonal antibodies and reduced incubation period. One such method is that of Thorns *et al.* (1992), who developed an ELISA test for the simultaneous detection of *E. coli* K99 and bovine coronavirus. Monoclonal antibodies that bound specifically to purified antigens in the direct binding ELISA were tested for their ability to detect antigen in diluted faeces captured by monoclonal antibodies bound to the solid phase.

Haemagglutination methodology

Erythrocyte agglutination in the presence of fimbriated bacteria is a rapid and inexpensive test for the classification of fimbrial types carried by a test strain. The two key factors which affect classification are the erythrocytes used and the culture conditions of the isolates under test. The most commonly used erythrocytes are those from guinea-pigs but to gain valid differential information a panel of erythrocytes from a range of sources is used. For example, Duguid *et al.* (1989) used 14 species of erythrocytes. Citrated, defibrinated blood is collected and red blood cells are separated by low speed centrifugation, washed in physiological saline and resuspended to 3% (v/v) in fresh saline or saline supplemented with D-mannose (2%,w/v). Immediate use is preferable but the erythrocyte suspension may be stored at 4°C for several days. Cultures may be grown on a variety of different media and under varying conditions of temperature and Po_2. The organisms are usually grown on solid media such as phosphate-buffered nutrient agar (Duguid *et al.*, 1989), colonization factor antigen agar (Evans *et al.*, 1977) and Minca medium (Guinee *et al.*, 1977), which are known to promote expression of fimbriae. Incubation is usually at 37°C or 18–20°C. Generally, incubation is aerobic but anaerobic or reduced Po_2 conditions may be used. The simplest form of the test is performed by using a loop to mix a heavy inoculum of a bacterial suspension with a small volume of prepared erythrocytes, with and without D-mannose, on a glass slide. Usually performed at room temperature, the slide is rocked gently and the time for agglutination recorded. A cut-off limit of 10 minutes at room temperature may be applied. Mechanized rocking devices may be employed and alternative temperatures used. If agglutination occurs in the absence of D-mannose only, haemagglutinating activity is mannose sensitive (MSHA).

Mannose-resistant haemagglutinating activity is determined by performing the test at 4 °C for 20 minutes followed by reading immediately upon removal from cold incubation. As the temperature is raised, bacteria may 'elute' off the erythrocytes. A more sophisticated agglutination involves the mixing of erythrocytes and bacteria in glass tubes or microtitre plate wells and incubating statically. Characteristic agglutinating clump settling patterns develop (Jones and Rutter, 1974).

With all the many variables described for these tests, interpretation of results may became ambiguous. Individual laboratories tend to develop their own 'in-house' protocols with standardized procedures. Complications arise in that an isolate may produce subclones which may or may not produce fimbriae. Others may produce multiple fimbriae of different types. Characterization of each type may require 'inactivation' of one adhesin by, for example, altering the temperature of incubation or blocking with D-mannose, heat treatment or formaldehyde. As the chemistry of receptors becomes better understood, alternative means of inhibiting adhesion with monoclonal antibodies or other means such as the Gal-Gal oligosaccharide which inhibits agglutination of human erythrocytes by P-fimbriated bacteria may be developed. For a fuller description of these methods, the reader is recommended to see Old (1985).

In vitro *attachment to intestinal villi*

A number of techniques have been used to demonstrate *in vitro* attachment such as isolated epithelial cells or brush border preparations, but these are difficult to prepare, to preserve and use. The technique of Girardeau *et al.* (1980) overcomes some of these difficulties. The villi are sampled from animals 1 week of age when their villi are long and easily removed by scraping. After slaughter the entire intestine is removed and placed in Kreb's buffer, pH 7.2, at 4 °C. It is then opened longitudinally, washed gently with Kreb's buffer at 4 °C, and the mucosa then scraped gently with a glass slide to detach the villi into the buffer. After settling, the villi are rinsed until a clear supernatant is obtained. The villi can then be preserved for months by freezing initially for 4 hours at −20 °C and then stored at −80 °C in Hanks-DMSO medium. For use the villi are thawed at room temperature and placed for 1 hour in Kreb's buffer containing 1% formaldehyde to stop autolysis. After rinsing, the preparation is ready for use. About 20 villi are transferred into 1.5 ml Kreb's buffer, pH 6.8; the bacterial suspension is added and the mixture is gently agitated for 20 minutes at room temperature. For observation the villi are transferred to a glass slide and cover slip.

Colisepticaemia

Colisepticaemia of calves, lambs and poultry is usually associated with a limited range of O groups. In calves and lambs colisepticaemia is associated with hypogammaglobulinaemia, which usually results from colostrum deprivation. Laboratory confirmation of septicaemic *E. coli* disease may be obtained by use of blood culture procedures to recover *E. coli* from blood. Blood culture media are available commercially. Culture of internal viscera following postmortem examination will yield profuse growth of the pathogenic *E. coli*. The samples should be taken shortly after death of the animal so as to avoid overgrowth by postmortem invaders.

Hypogammaglobulinaemia may be detected by the zinc sulfate turbidity test (Gay *et al.*, 1965). It may also be possible to examine heart blood from animals received for autopsy when the sodium sulfite test (Edwards, 1962) may give more accurate results with lysed blood.

Routinely, characterization of *E. coli* isolates from septicaemia is not carried out. However, determination of the OK serogroup and/or of putative virulence factors is sometimes done. This information may be useful in assessing whether a herd or flock problem is due to one or more than one type of *E. coli*.

Once the *E. coli* have been isolated, slide agglutination with OK sera will allow the recognition of the more common bacteraemic serogroups. In all species of farm animals, *E. coli* O78:K80 predominates and, in poultry, *E. coli* O1:K1 and O2:K1 are also frequent. A high percentage of invasive strains of *E. coli* produce the hydroxamate siderophore aerobactin and isolates from septicaemic disease may be tested for aerobactin production. It should be noted, however, that aerobactin is not produced by all bacteraemic strains and that it is produced by some non-invasive strains. A simple test for aerobactin is to test the ability of a strain to supply aerobactin to an aerobactin-dependent strain grown on iron-deficient medium. Other tests include the ferric perchlorate test (Atkin *et al.*, 1970) and DNA hybridization (Lafont *et al.*, 1987).

Fimbrial antigens have been associated with bacteraemic strains of *E. coli*. Contrepois *et al.* (1986) detected a surface antigen called 31A on bovine isolates, Harel *et al.* (1992) detected a P-like fimbrial antigen called F165 on porcine isolates and van der Bosch *et al.* (1993) detected F11 fimbriae on avian isolates which included O78:K80, O2:K1 and O1:K1 (Table 21.1). The significance of these antigens is not fully understood and their detection may be outside the capabilities of the diagnostic laboratory.

However, their presence on *E. coli* isolates may assist in arriving at a diagnosis.

E. coli Mastitis

Mastitis caused by *E. coli* is a common disease of cattle and pigs. No virulence determinants are associated with these isolates which appear to be simply opportunists arising from the faeces and the environment. Simple recovery of *E. coli* from suitable collected milk samples is all that is necessary for diagnosis.

Urinary Tract Infection

Colonization of the urinary tract by *E. coli* may or may not be accompanied by clinical signs and bacteriological data as well as other evidence must be considered in arriving at a diagnosis. Since collection of a urine sample for culture often results in contamination by *E. coli* or other bacteria in the lower part of the urinary tract, quantitative culture is necessary to assess the significance of any isolate. Collection of a urine sample by cystocentesis prevents contamination and eliminates the need for quantitative culture. In human medicine, a viable count of 10^5 or greater per millilitre of urine is interpreted as indicative of infection and 10^4 as suspicious. These values have arbitrarily been adopted in veterinary medicine but lower counts may be significant in dogs and cats.

Urine may be collected from animals by catheterization or by collection of a midstream sample. It may be necessary to use Lasix (Hoechst Animal Health) to induce urination. A number of commercial slides covered with culture media (dip-slides) are available for culture. A calibrated loop may be used to spread the urine on blood agar to obtain a rough estimate of the concentration of bacteria in the sample.

Routinely, virulence-associated factors are not determined for *E. coli* isolated from urine. However, it has been observed that a high percentage of isolates from urinary tract infections (UTI) are haemolytic, produce aerobactin, and are resistant to the bactericidal effects of serum. Also information is beginning to be obtained to show that specific fimbrial adhesins are associated with these types of *E. coli* implicated in disease in dogs. Garcia *et al.* (1988) showed that canine uropathogenic *E. coli* possess fimbrial antigens which are closely related to F12 and F13 identified on human uropathogenic *E. coli*. Senior *et al.* (1992) showed that type 1 fimbriae were frequently associated with canine uropathogenic *E. coli*.

Genetic Methods for the Detection of Toxin Genes of *E. coli*

Methods for the detection of the genes encoding the *E. coli* enterotoxins and verocytotoxins (Shiga-like toxins) by gene probing and the polymerase chain reaction are well established in many laboratories. However, these technologies are not used routinely by all front-line diagnostic laboratories due to the newness of the technology, the lack of simple commercial kits (although this is being remedied), and the availability of alternative traditional and new technologies. This section will give an overview of gene probing and polymerase chain reaction technologies, outlining potential diagnostic advantages that these methodologies confer.

A fundamental property of single-stranded DNA (and RNA) is that under suitable conditions it will form a double-stranded molecule by hydrogen bonding (i.e. hybridize), with another complementary single-stranded DNA (or RNA) molecule. This is the basis of gene probe technology. If a DNA or RNA molecule is labelled with, for example, a radioisotope such as ^{32}P or ^{35}S, the hybridization of the probe to a suitably treated sample in which the presence of the target organism is to be tested may be observed. The sensitivity of gene probes is generally about 10^3 organisms, assuming one gene copy per organism. The technique is comparatively quick and can be applied to a wide range of samples.

Toxin gene probes for ETEC and VTEC

Gene probe technology has advanced over recent years and there exists a number of potential options at each step in the hybridization process. Essentially, gene probing includes:

1. Preparation of probe (source, label, method of labelling).
2. Preparation of target sample.
3. The hybridization and posthybridization stringency washes.
4. Visualization of the result.

An overview of the options available is listed in Table 21.2; it will not be possible to cover each in depth.

To date, two major classes of toxin produced by *E. coli* have been described. These are the heat-labile and heat-stable enterotoxins and the verocytotoxins or Shiga-like toxins, the properties of which are described in Chapters 14 and 15. Over the past 10–15 years, the genes encoding these classes of toxin have been cloned and the deoxyribonucleotide sequences of each and numerous variants have been determined (Table 21.3). Gene probes derived from the toxin gene clones have been used widely for diagnosis of animal and human disease and procedures have been standardised (Hill and Payne, 1984). Here follows a brief description of the process involved and comments on more recent developments.

Table 21.2. Key features of gene probing.

Feature	Options
Source of probe	1. Prepared by restriction endonuclease cleavage of suitable recombinant plasmid 2. Prepared by PCR 3. Prepared as RNA from cloned plasmid with suitable promoter signal (e.g. SP6/7, T7) 4. Synthetic oligonucleotide (20 bp or more)
Labelling of probe	1. Nick translation 2. Random priming 3. PCR 4. RNA synthesis 5. Chemical addition to oligonucleotide
Type of label	1. Radioisotope (^{32}P, ^{33}P, ^{35}S) 2. Biotin 2. Digoxigenin 4. Chemiluminescent 5. Other innovative systems
Target sample	1. Culture lysed on filter membrane (nylon/nitrocellulose): a. pure culture lysed as colony, dot or slot blot; b. enriched culture from specimen; c. mixed culture direct from specimen 2. Treated specimen lysed on filter membrane 3. Biotrapping of organisms from specimen (e.g. with monoclonal ,antibody) 4. Total DNA extraction from sample
Hybridization	1. Solid phase (slow) 2. Liquid phase (fast)
Specificity washes (highly specific)	Proportional to hybridization conditions and stringency
Sensitivity (organisms)	Limit imposed by type of labelling method used (10^3 organisms)
Time	1. Solid phase hybridization – 8–10 hours 2. Liquid phase hybridization – 2 hours

Table 21.3. Sources of gene probes for ETEC and VTEC.

Toxin	Plasmid source[a]	Gene probe[b]	Reference
LTI	pEWD299	750 bp *Hin*dIII	Dallas *et al.* (1979) Lathe *et al.* (1980)
LTII	pSA-25	850 bp *Hin*cII	Pickett *et al.* (1986)
STI	pRIT10036	157 bp *Hin*fI	So and McCarthy (1979)
STII	pCHL6	460 bp *Hin*fI	Lee *et al.* (1983)
VT1 (SLTI)	pNTP705 pJN-10	530 bp *Hin*dIII/*Acc*I 1142 bp *Bam*HI	Willshaw *et al.* (1985b) Newland *et al.* (1985, 1987)
VT2/SLTII	pNM707 PM110ß18	660 bp *Eco*RV/*Hin*cII 842 bp *Sma*I/*Pst*I	Willshaw *et al.* (1987) Newland and Neill (1988)

[a] This list includes the most frequently cited probe sources but does not list probes for toxin variants which share significant homology with the original clones.
[b] The DNA fragments used as gene probes are shown as size (given in base pairs) and restriction endonucleases used to produce the desired fragment. There are many alternative fragments in the literature and only those most commonly used are cited.

Preparation of samples

Pure cultures are inoculated onto nylon or nitrocellulose membranes overlaid on solid medium and grown at 37°C for up to 6 hours. Alternatively, faecal or other clinical samples are resuspended in PBS, agitated and a small volume of the supernatant used to inoculate membranes overlaid on MacConkey agar and grown at 37°C for up to 16 hours. Positive and negative controls are also inoculated onto the same filters. The bacterial colonies are lysed by sequential transfer of the filter, colony side up, onto Whatman 3M paper saturated with sodium dodecyl sulfate (SDS) (5% w/v), denaturing solution (0.5M NaOH, 1.5M NaCl) and neutralizing solution (1.5M NaCl, 0.5M Tris, pH 8) for 5, 10 and 7 minutes, respectively. Excess cellular debris is removed by washing the filter in 2 × SSC (1 × SSC is 0.15M NaCl, 0.015M sodium citrate, pH 7). The filter is air dried and the single-stranded DNA bound to the filter either by UV transillumination if nylon membranes are used or by baking at 80°C for 2 hours. These methods follow those essentially described by Grunstein and Hogness (1975) and modified by Maas (1983).

Pure denatured DNA samples extracted from cultures or other sources may be applied to the filters directly; commercial DNA extraction columns are available and DNA may be prepared directly from clinical samples (see for example, Coll *et al.*, 1989).

Preparation of probe

The DNA to be used as gene probe is prepared commonly by restriction endonuclease digestion of a recombinant plasmid harbouring the cloned gene of interest (Table 21.3). Probes tend to be intragenic fragments which are resolved by gel electrophoresis through agarose using either Tris acetate or Tris borate buffers (Maniatis *et al.*, 1982). The desired DNA fragment is visualized by UV transillumination following staining of the gel with ethidium bromide. An agarose slice containing the desired DNA fragment is cut from the gel and the DNA is electroeluted. This procedure has been superseded largely by the use of low gelling agarose from which the DNA is either extracted by 'glass milk' binding systems available commercially or diluted with distilled water for later use. The DNA may be used directly for labelling by the many commercially available nick translation/random priming labelling systems. Nucleotides labelled at the alpha phosphate with ^{32}P are readily available. Many alternative non-radioisotopic labels such as biotinylated nucleotides are available also. Gene probes prepared with radioisotopes must be used before the isotope decays and reuse is limited, whereas non-radioisotopically labelled probes may be prepared in bulk and stored and reused many times. However these probes tend not to be as sensitive as isotopically labelled probes and usually result in more background signal.

Alternative methods for producing probes include polymerase chain reaction (PCR) (see below) in which the PCR amplification product is synthesized incorporating a modified nucleotide containing a suitable label. Synthetic oligonucleotides can be chemically manufactured with a suitable detection molecule attached such as biotin or alkaline phosphatase. Both these probe formats are used in the same way as conventionally prepared probes. If the gene of interest is cloned adjacent to a strong promoter (e.g. SP6/7 or T7), a single-stranded RNA molecule labelled to high specific activity may be produced and used as a gene probe.

Hybridization and posthybridization stringency washes

The test filter is placed in a minimal volume of hybridization solution, usually 2.5 ml per 10 cm^2 filter, which contains a suitable ionic environment (e.g. 6 × SSC) and a blocking agent to prevent non-specific binding of the probe when added. Denhardt (1966) demonstrated that a solution containing 0.02% each of Ficoll, polyvinylpyrrolidone and bovine serum albumin supplemented with an 'irrelevant' nucleic acid (e.g. tRNA, salmon sperm DNA) prevents non-specific binding. Other solutions are available from commercial sources which differ from that listed above and are used as alternatives depending upon the formulation of the gene probe. Prehybridization continues for up to 1 hour, after which the probe is added. Probes prepared from double-stranded templates are denatured at 94°C for 1 minute while single-stranded or synthetic oligonucleotide probes can be added directly without denaturation. It is not necessary to use fresh hybridization solution when adding the probe.

The temperature of hybridization is crucial for specificity; because the melting temperature of most double-stranded DNA molecules is around 72°C, incubation below this (65°C) permits hybridization of sequences sharing a high degree of complementarity. Handling hot solutions, especially if they contain radioisotopically labelled probes, is dangerous. Therefore hybridizations tend to be performed in sealable borosilicate glass bottles in contained rotating ovens. Furthermore, the stochastic reagent formamide may be added to the hybridization solution to a concentration of 50%, thus reducing incubation temperatures to 42°C without compromising specificity.

Hybridization continues for up to 16 hours although with probes labelled to a high specific activity this time may be reduced to as little as 4 hours. Upon completion of hybridization, the probe solution is removed. Non-radioisotopically labelled probes in solution may be recovered for later reuse. The filter is washed in a series of solutions of decreasing ionic strength and at a temperature commensurate with the specificity required. Usually, the final wash is in a solution comprising 0.2 × SSC supplemented with SDS (0.1% w/v) at a temperature of 65°C for 30 minutes. For radioisotopically labelled probes, the filters are air dried and exposed to X-ray film. Other wash and development systems are used for non-radioisotopically labelled probes. For example, biotinylated probes may be detected by streptavidin-linked alkaline phosphatase and digoxigenin-labelled probes may be detected by chemiluminescence methods.

The procedures described are termed solid-phase hybridization (that is the target DNA is fixed to a solid phase, namely the membrane, over which the probe solution washes) and is used widely because of its relative simplicity and the number of samples that can be loaded onto a single filter. Liquid phase hybridization (that is both target DNA and probe remain in solution during hybridization) is being developed largely for commercial gene probe kits with detection of the hybrid double-stranded DNA–DNA (or DNA–RNA) molecule by various capture systems.

Gene probes for the detection of ETEC

Probably the earliest paper recording the use of radioisotopically labelled gene probes specific for LT and ST to screen large numbers of potential ETEC in humans was by Moseley *et al.* (1983). The methods were as described above and since then there have been numerous publications using the same methods to detect ETEC from animal sources as well as food, and extending the range of gene probes (Patamoroj *et al.*, 1983; Hill and Payne, 1984; Lanata *et al.*, 1985; Bohnert *et al.*, 1988; Monckton and Hasse, 1988; Woodward *et al.*, 1990). The development and use of non-radioisotopically labelled probes and synthetic oligonucleotides have been described also by, for example, Hill *et al.* (1986), Bialkowski-Horbrzanska (1987) and Kumar *et al.* (1988).

Gene probes for the detection of VTEC

Since the initial cloning of the verocytotoxin (Shiga-like toxin) encoding genes by groups in the UK (Willshaw *et al.*, 1985, 1987) and North America (Newland *et al.*, 1985; Huang *et al.*, 1986), gene probes have been used extensively to study the epidemiology of VTEC. In particular, the presence of significant numbers of VTEC in healthy cattle and the recognition of the role of O157:H7 VTEC in haemorrhagic colitis and haemolytic uraemic syndrome in humans has been a stimulus to their development and use (see PCR below). The reader is referred to publications by, for example, Smith *et al.* (1988), Hales and Fletcher (1991), Woodward and Wray (1990) and Woodward *et al.* (1990). Synthetic oligonucleotide probes have been developed also (Karch and Meyer, 1989a). For a more comprehensive discussion the reader can consult a treatise on the many alternative gene probing strategies currently available, for example, Kricka (1992).

The principles of the polymerase chain reaction (PCR) amplification

Synthetic oligonucleotide probes bind specifically to their complementary target sequence under appropriate ionic and thermal conditions. This principle is exploited for the PCR in that a pair of synthetic oligonucleotide primers is designed based on known sequences (Table 21.4) following the principles of Innis and Gelfand (1990). The cycle commences by raising the temperature to denature or melt the target DNA into single strands. The temperature is then lowered sufficiently to allow specific hybridization of primers to their complementary target sequences. Under appropriate conditions the probes bind to either strand of the denatured double-stranded DNA target flanking the region to be amplified. The temperature is then raised to the optimum for DNA synthesis by a thermostable DNA polymerase using the available 3′-OH group of the hybridized oligonucleotide to prime the synthesis. Upon completion of the DNA synthesis, the DNA molecules are again denatured by raising the temperature for the next round of synthesis. After 30 or so cycles, many million copies of the sequence between the primers have been produced, hence the term

Table 21.4. Sources of deoxynucleotide sequences for synthetic oligonucleotides designed for priming polymerase chain reaction amplification.

Toxin	Sequence reference
LT-I	Spicer and Noble (1982) Yamamoto and Yokota (1983)
LT-IIa	Pickett *et al.* (1987)
LT-IIb	Pickett *et al.* (1989)
STIh	Moseley *et al.* (1983)
STIP	So and McCarthy (1980)
STII	Lee *et al.* (1983)
VT1/SLTI	Strockbine *et al.* (1988)
VT2/SLTIII	Jackson *et al.* (1987)
VT2e/SLTIIe (VT2v/SLTIIv)	Weinstein *et al.* (1988)
VT2d/SLTIId (VT2va/SLTII)	Gannon *et al.* (1990)
VT2vh/SLTIIvh	Ito *et al.* (1990)

amplification. This method was described first by Saiki *et al.* (1985) and has been developed subsequently as a very sensitive diagnostic tool. In principle, with appropriate primer design and optimized conditions, a single target sequence may be detected. Key features of the PCR are listed in Table 21.5.

PCR for ETEC and VTEC

The reaction mixture

Primers are designed to give amplified DNA products of between 250 base pairs (bp) and 1000 bp, although smaller and larger products may be produced if desired. There are numerous primer pairs cited in the literature (see below) that are not listed here. The reaction mixture (usually 50 μl or 100 μl final volume) comprises 50 mM KCl, 10 mM Tris-HCl, pH 8.4, 0.01% (w/v) gelatin, $MgCl_2$ titrated in a range 0.5–8.0 mM, 200 μM of each of the four nucleotides, 25 pM for each primer and 2.5 U of the thermostable DNA polymerase (usually called *Taq* polymerase because it was isolated from *Thermus aq*uaticus). The reaction mixture is overlaid with an equal volume of mineral oil to prevent evaporation during the cycling. The buffer described here is that originally used by Saiki *et al.* (1985) but

Table 21.5. Key features of the polymerase chain reaction.

Feature	Comments
Source of oligonucleotide sequence primers	1. Highly specific, designed on the basis of known gene 2. May include restriction endonuclease sites for cloning 3. May include additional sequences or residues for binding to capture system 4. May include non-radioisotopically labelled detection system such as biotin
Reaction conditions	1. Established for each primer pair 2. Minimal sample needed 3. Cycling and ramping times optimized to give up to 60 cycles in 3 hours or less
Target sample	1. Pure DNA 2. Treated clinical sample 2. Whole cells
Specificity	1. Absolute 2. Multiple systems
Sensitivity	1. Potentially one organism 2. Subject to contamination 3. Subject to inhibition with substances in the sample 4. Column purification systems desensitize
Confirmation	1. Agarose gel electrophoresis of PCR product 2. Confirmatory gene probe 3. ELISA type technologies 4. Potential for direct sequencing of product 5. Differentiation by restriction fragment length polymorphism (RFLP) analysis of PCR product and/or ligase chain reaction

other formulations exist. All reagents are commercially available as are wax replacements for the mineral oil and novel anticontamination reagents. Because of the extreme sensitivity of the PCR, these 'master' reaction mixtures are prepared in an isolated environment in which sterile operating procedures are used. Furthermore, it is normal practice to apply the PCR to all new reagents before incorporation of these reagents into routine testing to ensure freedom from contaminating sequences. All experiments require multiple negative controls.

Sample preparation

Purified DNA, washed whole cells and phenol–chloroform lysates of pure and mixed cultures may be used without impairing sensitivity or specificity of the reaction. The PCR may be used on relatively crude samples but clinical specimens may contain inhibitors. Haem and urine are known to inhibit the *Taq* polymerase so methods to extract target DNA from the samples are often required. The commercial availability of DNA purification columns has allowed the preparation of samples successfully from blood, serum, faeces, gut contents, urine, vaginal swabs, viscera and various food and drink sources. As little as 1–2 μl of final sample is added to the reaction mixture by filtered disposable tip through the mineral oil.

Thermal cycling

No one set of conditions is applicable to all primer pairs. Each is optimized by titrating thermal conditions against Mg^{2+} concentration. Using purified DNA, the presence of a single gene copy in up to 5 μg of heterologous DNA should yield a PCR product. Parameters for PCR are typically 94°C for 2 minutes, for 1 cycle, followed by 30 cycles of denaturation at 94°C for 1.5 minutes, hybridization at 60°C for 1.5 minutes, DNA polymerization at 72°C for 2 minutes, followed by a final extension by incubation at 72°C for 5 minutes. It is possible to enhance sensitivity and the speed of reaction by the use of sophisticated thermal cycling machines capable of instantaneous ramping between temperatures or rapid cycling of 30 seconds or less per temperature for 60 cycles. Multiplex PCR in which more than one pair of primers is incorporated in the reaction (Fraenkel *et al.*, 1989; Olsvik *et al.*, 1990) and quantitative PCR in which dilutions of a competing target sequence are added to a series of reactions are recent developments (Wang and Mark, 1990).

Detection and confirmation of final PCR amplified product

Samples (5–10 μl) from PCR reactions may be analysed by agarose gel electrophoresis, with the PCR product visualized by staining with ethidium bromide. The migration rate of the product is compared with that of standard molecular weight markers so an accurate sizing of the product is achieved. Whilst this is the commonest method for detection, the PCR product should be confirmed as encoding the predicted amplified sequence. This is usually achieved by probing with a synthetic oligonucleotide probe specific for a region within the amplified product. Rapid DNA hybridization procedures for probing PCR products have been developed (see above). Other methods for detection include monoclonal antibody capture of DNA/RNA hybrids, nested primers for second round PCR using a primer pair internal to the primary pair, or primer modification such that a recognition sequence is added to one primer. For example, the sequence (GCN)4 added to one primer permits capture of the PCR product by a column or suitably coated ELISA plate whilst biotin added to the other primer permits streptavidin-linked alkaline phosphatase detection using ELISA type technology. Incorporation of biotinylated nucleotides in the PCR reaction mixture permits streptavidin-alkaline phosphatase detection of biotinylated product.

PCR for ETEC and VTEC

The polymerase chain reaction is used widely for the detection of enterotoxin genes (Olive, 1989; Victor *et al.*, 1991) and verocytotoxin genes (Karch and Meyer, 1989b; Johnson *et al.*, 1990; Pollard *et al.*, 1990; Woodward *et al.*, 1992). Whilst the methods outlined above were used in principle by these workers, the reader is recommended to refer to the cited papers for the specific details of primer design and reaction conditions. The PCR is a rapid and versatile method. The potential exists to use the specific PCR to detect toxigenic *E. coli in situ* even in paraffin-wax-embedded thin sections (Nuovo *et al.*, 1991). Furthermore, primer design influences the range of toxin variants detected and their differentiation (Karch and Meyer, 1989b; Johnson *et al.*, 1990; Woodward *et al.*, 1992). Detailed discussions of the potential of PCR technology are presented by Innis and Gelfand (1990) and Birkenmeier and Mushahwar (1991).

Applications of gene probe and PCR technology

Panels of gene probes and PCR reagents specific for the enterotoxin and verocytotoxin genes are used widely. They detect as little as a single gene copy but a limitation of these tests is that they do not differentiate between live and dead organisms nor whether the detected genes are being expressed. The use of reverse transcriptase PCR may permit detection of the relevant mRNA species (Kawasaki, 1990). Additionally, experiments to detect the toxin of isolates known to encode a toxin gene have demonstrated a very high correlation between presence of gene and its expression (Vadivelu *et al.*, 1987; Carroll *et al.*, 1990).

Gene probes are also useful in determining whether toxin encoding genes have a chromosomal, plasmid or phage location (Bertin, 1992). The use of gene probes has also revealed the instability of some toxin genes (Karch *et al.*, 1992) and it is recommended that gene probing and PCR should be used directly on clinical samples or first isolations from clinical samples as subcultivation may result in gene loss.

Gene probes are being applied to newly described potential virulence factors such as CNF. The gene for CNF1 has been defined and the nucleotide sequence has been published (Falbo *et al.*, 1993).

The technology is sensitive and provides a powerful set of tools for diagnosis and epidemiological studies. The principle of gene probing and PCR amplification is applicable not only to toxin genes described above but also to other virulence determinants, such as F4 (K88), F5 (K99) and F6 (987P) fimbriae (Woodward and Wray, 1990). Recently, genes encoding the EPEC adherence factor (EAF) and the attaching and effacing factor (EAE), associated with the attaching and effacing phenotype of certain enteropathogenic and enterohaemorrhagic *E. coli* of human origin, have been cloned (Jerse *et al.*, 1990). An *eae* probe was developed for use against *E. coli* of human origin and has been used by Mainil *et al.* (1993) against *E. coli* of bovine origin. They found that, of 296 isolates tested, 70 were *eae* positive and, of these, 60 were VTEC. Gannon *et al.* (1993) have developed a PCR protocol to detect the *eae* gene and have demonstrated that some VTEC of porcine origin possess the gene also.

Concluding Remarks

In recent years there have been significant improvements in diagnostic tests for identification of *E. coli* implicated in disease. These tests have been designed primarily for *E. coli* in enteric diseases, because pathogenic isolates from the intestine need to be distinguished from *E. coli* which are normal flora and are unable to cause disease. Two major thrusts have developed. One is based on detection of fimbriae which are colonization factors and are good markers for enteric pathogens. Simple, rapid, and relatively inexpensive agglutination tests are now available commercially. The major drawback of these tests is that some types of fimbriae are not readily expressed *in vitro*. The second approach consists of gene-based tests involving hybridization or PCR amplification. Several such tests have been developed. They effectively overcome the problem associated with failure of expression of genes of interest, but have not yet been commercialized.

References

Acheson, D.W., Keusch, G.T., Lightowlers, M. and Donohue-Rolfe, A. (1990) Enzyme-linked immunosorbent assays for Shiga toxin and Shiga-like toxin II using Pl glycoprotein from hydatid cysts. *Journal of Infectious Diseases* 161, 134–137.

Aning, K.G., Thomlinson, J.R., Wray, C., Sojka, W.J. and Coulter, J. (1983) Adhesion factor distinct from K88, K99, F41, 987P, CFA1 and CFA2 in porcine *E. coli. Veterinary Record* 112, 251.

Atkin, C.L., Neilands, J.B. and Phaff, H.J. (1970) Rhodotorulic acid from species of *Leucosporidium*, *Rhodosporidium*, *Rhodotorula*, *Sproidiobolus* and *Sporobolomyces* and a new alanine-containing ferrichrome from *Cryptococcus melibiosium*. *Journal of Bacteriology* 103, 722–733.

Bertin, A. (1992) Plasmid content and localisation of the STaI (STaP) gene in enterotoxigenic *Escherichia coli* with a non-radioactive polynucleotide gene probe. *Journal of Medical Microbiology* 37, 141–147.

Bertschinger, H.U., Bachmann, M., Mettler, C., Popischil, A., Schraner, E.M., Stamm, M., Sydler, T. and Wild, P. (1990) Adhesive fimbriae produced *in vivo* by *Escherichia coli* O139:K12(B)HI associated with enterotoxaemia in pigs. *Veterinary Microbiology* 25, 267–281.

Bialkowski-Horbrzanska, H. (1987) Detection of enterotoxigenic *Escherichia coli* by dot blot hybridisation with biotinylated DNA probes. *Journal of Clinical Microbiology* 25, 338–343.

Birkenmeier, L.G. and Mushahwar, I.K. (1991) DNA probe amplification methods. *Journal of Virological Methods* 351, 117–126.

Bohnert, M.G., D'Hauteville, H.M. and Sansonetti, P.J. (1988) Detection of enteric pathotypes using six DNA probes. *Annals of the Institute of Pasteur, Microbiology* 138, 189–202.

Carroll, P.J., Woodward, M.J. and Wray, C. (1990) Detection of LT and STIa toxins by latex and EIA tests. *Veterinary Record* 127, 335–336.

Coll, P., Phillips, K. and Tenover, F.C. (1989) Evaluation of a rapid method of extracting DNA from stool samples for use in hybridisation assays. *Journal of Clinical Microbiology* 7, 2245–2248.

Contrepois, M., Dubourguier, H., Parodi, A.L., Girardeau, J.P. and Ollier, J.L. (1986) Septicaemic *Escherichia coli* and experimental infection of calves. *Veterinary Microbiology* 12, 109–118.

Dallas, W.S., Gill, D.M. and Falkow, S. (1979) Cistrons encoding *Escherichia coli* heat-labile toxin. *Journal of Bacteriology* 139, 850–858.

Dean, A.G., Ching, Y.-C., Williams, R.G. and Harden, L.B. (1972) Test for *Escherichia coli* enterotoxin using infant mice. Application in a study of diarrhoea in children in Honolulu. *Journal of Infectious Diseases* 15, 407–411.

Denhardt, D.T. (1966) A membrane-filter technique for the detection of complementary DNA. *Biochemical and Biophysical Research Communications* 23, 641–646.

Downes, F.P., Green, J.H., Greene, K., Strockbine, N., Wells, J.G. and Wachsmuth, I.K. (1989) Development and evaluation of enzyme-linked immunosorbent assays for detection of Shiga-like toxin I and Shiga-like toxin II. *Journal of Clinical Microbiology* 27, 1292–1297.

Duguid, J.P., Clegg, S. and Wilson, M.I. (1979) The fimbrial and nonfimbrial haemagglutinins of *Escherichia coli*. *Journal of Medical Microbiology* 12, 213–227.

Edwards, B.L. (1962) A simple test for deprivation of colostrum in piglets. *Veterinary Record* 74, 504–506.

Evans, D.G., Evans, D.J. and Tjoa, W. (1977) Haemagglutination of human group A erythrocytes by enterotoxigenic *Escherichia coli* isolated from adults with diarrhoea: correlation with colonisation factor. *Infection and Immunity* 18, 330–337.

Ewing, W.H. (1986) *Edwards and Ewing's Identification of Enterobacteriaceae*, 4th edn. Elsevier Science Publishers, New York.

Fairbrother, J., Lariviere, S. and Lallier, R. (1986) New fimbrial antigen F165 from *E. coli* serogroup O115 strains isolated from piglets with diarrhoea. *Infection and Immunity* 51, 10–15.

Falbo, V., Pace, T., Pilli, L., Pizzi, E. and Caprioli, A. (1993) Isolation and nucleotide sequence of the gene encoding cytotoxic necrotizing factor 1 of *Escherichia coli. Infection and Immunity* 61, 4909–4914.

Fraenkel, G., Giron, J.A., Valmassoi, J. and Schoolnik, G.K. (1989) Multigene amplification simultaneous detection of three virulence genes in diarrhoeal stool. *Molecular Microbiology* 3, 1729–1734.

Frantz, J.C. and Robertson, D.C. (1981) Immunological properties of *Escherichia coli* heat-stable enterotoxins: development of a radio-immunoassay specific for heat-stable enterotoxins with suckling mouse activity. *Infection and Immunity* 33, 193–198.

Gannon, V.P.J., Teerling, C., Massi, S.A. and Gyles, C.L. (1990) Molecular cloning and nucleotide sequence of another variant of the *Escherichia coli* Shiga-like toxin II family. *Journal of General Microbiology* 136, 1125–1135.

Gannon, V.P.J., Rashed, M., King, R.K. and Golsteyn-Thomas, E.J. (1993) Detection and characterisation of the *eae* gene of Shiga-like toxin producing *E. coli* using polymerase chain reaction. *Journal of Clinical Microbiology* 31, 1268–1274.

Garcia, E., Bergmans, H.E.N., van der Bosch, J.F., Ørskov, I., Zeijst, B.A.M. and Gaastra, W. (1988) Isolation and characterisation of dog uropathogenic *Escherichia coli* and their fimbriae. *Antonie van Leeuwenhoek* 54, 149–163.

Gay, C.C., Anderson, N., Fisher, E.W. and McEwan, A.D. (1965) Gamma-globulin levels and neonatal mortality in market calves. *Veterinary Record* 77, 148–149.

Giannella, R.A. (1976) Suckling mouse model for detection of heat-stable *Escherichia coli* enterotoxin: characteristics of the model. *Infection and Immunity* 14, 95–99.

Giannella, R.A., Drake, K.W. and Luttrell, M. (1981) Development of a radio-immunoassay for *Escherichia coli* heat-stable enterotoxin: comparison with the suckling mouse assay. *Infection and Immunity* 33, 186–192.

Girardeau, J.P., Dubourguier, M.C. and Contrepois, M. (1980) Attachement des *E. coli* entéropathogènes à muqueuse intestinale. *Cahiers Groupement Techniques Veterinaire 4B*, 190, 49–60.

Girardeau, J.P., Der Vartanian, M., Ollier, J.L. and Contrepois, M. (1988) CS31A; a new K88 related fimbrial antigen on bovine enterotoxigenic and septicaemic *Escherichia coli* strains. *Infection and Immunity* 56, 2180–2188.

Gross, R.J. and Rowe, B. (1985) Serotyping of *Escherichia coli*. In: Sussman, M. (ed.) *The Virulence of Escherichia coli*. Academic Press, London, pp. 345–363.

Grunstein, M. and Hogness, D.S. (1975) Colony hybridization: a method for the isolation of cloned DNAs that contain a specific gene. *Proceedings of the National Academy of Sciences of the United States of America* 72, 3961–3965.

Guinee, P.A.M., Veldkamp, J. and Jansen, W.H. (1977) Improved Minca medium for the detection of K99 antigen in calf enterotoxigenic strains of *Escherichia coli. Infection and Immunity* 15, 676–678.

Hales, B.A. and Fletcher, J.N. (1991) Incidence of common DNA sequences in bovine and porcine *Escherichia coli* strains causing diarrhoea. *Research in Veterinary Science* 50, 355–357.

Harel, J., Forget, C., St Amand, J., Daigle, F., Dubreuil, D., Jacques, M. and Fairbrother, J. (1992) Molecular cloning of a determinant coding for fimbrial antigen F165, a Prs-like fimbrial antigen from porcine septicaemic *E. coli. Journal of General Microbiology* 138, 1495–1502.

Hill, W.E. and Payne, W.L. (1984) Genetic methods for the detection of microbial pathogens. Identification of enterotoxigenic *Escherichia coli* by DNA colony hybridization. Collaborative study. *Journal of the Association of Official Analytical Chemists* 67, 801–807.

Hill, W.E., Wentz, B.A., Payne, W.L., Jagow, J.A. and Zon, G. (1986) DNA colony hybridization method using synthetic oligonucleotides to detect enterotoxigenic *Escherichia coli. Journal of the Association of Official Analytical Chemists* 69, 531–536.

Hitotsubashi, S., Fuji, Y., Yamanaka, H. and Okamoto, K. (1992) Some properties of *E. coli* heat-stable enterotoxin II. *Infection and Immunity* 60, 4468–4474.

Holland, R.E. (1990) Some infectious causes of diarrhoea in young farm animals. *Clinical Microbiology Reviews* 3, 345–375.

Huang, A., DeGrandis, S.A., Friesen, J., Karmali, M., Petric, M., Congi, R. and Brunton, J.L. (1986) Cloning and expression of the genes specifying Shiga-like toxin production in *Escherichia coli* H19. *Journal of Bacteriology* 166, 375–379.

Innis, M.A. and Gelfand, D.H. (1990) Optimization of PCRs. In: Innis, M.A., Gelfand, D.H., Sninsky, J.J. and White, T.J. (eds) *PCR Protocols: A Guide to Methods and Applications*. Academic Press, San Diego, pp. 3–12.

Ito, M., Terai, A., Kurazono, H., Takeda, Y. and Nishibuchi, M. (1990) Cloning and nucleotide sequencing of Verotoxin 2 variant genes from *Escherichia coli* O91:H21 isolated from a patient with the hemolytic uremic syndrome. *Microbial Pathogenesis* 8, 47–60.

Jackson, M.P., Neill, R.J., O'Brien, A.D., Holmes, R.K. and Newland, J.W. (1987) Nucleotide sequence analysis and comparison of the structural gene for Shiga-like toxin I and Shiga-like toxin II encoded by bacteriophages from *Escherichia coli* 933. *Federation of European Microbiological Societies Microbiological Letters* 44, 109–114.

Jerse, A.E., Yu, J., Tall, B.D. and Kaper, J.B. (1990) A genetic locus of enteropathogenic *E. coli* necessary for production of attaching and effacing lesions on tissue culture. *Proceedings of the National Academy of Sciences of the United States of America* 87, 7839–7843.

Johnson, W.M., Pollard, D.R., Lior, H., Tyler, D.S. and Rozee, K.R. (1990) Differentiation of genes encoding *E. coli* Verotoxin 2 and the verotoxin associated with porcine edema disease (VTe) by the polymerase chain reaction. *Journal of Clinical Microbiology* 28, 2351–2353.

Jones, G.W. and Rutter, J.M. (1974) The association of K88 antigen with haemagglutinating activity in porcine strains of *Escherichia coli. Journal of General Microbiology* 84, 135–144.

Karch, H. and Meyer, T. (1989a) Evaluation of oligonucleotide probes for identification of Shiga-like-toxin-producing *Escherichia coli*. *Journal of Clinical Microbiology* 27, 1180–1186.

Karch, H. and Meyer, T. (1989b) Single primer pair for amplifying segments of distinct Shiga-like toxin genes by polymerase chain reaction. *Journal of Clinical Microbiology* 27, 2750–2757.

Karch, H., Strockbine, N.A. and O'Brien, A.D. (1986) Growth of *Escherichia coli* in the presence of trimethoprim-sulphamethoxazole facilitates detection of Shiga-like toxin producing strains by colony blot assays. *Federation of European Microbiological Societies Microbiological Letters* 35, 141–145.

Karch, H., Meyer, T., Russman, H. and Heesemann, J. (1992) Frequent loss of Shiga-like toxin genes in clinical isolates of *Escherichia coli* upon subcultivation. *Infection and Immunity* 60, 3464–3467.

Karmali, M.A., Steele, B.T., Petric, M. and Lim, C. (1983) Sporadic cases of haemolytic uraemic syndrome associated with faecal cytotoxin and cytotoxin-producing *Escherichia coli* in stools. *Lancet* i, 619–620.

Kawasaki, E.S. (1990) Amplification of RNA. In: Innis, M.A., Gelfand, D.H., Sninsky, J.J. and White, T.J. (eds) *PCR Protocols: A Guide to Methods and Applications*. Academic Press, London, pp. 21–27.

Kennan, R.M. and Monckton, R.P. (1990) Adhesive fimbriae associated with porcine enterotoxigenic *Escherichia coli* of the O141 group. *Journal of Clinical Microbiology* 28, 2006–2011.

Kricka, L.J. (ed.) (1992) *Nonisotopic DNA Probe Techniques*. Academic Press, London.

Kumar, A., Contrepois, M., Tchen, P. and Cohen, J. (1988) Non-radioactive oligonucleotide probe for the detection of clinical enterotoxigenic *Escherichia coli* isolates of bovine origin. *Annals of the Institute of Pasteur, Microbiology* 139, 315–323.

Lafont, J.P., Dho, M., D'Hauteville, H.M., Bree, A. and Sansonetti, P.J. (1987) Presence and expression of aerobactin genes in virulent avian strains of *E. coli*. *Infection and Immunity* 55, 193–197.

Lanata, C.F., Kaper, J.B., Baldini, M.M., Black, R.E. and Levine, M.M. (1985) Sensitivity and specificity of DNA probes with stool blot technique for detection of *Escherichia coli* enterotoxins. *Journal of Infectious Diseases* 152, 1087–1090.

Lathe, R., Hirth, P., DeWilde, M., Harford, N. and Lecocq, J.-P. (1980) Cell-free synthesis of enterotoxin of *E. coli* from a cloned gene. *Nature (London)* 284, 483–474.

Law, D., Ganguli, L.A.A., Donohue-Rolfe, A. and Acheson, D.W.K. (1992) Detection by ELISA of low numbers of Shiga-like toxin producing *E. coli* in mixed-culture after growth in the presence of mitomycin C. *Journal of Medical Microbiology* 36, 198–202.

Lee, C.H., Moseley, S.L. and Moon, H.W. (1983) Characterization of the gene encoding heat-stable toxin II and preliminary molecular epidemiological studies of enterotoxigenic *Escherichia coli* heat-stable II producers. *Infection and Immunity* 42, 264–268.

Maas, R. (1983) An improved colony hybridization method with significantly increased sensitivity for detection of single copy genes. *Plasmid* 10, 296–298.

Mainil, J.G., Jacquemin, E.R., Kaekenbeeck, A.E. and Pohl, P.H. (1993) Association between the effacing (*eae*) gene and the Shiga-like toxin-encoding genes in *E. coli* isolates from cattle. *American Journal of Veterinary Research* 54, 1064–1068.

Maniatis, T., Fritsch, C.F. and Sambrook, J. (1982) *Molecular Cloning: A Laboratory Manual*. Cold Spring Harbor Laboratory, Cold Spring Harbor, New York.

McLaren, I. and Wray, C. (1986) Another animal *E. coli* cytopathic factor. *Veterinary Record* 119, 576–577.

Mills, K.W., Tietze, K.L. and Phillips, R.M. (1983) Use of ELISA for detection of K88 pili in faecal specimens from swine. *American Journal of Veterinary Research* 44, 2188–2189.

Monckton, R.P. and Hasse, D. (1988) Detection of enterotoxigenic *Escherichia coli* in piggeries in Victoria by DNA hybridization using K88, K99, LT, ST1 and ST2 probes. *Veterinary Microbiology* 16, 273–281.

Moseley, S.L., Hardy, J.W., Huq, M.I., Echeverria, P. and Falkow, S. (1983) Isolation and nucleotide sequence determination of a gene encoding a heat-stable enterotoxin of *Escherichia coli. Infection and Immunity* 39, 1167–1174.

Mundell, D.H., Anselmo, C.R. and Wishnow, R.M. (1976) Factors influencing heat-labile *Escherichia coli* enterotoxin activity. *Infection and Immunity* 14, 383–388.

Nagy, B., Arp, L.H., Moon, H.W. and Casey, T.A. (1992) Colonisation of the small intestine of weaned pigs by enterotoxigenic *Escherichia coli* that lack known colonisation factors. *Veterinary Pathology* 29, 239–246.

Newland, J.W. and Neill, R.J. (1988) DNA probes for Shiga-like toxins I and II and toxin-converting bacteriophages. *Journal of Clinical Microbiology* 26, 1292–1297.

Newland, J.W., Strockbine, N.A., Miller, S.F., O'Brien, A.D. and Holmes, R.K. (1985) Cloning of the Shiga-like toxin structural genes from a toxin-converting phage of *Escherichia coli. Science* 230, 179–181.

Newland, J.W., Strockbine, N.A. and Neill, R.J. (1987) Cloning of genes for production of *Escherichia coli* Shiga-like toxin type II. *Infection and Immunity* 55, 2675–2680.

Nuovo, G.J., MacConnell, P., Forde, A. and Delvenne, P. (1991) Detection of human papillomavirus DNA in formalin fixed tissues by *in situ* hybridisation after amplification by polymerase chain reaction. *American Journal of Pathology* 139, 847–854.

Old, D.C. (1985) Haemagglutination methods in the study of *Escherichia coli*. In: Sussman, M. (ed.) *The Virulence of Escherichia coli*. Academic Press, London, pp. 287–313.

Olive, D.M. (1989) Detection of enterotoxigenic *Escherichia coli* after polymerase chain reaction amplification with thermostable DNA polymerase. *Journal of Clinical Microbiology* 27, 261–265.

Olsvik, O., Rimstad, E., Wasteson, Y., Hornes, E. and Strockbine, N. (1990) Detection of Shiga-like toxin genes by magnetic separation and quantitation of triple primer PCR products. In: *Abstracts of the 90th Annual Meeting of the American Society for Microbiology*. American Society for Microbiology, Washington, DC, Abstr. D-49, p. 88.

Patamoroj, U., Seriwatana, J. and Echeverria, P. (1983) Identification of enterotoxigenic *Escherichia coli* isolated from swine with diarrhoea in Thailand by colony hybridization, using three enterotoxin gene probes. *Journal of Clinical Microbiology* 18, 1429–1431.

Pickett, C.L., Twiddy, E.M., Belisle, B.W. and Holmes, R.K. (1986) Cloning of genes that encode a new heat-labile enterotoxin of *Escherichia coli. Journal of Bacteriology* 165, 348–352.

Pickett, C.L., Weinstein, D.L. and Holmes, R.K. (1987) Genetics of type IIa heat-labile enterotoxin of *Escherichia coli*: operon fusions, nucleotide sequence and hybridization studies. Journal of Bacteriology 169, 5180–5187.

Pickett, C.L., Twiddy, E.M., Coker, C. and Holmes, R.K. (1989) Cloning, nucleotide sequence and hybridization studies of type IIb heat-labile enterotoxin gene of *Escherichia coli. Journal of Bacteriology* 171, 4945–4952.

Pohl, P., Lintermans, P., Van Muylem, K. and Schotte, M. (1982) Colibacilles entérotoxigènes du veau possédent un antigène d'attachement diférent de l'antigène K99. *Annales de Medecin Veterinaire* 126, 569–571.

Pohl, P., Mainil, J., Devriese, L., Haesebrouck, F., Broes, A., Linterman, P. and Oswald, E. (1992) *Escherichia coli* productices de la toxine cytotoxique nécrosant de type 1 (CNF1) isolées à partir de processus pathologiques chez des chats et des chiens. *Annales de Medicine Veterinaire* 137, 21–25.

Pollard, D.R., Johnson, W.M., Lior, H., Tyler, S.D. and Rozee, K.R. (1990) Rapid and specific detection of verotoxin genes in *Escherichia coli* by the polymerase chain reaction. *Journal of Clinical Microbiology* 28, 540–545.

Saiki, R.J., Scharf, S., Faloona, F., Mullis, K.B., Horn, G.T., Erlich, H.A. and Arnheim N. (1985) Enzymatic amplification of β-globin genomic sequences and restriction site analysis for diagnosis of sickle cell anemia. *Science* 23, 1350–1354.

Salajka, E., Salajkova, Z., Alexa, P. and Hornich, M. (1992) Colonisation factor different from K88, K99, F41 and 987P in enterotoxigenic *Escherichia coli* strains isolated from post weaning diarrhoea in pigs. *Veterinary Microbiology* 32, 163–175.

Semjen, G., Ørskov, I. and Ørskov, F. (1977) K-antigen determination of *Escherichia coli* by counter-immunoelectrophoresis (CIE). *Acta Pathologica Microbiologica Scandinavica Sect. B.* 85, 103–107.

Senior, D.F., de Man, P. and Svanborg, C. (1992) Serotype haemolysin production and adherence characteristics of strains of *E. coli* causing urinary tract infection in dogs. *American Journal of Veterinary Research* 53, 494–498.

Smith, H.R., Scotland, S.M., Willshaw, G.A., Wray, C., McLaren, I.M., Cheasty, T. and Rowe, B. (1988) Verocytotoxin production and presence of VT genes in *Escherichia coli* strains of animal origin. *Journal of General Microbiology* 134, 829–834.

So, M. and McCarthy, B.J. (1980) Nucleotide sequence of bacterial transposon Tn1681 encoding a heat stabile toxin (ST) and its identification in enterotoxigenic *E. coli* strains. *Proceedings of the National Academy of Sciences of the United States of America* 77, 4011–4015.

Sojka, W.J. (1965) *Escherichia coli in Domestic Animals and Poultry*. Commonwealth Agriculture Bureaux, Farnham Royal, UK.

Sojka, W.J. (1971) Enteric diseases in new-borne piglets, calves and lambs due to *Escherichia coli* infection. *Veterinary Bulletin* 41, 509–522.

Spicer, E.K. and Noble, J.A. (1982) *Escherichia coli* heat-labile enterotoxin:

nucleotide sequence of the A subunit gene. *Journal of Biological Chemistry* 257, 5716–5721.

Strockbine, N.A., Marques, L.R.M., Holmes, R.K. and O'Brien, A.D. (1985) Characterization of monoclonal antibodies against Shiga-like toxin from *Escherichia coli. Infection and Immunity* 50, 695–700.

Strockbine, N.A., Jackson, M.P., Sung, L.M., Holmes, R.K. and O'Brien, A.D. (1988) Cloning and sequencing of the genes for Shiga toxin from *Shigella dysenteriae* type 1. *Journal of Bacteriology* 170, 1116–1122.

Thorns, C.J., Sojka, M.G. and Roeder, P.L. (1989) Detection of fimbrial adhesin of enterotoxigenic *Escherichia coli* using monoclonal antibody-based latex reagents. *Veterinary Record* 125, 91–92.

Thorns, C.J., Bell, M.M., Chasey, D., Chesham, J. and Roeder, P.L. (1992) Development of monoclonal antibody ELISA for simultaneous detection of bovine coronavirus, rotavirus serogroup A and *Escherichia coli* K99 antigen in feces of calves. *American Journal of Veterinary Research* 53, 36–43.

Urban, R.G., Pipper, E.M., Dreyfus, L.A. and Whipp, S.C. (1990) High-level production of *Escherichia coli* STb heat-stable enterotoxin and quantification by a direct enzyme-linked immunosorbent assay. *Journal of Clinical Microbiology* 28, 2383–2388.

Vadivelu, J., Dunn, D.T., Feachem, R.G., Drasar, B.S., Cox, N.P., Harrison, T.J. and Lloyd, B.J. (1987) Comparison of five assays for the heat-labile enterotoxin of *E. coli. Journal of Medical Microbiology* 23, 221–226.

van der Bosch, J.F., Hendriks, J.H.I.M., Gladigau, I., Willems, H.M.C., Stom, P.K. and de Graaf, F.K. (1993) Identification of Fll fimbriae on chicken *E. coli* strains. *Infection and Immunity* 61, 800–806.

van der Heijden, P.J. (1981) Laboratory diagnosis in neonatal calf and pig diarrhoea.In: de Leeuw, P.W. and Guinée, P.A.M. (eds) *Current Topics in Veterinary and Animal Science*, Vol. 13. Martinus Nijhoff Publishers, The Haque, pp. 175–181.

Varga, J. (1991) Characterisation of a new fimbrial antigen present in *Escherichia coli* strains isolated from calves. *Journal of Veterinary Medicine B* 38, 689–700.

Victor, T., Du Toit, R., Van Zyl, J., Bestel, A.J. and Van Helden, P.D. (1991) Improved method for the routine identification of toxigenic *Escherichia coli* by DNA amplification of a conserved region of the heat labile toxin A subunit. *Journal of Clinical Microbiology* 29, 158–161.

Wang, A.M. and Mark, D.F. (1990) Quantitative PCR. In: Innis, H.A., Gelford, D.H., Sninsky, J.J. and White, T.J. (eds) *PCR Protocols, A Guide to Methods and Applications*. Academic Press, London, pp. 70–75.

Weinstein, D.L., Jackson, M.P., Samuel, J.E., Holmes, R.K. and O'Brien, A.D. (1988) Cloning and sequencing of a Shiga-like toxin type II variant from an *Escherichia coli* strain responsible for edema disease of swine. *Journal of Bacteriology* 170, 4223–4230.

Whipp, S.C. (1990) Assay for enterotoxigenic *Escherichia coli* heat-stable toxin b in rats and mice. *Infection and Immunity* 58, 930–934.

Willshaw, G.A., Smith, H.R., Scotland, S.M. and Rowe, B. (1985) Cloning genes determining the production of Vero Cytotoxin by *Escherichia coli. Journal of General Microbiology* 131, 3047–3053.

Willshaw, G.A., Smith, H.R., Scotland, S.M., Field, A.M. and Rowe, B. (1987)

Heterogeneity of *Escherichia coli* phages encoding Vero cytotoxin: comparison of clones sequences determining VT1 and VT2 and development of specific gene probes. *Journal of General Microbiology* 133, 1309–1317.

Woodward, M.J. and Wray, C. (1990) Nine DNA probes for detection of toxin and adhesin genes in *Escherichia coli* isolated from diarrhoeal disease in animals. *Veterinary Microbiology* 25, 55–65.

Woodward, M.J., Kearsley, R., Wray, C. and Roeder, P.L. (1990) DNA probes for detection of toxin genes in *Escherichia coli* isolated from diarrhoeal disease in cattle and pigs. *Veterinary Microbiology* 22, 277–290.

Woodward, M.J., Carroll, P.J. and Wray, C. (1992) Detection of entero- and verocytotoxin genes in *Escherichia coli* from diarrhoeal disease in animals using the polymerase chain reaction. *Veterinary Microbiology* 31, 251–261.

Yamamoto, T. and Yokota, T. (1983) Sequence of heat-labile enterotoxin of *Escherichia coli* pathogenic for humans. *Journal of Bacteriology* 155, 728–733.

Yano, T., Leite, D.S., de Carmargo, I.J.B. and de Castro, A.F.P. (1986) A probable new adhesive factor (F42) produced by enterotoxigenic *Escherichia coli* isolated from pigs. *Microbiology and Immunology* 30, 495–508.

Vaccines Against *Escherichia coli* Diseases

22

R.E. ISAACSON
Department of Veterinary Pathobiology, University of Illinois, College of Veterinary Medicine, Urbana, Illinois 61801, USA

Introduction

Diseases caused by *E. coli* are a primary cause of morbidity and mortality in young animals. The most common type of disease is diarrhoea. In a recent survey of swine production in the USA, it was estimated that 7% of piglets between the ages of 0 and 4 days of age exhibited diarrhoea, with the greatest portion being caused by *E. coli* (USDA, 1991). Fifty per cent of those animals died. Because *E. coli* is a major cause of infectious diseases in domestic animals, strategies to reduce the incidence and severity of disease have been considered important priorities to reduce the large economic losses resulting from these diseases (Moon and Bunn, 1993). The principle of vaccination, discovered in 1796 by Jenner, has provided the means to effectively reduce diseases caused by pathogenic *E. coli*. In particular, there are numerous commercial vaccines for the prevention of neonatal diarrhoea in pigs, calves, and lambs. While vaccines have had a major impact on disease, other management strategies that employ improved sanitation, the use of antibiotics, and the assurance that neonates receive colostrum early in life also are important in the reduction of disease and will remain an integral part of disease prevention.

The major diseases caused by *E. coli* in domesticated animals include diarrhoea (neonatal and weanling), oedema disease in pigs, septicaemia and mastitis. Commercial vaccines for the prevention of neonatal diarrhoea in pigs, lambs and calves by enterotoxigenic *E. coli* (ETEC) are readily available worldwide. The manufacturers of some of these vaccines also claim efficacy against weanling diarrhoea. The objective of this chapter is to discuss established vaccination approaches within the context of the rationale behind their development, the research demonstrating protective effects, and the limitations of such approaches. Since the primary target of vaccines against *E. coli*-induced diseases has been neonatal diarrhoea, the strategies being employed for the development of newer generation vaccines will also be discussed. The rationale for much of what will be discussed is based on the mechanisms that *E. coli* pathogens employ to cause disease. However, the scope of this chapter does not include a detailed description of pathogenesis. Readers are urged to review chapters in Part II of this book, which are devoted to various aspects of pathogenesis.

Neonatal Diarrhoea Due to Enterotoxigenic *E. coli*

Enterotoxigenic *E. coli* (ETEC) are probably the most common cause of diarrhoea in animals during the first week of life and again around the time of weaning. Because of the incidence and severity of the disease and the potential for large economic losses, ETEC have been the subject of intensive study. As a result, the pathogenesis of diseases caused by ETEC is well understood and vaccines have been developed to prevent diarrhoeal disease during the first week of life (Moon *et al.*, 1979; Gaastra and de Graaf, 1982; Levine *et al.*, 1983; Acres, 1985; Isaacson, 1988). Since disease occurs at such an early age, it is not possible to induce active immunity in the animals at risk, and the vaccination strategy that has been adopted has been passive immunity through the stimulation of lacteal immunity in the dam. Animals suckling vaccinated dams are protected by *E. coli*-specific antibodies in colostrum and milk.

Empirical vaccines

Two general approaches for the development of vaccines have been employed: empirical and mechanism based. In the empirical approach, killed or live whole cell preparations are used as the vaccine. The rationale of this approach is that the entire *E. coli* cell is likely to contain antigens important for disease and survival *in vivo* and may elicit antibody responses to several bacterial structures and products. The advantage of the empirical vaccine is that knowledge of specific mechanisms of disease pathogenesis is not required. This approach, however, makes the assumptions that all pathogenic *E. coli* produce the same set of antigens that stimulate the production of protective antibodies, that the production of these antigens (although unknown) is consistent from culture to culture, and that pathogenic *E. coli* can be distinguished from non-pathogenic *E. coli*. Indeed, we now know that there are unique strains of *E. coli* that are pathogenic. These strains produce several surface antigens and enterotoxins that are important in disease. These antigens vary amongst pathogenic strains and are not produced by non-pathogenic strains. One potential set of targets for vaccination are the O and K antigens since they are present on the surface of the cell. However, since there are nearly 200 different O antigens and close to 100 different K antigens, creating thousands of OK serogroups, the best that could be expected if O and K antigens were protective is that many strains would have to be included in the vaccine. This approach would be feasible if only a few serotypes were important, otherwise protection would only be correlated with homology of antigens used to vaccinate and with those produced by the infecting organism. To obtain broad-spectrum protection a mixture of all of the relevant serotypes would be required. This is probably not realistic.

Beginning in 1971, data demonstrating the protective effects of vaccinating sows with whole cells or cell lysates from ETEC were published (Kohler and Cross, 1971). In one study, for example, serum collected from pigs vaccinated parenterally with a whole cell lysate of an ETEC was fed to piglets. These piglets were protected from disease caused by the same ETEC. Piglets which consumed serum from non-vaccinated pigs or pigs vaccinated with a non-enterotoxigenic *E. coli* were not protected when they were challenged with an ETEC. While this approach was empirical in that the protective antigens were not known, it demonstrated that orally administered serotype-specific antibodies against ETEC could prevent disease. It also demonstrated that protection only correlated with homology of challenge organism and organism used to produce the vaccine.

A logical extension from this concept was to provide the protective antibodies via colostrum. Thus, when killed cultures of *E. coli* were used to vaccinate pregnant sows, *E. coli*-specific antibodies were found in colostrum (Kohler, 1974; Kohler *et al.*, 1975). Piglets consuming this colostrum were protected against disease caused by ETEC used to vaccinate the dams. A second extension of this concept was to use ETEC isolated from within the herd as the vaccine strain(s). Since there are many serotypes of ETEC, this latter extension increased the probability that the vaccine would contain the relevant antigens for the organism(s) causing disease in a specific herd. To accomplish this objective, however, it was important that pathogenic strains (i.e. ETEC) were used. This required the use of tests to identify strains of *E. coli* that produced enterotoxins (Dean *et al.*, 1972; Donta *et al.*, 1974). This ultimately led to the successful implementation of a vaccination strategy using 'autogenous' vaccines (Kohler, 1978). A third extension of this concept was to use live *E. coli* rather than killed organisms and to vaccinate orally. ETEC were fed to pregnant sows on 3 successive days approximately 2 weeks prior to parturition. The number of organisms per dose was approximately 10^{11}. Piglets consuming colostrum from these animals were protected against disease caused by the same ETEC. The use of live oral autogenous vaccines has been successfully implemented in many herds and leads to a high level of protection (Kohler, 1978).

While it is not known what the protective mechanism (antigens) were for these empirical vaccines, they probably worked because the preparations contained antigens that were essential for the virulence or viability of the infecting pathogen. In the approaches described below, these antigens have been identified and directly exploited to elicit protective immunity.

Vaccines based on virulence factors

ETEC-induced diarrhoeal disease is dependent on the expression of two classes of virulence factors: adhesins that facilitate the attachment of ETEC to small intestines and enterotoxins that cause the secretion of water into the lumen of small intestines (Acres, 1985; Isaacson, 1988). The hypothesis that these virulence factors are essential for disease and that inhibiting one or both classes would prevent disease was the basis for testing new vaccines. Both of these classes of virulence attributes have been exploited as vaccine candidates.

Pilus-adhesins

In order for ETEC to cause disease, they must colonize the small intestines of the infected animal (Moon *et al.*, 1979; Gaastra and de Graaf, 1982; Isaacson, 1988). Host clearance mechanisms such as peristalsis, villus pumping, and mucus secretion serve to reduce the number of contaminating bacteria in the small intestines. ETEC possess specific adhesins that allow them to attach firmly to the mucosal surface of the small intestines and thereby resist host clearance. Antibodies that specifically neutralize the adhesive activity of the pilus-adhesin should prevent attachment, colonization and disease. The structures that serve as adhesins on ETEC are morphologically distinguishable, being long filamentous appendages termed pili or fimbriae. Pili that serve as adhesins are called pilus-adhesins. The pili are composed of highly antigenic, repeating protein subunits that are polymerized into filamentous structures (Isaacson, 1988). These surface appendages are readily recognized by cells of the immune system and are therefore excellent targets for vaccination. It is not surprising that the vaccination approach that has generally shown the greatest efficacy has been based on inducing antibodies that combine with the pilus-adhesins.

The first demonstration that this approach was viable was provided by Rutter and Jones (Rutter, 1973; Rutter and Jones, 1975). They vaccinated pregnant gilts by the intramammary route with purified K88 pili, which are important in the colonization of swine small intestines by certain ETEC (Smith and Linggood, 1971a). The newborn piglets were allowed to consume colostrum and were then challenged with a virulent $K88^+$ ETEC. Mortality in non-vaccinated litters was 69% compared to 13% in vaccinated litters. From this experiment, it was concluded that passive, lacteal immunity directed against the pilus-adhesin (in this case K88) could effectively reduce morbidity and mortality. In addition to K88, other pilus-adhesins have been identified and characterized that are important in ETEC that cause disease in animals. These other structures include K99 (pigs, calves, and lambs: Smith and Linggood, 1971b; Moon *et al.*, 1977), 987P (pigs: Nagy *et al.*, 1977; Isaacson and Richter, 1981) and F41 (pigs, calves, and lambs: de Graaf and Roorda, 1982; Morris *et al.*, 1982). Nagy *et al.* (1978) demonstrated that the 987P pilus-adhesin was protective against disease caused by $987P^+$ ETEC. These results confirmed and extended the concept that pilus-adhesins could serve as effective vaccines against ETEC-induced disease first demonstrated with K88.

Each of these pilus-adhesins is unique and antigenically unrelated to other pilus-adhesins. Therefore, protection conferred by vaccination with a single type of pilus-adhesin should not extend to ETEC strains producing a different pilus-adhesin. Morgan *et al.* (1978) demonstrated that a mixture of two different pilus-adhesins generated protection against ETEC producing either of the pilus-adhesins and that protection was likely a result of pilus-adhesin-specific antibodies. In these experiments, purified 987P and K99 were mixed together and used to vaccinate pregnant sows. Following consumption of colostrum, piglets were challenged with the ETEC used to prepare the 987P or K99, or with a $987P^+$ ETEC that had O and K antigens different from those of the vaccine strain. As shown in Table 22.1, piglets from vaccinated dams were protected against disease and mortality while pigs vaccinated with saline were not. Protection was also elicited against the $987P^+$ ETEC, although its O and K antigens were different from those of the vaccine organism. Since the only surface antigens in common between the strain used to produce the vaccine and the $987P^+$ challenge strain was 987P, it was concluded that protection was mediated by 987P (and not other major surface antigens).

Moon and Isaacson (1978, 1980) showed that protection could be mediated by pilus-specific antibodies induced by oral vaccination of gilts

Table 22.1. Protective effects of purified pili against ETEC-induced diarrhoea in neonatal pigs.

	Serogroup of challenge ETEC		
Vaccine	O9:K103, 987P	O20:K101, 987P	O101:K30, K99
987P	0/38[a] (0)[b]	1/37 (0.02)	9/30 (30)
K99	7/41 (17)	7/39 (18)	0/41 (0)
Control (saline)	12/44 (27)	5/34 (15)	14/35 (40)

[a] Deaths/number challenged.
[b] Per cent mortality in parentheses.

with live, piliated *E. coli.* To prove that protection was due to the pilus-specific antibodies, piglets were challenged with a strain of ETEC, which had only the pilus-adhesin antigen in common with the vaccine organism.

Generally, oral immunization has been used to elicit a mucosal (local) immune response. This practice is important for the prevention of infections on mucosal surfaces. In the case of ETEC diarrhoea, the objective is to get antibodies to the mucosal surface of the small intestines. It is likely that oral vaccination with pili or other *E. coli* induces local immunity. However, because it is important to vaccinate neonates and yet it is not possible to elicit an active mucosal response within the narrow window of susceptibility to disease in these animals, the only effective means to protect them is by passive transfer of antibodies in colostrum and milk. Protection is independent of the class of antibody. Both oral and parenteral vaccinations have been shown to induce specific antibodies in colostrum and milk and, therefore, the route of vaccination is not critical for protective immunity.

Numerous other studies have confirmed that pili are effective immunogens and demonstrated that mixtures of K88, K99 and 987P were effective vaccines to prevent ETEC-induced diarrhoea in livestock (Rutter and Jones, 1973; Rutter 1975; Morgan *et al.*, 1978; Nagy *et al.*, 1978; Acres *et al.*, 1979; Snodgrass *et al.*, 1982; Moon and McDonald, 1983; Avila *et al.*, 1986; Gyimah *et al.*, 1986; Runnels *et al.*, 1987; Greenwood *et al.*, 1988; Valente *et al.*, 1988; Francis and Willgohs, 1991; Mouricout, 1991). Currently, most commercial vaccines used to protect against neonatal diarrhoea contain pilus-adhesins (either in a purified form or associated with bacteria or bacterial fractions-bacterins). Since K99 is the pilus type found on almost all bovine ETEC, this pilus is generally all that is needed in a vaccine to stimulate protective antibodies in the colostrum and milk of cows. Because F41 is found on some bovine ETEC, it is sometimes included.

Most commercial vaccines for use in pigs currently contain K88, K99, 987P and F41 pili. As described above, these antigens can confer a high degree of protection against disease in neonates. These antigens are either provided as cell-free products or attached to killed cells. In some instances, the cell-free antigens have been prepared from *E. coli* strains engineered using recombinant DNA techniques (Simonson *et al.*, 1983; Greenwood *et al.*, 1988). The use of cloned products has the advantages of increased and reproducible yield in preparation of the vaccine antigen and a reduction of the amount of contaminating endotoxin present in the vaccine. Endotoxin has many adverse biological properties that are relevant to the target animals, particularly the ability to induce abortions. Other antigens that have been included in some vaccines are heat labile enterotoxin, type I pili, and O and K surface antigens (generally as whole, killed cells).

Other surface antigens

Other surface antigens have been tested as possible vaccine candidates. For example, Moon and Runnels (1983) attempted to determine whether somatic O antigen or capsular K antigens would elicit protective immunity against ETEC possessing the same antigens. They demonstrated that vaccination with the O101 antigen did not elicit a protective immune response in pigs even against an acapsular, virulent ETEC strain producing O101. On the other hand, vaccination against the K30 capsular antigen did evoke a protective response as long as the challenge ETEC strain also produced K30. This protection was independent of a response to the pilus-adhesin. While the results demonstrated that capsular antigens could elicit a protective immune response, the use of capsules as broad-spectrum vaccines is limited by the need to include antigens from all of the relevant capsules types on ETEC that produce disease in newborn pigs. Furthermore, capsular K antigens do not elicit strong immune responses. To produce a broadly protective vaccine would, therefore, require the preparation of a mixture of strains producing all of the relevant capsules and probably would require the administration of large amounts of this material. While this is possible, because there are only a few pilus-adhesins that are relevant in diarrhoeal disease of animals, the preparation of an appropriate mixture of pili is more economical and provides good protection.

Enterotoxins

The other major class of virulence attributes is enterotoxin. ETEC can produce two, antigenically unrelated classes of enterotoxins: heat labile (LT) and heat stable (ST). ETEC can produce one or both of these classes of enterotoxins: LT, LT-ST, ST. LT is structurally, genetically and antigenically related to cholera toxin (Yamamoto *et al.*, 1984). LT is a classical A/B toxin that functions by enzymatically adding an ADP-ribosyl group to a G_s protein that regulates adenylate cyclase (Moss and Richardson, 1978). Being a multiple subunit protein toxin, LT can induce a good humoral immune response. In several trials using LT, this immune response has been shown to be protective if the challenge strain produces LT and does not produce ST (Frantz and Mellencamp, 1983). Vaccination with LT does not affect colonization. Protection does not extend to strains producing ST. There are two varieties of ST: ST_a and ST_b (also known as STI and STII, respectively). Both can be produced by ETEC that cause disease in pigs. ETEC from calves typically produce ST_a only. Neither ST_a nor ST_b is inherently antigenic. The chemical coupling of ST_a to a protein carrier can induce an antitoxin response (Frantz *et al.*, 1987), but antitoxin does not protect against disease. Therefore, while vaccination against LT appears to be possible, protection from ST_a and ST_b is not effected and, thus, an antienterotoxin approach is limited.

Oral administration of specific antibodies

Since vaccination against ETEC-induced diarrhoea is via passive immunity, one additional strategy to provide protection is by the oral administration of specific antibodies to neonates. For example, monoclonal antibodies produced against K99 were shown to confer protection to calves challenged with a $K99^+$ ETEC (Sherman *et al.*, 1983). Other antigen specificities could be included in a cocktail to prevent disease caused by other pilus types. The limitation to this approach is that the antibody must be present at the time of infection or shortly after exposure. Therefore, the on-farm use of specific antibody cocktails is dependent upon the identification of animals that are at risk of infection. The use of antibody cocktails could be of use in weanling diarrhoea in pigs (see below). Attempts to use dried whey powders from cows exposed to K99 have been undertaken to protect calves against disease. This approach has had limited success.

Weanling Diarrhoea in Swine

This disease occurs at the time of weaning and is caused by ETEC. Unlike strains that cause disease in neonates, not all of the virulence factors of these ETEC have been identified. Some strains produce K88 and it is presumed that this adhesin is important in disease. However, many ETEC associated with weanling diarrhoea do not produce K88 and, therefore, it has been concluded that other bacterial adhesins must be important in this disease. None of the ETEC that cause weanling diarrhoea produce K99, 987P or F41. Nagy *et al.* (1992a, b) have identified a pilus on several ETEC strains that have been shown to cause weanling diarrhoea. It has been hypothesized that this pilus, which has been given a provisional name of 2134P, is an important adhesin. The distribution of this pilus on ETEC that cause weanling diarrhoea has not been determined and, therefore, its relative importance has not been established.

The potential to use K88 pili and the pili of strain 2134 or other pilus-adhesins as vaccines in a manner patterned after the vaccines for neonatal diarrhoea is obvious. However, there are logistical considerations that are important for the success of this strategy. Of primary importance is the development of methods to elicit an antibody response to these antigens within a limited time frame. Because these animals are no longer receiving maternal antibodies, active immunity is required for protection against this disease. In the USA, pigs are generally weaned 3–4 weeks after birth, with the trend towards earlier weaning. This limits the period of time to elicit a protective, active immune response in these animals. Furthermore, since this disease is caused by strains that colonize the mucosal surface of small intestines, secrete an enterotoxin and do not invade, it is necessary to stimulate a local (mucosal) immune response. Thus, the challenges for the development of an effective vaccine against weanling diarrhoea include:

1. Identification of the important adhesins/virulence factors for these strains.
2. A means to stimulate a local immune response.
3. The ability to stimulate this response during the narrow window of time between birth and weaning.

Superimposed on these challenges is whether neonates will even be receptive to these antigens when administered orally. In order to elicit a protective immune response against organisms that cause weanling diarrhoea, vaccination would have to occur shortly after birth. If the dam had been exposed to ETEC that cause weanling diarrhoea, it is likely that ETEC-specific antibodies will be present in the colostrum and milk. The presence of these antibodies may suppress an immune response in the weanling pigs. This may be due to the reaction of vaccine antigen with maternal antibodies and rapid clearance from the intestines, thereby preventing processing by cells of the immune system. Moreover, exposure of neonates to antigens in the vaccine during the first day or so of life may further suppress the ability to elicit an appropriate antibody response to these antigens and result in immune tolerance. It is clear that there are several major hurdles that must be cleared before an effective vaccine for weanling diarrhoea will be available. Even empirical approaches that negate the need to understand the mechanism of pathogenesis will still require an effective strategy to stimulate the protective response and requires the identification of relevant antigens on strains of ETEC that cause weanling diarrhoea. The use of cocktails containing ETEC-specific antibodies administered orally to susceptible pigs may be an effective tool in the prevention of weanling diarrhoea.

One other strategy that may overcome these hurdles is to use genetically engineered live *Salmonella* cells as carriers of the protective antigens (Dougan *et al.*, 1987). Attenuated strains of *S. typhimurium* have been prepared by creating mutations in genes such as *gal*E, *aro*A or *cya* and *crp*. These strains retain the ability to invade the mucosa of the small intestines including Peyer's patches, but do not replicate or survive in sites beyond the small intestines. Consequently, they remain locally in the small intestines and stimulate a local immune response. A local protective immune response to ETEC may be obtained by inserting and expressing ETEC genes that encode relevant antigens in one of these attenuated strains of *S. typhimurium*.

Colisepticaemia

This disease is characterized by invasion of *E. coli* through the intestinal mucosa of young animals with widespread dissemination throughout the body. In mammals, this disease occurs in neonates and is associated with animals that do not absorb sufficient quantities of colostral immunoglobulins (Chapter 3). The mechanism of disease pathogenesis is not well characterized but probably results from the attachment and colonization of the pathogen in the intestinal tract followed by invasion through the mucosa. It is assumed that endotoxin is the major factor eliciting clinical signs. The production of a siderophore, usually aerobactin, is also necessary to acquire iron after invasion. The siderophore is required for survival of the organism after it has spread systemically.

Several surface structures have been identified on strains of *E. coli* that cause colisepticaemia. The capsule (V165) and pili (F165) of *E. coli* strain 165 have both been shown to play important roles in the pathogenesis of disease in pigs (Fairbrother *et al.*, 1988; Dubreuil and Fairbrother, 1992; Harel *et al.*, 1992a, b; Ngeleka *et al.*, 1992, 1993). Mutants lacking the ability to produce either of these structures are of reduced virulence. Likewise, CS31A, a pilus found on some strains of *E. coli* that cause colisepticeamia in calves, has been proposed as an important adhesin in calves (Girardeau *et al.*, 1988, 1991; Martin *et al.*, 1991; Contrepois *et al.*, 1993). CS31A has DNA sequence homology with K88 and with some of the accessory genes of F41. These surface structures provide a source of antigen that could be used for vaccination.

Disease appears to be correlated with insufficient consumption of colostrum. This observation suggests two viable approaches to elicit protection. The first is through effective management practices that ensure consumption of sufficient amounts of colostrum. The second is to increase the amount of *E. coli*-specific antibodies present in colostrum through vaccination. These antibodies will bathe the mucosal surface of the gastrointestinal tract and prevent colonization by pathogenic *E. coli* in a manner analogous to the vaccines used to protect against neonatal diarrhoea. For a period of time after birth, the epithelial cells of the small intestines actively transport macromolecules from the intestinal lumen. Antibodies that are present in the lumen eventually show up in blood and other tissues in an unaltered form as a result of this transport process. As a result, *E. coli*-specific antibodies will be available in the lumen of the intestines to prevent colonization and invasion and systemically to prevent disease caused by invasive *E. coli*.

A major deficiency in this targeted approach for vaccination lies with the lack of sufficient epidemiological data regarding the prevalence of relevant pilus antigens on *E. coli* strains that cause septicaemia. In order to induce a broad-spectrum protective immune response it will be necessary to include antigens representative of all the strains that cause disease. As is the case with ETEC, it is likely that only a few adhesins exist on the strains that cause colisepticaemia. This would make an anti-adhesive approach plausible if the logistics of timing can be solved.

Colisepticaemia is one of the syndromes referred to as colibacillosis in chickens and turkeys (Chapter 11). Obviously, maternal immunity is not important. Strains of *E. coli* that cause colibacillosis in birds fall largely into a restricted number of O serogroups: O1, O2, O35 and O78. Pyelonephritis associated pili (pap), type 1 pili and F11 pili have been frequently identified on these strains (Gyimah *et al.*, 1986). The role of these pili, however, remains undefined in the disease in birds.

Two strategies for vaccination of birds are apparent and have been tested. Since the number of O serogroups of these strains is restricted it is possible that these strains represent unique clonal descendants (lines or strains). If this is true, vaccination with a mixture of whole killed or modified live organisms representing each serogroup is possible. Such an approach would elicit antibodies specific to this class of organisms and it is likely that several of the surface antigens on these organisms will elicit a protective immune response. Melamed *et al.* (1991) have shown that this approach is viable. They used ultrasonically treated ultraviolet-irradiated *E. coli* to vaccinate chickens. This vaccine led to a protective immune response. In another study, outer membrane proteins induced by iron starvation were used to vaccinate chickens (Bolin and Jensen, 1987). This vaccine was also protective.

The second strategy is to use the pili identified on avian septicaemic strains for vaccination in a manner similar to the pilus vaccines that have been developed for use against ETEC in pigs, calves and lambs. In a somewhat empirical approach, the pili from O1, O2 and O78 *E. coli* were collected and used to vaccinate chickens (Gyimah *et al.*, 1986). Vaccination resulted in decreased mortality and disease when chickens were challenged with the *E. coli* strains used to produce the vaccine. Whether protection against other strains would occur has not been tested. However, the use of pili for colibacillosis in birds does appear to be a viable approach.

Oedema Disease

This disease of weaned pigs is associated with widespread oedema, neurological dysfunction and death. *E. coli* that cause oedema disease generally fall into the serogroups O138, O139 and O141 (Karmali, 1989) and produce a toxin that is a variant of Shiga-like toxin II (SLT-II_v) (Marques *et al.*, 1986) (now called SLT-IIe or VT2e). The toxin is essential for disease and the signs and lesions of oedema disease have been reproduced by intravenous injection of SLT II_v into weaned pigs (MacLeod *et al.*, 1991).

The toxin is a classical A/B protein toxin that functions as a specific *N*-glycosidase that is targeted at 28S rRNA (OBrien and Holmes, 1987; Endo *et al.*, 1988). Thus, antibodies that neutralize the toxin should result in decreased morbidity and mortality. However, the toxin is inherently very toxic and, thus, would have to be inactivated to be used as a vaccine. Genetic techniques have been employed to reduce the cytotoxic activity of SLT II_v while retaining its immunogenic activity. In one study, the replacement of the amino acid at position 167 of the A subunit by glutamine resulted in a 10^6-fold reduction of cytotoxic activity (Gordon *et al.*, 1992). Pigs vaccinated with this mutant toxin responded by producing neutralizing antibodies. No lesions of oedema disease were produced in these animals, confirming that the toxin had been attenuated and is safe. At this time pigs vaccinated with this product have not been challenged to assess the protective value of the antibodies against the toxin in the prevention of disease.

There have been a number of studies to show that antitoxic immunity is likely to be effective in protecting against oedema disease. MacLeod and Gyles (1991) inactivated purified SLT-II_v by treating with glutaraldehyde and demonstrated that pigs that were actively immunized by parenteral inoculation or passively immunized by intraperitoneal injection of antitoxin antibodies were highly protected against a lethal challenge dose of purified toxin. Awad-Masalmeh *et al.* (1989) used crude toxin preparations to elicit protection in weaned pigs against oral challenge with an oedema disease producing strain of *E. coli*.

Mastitis

E. coli is one of the most common causes of mastitis in cows. Infection generally proceeds by contamination of the teats with *E. coli* found in faeces. Pathogenesis of disease appears to depend on endotoxin which elicits an intense inflammatory response. Other factors that contribute to virulence have not been identified. Indeed, all the evidence indicates that no special virulence properties are required (Chapter 5).

Because colostrum and milk naturally contain antibodies, strategies to get protective antibodies to the site of infection are not difficult and can be accomplished by parenteral or oral vaccination protocols. However, since specific virulence factors do not appear to be required to cause disease, empirical approaches have been applied to this problem. The most intensively studied approach has been to vaccinate with a rough strain of *E. coli*. The outer membrane of Gram-negative bacteria contains a unique molecule called lipopolysaccharide (Chapter 17). This molecule is found on the outer leaflet of the outer membrane and is divided into three regions: O antigen found on the outside, the core, and lipid A found associated with the membrane. The O antigen, which is composed of repeating oligosaccharide units, is responsible for the smooth surface antigen in *E. coli*. There are close to 200 unique O antigens that can be used to distinguish various strains. Unlike other *E. coli* pathogens discussed in this chapter, mastitis can probably be caused by any serotype. Since there is such a diversity of O antigens, vaccination with O antigen only would lead to immunity against strains possessing the same O antigens as are in the vaccine (if the antibodies were protective at all). Thus, this probably is not a viable strategy for vaccination against mastitis. The core region is composed of carbohydrate and contains several unique sugars: KDO and heptose. The core region is conserved among most Gram-negative organisms. Although the core region is small compared with the O antigen and other proteins, if an antibody response could be elicited against it, it would have broad-spectrum protective value. The third region of LPS consists of lipid and carbohydrate and is inserted in the outer membrane. The lipid component is responsible for endotoxic activity.

An *E. coli* strain designated J5 is a rough mutant that resulted from the loss in the ability to produce the enzyme uridine diphosphate galactose 4-epimerase (Elbein and Heath, 1965). This enzyme is required for the synthesis of complete O antigen. As a result, the core antigens in this strain are exposed and when used to vaccinate animals, the animals produce antibodies to the core region.

E. coli strain J5 has been used in several trials to determine its efficacy against *E. coli*-induced mastitis in cows. Gonzalez *et al.* (1989) tested *E. coli* J5 as a vaccine to prevent naturally occurring mastitis in an open field trial. They concluded that vaccination caused a significant decrease in the incidence of mastitis. Of particular interest was their observation that the J5 vaccine not only reduced the incidence of *E. coli*-induced mastitis, but also reduced the incidence of mastitis caused by other members of Enterobacteriaceae. This cross-protection was presumed to occur as a result of the commonality of the core region of LPS among these different organisms. While the results obtained from this vaccination trial and others using J5 are encouraging, some studies have not been as successful (Daigneault *et al.*, 1991; Hill, 1991; Hogan *et al.*, 1992a, b).

Other *E. coli* Diseases

E. coli is responsible for a number of other diseases, including urogenital infections in dogs and haemorrhagic colitis in calves. Presently, there is very little impetus for vaccine development against these diseases. Although probable virulence factors, including pilus types, have been identified for *E. coli* implicated in both conditions, multiplicity of antigenic types in both cases and the low frequency of disease in the case of haemorrhagic colitis in calves make it unlikely that vaccines will be developed.

Concluding Remarks

Vaccination has played and will continue to play an important role in the prevention of *E. coli*-induced diseases in animals. Currently, licensed vaccines are available for ETEC-induced diarrhoea and, to a lesser extent, $K88^+$ weanling diarrhoea. These vaccines were developed by rational design and attack the disease process at the level of attachment and colonization. Whether, this approach to prevention of other *E. coli* diseases will be successfully applied will require further investigations. Because ETEC-induced diarrhoea has significant economic effects on the production of food animals, there has been a strong motivation to understand the disease processes. These studies ultimately lead to the discovery of the vaccines that are available. The application of these general principles of pathogenesis and the technology used to develop the vaccines may accelerate our understanding of other *E. coli*-induced diseases and should lead to the development of additional vaccines for the prevention of non-$K88^+$ weanling diarrhoea, oedema disease, colisepticaemia and mastitis.

References

Acres, S.D. (1985) Enterotoxigenic *Escherichia coli* infections in newborn calves: a review. *Journal of Dairy Science* 68, 229–256.

Acres, S.D., Isaacson, R.E., Babuik, L.A. and Kapitany, R.A. (1979) Immunization of calves against enterotoxigenic colibacillosis by vaccinating dams with purified K99 antigen and whole cell bacterins. *Infection and Immunity* 25, 121–126.

Avila, F.A., Avila, S.H.P., Schocken-Iturrino, R.P. and Marques, M.A. (1986) Evidence of pili K88 and K99 as protecting antigens: immunization against enteric swine colibacillosis by sow vaccination. Revue D'Elevage et de Medicine Veterinaire des Pays. *Tropicaux* 39, 293–296.

Awad-Masalmeh, M., Schuh, M., Köfer, J. and Quakyi, E. (1989) Unerprüfung der schutzwirkung eines toxoidimpfstoffes gegen die odemkrankheit des absetzferkels im imfektionsmodell. *Deutsche Tierärztliche Wochenschrift* 96, 397–432.

Bolin, C.A. and Jensen, A.E. (1987) Passive immunization with antibodies against iron-regulated outer membrane proteins protects turkeys from *Escherichia coli* septicemia. *Infection and Immunity* 55, 1239–1242.

Contrepois, M., Bertin, Y., Girardeau, J.P., Picard, B. and Goullet, P. (1993) Clonal relationships among bovine pathogenic *Escherichia coli* producing surface antigen-CS31A. *Federation of European Microbiological Societies Microbiology Letters* 106, 217–222.

Daigneault, J., Thurmond, M., Anderson, M., Tyler, J., Picanso, J. and Cullor, J. (1991) Effect of vaccination with the R mutant *Escherichia coli* (J5) antigen on morbidity and mortality of dairy calves. *American Journal of Veterinary Research* 52, 1492–1496.

Dean, A.G., Ching, Y.-C., Williams, R.G. and Harden, L.B. (1972) Test for *Escherichia coli* enterotoxin using infant mice: application in a study of diarrhea in children in Honolulu. *Journal of Infectious Diseases* 125, 407–411.

de Graaf, F.K. and Roorda, I. (1982) Production, purification, and characterization of the fimbrial adhesive antigen F41 isolated from calf enteropathogenic *Escherichia coli* strain B41M. *Infection and Immunity* 36, 751–758.

Donta, S.T., Moon, H.W. and Whipp, S.C. (1974) Detection of heat-labile *Escherichia coli* enterotoxin with the use of adrenal cells in tissue culture. *Science* 185, 334–335.

Dougan, G., Hormaeche, C.E. and Maskell, D.J. (1987) Live oral *Salmonella* vaccines: potential use of attenuated strains as carriers of heterologous antigens to the immune system. *Parasite Immunology* 9, 151–160.

Dubreuil, J.D. and Fairbrother, J.M. (1992) Biochemical and serological characterization of *Escherichia coli* fimbrial antigen-F165$_2$. *Federation of European Microbiological Societies Microbiology Letters* 95, 219–224.

Elbein, A.D. and Heath, E.C. (1965) The biosynthesis of cell wall lipopolysaccharides in *Escherichia coli*. I. The biochemical properties of uridine diphosphate galactose-4-epimeraseless mutant. *Journal of Biological Chemistry* 240, 1919–1925.

Endo, Y., Tsurugi, K., Yutsudo, T., Takeda, Y., Ogasawara, K. and Igarashi, K. (1988) Site of action of a verotoxin (VT2) from *Escherichia coli* O157 : H7 and shiga toxin on eukaryotic ribosomes. *European Journal of Biochemistry* 171, 45–50.

Fairbrother, J.M., Lallier, R., Leblanc, L., Jacques, M. and Lariviere, S. (1988). Production and purification of *Escherichia coli* fimbrial antigen F165. *Federation of European Microbiological Societies Microbiology Letters* 56, 247–252.

Francis, D.H. and Willgohs, J.A. (1991) Evaluation of a live avirulent *Escherichia coli* vaccine from K88$^+$, LT$^+$ enterotoxigenic colibacillosis in weaned pigs. *American Journal of Veterinary Research* 52, 1051–1055.

Frantz, J.C. and Mellencamp, M.W. (1983) Production and testing of *Escherichia coli* (LTb) toxoid. In: Acres, S. (ed.) *Fourth International Symposium on Neonatal Diarrhea, Saskatoon.* Veterinary Infectious Disease Organization, Saskatoon, Saskatchewan, pp. 500–517.

Frantz, J.C., Bhatnagar, P.K., Brown, A.L., Garrett, L.K. and Hughes, J.L. (1987) Investigation of synthetic *Escherichia coli* heat-stable enterotoxin as an immunogen for swine and cattle. *Infection and Immunity* 55, 1077–1084.

Gaastra, W. and de Graaf, F.K. (1982) Host-specific fimbrial adhesins of noninvasive enterotoxigenic *Escherichia coli* strains. *Microbiological Reviews* 46, 1129–1161.

Girardeau, J.P., Der Vartanian, M., Ollier, J.L. and Contrepois, M. (1988) CS31A, a new K88-related fimbrial antigen on bovine enterotoxigenic and septicaemic *Escherichia coli* strains. *Infection and Immunity* 56, 2180–2188.

Girardeau, J.P., Bertin, Y., Martin, C., Vartanian, M.D. and Boeuf, C. (1991) Sequence analysis of the *clp*G gene, which codes for surface antigen-CS31A subunit – evidence of an evolutionary relationship between CS31A, K88, and F41 subunit genes. *Journal of Bacteriology* 173, 7673–7683.

Gonzalez, R.N., Cullor, J.S., Jasper, D.E., Farver, T.B., Bushnell, R.B. and Oliver, M.N. (1989) Prevention of clinical coliform mastitis in dairy cows by a mutant *Escherichia coli* vaccine. *Canadian Journal of Veterinary Research* 53, 301–305.

Gordon, V.M., Whipp, S.C., Moon, H.W., O'Brien, A.D. and Samuel, J.E. (1992) An Enzymatic mutant of Shiga-like toxin-II variant is a vaccine candidate for oedema disease of swine. *Infection and Immunity* 60, 485–490.

Greenwood, P.E., Clark, S.J., Cahill, A.D., Trevallyn-Jones, J. and Tzipori, S. (1988) Development and protective efficacy of a recombinant-DNA derived fimbrial vaccine against enterotoxic colibacillosis in neonatal piglets. *Vaccine* 6, 389–392.

Gyimah, J.E., Panigrahy, B. and Williams, J.D. (1986) Immunogenicity of an *Escherichia coli* multivalent pilus vaccine in chickens. *Avian Diseases* 30, 687–689.

Harel, J., Forget, C., Ngeleka, M., Jacques, M. and Fairbrother, J.M. (1992a) Isolation and characterization of adhesin-defective TnphoA mutants of septicaemic porcine *Escherichia coli* of serotype O115:K:F165. *Journal of General Microbiology* 138, 2337–2345.

Harel, J., Forget, C., Saintamand, J., Daigle, F., Dubreuil, D., Jacques, M. and Fairbrother, J. (1992b) Molecular cloning of a determinant coding for fimbrial antigen F165-1, a Prs-like fimbrial antigen from porcine septicaemic *Escherichia coli. Journal of General Microbiology* 138, 1495–1502.

Hill, A.W. (1991) Vaccination of cows with rough *Escherichia coli* mutants fails to protect against experimental intramammary bacterial challenge. *Veterinary Research Communications* 15, 7–16.

Hogan, J.S., Smith, K.L., Todhunter, D.A. and Schoenberger, P.S. (1992a) Field trial to determine efficacy of an *Escherichia coli* J5 mastitis vaccine. *Journal of Dairy Science* 75, 78–84.

Hogan, J.S., Weiss, W.P., Todhunter, D.A., Smith, K.L. and Schoenberger, P.S. (1992b) Efficacy of an *Escherichia coli* J5 mastitis vaccine in an experimental challenge trial. *Journal of Dairy Science* 75, 415–422.

Isaacson, R.E. (1988) Molecular and genetic basis of adherence for enteric *Escherichia coli* in animals. In: Roth, J. (ed.) *Virulence Mechanisms.* American Society for Microbiology, Washington, DC, pp. 28–44.

Isaacson, R.E. and Richter, P. (1981) *Escherichia coli* 987P pilus: purification and partial characterization. *Journal of Bacteriology* 146, 784–789.

Karmali, M.A. (1989) Infection by verocytotoxin-producing *Escherichia coli. Clinical Microbiology Reviews* 2, 15–38.

Kohler, E.M. (1974) Protection of pigs against neonatal enteric colibacillosis with colostrum and milk from orally vaccinated sows. *American Journal of Veterinary Research* 35, 331–338.

Kohler, E.M. (1978) Results of 1976 field trials with oral *Escherichia coli* vaccination of sows. *Veterinary Medicine/Small Animal Clinician* 73, 352–356.

Kohler, E.M. and Cross, R.F. (1971) Feeding bacteria-free whole cell lysates of *Escherichia coli* to gnotobiotic pigs and the effects of giving antiserums. *American Journal of Veterinary Research* 32, 739–748.

Kohler, E.M., Cross, R.F. and Bohl, E.H. (1975) Protection against neonatal enteric colibacillosis in pigs suckling orally vaccinated sows. *American Journal of Veterinary Research* 36, 757–764.

Levine, M.M., Kaper, J.B., Black, R.E. and Clements, M.L. (1983) New knowledge on pathogenesis of bacterial enteric infections as applied to vaccine development. *Microbiological Reviews* 47, 510–550.

MacLeod, D.L. and Gyles, C.L. (1991) Immunization of pigs with a purified Shiga-like toxin II variant toxoid. *Veterinary Microbiology* 29, 309–318.

MacLeod, D.L., Gyles, C.L. and Wilcock, B.P. (1991) Reproduction of edema disease of swine with purified shiga-like toxin-II variant. *Veterinary Pathology* 28, 66–73.

Marques, L.R.M., Moore, M.A., Wells, J.G., Wachsmuth, I.K. and O'Brien, A.D. (1986) Production of shiga-like toxin by *Escherichia coli. Journal of Infectious Diseases* 154, 338–341.

Martin, C., Boeuf, C. and Bousquet, F. (1991) *Escherichia coli* CS31A fimbriae – molecular cloning, expression and homology with the K88-determinant. *Microbial Pathogenesis* 10, 429–442.

Melamed, D., Leitner, G. and Heller, E.D. (1991) A vaccine against avian colibacillosis based on ultrasonic inactivation of *Escherichia coli. Avian Diseases* 35, 17–22.

Moon, H.W. and Bunn, T.O. (1993) Vaccines for preventing enterotoxigenic *Escherichia coli* infections in farm animals. *Vaccine* 11, 213–220.

Moon, H.W. and Isaacson, R.E. (1978). Immunization against enterotoxigenic *Escherichia coli*: response of piglets suckling dams given live piliated or non-piliated *Escherichia coli* vaccines orally. In: *Symposium on Cholera, Karatsu, Japan*, pp. 90–93.

Moon, H.W. and Isaacson, R.E. (1980). Pili of enterotoxigenic *E. coli* as protective antigens in live oral vaccines. In: *Symposium on Cholera, Gifu, Japan*, pp. 335–341.

Moon, H.W. and McDonald, J.S. (1983) Antibody response of cows to *Escherichia coli* pilus antigen K99 after oral vaccination with live or dead bacteria. *American Journal of Veterinary Research* 44, 493–496.

Moon, H.W. and Runnels, P.L. (1983). Trials with somatic (O) and capsular (K) antigens in vaccines for swine. In: Acres, S. (ed.) *Fourth International Symposium on Neonatal Diarrhea, Saskatoon.* Veterinary Infectious Disease Organization, Saskatoon, Saskatchewan, pp. 558–569.

Moon, H.W., Nagy, B., Isaacson, R.E. and Ørskov, I. (1977) The occurrence of K99 antigen of *Escherichia coli* isolated from pigs and colonization of pig ileum by $K99^+$ enterotoxigenic *E. coli* from calves and pigs. *Infection and Immunity* 15, 614–620.

Moon, H.W., Isaacson, R.E. and Pohlenz, J. (1979) Mechanisms of association of enteropathogenic *Escherichia coli* with intestinal epithelium. *American Journal of Clinical Nutrition* 32, 1119–1127.

Morgan, R.L., Isaacson, R.E., Brinton, C.C. and Moon, H.W. (1978) Immunization of neonatal suckling pigs against enterotoxigenic *Escherichia coli* diarrhea by vaccinating dams with purified 987 or K99 pili: protection correlates with pilus homology of vaccine and challenge. *Infection and Immunity* 22, 771–777.

Morris, J.A., Thorns, C., Scott, A.C., Sojka, W.J. and Wells, G.A. (1982) Adhesion *in vitro* and *in vivo* associated with an adhesive antigen (F41) produced by a K99 mutant of the reference strain *Escherichia coli* B41. *Infection and Immunity* 36, 1146–1153.

Moss, J. and Richardson, S.H. (1978) Activation of adenylate cyclase by *Escherichia coli* enterotoxin. Evidence for ADP-ribosyl transferase activity similar to that of choleragen. *Journal of Clinical Investigations* 62, 281–285.

Mouricout, M. (1991) Swine and cattle enterotoxigenic *Escherichia coli* mediated diarrhea. Development of therapies based on inhibition of bacteria–host interactions. *European Journal of Epidemiology* 7, 588–604.

Nagy, B., Moon, H.W. and Isaacson, R.E. (1977) Colonization of porcine intestines by enterotoxigenic *Escherichia coli*: selection of piliated forms *in vivo*, adhesion of piliated forms to epithelial cells *in vitro*, and incidence of a pilus antigen among porcine enteropathogenic *E. coli*. *Infection and Immunity* 16, 344–352.

Nagy, B., Moon, H.W., Isaacson, R.E. and Brinton, C.C. (1978) Immunization of suckling pigs against enterotoxigenic *Escherichia coli* infection by vaccinating dams with purified pili. *Infection and Immunity* 21, 269–274.

Nagy, B., Arp, L.H., Moon, H.W. and Casey, T.A. (1992a) Colonization of the small intestine of weaned pigs by enterotoxigenic *Escherichia coli* that lack known colonization factors. *Veterinary Pathology* 29, 239–246.

Nagy, B., Casey, T.A., Whipp, S.C. and Moon, H.W. (1992b) Susceptibility of porcine intestine to pilus-mediated adhesion by some isolates of piliated enterotoxigenic *Escherichia coli* increases with age. *Infection and Immunity* 60, 1285–1294.

Ngeleka, M., Harel, J., Jacques, M. and Fairbrother, J.M. (1992) Characterization of a polysaccharide capsular antigen of septicemic *Escherichia coli* O115:K 'V165':F165 and evaluation of its role in pathogenicity. *Infection and Immunity* 60, 5048–5056.

Ngeleka, M., Martineau-Doizé, M.J.B., Daigle, F., Harel, J. and Fairbrother, J.M. (1993) Pathogenicity of an *Escherichia coli* O115:K 'V165' mutant negative for $F165_1$-fimbriae in septicemia of gnotobiotic pigs. *Infection and Immunity* 61, 836–843.

O'Brien, A.D. and Holmes, R.K. (1987) Shiga and shiga-like toxins. *Microbiological Reviews* 51, 206–220.

Runnels, P.L., Moseley, S.L. and Moon, H.W. (1987) F41 pili as protective antigens of enterotoxigenic *Escherichia coli* that produce F41, K99, or both pilus antigens. *Infection and Immunity* 55, 555–558.

Rutter, J.M. (1975) *Escherichia coli* infections in piglets: pathogenesis, virulence and vaccination. *Veterinary Record* 96, 171–175.

Rutter, J.M. and Jones, G.W. (1973) Protection against enteric disease caused by *Escherichia coli* – a model for vaccination with a virulence determinant. *Nature (London)* 242, 531–532.

Sherman, D.M., Acres, S.D., Sadowski, P.L., Springer, J.A., Bray, B., Raybould, T.J.G. and Muscoplat, C.C. (1983) Protection of calves against fatal enteric colibacillosis by orally administered *Escherichia coli* K99-specific monoclonal antibodies. *Infection and Immunity* 42, 653–658.

Simonson, R.R., Isaacson, R.E., Jacob, C.R. and Newman, K.Z. (1983). The class specific antibody in passive protection against *Escherichia coli* diarrhea using a subunit genetically engineered pili vaccine. In: Acres, S. (ed.) *Fourth International Symposium on Neonatal Diarrhea, Saskatoon.* Veterinary Infectious Disease Organization, Saskatoon, Saskatchewan, pp. 548–557.

Smith, H.W. and Linggood, M.A. (1971a) Observations on the pathogenic properties of the K88, Hly, and Ent plasmids of *Escherichia coli* with particular reference to porcine diarrhea. *Journal of Medical Microbiology* 4, 467–485.

Smith, H.W. and Linggood, M.A. (1971b) Further observation on *Escherichia coli* enterotoxins with particular regard to those produced by atypical piglet strains and by calf and lamb strains: the transmissible nature of these enterotoxins and of a K antigen possessed by calf and lamb strains. *Journal of Medical Microbiology* 5, 243–250.

Snodgrass, D.R., Nagy, L.K., Sherwood, D. and Campbell, I. (1982) Passive immunity in calf diarrhea: vaccination with K99 antigen of enterotoxigenic *Escherichia coli* and rotavirus. *Infection and Immunity* 37, 586–591.

United States Department of Agriculture (1991) *Preweaning Morbidity and Mortality: National Animal Health Monitoring System.* USDA, APHIS. Washington, DC.

Valente, C., Fruganti, G., Tesei, B., Ciorba, A., Cardaras, P., Floris, A. and Bordoni, E. (1988) Vaccination of pregnant cows with K99 antigen of enterotoxigenic *Escherichia coli* and protection by colostrum in newborn calves. *Comparative Immunology, Microbiology and Infectious Diseases* 11, 189–198.

Yamamoto, T., Tamura, T. and Yokota, T. (1984) Primary structure of heat-labile enterotoxin produced by *Escherichia coli* pathogenic for humans. *Journal of Biological Chemistry* 259, 5037–5044.

Index